MW00845468

FALL PREVENTION
AND PROTECTION

Principles, Guidelines, and Practices

Human Factors and Ergonomics Series

FALL PREVENTION
AND PROTECTION

Principles, Guidelines, and Practices

edited by **Hongwei Hsiao**

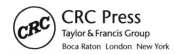

CRC Press
Taylor & Francis Group
Boca Raton London New York

CRC Press is an imprint of the
Taylor & Francis Group, an **informa** business

CRC Press
Taylor & Francis Group
6000 Broken Sound Parkway NW, Suite 300
Boca Raton, FL 33487-2742

© 2017 by Taylor & Francis Group, LLC
CRC Press is an imprint of Taylor & Francis Group, an Informa business

No claim to original U.S. Government works

Printed on acid-free paper
Version Date: 20160815

International Standard Book Number-13: 978-1-4822-1714-8 (Hardback)

Visit the Taylor & Francis Web site at
http://www.taylorandfrancis.com

and the CRC Press Web site at
http://www.crcpress.com

Printed and bound in the United States of America by Edwards Brothers Malloy on sustainaly sourced paper.

Contents

Section III   Research on Slips, Trips, and Falls

Section IV   Practical Applications of Prevention and Protection Tools and Methods

Section V   Fall Incident Investigation and Reconstruction

Section VI   Knowledge Gaps, Emerging Issues, and Recommendations for Fall Protection Research and Fall Mitigation

Preface

The most recent report on fatal occupational injuries showed that there were 699 slip, trip, and fall (STF)-related fatalities in 2013 in the United States, which accounted for 16% of the overall occupational fatality cases. In addition, there were 296,140 STF-related non-fatal occupational injuries resulting in days away from work in 2013, which accounted for about 25.5% of all occupational injuries in that year. Many countries are facing the same challenges as the United States with STF injury problems in the workplace. Aside from workplace incidents, STFs were prevalent in U.S. homes and communities, resulting in 30,208 fatalities and 8.8 million injuries in 2013. Elderly individuals were particularly at risk. More than 3.4 million nonfatal fall injuries among older adults (55–85+ years old) were recorded in emergency departments in 2013. Often, residents fall from ladders or on stairs, uneven surfaces, or wet areas at home. Similar concerns are also seen worldwide.

The etiology of STFs as injury-producing events is multifactorial and encompasses multiple mechanisms of exposure. Working at height presents different fall risks than those found on work surfaces and floors. The different exposures represent serious safety risks in both cases and can result in fatal and serious nonfatal injury. To address the various causes of multifactorial events such as these, there needs to be wide-ranging and multi-disciplinary injury-mitigation research and translational efforts to provide safety professionals, workers, citizens, and caregivers with validated research findings, methods, and recommendations for safe practices.

This book covers a wealth of knowledge from experts and informed stakeholders on the best ways to understand, prevent, and control fall-related risk exposures. Featured are subjects on (1) a public health view of fall problems and strategic goals; (2) the sciences behind human falls and injury risk; (3) research on STFs; (4) practical applications of prevention and protection tools and methods in industrial sectors and homes/communities; (5) fall incident investigation and reconstruction; and (6) knowledge gaps, emerging issues, and recommendations for fall protection research and fall mitigation.

Chapters in the book also address topics including (1) injury and fatality data, vulnerable groups, falls among aging workforces, and global strategic goals for fall prevention and protection; (2) human balance control, vision, lighting, behavior, physics, environments, and tribology; (3) roofing, ladder use, scaffolding, aerial platforms, and fall arrest and rescue; (4) risk recognition, hazard control, training, and practitioners' manuals; (5) fall prevention applications in construction, health service, wholesale and retail trade, public safety, manufacturing sectors, and homes and community settings; (6) fall forensics, investigation methods, and case examples; and (7) knowledge gaps and emerging issues in protective technologies, vulnerable populations, fall prevention management, and effective implementation evaluation.

Publishing a book on fall prevention and injury protection is a timely action to inform the scientific community, corporate managers, and safety professionals about new findings and best practices that will advance professional and scholarly knowledge in the field. It is expected that the book will bring attention to novel fall prevention research and practice methods in the international community. It will serve to bring together disparate communities of interest that work to prevent and ameliorate fall-related injuries and will spur efforts that will continue in the form of joint and supported research investigations, research consortia, and informed dialogue in support of a common goal.

Hongwei Hsiao
National Institute for Occupational Safety and Health

Editor

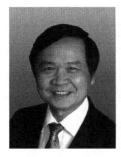

Dr. Hongwei Hsiao serves as chief of the Protective Technology Branch at the National Institute for Occupational Safety and Health (NIOSH). He received his degrees from Cornell University and the University of Michigan and has held engineering and management positions in both the manufacturing industry and the U.S. Government. He also has taught engineering and public health in academia.

Dr. Hsiao has coordinated numerous large-scale programs and projects in the areas of safety research and human factors engineering, including fall prevention, equipment safety, and protective technologies for special populations, which have had significant public health and occupational safety impacts. An internationally recognized scientist for occupational fall prevention, he is involved in the development of international fall prevention strategic goals and fall protection safety standards. He coordinated and chaired the 1st International Conference on Fall Prevention and Protection in 2010.

Dr. Hsiao currently manages nine laboratories for NIOSH, including the Virtual Reality Lab, Human Factors Lab, Anthropometry Research Lab, and Vehicle Safety Lab, among others. An editorial board member for 10 scientific journals, Dr. Hsiao has also authored more than 160 publications and holds patents in engineering innovation for injury control. He also edited two journal special issues on fall prevention and protection. With more than 25 years of program management and safety research experience, he has been frequently invited to be an international speaker on fall prevention research and practice and strategic planning for industrial safety. He is a recipient of 20 prestigious service, science, and innovation awards. Among his most recent honors are the Public Health Service Engineer of the Year from the U.S. Government (2011), the Human Factors Prize from the Human Factors and Ergonomics Society (2012), the Alice Hamilton Award (2013), the Bullard-Sherwood Transfer of Knowledge Award (2014), and the Federal Health Information Technology Innovation Award from the Digital Health Xchange (2015).

Dr. Hsiao was elected as a fellow of the Institute of Ergonomics and Human Factors (United Kingdom) in 2003 and an Honorary Fellow of the Human Factors and Ergonomics Society (United States) in 2005. In 2003, he was credentialed by the U.S. Government Centers for Disease Control and Prevention (CDC) Executive Resources Board as a Silvio O. Conte Senior Biomedical Research Service Fellow and was named a CDC Distinguished Consultant.

Contributors

Anil Adisesh
Dalhousie University
Department of Medicine
New Brunswick, Canada

Grant T. Baldwin
National Center for Injury Prevention and
    Control (NCIPC)
Atlanta, Georgia

Jennifer L. Bell
National Institute for Occupational Safety
    and Health (NIOSH)
Washington, DC

Kurt E. Beschorner
Department of Bioengineering
University of Pittsburgh
Pittsburgh, Pennsylvania

Amit Bhattacharya
Department of Bioengineering
University of Cincinnati
Cincinnati, Ohio

Don Bloswick
Department of Mechanical Engineering
University of Utah
Salt Lake City, Utah

Christine M. Branche
Office of Construction Safety and Health
National Institute for Occupational Safety
    and Health (NIOSH)
Washington, DC

Chris Trahan Cain
CPWR-The Center for Construction
    Research and Training (CPWR),
Silver Spring, Maryland

Wen-Ruey Chang
Liberty Mutual Research Institute for Safety
Hopkinton, Massachusetts

Chia-Fen Chi
Department of Industrial Management
National Taiwan University of Science and
    Technology
Taipei, Taiwan

Sharon S. Chiou
National Institute for Occupational Safety
    and Health (NIOSH)
Morgantown, West Virginia

H. Harvey Cohen
Error Analysis, Inc.
San Diego, California

Joseph Cohen
Error Analysis, Inc.
San Diego, California

James W. Collins
National Institute for Occupational Safety
    and Health (NIOSH)
Washington, DC

Xiuwen Sue Dong
CPWR-The Center for Construction
    Research and Training (CPWR),
Silver Spring, Maryland

Kari Dunning
Department of Rehabilitation
University of Cincinnati
Cincinnati, Ohio

G. Scott Earnest
Office of Construction Safety and Health
National Institute for Occupational Safety
    and Health (NIOSH)
Washington, DC

Sue Hignett
Loughborough Design School
Loughborough University
Loughborough, United Kingdom

Gavin Horn
University of Illinois at
  Urbana-Champaign
Illinois Fire Service Institute
Champaign, Illinois

David Hostler
Department of Exercise and Nutrition
  Sciences
Center for Research and Education in
  Special Environments
University at Buffalo
Buffalo, New York

Hongwei Hsiao
Protective Technology Branch
National Institute for Occupational Safety
  and Health (NIOSH)
Washington, DC

Yu-Hsiu Hung
Department of Industrial Design
National Cheng Kung University
Tainan, Taiwan

Daniel Johnson
Daniel A. Johnson, Inc.
Olympia, Washington

Paul R. Keane
National Institute for Safety and Health
  (NIOSH)
Morgantown, West Virginia

K. Han Kim
University of Michigan Transportation
  Research Institute
University of Michigan
Ann Arbor, Michigan

Philippe Lacherez
School of Psychology and Counselling
Queensland University of Technology
Brisbane, Australia

Julie A. Largay
CPWR-The Center for Construction
  Research and Training (CPWR)
Silver Spring, Maryland

Sylvie Leclercq
French National Research and Safety
  Institute (INRS)
Paris, France

Bruce Lippy
CPWR-The Center for Construction
  Research and Training (CPWR)
Silver Spring, Maryland

Stephen R. Lord
NeuRA
University of New South Wales
Sydney, Australia

Ashutosh Mani
Department of Environmental Health
University of Cincinnati
Cincinnati, Ohio

Loui McCurley
Vertical Rescue Solutions
Pigeon Mountain Industries
Denver, Colorado

Timothy Merinar
National Institute for Occupational Safety
  and Health (NIOSH)
Washington, DC

Andrew Merryweather
Department of Mechanical Engineering
University of Utah
Salt Lake City, Utah

Janice Morse
College of Nursing
University of Utah
Salt Lake City, Utah

Hisao Nagata
The Ohara Memorial Institute for Science
  of Labour
Tokyo, Japan

Rita K. Noonan
National Center for Injury Prevention and
  Control (NCIPC)
Atlanta, Georgia

Christopher S. Pan
National Institute for Occupational Safety
    and Health (NIOSH)
Washington, DC

Steven Di Pilla
ESIS Inc.
Philadelphia, Pennsylvania

James W. Platner
CPWR-The Center for Construction
    Research and Training (CPWR)
Silver Spring, MD

Mark S. Redfern
Department of Bioengineering
University of Pittsburgh
Pittsburgh, Pennsylvania

Matthew P. Reed
University of Michigan Transportation
    Research Institute
University of Michigan
Ann Arbor, Michigan

Rosalba Arauz Rivera
Donald W. Reynolds Department of
    Geriatric Medicine
University of Oklahoma College of
    Medicine
Oklahoma City, Oklahoma

Laurence Z. Rubenstein
Donald W. Reynolds Department of
    Geriatric Medicine
University of Oklahoma College of
    Medicine
Oklahoma City, Oklahoma

Peter Simeonov
National Institute for Occupational Safety
    and Health (NIOSH)
Washington, DC

David A. Sleet
National Center for Injury Prevention and
    Control (NCIPC)
Atlanta, Georgia

Christina Socias
National Institute for Occupational Safety
    and Health (NIOSH)
Washington, DC

Erich Pete Stafford
CPWR-The Center for Construction
    Research and Training (CPWR)
Silver Spring, Maryland

Judy A. Stevens
National Center for Injury Prevention and
    Control (NCIPC)
Atlanta, Georgia

Ellen Taylor
Center for Health Design
Concord, California

Xuanwen Wang
CPWR-The Center for Construction
    Research and Training (CPWR)
Silver Spring, MD

Laurie Wolf
Barnes Jewish Hospital
St. Louis, Missouri

Section I

A Public Health View of Fall Problems and Strategic Goals

1

Fall Prevention and Protection: A Public Health Matter

Hongwei Hsiao

CONTENTS

ABSTRACT Slips, trips, and falls (STF) represent a serious hazard to workers and occupants in many industries, homes, and communities. Countering STF hazards and risks through all aspects of control measures is a public health matter, a challenging yet tangible undertaking. This chapter describes a public health approach to STF prevention. It summarizes the industries, occupations, and special population groups that are at increased STF risk due to their high STF-related fatality or nonfatal injury counts (or rates). The chapter also suggests critical research topics for global STF control, which correspond to the overall structure of this book—from fall injury risk factors to fall prevention research, evidence-based fall prevention practices, fall injury case studies, and emerging issues in fall prevention and protection.

KEY WORDS: *falls, construction, healthcare, trade, aging, human characteristics, public health, control measure.*

1.1 Introduction

The most recent report on fatal occupational injuries showed that slips, trips, and falls (STF) took the lives of 699 workers in the United States in 2013 (BLS, 2014a), which accounted for 16% of all occupational fatality cases. In addition, there were 296,140 STF-related nonfatal occupational injuries resulting in days away from work in 2013, which accounted for about 25.5% of all occupational injuries in that year (BLS, 2015a). The construction industry continued to have the highest count of STF-related fatalities (BLS, 2014a). The health-care and social assistance sector, retail trade, and accommodation and food services have the highest number of nonfatal STF-related injuries (BLS, 2015b). In addition, transportation and warehousing, agriculture and the forestry industry, and the construction sector have the highest rate (per 10,000 full-time workers) of nonfatal STF-related injuries (BLS, 2015c). Many countries are facing the same challenges as the United States with STF injury problems in the workplace (NIOSH, 2011a).

Aside from workplace incidents, STFs are the second leading cause of unintentional death in homes and communities, resulting in more than 27,100 fatalities in 2012 (NSC, 2014). In addition, falls were the leading cause of nonfatal injuries among the general population in the United States in 2013 for all age groups from <1 to 85+, except for the 10–24 age group, who had more struck-by-related injuries than falls (NCIPC, 2015). Often, inhabitants fall from ladders, from stairs, on uneven surfaces, or in wet areas at home. Elderly individuals are particularly at risk. In 2013, more than 3.4 million nonfatal fall injuries among older adults (55–85+ years old) were recorded in emergency departments (NCIPC, 2015). Similar concerns are seen worldwide (WHO, 2007).

Given the prevalence of STF problems, an organized national and global prevention research and practice effort is warranted. Considering STF control as a public health matter, we can prioritize our resources for STF prevention actions on industries and populations with the highest counts or rates of STF-related fatalities and injuries. We can also focus on the most compelling STF-related risks facing workers across all industry sectors and citizens in homes and communities to effectively reduce STF-related injuries and deaths. This book is organized around the public health concept and includes information on fall injury data, fall injury risk factors, fall prevention and protection research, evidence-based fall -prevention practices, fall injury investigation and case studies, and emerging issues in fall prevention and protection. This chapter describes the public health view on STF prevention.

1.2 Public Health View on Slip, Trip, and Fall Prevention

1.2.1 Public Health Approach

To effectively reduce national or global STF-related injuries and deaths, a focused effort that considers high-quality research, active partnerships, and research-to-practice actions is necessary. High-quality research refers to organized explorations with meaningful impacts. The public health approach provides a means to prioritize national and global efforts and assess impacts. The public health approach includes incident surveillance, risk identification, intervention, and implementation (Figure 1.1; Hsiao, 2014). Incident surveillance identifies the magnitude and severity of problems. Often, injury data systems and

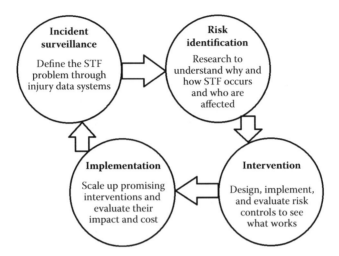

FIGURE 1.1
Public health approach for slip, trip, and fall prevention. (From Hsiao, H., *Industrial Health*, 52, 381–392, 2014.)

fatality reports reveal trends or changes in STF problems. Risk identification characterizes risks and causes. It is a step toward understanding why and how STF occurs and who is affected. Intervention refers to the design and evaluation of risk controls. Both field and laboratory studies can be performed to understand what mechanisms work and their levels of effectiveness. Implementation promotes promising interventions and evaluates their impact and cost-effectiveness; the idea of implementation is to bring STF prevention measures to a broad segment of the population and reduce STF at a population level. The public health approach is a continuing process to understand the causes and sources for STF prevention and policy/strategy interventions.

1.2.2 Incident Surveillance

While most current injury data systems do not include detailed information on how a fatality or injury incident happened, some systems provide sufficient consolidated information on STF incidents by industry, occupation, population, age, and other parameters for national strategic goal-planning purposes. Among the available databases are the Census of Fatal Occupational Injuries and Nonfatal Occupational Injuries and Illnesses from the Survey of Occupational Injuries and Illnesses by the Bureau of Labor Statistics (BLS, 2014a, 2015a) and the Web-based Injury Statistics Query and Reporting System (WISQARS) by the National Center for Injury Prevention and Control (NCIPC, 2015).

The Census of Fatal Occupational Injuries (Table 1.1; BLS, 2014a) reported that the construction sector had the highest count of STF-related fatalities in 2013, followed by the waste-management sector. The same database (Table 1.2; BLS, 2015d) indicated that construction and extraction occupations encountered the highest number of STF-related fatalities, followed by the building- and grounds-cleaning/maintenance occupations; installation, maintenance, and repair occupations; and transportation and material-moving occupations. Most of these incidents (574 out of 699) were falls to a lower level, and of the cases where the height of the fall was known (466 cases), three out of every five were falls of 20 ft or less (BLS, 2014b).

The Survey of Occupational Injuries and Illnesses (Table 1.3; BLS, 2015b) showed that the health-care and social assistance sector had the highest *count* of STF-related nonfatal

TABLE 1.1

Fatal Occupational Falls by Industry in the United States in 2013

Industry	NAICS Code	Total STF Count (699)
Agriculture, forestry, fishing and hunting	11	30
Mining	21	19
Construction	23	294
Manufacturing	31, 32, 33	41
Wholesale trade	42	23
Retail trade	44, 45	31
Transportation and warehousing	48, 49	35
Information	51	10
Finance and insurance	52	0
Real estate and rental and leasing	53	13
Professional, scientific, and technical services	54	7
Management of companies and enterprises	55	0
Administrative, support, waste management, remediation	56	78
Education services	61	3
Health-care and social assistance	62	10
Art, entertainment, and recreation	71	8
Accommodation and food services	72	15
Other services, except public administration	81	27
Federal government		13
State government		6
Local government		31

Source: BLS, Fatal occupational injuries by industry and event or exposure, All U.S., 2013, (Table A.1), 9/11/2014. US Bureau of Labor Statistics, Washington, DC, 2014a. http://www.bls.gov/iif/oshwc/cfoi/cftb0277. pdf.

injuries, followed by the retail trade and the accommodation and food services sector. The transportation and warehousing sector had the highest *rate* (per 10,000 full-time workers) of STF-related nonfatal injuries (Table 1.3; BLS, 2015c), followed by the agriculture, forestry, fishing, and hunting sector and the construction sector. The same database revealed that transportation and material-moving occupations had the highest *number* of STF-related nonfatal injuries (Table 1.4; BLS, 2015e), followed by the food preparation and serving occupations and the construction and extraction occupations. The building- and grounds-cleaning and maintenance occupations had the highest *rate* of STF-related nonfatal injuries, followed by the transportation and material-moving occupations and the construction and extraction occupations (Table 1.4; BLS, 2015f).

Data from WISQARS showed 31,240 fall deaths among the general population in the United States in 2013 (Table 1.5; NCIPC, 2015), which is equivalent to 9.88 cases per 100,000 citizens. Of the cases, 51% (N = 15,957) were males and 49% (N = 15,283) were females. For males, about 85% (N = 13,527) of the deaths were at age 55–85+. For females, about 95% (N = 14,501) of the deaths were in the same age category. The same system reported that there were 8,790,337 STF-related nonfatal injuries among the general population in 2013 (Table 1.6; NCIPC, 2015). Among them, 45% (N = 3,960,046) were male and 55% (N = 4,830,224) were female; there were 66 cases in which gender was not recorded. Older groups, aged 55–85+, had higher fall injury rates than the younger groups.

TABLE 1.2

Fatal Occupational Falls by Occupation in the United States in 2013

Occupation	Occupation Code	Total STF Count (699)
Management occupations	11	39
Business and financial operations	13	3
Computer and mathematical occupations	15	0
Architecture and engineering	17	6
Life, physical, and social science	19	0
Community and social service	21	3
Legal occupations	23	4
Education, training, and library	25	5
Arts, design, entertainment, sports, and media	27	8
Health-care practitioners and technical occupations	29	3
Health-care support occupations	31	1
Protective service occupations	33	12
Food preparation and serving-related occupations	35	12
Building and grounds cleaning and maintenance	37	76
Personal care and service occupations	39	6
Sales and related occupations	41	20
Office and administrative support occupations	43	17
Farming, fishing, and forestry occupations	45	10
Construction and extraction occupations	47	293
Installation, maintenance, and repair occupations	49	70
Production occupations	51	38
Transportation and material-moving occupations	53	66
Military-specific occupations	—	4

Source: BLS, Table A.5. Fatal occupational injuries by occupation and event or exposure, All U.S., 2013. US Bureau of Labor Statistics, Washington, DC, 2015d. http://www.bls.gov/iif/oshwc/cfoi/cftb0281.pdf.

1.2.3 Risk Identification

The incident surveillance data mentioned in the previous section provide a direction for organizations that are in charge of or interested in fall prevention strategic planning to effectively organize resources for the greatest impact. In addition to the data, the next key step for successful STF control is to identify risk factors. STFs occur as a result of a complex interaction of risk factors, which can be organized into three categories: personal, environmental, and task-related factors (Table 1.7; Hsiao and Simeonov, 2001).

The personal factors include individual differences: age, gender, race, body size, work experience, chronic illness, physical strength, substance use, cognitive capacities, constraints of personal protective equipment (PPE), visual acuity, contrast sensitivity, discrepant vision between the eyes, and expiratory flow rate (WHO, 2007; Hsiao and Simeonov, 2001; Knudtson et al., 2009; Gauchard et al., 2001; Tinetti and Speechley, 1989; Mesure et al., 1997; Robertson et al., 1994; Black et al., 1993). The environmental factors concern the properties of environments as well as information available from visual and physical interactions with environments, including elevation perception, moving visual scenes, depth perception, visual ambiguity, visual detection of obstacles and their properties, restricted support surfaces, inclination of support surfaces, lighting, building design, and material properties of support surfaces (e.g., friction, contaminants, evenness, loose fixtures, and firmness) (Hsiao and Simeonov, 2001; Gauchard et al., 2001; Bles et al., 1980; Brandt et al.,

TABLE 1.3

Nonfatal Occupational Falls by Industrial Sector in Private Industry in the United States in 2013

Nonfatal Occupational Falls by Industry (Private Industry) Industry	NAICS Code	Number[a]				Rate per 10,000 Workers[b]			
		Total STF	Fall to Lower Level	Fall on Same Level	Slips or Trips without Fall	Total STF	Fall to Lower Level	Fall on Same Level	Slips or Trips without Fall
Agriculture, forestry, fishing and hunting	11	5,030	1,960	2,310	600	52.1	20.3	23.9	6.2
Mining	21	1,550	470	780	210	18.1	5.5	9.2	2.4
Construction	23	21,890	9,560	8,560	3,010	41.3	18	16.1	5.7
Manufacturing	31–33	21,430	4,370	12,730	3,790	18	3.7	10.7	3.2
Wholesale trade	42	12,640	3,390	6,430	2,100	22.4	6	11.4	3.7
Retail trade	44, 45	29,690	5,810	19,680	3,660	26	5.1	17.2	3.2
Transportation and warehousing	48, 49	21,970	4,890	11,460	4,140	54.3	12.1	28.3	10.2
Information	51	4,850	920	2,640	1150	19.5	3.7	10.6	4.6
Finance and insurance	52	4,620	490	3,610	500	8.6	0.9	6.7	0.9
Real estate and rental and leasing	53	4,430	1440	1,920	720	24.8	8.1	10.7	4.1
Professional, scientific, and technical services	54	4,280	980	2,360	870	5.7	1.3	3.1	1.1
Management of companies and enterprises	55	2,170	370	1,600	200	11.3	1.9	8.3	1
Administrative, support, waste management	56	12,850	2,840	7,540	2,290	27	6	15.9	4.8
Education services	61	3,930	510	2,910	450	21.2	2.8	15.7	2.4
Health care and social assistance	62	43,820	3,890	33,290	6,340	32.9	2.9	25	4.8
Art, entertainment, and recreation	71	4,310	620	2,920	620	33.4	4.8	22.7	4.8
Accommodation and food services	72	22,810	2,610	17,100	2,800	29.3	3.4	22	3.6
Other services, except public administration	81	5,860	1,690	2,710	1,280	19.3	5.6	8.9	4.2

[a] BLS, Table R4. Number of nonfatal occupational injuries and illnesses involving days away from work by industry and selected events or exposures leading to injury or illness, private industry, 2013. US Bureau of Labor Statistics, Washington, DC. 2015b. http://www.bls.gov/iif/oshwc/osh/case/ostb3985.pdf.

[b] BLS, Table R8. Incidence rates for nonfatal occupational injuries and illnesses involving days away from work per 10,000 full-time workers by industry and selected events or exposures leading to injury or illness, private industry, 2013. US Bureau of Labor Statistics, Washington, DC. 2015c. http://www.bls.gov/iif/oshwc/osh/case/ostb3989.pdf.

TABLE 1.4

Nonfatal Occupational Falls by Occupation in Private Industry in the United States in 2013

Nonfatal Occupational Falls by Occupation (Private Industry) / Industry	Occup. Code	Number[a]				Rate Per 10,000 Workers[b]			
		Total STF	Fall to Lower Level	Fall on Same Level	Slips or Trips without Fall	Total STF	Fall to Lower Level	Fall on Same Level	Slips or Trips without Fall
Management occupations	11	7,960	1,530	5,180	1,170	14	2.7	9.1	2.1
Business and financial operations	13	3,390	490	2,650	230	6.8	1	5.4	0.5
Computer and mathematical occupations	15	720	180	460	70	2.4	0.6	1.5	0.2
Architecture and engineering	17	720	140	450	110	3.7	0.7	2.3	0.6
Life, physical, and social science	19	510	150	280	20	8.4	2.5	4.5	0.4
Community and social service	21	2,470	350	1,770	330	26.5	3.8	19	3.6
Legal occupations	23	310	30	270	0	4.3	0.4	3.7	0
Education, training, and library	25	2,830	220	2,100	470	20	1.5	14.9	3.3
Arts, design, entertainment, sports, and media	27	1,540	250	860	340	12.5	2	7	2.8
Health-care practitioners and technical occupations	29	13,830	950	10,480	2,290	25.7	1.8	19.4	4.3
Health-care support occupations	31	11,770	850	9,190	1,660	43.1	3.1	33.6	6.1
Protective service occupations	33	3,810	630	2,530	550	41.1	6.8	27.3	5.9
Food preparation and serving	35	20,530	1,570	16,300	2,470	27.6	2.1	21.9	3.3
Building and grounds cleaning and maintenance	37	16,290	3,460	9,840	2,390	60.6	12.9	36.6	8.9
Personal care and service	39	5,710	840	3,830	980	23.5	3.5	15.8	4.1
Sales and related occupations	41	17,440	3,800	11,010	2,270	16.1	3.5	10.2	2.1
Office and administrative support	43	19,640	2,360	14,210	2,850	13.7	1.6	9.9	2
Farming, fishing, and forestry	45	4,140	1,590	1,890	560	46.4	17.8	21.2	6.3
Construction and extraction	47	20,250	8,760	8,040	2,720	48.7	21.1	19.4	6.5
Installation, maintenance, and repair	49	16,570	6,010	6,970	2,960	38.9	14.1	16.4	6.9
Production occupations	51	17,490	2,950	10,920	3,170	22.6	3.8	14.1	4.1
Transportation and material-moving occupations	53	40,760	9,970	21,420	7,340	56.5	13.8	29.7	10.2

[a] BLS, Table R12. Number of nonfatal occupational injuries and illnesses involving days away from work by occupation and selected events or exposures leading to injury or illness, private industry, 2013. US Bureau of Labor Statistics, Washington, DC. 2015e. http://www.bls.gov/iif/oshwc/osh/case/ostb3993.pdf.

[b] BLS, Table R100. Incidence rates for nonfatal occupational injuries and illnesses involving days away from work per 10,000 full-time workers by occupation and selected events or exposures leading to injury or illness, 2013. US Bureau of Labor Statistics, Washington, DC. 2015f. http://www.bls.gov/iif/oshwc/osh/case/ostb4081.pdf.

TABLE 1.5

Fall Deaths among General Population in the United States in 2013

Fall Deaths	Males (N = 15,957)			Females (N = 15,283)		
Age Group	Number of Deaths	Population	Rate Per 100,000	Number of Deaths	Population	Rate Per 100,000
0–9	32	20,661,392	0.15	20	19,777,277	0.10
10–19	93	21,398,713	0.43	35	20,410,705	0.17
20–24	197	11,678,965	1.69	51	11,116,473	0.46
25–29	223	10,959,879	2.03	39	10,620,319	0.37
30–34	204	10,681,612	1.91	58	10,582,777	0.55
35–39	211	9,785,269	2.16	59	9,818,501	0.60
40–44	310	10,359,992	2.99	100	10,488,928	0.95
45–49	475	10,498,118	4.52	167	10,710,188	1.56
50–54	684	11,070,966	6.18	252	11,488,260	2.19
55–59	783	10,282,382	7.61	329	10,912,048	3.02
60–64	893	8,674,373	10.29	430	9,447,628	4.55
65–69	1054	6,913,190	15.25	560	7,695,527	7.28
70–74	1178	4,884,452	24.12	861	5,723,597	15.04
75–79	1684	3,390,347	49.67	1379	4,287,534	32.16
80–84	2511	2,370,170	105.94	2444	3,398,468	71.91
85 and up	5424	2,041,782	265.65	8498	3,999,007	212.50

TABLE 1.6

Nonfatal Fall Injuries among the General Population in the United States in 2013

Fall Injuries	Males			Females		
Age Group	Number of Injuries	Population	Rate per 100,000	Number of Injuries	Population	Rate per 100,000
0–9	915,912	20,661,392	4432.96	696,791	19,777,277	3523.19
10–19	543,167	21,398,713	2538.32	425,791	20,410,705	2086.12
20–24	208,626	11,678,965	1786.34	201,749	11,116,473	1814.87
25–29	182,695	10,959,879	1666.94	191,746	10,620,319	1805.46
30–34	176,944	10,681,612	1656.53	195,617	10,582,777	1848.45
35–39	151,875	9,785,269	1552.08	190,946	9,818,501	1944.76
40–44	164,931	10,359,992	1592.00	199,357	10,488,928	1900.64
45–49	185,302	10,498,118	1765.10	232,901	10,710,188	2174.57
50–54	221,028	11,070,966	1996.47	277,180	11,488,260	2412.72
55–59	205,777	10,282,382	2001.26	288,244	10,912,048	2641.52
60–64	172,517	8,674,373	1988.81	264,954	9,447,628	2804.45
65–69	158,611	6,913,190	2294.32	259,089	7,695,527	3366.75
70–74	148,605	4,884,452	3042.41	238,223	5,723,597	4162.12
75–79	139,697	3,390,347	4120.43	259,104	4,287,534	6043.19
80–84	150,821	2,370,170	6363.30	300,292	3,398,468	8836.10
85 and up	233,265	2,041,782	11424.58	608,099	3,999,007	15206.25
Unknown	276			141		

TABLE 1.7

Risk Factors Associated with Slips, Trips, and Falls

Model	Primary Factors	Elements
 There are intersections of some elements under each of the three primary factors between or among primary factors, although they are classified as belonging to a single primary factor	Personal factors	Age, gender, race, body size, work experience, physical strength, chronic illness, substance use, cognitive capacities, constraints of PPE, visual acuity, contrast sensitivity, discrepant vision between the eyes, and expiratory flow rate
	Environmental factors	Restricted support surfaces, inclination of support surfaces, lighting, building design, material properties of support surfaces (e.g., friction, contaminants, evenness, loose fixtures, and firmness), elevation perception, moving visual scenes, depth perception, visual ambiguity, and visual detection of obstacles and their properties
	Task-related factors	Load handling, physical exertion and fatigue, footwear, complexity of tasks, social interactions, and community resources

Source: Hsiao H. and Simeonov P., *Ergonomics*, 44 (5), 537–561, 2001.

1980; Paulus et al., 1984; Peterka and Benolken, 1995; Clark et al., 1996; Lasley et al., 1991). The task-related factors include load handling, physical exertion and fatigue, footwear, complexity of tasks, social interactions, and community resources (WHO, 2007; Hsiao and Simeonov, 2001; Commissaris and Toussaint, 1997; Seliga et al., 1991; Zohar, 1978; Patla, 1997). Many of the above-mentioned elements within each of the primary factors relate to the interaction between or among primary factors, although they are classified as belonging to only a single primary factor.

National and global research efforts to prevent STF vary among government agencies, professional societies, and individual safety and health research organizations. Many of the entities have focused on certain aspects of research topics and applications, such as occupational issues, biomarkers, forensics, and elderly falls. As national and global communities are moving to improve workplace safety and quality of life as a whole, countering fall hazards and risks faced by community dwellers and workers on the job, at home, and in the public area becomes more inseparable. Workers use ladders at work. People use ladders in their homes for household chores as well. Community members access building floors through stairways at home as well as at workplaces and public facilities. Adequate material properties of walkways and proper lighting are equally critical at work and at home for walkway-related fall control. Moreover, an STF injury typically affects a person's ability to perform tasks at the workplace and in the home; it may diminish a person's social capacity in the community as well. The settings may differ, but the scientific basis, risk assessment tools, and control strategies for STF are similar. Global entities, whether their specific foci are on workplace safety, home safety, or public safety, can integrate current knowledge and research efforts among all aspects to advance the identification of risk factors and innovations for STF control, and transfer realistic and effective STF interventions into practice.

1.2.4 Intervention and Implementation

In STF prevention using the public health approach, *intervention* refers to the design and evaluation of risk-factor controls to understand what works and the level of effectiveness.

Implementation refers to bringing STF prevention measures to a broad segment of the population and reducing STF at a population level. Both intervention and implementation require active partnerships and research-to-practice engagements for their effective impact. *Active partnerships* refers to collaborative partnerships among labor, industry, government agencies, academic institutions, and other stakeholders. Collaborative partnerships ensure the input from partners at all stages of the public health model to facilitate the linkage of research with the development of practical injury-control solutions. *Research-to-practice actions* refers to the transfer and translation of research findings into effective use. Organizations may focus their efforts on knowledge or technology transfer to achieve an impact on reducing fall risks, injuries, and deaths among workers or the general population.

1.3 Strategic Goals to Address Global STF Burden

The incident surveillance data described in Section 1.2.2 provide a means to highlight program activities and directions that are likely to have the greatest impact on preventing fall injuries and deaths among high-risk industries, occupations, and population groups. Some industry targets indicated by the surveillance data are the construction industry, the retail trade, and the health services industry. Occupational targets include the transportation and material-moving occupations. General population targets include focusing on fundamental knowledge and practical solutions for STF prevention in homes and communities, especially for older populations. These primary STF prevention targets are further elaborated in this chapter, and this book is organized around these subjects.

1.3.1 Reducing STF in the Construction Industry and among Construction Trade Workers

The construction industry has the highest count of STF-related fatalities of all industries in the United States, and the construction, building- and grounds-cleaning, and installation and repair occupations have encountered the highest number of STF-related fatalities. Efforts that can be made to address the burden include (1) inventory of existing fall protection technologies and identification of gaps where technical engineering guidance needs to be developed or modified further for fall prevention and protection (such as fall protection anchorage systems); (2) development and evaluation of engineering interventions and guidelines to address fall prevention gaps (such as aerial lift safety guidelines); (3) partnership with insurance companies and consultation organizations to identify the implementation obstacles to small contractors associated with existing fall prevention and protection measures (such as fall prevention in residential construction); (4) inventory of existing research, regulations, guidance, and practitioner materials on ladders, scaffolds, and roofing safety, and identification of key gaps and needs (such as graphic-based ladder safety guidelines); and (5) conducting and evaluating national or regional construction fall prevention campaigns.

1.3.2 Fall Injury Control in the Health Services Industry

The health-care and social assistance sector has the highest count of nonfatal STF-related injuries among industrial sectors. Health-care practitioners and health-care support technical occupations together are among the groups with the highest rates of falls on the same level. The literature has reported STF control strategies for the health services industry, and many of them have been adopted by the industry. In addition, STF prevention toolkits for the health-care sector are being developed and adopted by many hospitals in the United States. There is a need for the health services industry, insurance companies, occupational safety professionals, safety equipment manufacturers, government, and fall prevention research organizations to promote widespread implementation of comprehensive STF prevention programs in health-care settings.

1.3.3 Reducing STF in Retail Trade Settings

The retail trades have the second highest nonfatal STF injury counts among industrial sectors after the health-care industry. Their associated food preparation and serving occupations account for the second highest number of STF injuries, following the transportation and material-moving occupations. The retail trades are known to have some unique STF issues. Organized efforts toward STF research and prevention among the retail trades, however, are not well reported in the literature. The implementation of effective, evidence-based fall prevention and protection designs, technologies, programs, and communication materials for the handling, storage, and retrieval of merchandise is needed. Among the critical topics are (1) developing and evaluating innovative fall preventive/protective solutions (strategy, technology, or PPE) addressing merchandise storage and retrieval-associated fall incidents; (2) testing the feasibility of advanced technologies for integration into existing elevation-access devices; (3) transferring fall prevention innovations (or existing effective fall prevention solutions) and the related fall prevention knowledge into industrial practices in the retail trade, such as trucking/transporting and goods retrieval practices; and (4) providing scientific evidence and business case support for comprehensive STF prevention programs to reduce STF injuries among food service workers.

1.3.4 Reducing Fall Injuries among Transportation and Material-Moving Occupations

Transportation and material-moving occupations account for the highest number of non-fatal STF injuries among all occupations. Vehicle and equipment manufacturers, standards committees, occupational safety professionals, and government agencies can work together to improve the design of delivery trucks and material-moving procedures to reduce the risk of injuries and fatalities associated with falls from these vehicles and falls during the material-moving process. Among the main topics are (1) evaluating vehicle configuration and access system designs of delivery trucks, and working with equipment manufacturers to review and consider design enhancement; (2) working with national standards groups to update or develop vehicle configuration and access system standards for delivery vehicles; (3) developing and disseminating guidelines for vehicle configuration, access system use, and material-movement assistance systems to reduce STFs among truck drivers and material-moving workers.

1.3.5 Fall Injury Control among Vulnerable Populations

Workers of specific age, social, and economic characteristics may have unique vulnerabilities to fall injury. It is important to focus on these populations, particularly as they have been largely underserved in the past. One example is the study of the constraints on aging workforces in coping with injury risks. Injury data systems have shown that 42%

of fatal STF victims in the workplace in 2013 were aged 55 and above (BLS, 2015g). Data on fall deaths among the general population in the United States in 2013 also showed disproportional STF fatalities in the 55–85+ age category, accounting for 85% of male and 95% of female victims (NCIPC, 2015). One topic would be to study older workers' physical and psychosocial characteristics associated with falls and the mechanisms through which older citizens are at increased risk for fall injury, and develop guidance to address risks for falls among older populations.

1.3.6 Fall Injury Protection among Diverse Populations

Populations of a given age, gender, ethnicity, and occupation may have unique body size and shape compositions. Workplaces, community environments, and PPE need to be adequately designed to accommodate diverse populations. Developing improved protective gear, better home and community environments, and user-friendly assist devices for fall prevention that fit diverse population groups is a significant agenda for the research community. In addition, safety research organizations, trade associations, insurance companies, and employers can identify, characterize, and reduce fatal and serious injuries associated with falls to a lower level among Hispanic construction workers. Hispanic workers have disproportional STF-related fatalities in the construction industry (Dong et al., 2009).

1.3.7 Understanding Human Characteristics for Effective Fall Control Measures

The majority of human falls can be regarded as loss-of-balance incidents. Factors that may lead to disruption of balance include lack of adequate visual cues, inadequate lighting or visual information in the work environment, narrow and inclined support surfaces, unexpected changes in surface properties, load handling, physical exertion, fatigue, task complexity that diverts workers' attention, individual differences, lack of work experience and training, and the physiological and mental load imposed by PPE (Hsiao and Simeonov, 2001). Understanding human characteristics, social-organizational characteristics, and biotechnology-based fall control measures will generate fundamental knowledge and practical solutions for STF prevention in the workplace, the home, and the community. Research organizations can identify human biomarkers, social-organizational characteristics, and human–system interface traits that are common precursors to fall incidents, and use them to design out fall risk factors or craft engineering solutions and organizational interventions to reduce the incidence of STF. Accordingly, manufacturers can produce improved fall protection devices and systems that effectively reduce the forces on the human body during fall arrest and fall impact. Furthermore, safety professionals and researchers can develop and use comprehensive digital models of human fall dynamics to evaluate new fall prevention and protection technologies, products, and methods as well as to conduct fall injury investigations and verify solutions. Among the important topics are (1) exploring the effects of physical variations, neurological traits, cognition processes, social-organizational and cultural factors, and safety attitudes on fall risk; (2) publishing information on the effectiveness of new strategies, technologies, and sensory-enhancement approaches to reduce fall-initiation risk; (3) transferring recommendations to industrial practice on improved sizing systems and configurations of fall protection devices to accommodate current worker populations; (4) developing improved devices or accessories for impact energy or stress relief (such as swing falls and suspension-trauma relief during and after a fall incident) and establishing rescue guidelines to further protect workers; (5) developing knowledge databases for improving digital human models on fall dynamics, including the phases of fall initiation and fall termination, for use in efficient evaluation of new fall prevention and protection methods and strategies, in fall incident investigations (reconstruction), and in workers' hazard-recognition training; and (6) transferring knowledge databases to digital model developers to develop scientifically comprehensive yet easy-to-use digital modeling modules for use in workplace planning for fall prevention, workers' hazard recognition training, and fall incident investigations.

1.3.8 Emerging Issues in Fall Injury Control

In this new era of changing technology, there are unique issues in the booming green energy and digital communication businesses in which fall protection measures are important (e.g., safe erection of wind turbines and communication towers). Preplanned fall protection measures are necessary for both erection and maintenance stages. Next, smartphone-based safety software applications (apps) represent an emerging area of education and communication for STF control. Many STF risk exposure assessment tools and safety guidelines can be developed into mobile apps for STF prevention in workplaces and homes. The National Institute for Occupational Safety and Health (NIOSH) ladder safety mobile app is a successful example (Simeonov et al., 2013). Furthermore, a paradigm shift by adopting technology from other fields may offer a creative solution for STF control. For instance, the concept of wearable airbags may be useful to combat fall injuries. With advancements in durability and reduction in cost, wearable airbags to reduce fall-related injuries may become an integral part of worker fall protection systems in the near future. The notion is equally valuable in protecting inhabitants during household chore activities (e.g., window cleaning) and reducing resident and worker fall injury risk in health-care or home care settings during daily activities.

1.4 Summary

STF research has long been recognized as one of the most important and necessary areas of occupational and nonoccupational injury prevention research. The complex and multifactorial nature of STFs in workplaces, homes, and communities demands a proactive and systematic approach to prevention. Considering STF prevention as a public health matter offers an opportunity to integrate science-based information to publicize the importance of fall prevention and further STF risk factor identification and control. It also facilitates practical and effective STF innovations and implementation in the community. To maximize the benefits of this opportunity, collaborations should be actively implemented among national and international government entities, medical institutes, technology firms, STF control assist-device developers, and research centers to develop global research agendas, promote knowledge exchange, and conduct joint research. This chapter describes injury data, critical research topics, and practical suggestions for global STF control, which correspond to the overall organization of this book: from fall injury risk factors to fall prevention research, evidence-based fall prevention practices, fall injury case studies, and emerging issues in fall prevention and protection in homes, communities, and workplaces.

1.5 Disclaimer

The findings and conclusions in this chapter are those of the author and do not necessarily represent the views of the NIOSH. Mention of company names or products does not constitute endorsement by NIOSH.

References

Black S. E., Maki B. E. and Fernie G. R. (1993). Aging, imbalance, and falls, in J. A. Sharpe and H. O. Barber (eds.), *The Vestibulo-Ocular Reflex and Vertigo* (New York: Raven Press), 317–335.

Bles W., Kapteyn T. C., Brandt T. and Arnold F. (1980). The mechanism of physiological height vertigo, II. Posturography, *Acta Oto-laryngologica*, 89, 534–540.

BLS (2014a). Fatal occupational injuries by industry and event or exposure, All U.S., 2013, (Table A.1), 9/11/2014. Washington DC: US Bureau of Labor Statistics. Retrieved March 13, 2015, from http://www.bls.gov/iif/oshwc/cfoi/cftb0277.pdf.

BLS (2014b). Fatal falls to lower level by height of fall, 2013. Washington DC: US Bureau of Labor Statistics. Retrieved March 30, 2015, from http://www.bls.gov/iif/oshwc/cfoi/cfch0012.pdf.

BLS (2015a). 2013 Nonfatal occupational injuries and illnesses: cases with days away from work, January 2015. Washington DC: US Bureau of Labor Statistics. Retrieved March 13, 2015, from http://www.bls.gov/iif/oshwc/osh/case/osch0053.pdf.

BLS (2015b). Table R4. Number of nonfatal occupational injuries and illnesses involving days away from work by industry and selected events or exposures leading to injury or illness, private industry, 2013. Washington DC: US Bureau of Labor Statistics. Retrieved March 30, 2015, from http://www.bls.gov/iif/oshwc/osh/case/ostb3985.pdf.

BLS (2015c). Table R8. Incidence rates for nonfatal occupational injuries and illnesses involving days away from work per 10,000 full-time workers by industry and selected events or exposures leading to injury or illness, private industry, 2013. Washington DC: US Bureau of Labor Statistics. Retrieved March 30, 2015, from http://www.bls.gov/iif/oshwc/osh/case/ostb3989.pdf.

BLS (2015d). Table A.5. Fatal occupational injuries by occupation and event or exposure, All U.S., 2013. Washington DC: US Bureau of Labor Statistics. Retrieved March 30, 2015, from http://www.bls.gov/iif/oshwc/cfoi/cftb0281.pdf.

BLS (2015e). Table R12. Number of nonfatal occupational injuries and illnesses involving days away from work by occupation and selected events or exposures leading to injury or illness, private industry, 2013. Washington DC: US Bureau of Labor Statistics. Retrieved March 30, 2015, from http://www.bls.gov/iif/oshwc/osh/case/ostb3993.pdf.

BLS (2015f). Table R100. Incidence rates for nonfatal occupational injuries and illnesses involving days away from work per 10,000 full-time workers by occupation and selected events or exposures leading to injury or illness, private industry, 2013. Washington DC: US Bureau of Labor Statistics. Retrieved March 30, 2015, from http://www.bls.gov/iif/oshwc/osh/case/ostb4081.pdf.

BLS (2015g). Table A.8. Fatal occupational injuries by event or exposure and age, All U.S., 2013. Washington DC: US Bureau of Labor Statistics. Retrieved March 30, 2015, from http://www.bls.gov/iif/oshwc/cfoi/cftb0284.pdf.

Brandt T., Arnold F., Bles W. and Kapteyn T. S. (1980). The mechanism of physiological height vertigo, I. Theoretical approach and psychophysics, *Acta Oto-laryngologica*, 89, 513–523.

Clark M., Jackson P. and Cohen H. H. (1996). What you don't see can hurt you: Understanding the role of depth perception in slip, trip, and fall incidents, *Ergonomics in Design*, 4 (3), 16–21.

Commissaris D. A. and Toussaint H. M. (1997). Load knowledge affects low-back loading and control of balance in lifting tasks, *Ergonomics*, 40, 559–575.

Dong X. S., Fujimoto A., Ringen K. and Men Y. (2009). Fatal falls among Hispanic construction workers, *Accident Analysis and Prevention* 41 (5), 1047–1052.

Gauchard G., Chau N., Mur J. M. and Perrin P. (2001). Falls and working individuals: Role of extrinsic and intrinsic factors, *Ergonomics*, 44 (14), 1330–1339.

Hsiao H. (2014). Fall prevention research and practice: A total worker safety approach, *Industrial Health*, 52 (3), 381–392.

Hsiao H. and Simeonov P. (2001). Preventing falls from roofs: A critical review, *Ergonomics*, 44 (5), 537–561.

Knudtson M. D., Klein B. and Klein R. (2009). Biomarkers of aging and falling: The Beaver Dam eye study, *Archives of Gerontology Geriatrics*, 49 (1), 22–26.

Lasley D. J., Hamer R. D., Dister R. and Cohn T. E. (1991). Postural stability and stereo-ambiguity in man-designed visual environments, *IEEE Transactions on Biomedical Engineering*, 38, 808–813.

Mesure S., Amblard B. and Cremieux J. (1997). Effect of physical training on head-hip coordinated movements during unperturbed stance, *NeuroReport*, 8, 3507–3512.

NCIPC (2015). Leading causes of nonfatal injury reports, 2001–2013, WISQARS. Atlanta, GA: National Center for Injury Prevention and Control, Centers for Disease Control and Prevention. Retrieved March 21, 2015, from http://webappa.cdc.gov/sasweb/ncipc/nfilead2001.html.

NIOSH (2011a). *Research and practice for fall injury control in the workplace*, DHHS Publication No. 2012-103. Morgantown, WV: National Institute for Occupational Safety and Health.

NIOSH (2011b). *Slip, trip, and fall prevention for healthcare workers*, NIOSH Publication No. 2011-123. Morgantown, WV: National Institute for Occupational Safety and Health.

NSC (2014). *Injury Facts*, Itasca, IL: National Safety Council (page 134).

Patla A. E. (1997). Understanding the role of vision in the control of human locomotion, *Gait and Posture*, 5, 54–69.

Paulus W. M., Straube A. and Brandt T. (1984). Visual stabilization of posture. Physiological stimulus characteristics and clinical aspects, *Brain*, 107, 1143–1163.

Peterka R. J. and Benolken M. S. (1995). Role of somatosensory and vestibular cues in attenuating visually induced human postural sway, *Experimental Brain Research*, 105, 101–110.

Robertson S., Collins J., Elliott D. and Starkes J. (1994). The influence of skill and intermittent vision on dynamic balance, *Journal of Motor Behavior*, 26, 333–339.

Seliga R., Bhattacharya A., Succop P., Wickstrom R., Smith D. and Willeke K. (1991). Effect of work load and respirator wear on postural stability, heart rate, and perceived exertion, *American Industrial Hygiene Association Journal*, 52, 417–422.

Simeonov P., Hsiao H., Kim I-J., Powers J., Kau T. and Weaver D. (2013). Research to improve extension ladder angular positioning, *Applied Ergonomics*, 44 (3), 496–502.

Tinetti M. E. and Speechley M. (1989) Prevention of falls among the elderly, *New England Journal of Medicine*, 320, 1055–1059.

WHO (2007). *WHO Global Report on Falls Prevention in Older Age*. Geneva, Switzerland: World Health Organization.

Zohar D. (1978). Why do we bump into things while walking? *Human Factors*, 20, 671–679.

2

The Epidemiology and Risk Factors for Falls among Older Adults

Judy A. Stevens, David A. Sleet, Grant T. Baldwin, and Rita K. Noonan

CONTENTS

2.1 Introduction

The U.S. population is aging rapidly due to increasing life expectancies combined with declining birth rates. At present, 35 million people—one-eighth of the U.S. population—are over 64 years of age, and by 2020 this number is expected to reach 77 million. The aging process often results in physiological changes that can make older adults (those aged 65 years and older) particularly susceptible to falling (Peel et al., 2007).

Falls among older adults are a major public health problem. More than a third of older adults fall annually (Morrison et al., 2013), and those who fall are two to three times more likely to fall again within a year (Teno et al., 1990). Although many falls do not result in injury, about 20% cause serious injuries such as head trauma, lacerations, and fractures (Rubenstein and Josephson, 2002)—injuries that can limit mobility, diminish quality of life, and increase the risk of premature death (Alexander et al., 1992).

This chapter describes the magnitude of this health issue and briefly summarizes the epidemiology and risk factors for falls among older adults.

2.2 Public Health Burden

Falls are the leading cause of both fatal and nonfatal injuries among people aged 65 and older (Centers for Disease Control and Prevention [CDC], 2014). In 2013, there were 45,900 unintentional injury deaths among older adults, of which 55% were the result of falls. But fall deaths represent only the "tip of the iceberg." In the same year, 3.9 million nonfatal unintentional injuries among older adults were treated in emergency departments, of which 2.5 million (63%) were due to falls. Of these fall injuries, 63% were sustained by women (Figure 2.1).

One of the most serious fall outcomes is a hip fracture. This injury often results in long-term functional impairment, nursing home admission, and increased mortality (Stevens, 2005). More than 95% of all hip fractures in older adults are caused by falls (Parkkari et al., 1999), usually by falling sideways onto the hip from a standing height (Hayes et al., 1993). In 2010, there were 258,000 hospital admissions for hip fractures, and about three-quarters of these injuries were sustained by women (National Hospital Discharge Survey, 2010).

In addition to physical injuries, falls can have significant psychological and social consequences. Many people who fall, whether or not they sustain injuries, develop a fear of falling. It is estimated that between 21% and 85% of older adults are afraid of falling (Vellas et al., 1997; Friedman et al., 2002; Scheffer et al., 2008). This fear can cause people to restrict their activities, leading to reduced mobility, muscle weakness, and a subsequent increased fall risk (Vellas et al., 1997).

The financial burden of falls is also substantial. Adjusted for inflation, the direct medical costs of fall injuries among adults 65 years and older exceed $30 billion (Stevens et al., 2006). Furthermore, about two-thirds of these costs were for people who were hospitalized. The public health burden also varies by setting. Next, we describe some setting-specific characteristics of falls.

2.2.1 Community Settings

Approximately 96% of the 35 million adults aged 65 and older live independently in the community. In a 2006 national survey, an estimated 5.8 million (15.9%) community-dwelling older adults reported having fallen at least once in the preceding three months

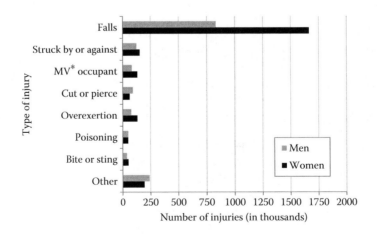

FIGURE 2.1
Leading causes of unintentional nonfatal injuries among men and women aged 65+, United States, 2013. * Motor vehicle. (Data from www.cdc.gov/ncipc/wisqars. Accessed January 29, 2014.)

(Stevens et al., 2008). Of those who said they had fallen, 23.1% reported falling three or more times. People who fall repeatedly are at a greatly increased risk of sustaining a serious injury (Nevitt et al., 1991). Between one-half and two-thirds of all falls happen in or around the home (Deprey, 2009), and most people fall on the same level and from a standing height (e.g., by slipping or tripping while walking) (Ellis and Trent, 2001).

2.2.2 Nursing Homes

Nursing-home residents are particularly vulnerable to falls and fall-related injuries. The fall rate among nursing-home residents is two to three times the rate for older adults living in the community, with an average incidence of 1.5 falls per bed per year (Rubenstein et al., 1994). At least half of nursing-home residents fall annually, and the proportion is higher among certain high-risk groups such as people with dementia, where the incidence is 70%–80% (Shaw, 2007). Compared with older adults living in the community, people in nursing homes are older, more likely to be cognitively impaired, have a greater number and more severe chronic conditions, and have more functional limitations—all factors that are associated with falling (Ejaz et al., 1994).

2.2.3 Hospitals

Fall rates among hospital patients vary by patient population, type of hospital, and reasons for hospitalization. The highest rates are seen among the oldest patients and, within the geriatric population, rates of 8.9–17.1 falls per 1000 patient-days have been reported for neuroscience, rehabilitation, and psychiatry departments (Nyberg et al., 1997; Rhode et al., 1990).

2.3 Epidemiology

2.3.1 Fatal Falls

In 2013, 25,464 older adults died from fall injuries (CDC, 2014). This is an average of one death every 21 min (CDC, 2014). Rates differ by both sex and race. Whites have the highest fall death rates, followed by the rates for Asians and blacks (Stevens and Dellinger, 2002). Men are more likely than women to die from a fall. In 2013, the age-adjusted fall death rate for men (67.9 per 100,000 of population) was 39% higher than the rate for women (48.7 per 100,000). Rates for both men and women increased sharply with age, with the greatest rate increase occurring after age 80 (CDC, 2014).

National data show that from 2000 to 2013, age-adjusted fall death rates increased 76% in men and 99% in women (CDC, 2014) (Figure 2.2). Reasons for this increase are unclear. One possible explanation is that the U.S. population is living longer with chronic conditions such as diabetes, arthritis, and cardiovascular disease. In addition, the quality of these data depends on the training and/or experience of the physician or medical examiner filling out the death certificate, and falls may be undercounted if a fall did not occur close to the time of death.

2.3.2 Nonfatal Falls

In 2013, 2.5 million nonfatal falls among people aged 65 and older were treated in hospital emergency departments (CDC, 2014). About 69% of patients were treated and released

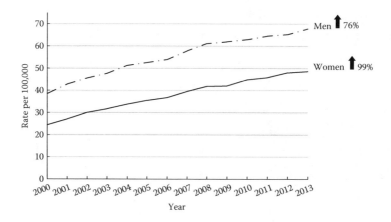

FIGURE 2.2
Trends in age-adjusted fall death rates for men and women aged ≥65, United States, 2000–2013. (Data from www.cdc.gov/ncipc/wisqars. Accessed January 29, 2014.)

while about 30% was subsequently hospitalized. Women are disproportionately affected by nonfatal fall injuries. In 2013, after adjusting for age, the fall injury rate for women was 43% higher than the rate for men (CDC, 2014).

Women were more likely to sustain serious injuries such as fractures and head injuries that required hospitalization. Compared to men, injury rates for women were 2.2 times higher for fractures, 70% higher for contusions or abrasions, and 10% higher for lacerations (Stevens and Sogolow, 2005).

Much of the observed gender disparity is due to women's greater susceptibility to hip fracture, an extremely serious fall injury that can result in disability, nursing-home admission, and increased mortality (Wolinsky et al., 1997; Hall et al., 2000; Braithwaite et al., 2003). White women are much more likely to sustain hip fractures than are African-American or Asian women (Ellis and Trent, 2001). Although most hip fractures are caused by falls (Parkkari et al., 1999), usually by falling sideways onto the hip from a standing height (Hayes et al., 1993), an important contributing factor is osteoporosis, a metabolic disease that makes bones porous and susceptible to fracture, and which most often affects postmenopausal women and men over age 80 (National Osteoporosis Foundation, 2010).

2.3.3 Fall Risk Factors

Epidemiological studies have identified numerous fall risk factors, and the prevalence of many of these increases with age. Risk factors frequently are classified as intrinsic or biological (i.e., originating within the body), extrinsic or environmental (i.e., originating outside the body), and behavioral. Selected fall risk factors are shown in Table 2.1.

2.3.4 Risk Factor Interactions

Most falls are the result of interactions among multiple risk factors (Rubenstein and Josephson, 2006) (see Figure 2.3). In an early study of community-dwelling older adults, Tinetti et al. (1986) found that the likelihood of falling increased with the number of risk factors present. The proportion of people who fell increased rapidly, from 27% for those with one risk factor to 32% for those with two risk factors, to 60% for those with three risk factors, to 78% for those with four or more risk factors.

TABLE 2.1

Selected Fall Risk Factors

Biological	Environmental	Behavioral
Advanced age	Lack of stair handrails	Multiple medications
Previous falls	Poor stair design	Psychoactive medications
Female gender	Lack of bathroom grab bars	Inactivity
Muscle weakness	Dim lighting or glare	Risk-taking behaviors
Poor balance and coordination	Obstacles and tripping hazards	Fear of falling
Gait disorders	Slippery or uneven surfaces	Improper or inappropriate use
Poor vision	Poor building design and/or	of mobility aids
Chronic conditions: arthritis,	maintenance	Poor nutrition or hydration
diabetes, stroke, Parkinson's	Poorly designed or maintained	Inappropriate footwear
disease, incontinence, dementia	public spaces	Alcohol use

Source: Data adapted from Scott, V., Prevention of falls and injuries among the elderly. Vancouver, BC: British Columbia—Office of the Provincial Health Officer, 2004; and Rubenstein L.Z. et al., *Med Clin North Am* 90(5), 807–824, 2006.

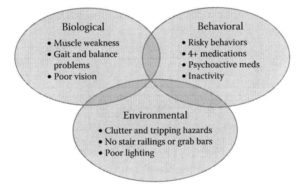

FIGURE 2.3
Multifactorial fall interventions.

2.4 Fall Prevention Interventions

Fall prevention efforts have focused on a number of potentially modifiable risk factors. These include muscle weakness in the legs, gait and balance problems, psychoactive medication use, poor vision, and environmental hazards (Rubenstein and Josephson, 2002). In addition, identifying and treating the symptoms of chronic conditions may reduce fall risk (AG/BGS, 2010).

Effective interventions may involve a single strategy or be multifactorial. The most effective single strategy involves exercise or physical therapy to improve gait, balance, and strength (Stevens et al., 2010). Multifactorial interventions include components that address a number of fall risk factors. An example is a clinical intervention that includes fall risk factor assessment, treatment, and/or referrals to specialists. Community-based multifactorial interventions usually include education about fall risk factors, an exercise program, medication review and modification, and other elements such as vision correction and/or home hazard reduction. Effective home-based interventions are implemented by occupational therapists and include home modification coupled with behavioral changes (Stevens, 2010).

2.5 Future Directions

As we move forward, we will need to refine these proven interventions to broaden their use across diverse populations, create an infrastructure to train implementers how to use proven strategies, disseminate effective fall prevention programs, and support widespread adoption at the local level.

Incorporating research findings into practice remains a challenge due to limited time for implementation, poor motivation of the target population, and insufficient cooperation among health care providers (Hester and Wei, 2013). Evidence exists to demonstrate that it is possible to scale up an effective health-related fall prevention program in a community of older adults with differing cultural backgrounds, provided the intervention adheres to three conditions:

1. The intervention is translated and delivered in the *participants' native language.*
2. The intervention is *implemented by a broadly embedded community organization,* such as an Area Agency on Aging.
3. The intervention is delivered with *fidelity to specific research-tested protocols* (Sleet and Baldwin, 2014).

Such a multifaceted approach would support the broad implementation of effective fall interventions and would reduce the personal and societal burden associated with falls among older adults.

Interventions that focus on changing individual behavior can produce population-level change when scaling up is feasible, cost-effective, and sustainable. It is possible to broadly implement effective adult fall prevention programs when these are fully integrated and leverage existing infrastructure, such as through Area Agencies on Aging, YMCAs, and other community outlets.

Efforts like Stopping Elderly Accidents, Deaths, and Injuries (STEADI)—a toolkit to support decision making—can help simplify, standardize, and automate evidence-based practice protocols. The result will be improved screening, treatment, and outcomes. STEADI will also help health care practitioners utilize clinical guidelines, reduce barriers to care and foster public/private insurance mechanisms to incentivize best practices using innovative reimbursement methods. Straightforward clinical interventions like modifying older adult patients' medications and encouraging them to take at least 800 IU Vitamin D daily can reduce the risk of falling (Kalyani et al., 2010; Murad et al., 2011; Gillespie et al., 2012; Hill and Wee, 2012). Integrating best practices in public health using electronic health records or other health information technologies offers a promising solution.

Finally, greater efforts can be made to engage those who are most integrated into the social life of older adults—caregivers. Although caregivers have been largely ignored in fall prevention efforts, but they act as a health "gatekeepers." They can mitigate fall risk factors by accompanying the older adult to medical appointments and requesting a fall risk assessment; supporting exercise to help the older adult improve lower body strength and balance; encouraging medication reviews and providers to conduct vision assessments; and engaging an occupational therapist or a certified Aging-in-Place specialist to conduct a home safety assessment (Roldos et al., 2013).

2.6 Conclusion

Falls and fall injuries are age-related problems, and the U.S. population is aging rapidly. People over 85 represent the fastest growing segment of the older population (Bureau of Census, 2010) and have the highest fall injury rate (CDC, 2014). In the future, a greater number of older adults will be affected by these injuries unless we take preventive action—including educating older adults, caregivers, health-care providers, and senior services providers about fall risk factors and effective prevention strategies. Public health and clinical medicine can be partners in reducing the societal burden of fall injuries and improving the health and quality of life for older adults.

2.7 Disclaimer

The findings and conclusions in this chapter are those of the author and do not necessarily represent the views of the Centers for Disease Control and Prevention (CDC). Mention of company names or products does not constitute endorsement by CDC.

References

AGS/BGS Clinical Practice Guideline: Prevention of Falls in Older Persons. The American Geriatrics Society. (2010). Retrieved July 18, 2016 from http://www.americangeriatrics.org/health_care_professionals/clinical_practice/clinical_guidelines_recommendations/prevention_of_falls_summary_of_recommendations.

Alexander, B.H., Rivara, F.P., and Wolf, M.E. (1992). The cost and frequency of hospitalization for fall-related injuries in older adults. *Am J Pub Health*, 82(7), 1020–1023.

Braithwaite, R.S., Co, N.F., and Wong, J.B. (2003). Estimating hip fracture morbidity, mortality and costs. *J Am Geriatr Soc*, 51, 364–370.

Bureau of the Census (US). (2014). Population Projections: 2008 National Population Projections, Summary Tables. Retrieved July 18, 2016 from http://www.census.gov/population/projections/data/national/2008.html.

Centers for Disease Control and Prevention (CDC). (2014). Web-based Injury Statistics Query and Reporting System (WISQARS). National Center for Injury Prevention and Control, Centers for Disease Control and Prevention (producer) (online). Retrieved July 18, 2016 from http://www.cdc.gov/injury/wisqars/index.html.

Deprey, S.M. (2009). Descriptive analysis of fatal falls of older adults in a Midwestern county in the year 2005. *J Geriatr Phys Ther*, 32(2), 23–28.

Ejaz, F.K., Jones, J.A., and Rose, M.S. (1994). Falls among nursing home residents: An examination of incident reports before and after restraint reduction programs. *J Am Geriatr Soc*, 42(9), 960–964.

Ellis, A.A. and Trent, R.B. (2001). Hospitalized fall injuries and race in California. *Inj Prev*, 7, 316–320.

Friedman, S.M., Munoz, B., West, S.K., Rubin, G.S., and Fried, L.P. (2002). Falls and fear of falling: Which comes first? A longitudinal prediction model suggests strategies for primary and secondary prevention. *J Am Geriatr Soc*, 50(8), 1329–1335.

Gillespie, L.D., Robertson, M.C., Gillespie, W.J, Sherrington, C., Gates, S., Clemson, L.M., and Lamb, S.E. (2012). Interventions for preventing falls in older people living in the community. *Cochrane Database Syst Rev*, 9, CD007146.

Hall, S.E., Williams, J.A., Senior, J.A., Goldswain, P.R., and Criddle, R.A. (2000). Hip fracture outcomes: Quality of life and functional status in older adults living in the community. *Aust NZ J Med*, 30(3), 327–332.

Hayes, W.C., Myers, E.R., Morris, J.N., Gerhart, T.N., Yett, H.S., and Lipsitz, L.A. (1993). Impact near the hip dominates fracture risk in elderly nursing home residents who fall. *Calcif Tissue Int*, 52, 192–198.

Hester, A.L. and Wei, F. (2013). Falls in the community: State of the science. *Clin Interv Aging*, 8, 675–679.

Hill, K.D. and Wee, R. (2012). Psychotropic drug-induced falls in older people: A review of interventions aimed at reducing the problem. *Drugs Aging*, 29(1), 15–30.

Kalyani, R.R., Stein, B., Valiyil, R., Manno, R., Maynard, J.W., and Crews, D.C. (2010). Vitamin D treatment for the prevention of falls in older adults: Systematic review and meta-analysis. *J Am Geriatr Soc*, 58(7), 1299–1310.

Murad, M.H., Elamin, K.B., Abu Elnour, N.O., Elamin, M.B., Alkatib, A.A., Fatourechi, M.M., Almandoz, J.P., et al. (2011). Clinical review: The effect of vitamin D on falls: A systematic review and meta-analysis. *J Clin Endocrinol Metab*, 96(10) 2997–3006.

Morrison, A., Fan, T., Sen, S.S., and Weisenfluh, L. (2013). Epidemiology of falls and osteoporotic fractures: A systematic review. *Clinicoecon Outcomes Res*, 5, 9–18.

National Hospital Discharge Survey (NHDS). (2010). National Center for Health Statistics. Retrieved January 16, 2014 from http://www.cdc.gov/nchs/hdi.htm.

National Osteoporosis Foundation (NOF). (2010). Clinician's guide to prevention and treatment of osteoporosis. Retrieved July 18, 2016 from http://www.natap.org/2008/HIV/NOF_Clinicians_Guide-1.pdf.

Nevitt, M.C., Cummings, S.R., and Hudes, E.S. (1991). Risk factors for injurious falls: A prospective study. *J Geront Med Sci*, 46(5), M164–170.

Nyberg, L., Gustafson, Y., Janson, A., Sandman, P-O., and Eriksson, S. (1997). Incidence of falls in three different types of geriatric care. *Scand J Soc Med*, 25(1), 8–13.

Parkkari J., Kannus, P., Palvanen, M., Natri, A., Vainio J., Aho, H., Vuori, I., and Järvinen, M. (1999). Majority of hip fractures occur as a result of a fall and impact on the greater trochanter of the femur: A prospective controlled hip fracture study with 206 consecutive patients. *Calcif Tissue Int*, 65, 183–187.

Peel, N.M., McClure, R.J., and Hendrikz, J.K. (2007). Psychosocial factors associated with fall-related hip-fractures. *Age Ageing*, 36, 145–151.

Rhode, J.M., Myers, A.H., and Vlahov, D. (1990). Variation in risk for falls by clinical department: Implications for prevention. *Infect Control Hosp Epidemiol*, 11(10), 521–524.

Roldos, I., Noonan, R.K., and Beattie, L. (2013). Strengthening the role of caregivers in promoting fall-risk screening for older adults during the wellness visit. *Perspect Public Health*, 133(5), 246–247.

Rubenstein, L.Z. and Josephson, K.R. (2002). The epidemiology of falls and syncope. *Clin Geriatric Med*, 18(2), 141–158.

Rubenstein, L.Z. and Josephson, K.R. (2006). Falls and their prevention in elderly people: What does the evidence show? *Med Clin North Am*, 90(5), 807–824.

Rubenstein, L.Z., Josephson, K.R., and Robbins, A.S. (1994). Falls in the nursing home. *Ann Intern Med*, 121, 442–451.

Scheffer, A.C., Schuurmans, M.J., Van Dijk, N., and Van Der Hoof, T. (2008). Fear of falling: Measurement strategy, prevalence, risk factors and consequences among older persons. *Age Ageing*, 37, 19–24.

Scott, V. (2004). Prevention of falls and injuries among the elderly. Vancouver, BC: British Columbia—Office of the Provincial Health Officer.

Shaw, F.E. (2007). Prevention of falls in older people with dementia. *J Neural Trans*, 114, 1259–1264.

Sleet, D.A. and Baldwin, G.T. (2014). Can an evidence-based fall prevention program be translated for use in culturally diverse communities? *J Sport Health Sci*. (online: http://dx.doi.org/10.1016/j.jshs.2013.11.001).

Stevens, J.A. (2005). Falls among older adults: Risk factors and prevention strategies. In: *Falls Free: Promoting a National Falls Prevention Action Plan: Research Review Papers*. NCOA Center for Healthy Aging, 3–18.

Stevens, J.A. (2015). A CDC compendium of effective fall interventions: What works for community-dwelling older adults. Atlanta, GA: Centers for Disease Control and Prevention, National Center for Injury Prevention and Control. Retrieved July 18, 2016 from http://www.cdc.gov/homeandrecreationalsafety/falls/pubs.html.

Stevens, J.A., Corso, P.S., Finkelstein, E.A. and Miller, T.R. (2006). Cost of fatal and nonfatal falls among older adults. *Inj Prev*, 12(5), 290–295.

Stevens, J.A. and Dellinger, A.M. (2002). Motor vehicle and fall related deaths among older Americans 1990–98: Sex, race, and ethnic disparities. *Inj Prev*, 8, 272–275.

Stevens, J.A., Mack, K.A., Paulozzi, L.J., and Ballesteros, M.F. (2008). Self-reported falls and fall-related injuries among persons aged≥65 years—United States, 2006. *J Safety Res*, 39, 345–349.

Stevens, J.A., Noonan, R.K., and Rubenstein, L.Z. (2010). Older adult fall prevention: Perceptions, beliefs, and behaviors. *Am J Lifestyle Med*, 4(1), 16–20.

Stevens, J.A. and Sogolow, E.D. (2005). Gender differences for non-fatal unintentional fall related injuries among older adults. *Inj Prev*, 11(2), 115–119.

Teno, J., Kiel, D.P., and Mor, V. (1990). Multiple stumbles: A risk factor for falls in community-dwelling elderly. A prospective study. *J Am Geriatr Soc*, 38, 1321–1325.

Tinetti, M.E., Williams, T.F., and Mayewski, R. (1986). Fall risk index for elderly patients based on number of chronic disabilities. *Am J Med*, 80, 429–434.

Vellas, B.J., Wayne, S.J., Romero, L.J., Baumgartner, R.N., and Garry, P.J. (1997). Fear of falling and restriction of mobility in elderly fallers. *Age Ageing*, 26, 189–193.

Wolinsky, F.D., Fitzgerald, J.F., and Stump, T.E. (1997). The effect of hip fracture on mortality, hospitalization, and functional status: A prospective study. *Am J Pub Health*, 87(3), 398–403.

3

Fall Prevention in Nursing Homes

Laurence Z. Rubenstein and Rosalba Arauz Rivera

CONTENTS

3.1 Introduction

Nursing homes (NHs) are places where frail and vulnerable people reside, and falls are extremely common therein. Falls in NHs produce high rates of morbidity, mortality, hospitalizations, lawsuits, and excess expenses. Controlled studies have shown many strategies to be effective in reducing falls among older persons in a variety of locations, although fewer strategies have been shown to be effective in NHs because of the frailty of the NH population. The key to preventing falls in NHs involves a systematic approach that identifies risk factors and arranges interventions to reduce them, both among residents who have fallen as well as among those who have not yet fallen.

3.2 Epidemiology

The incidence of falls in older adults and the severity of complications increase with age, morbidity, and physical disability. Unintentional injuries are among the top causes of death in older adults, and falls account for two-thirds of such deaths (Rubenstein, 2006).

In NHs, fall rates are more than twice as high as in the community. The mean fall incidence calculated from several large NH studies is two to three times the rate for community-living elderly persons (mean, 1.5 falls/bed per year), related to both the more frail nature of persons living in NHs and to more accurate reporting of falls in institutions

(Rubenstein and Josephson 2002) (http://www.cdc.gov/homeandrecreationalsafety/falls/nursing.html).

In 2003, 1.5 million people in the United States aged 65 years and older lived in NHs (National Center for Health Statistics, 2005). If current rates continue, by 2030 this number will have risen to about 3 million (Sahyoun et al., 2001). While only about 5% of adults aged 65 and older live in NHs, about 20% of deaths in those aged 65 and older occur in NHs. Each year, a typical NH with 100 beds reports 100–200 falls, and many less serious falls go unreported (Rubenstein et al., 1994). Each year, about 1800 people living in the United States NHs die from falls. About 10%–20% of NH falls cause serious injuries; 2%–6% cause fractures (Rubenstein et al., 1988). About 35% of fall injuries in NHs occur among residents who cannot walk (Thapa et al., 1996).

In addition to causing injuries, falls can have serious consequences for physical functioning and quality of life. Loss of function can result from both fracture-related disability as well as self-imposed functional limitations caused by fear of falling and "post-fall anxiety syndrome." Decreased confidence in the ability to ambulate safely can lead to further functional decline, depression, feelings of helplessness, and social isolation. In addition, the use of physical or chemical restraints by institutional staff to prevent high-risk persons from falling also has negative effects on functioning.

3.3 Causes and Risk Factors for NH Falls

Frail, high-risk persons living in institutions tend to have a higher incidence of falls caused by gait disorders, weakness, dizziness, and confusion, whereas falls among community-living persons tend to be more related to environmental or situational hazards (Rubenstein et al., 1994).

A large study in 528 German NHs found that about 75% of falls occurred in the resident's rooms or in the bathrooms, with transfers and walking responsible for 41% and 36% of all falls, respectively. Most falls were observed between 10 a.m. and midday and between 2 p.m. and 8 p.m. (Rapp et al., 2012).

The prevalence of risk factors for falls is higher in NHs than in the community, and most residents have more than one risk factor. In the long-term care (LTC) setting, well recognized risk factors are muscular weakness, balance and gait deficits, poor vision, delirium, cognitive and functional impairment, orthostatic hypotension (OH), urinary incontinence, medications (number of drugs, antidepressants, antipsychotics, sedatives, nonsteroidal anti-inflammatory drugs, vasodilators) and comorbidities (depression, stroke, Parkinson's disease, arthritis) (Becker et al., 2010).

Data from a survey on a probabilistic sample of residents in a Spanish NH showed a fall rate of 2.4 falls per person year (95% confidence interval [CI], 2.04–2.82). The strongest risk factor was the number of diseases, with an adjusted rate ratio (RR) of 1.32 (95% CI, 1.17–1.50) for each additional diagnosis. Other variables associated with falls were urinary incontinence (RR = 2.56 [95% CI, 1.32–4.94]); antidepressant use (RR = 2.32 [95% CI, 1.22–4.40]); arrhythmias (RR = 2.00 [95% CI, 1.05–3.81]); and polypharmacy (RR = 1.07[95% CI, 0.95–1.21] for each additional medication). The attributable fraction for number of diseases (with reference to those with ≤1 condition) was 84% (95% CI, 45%–95%) (Damian et al., 2013).

A systematic review and meta-analysis from 2013 aimed to provide a comprehensive and quantitative understanding of risk factors for falls in older people in NHs and hospitals. Twenty-four studies met the inclusion criteria. Eighteen risk factors for NH residents and six for older hospital inpatients were considered, including sociodemographics, mobility, sensory impairments, medical factors, and medication use. For NH residents, the strongest associations were with history of falls (OR = 3.06), walking-aid use (OR = 2.08), and moderate disability (OR = 2.08). A few other medical conditions and medications were also associated with a moderately increased risk. For some important factors (e.g., balance and muscle weakness), a summary estimate was not computed because the measures used in various studies were not comparable. The authors concluded that falls among institutionalized older people have multifactorial etiologies. A history of falls, use of walking aids, and disability are strong predictors of future falls (Deandrea et al., 2013).

One recent study analyzed real-life falls in LTC captured on video and found that the most frequent cause of falling was incorrect weight shifting, which accounted for 41% of falls, followed by trip or stumble (21%), hit or bump (11%), loss of support (11%), and collapse (11%). Slipping accounted for only 3% of falls. The three activities associated with the highest proportion of falls were forward walking (24%), standing quietly (13%), and sitting down (12%) (Robinovitch et al., 2013).

As people age, risk factors for falls become more common. For example, bone density decreases, joints become stiffer and less flexible, and cartilage degenerates. Muscles atrophy, have less tone, and contract less efficiently. The prevalence of most diseases increases.

Nonspecific symptoms also increase with age. For example, dizziness, vertigo, and disequilibrium are common symptoms with age and can result from many factors, including a peripheral or central vestibular disorder, drug side effects, postural hypotension, and vascular insufficiency, to name but a few. Dizziness is commonly reported by elderly persons who have fallen; however, it is often difficult to evaluate this symptom because it means different things for different people and has several causes. Symptoms described as "imbalance on walking" often stem from a gait disorder. Many residents describe a vague light-headedness that may reflect cardiovascular problems, hyperventilation, OH, drug side effects, anxiety, or depression (Rubenstein et al., 1994).

Syncope (a sudden loss of consciousness with spontaneous recovery) is a major cause of falls. However, it is relatively uncommon in most fall studies (0.3%–5%) (Rubenstein et al., 2002), which is likely because many clinical trials exclude patients with this diagnosis. Also, it is often difficult to diagnose syncope because it is typically not witnessed, and many patients present with retrograde amnesia and may confuse syncope with drop attacks (sudden falls without loss of consciousness and without dizziness) (Rubenstein et al., 1994).

Framingham data show that the incidence of syncope rises sharply after 70 years of age, from 5.5 events per 1000 person years between the ages of 60 and 69, to 11.1 between 70 and 79 years (Soteriades et al., 2002). A study of institutionalized patients 75 years of age and older reported a 6% annual incidence of syncope, with a recurrence rate of 30% (Lipsitz et al., 1985).

Some syncope arises from disorders of maintaining adequate blood pressure (BP), such as OH, postprandial hypotension, or vasovagal hypotension. Patients with vasovagal or neurogenic OH can present with light-headedness, presyncope, or syncope resulting from systemic hypotension. The ability to maintain an upright posture without syncope requires the coordinated actions of an intact autonomic nervous system. Both exaggerated autonomic reflexes, as seen in vasovagal syncope; or autonomic nerve damage and hypofunction of the autonomic nervous system, as seen in neurogenic OH, can result in syncope (Raj et al., 2013).

Postprandial hypotension, or fall in BP after a meal, is a syndrome that is well described in NH patients but is still under-recognized. Patients with Parkinson's disease and autonomic failure are at particularly high risk (Luciano et al., 2010). One study showed that the biggest drop in systolic and diastolic blood pressure occurred 45 min after a meal, without a significant change in pulse rate. The authors concluded that nurses caring for NH patients should be on the alert for drops in postprandial blood pressure so as to reduce the risk of falls, syncope, and stroke (Son et al., 2002).

Estimates of the prevalence of OH have been as high as 70% in LTC facilities. OH has been shown in numerous studies to represent an intrinsic risk factor for falls in older adults, with an associated odds ratio of about 2.2. One study concluded that OH is an independent risk factor for recurrent falls among NH residents (Gangavati et al., 2011; Heitterachi et al., 2002; Ooi et al., 2000; Tinetti et al., 1994).

The 1996 American Autonomic Society and American Academy of Neurology Consensus criteria defined OH as sphygmomanometer-measured drops in systolic blood pressure (SBP) of 20 mmHg and diastolic blood pressure (DBP) of 10 mmHg during active standing or head up tilt. This consensus was updated in 2011, which included a definition for "initial OH" (>40 mmHg drop SBP, >20 mmHg drop DBP), a requirement for a larger drop in people with hypertension (>30 mmHg SBP), and the addition of the term *sustained drop* to the previous diagnostic criteria of OH (Freeman et al., 2011; Consensus Committee of the American Autonomic Society and the American Academy of Neurology, 1996). Although the benefit of treating OH will require further study, a prudent approach seems to be to identify high-risk residents and institute precautionary measures (Ooi et al., 2000; Frith et al., 2014).

Medications have long been associated with falls. The strongest risk associations occur with psychotropic medications, antihypertensives, and polypharmacy (defined variably as taking more than 4, 5, or 6 medications) (Kim et al., 2001; Tinetti et al., 2014; Panel on Prevention of Falls in Older Persons, American Geriatrics Society and British Geriatrics Society, 2011).

Several studies have shown that despite consensus recommendations and prescribing guidelines, potentially inappropriate psychoactive medications continue to be frequently prescribed to elderly NH residents and to be associated with falls (Agashivala and Wu, 2009). In one recent study, the most unsafe profile was detected for long-half-life benzodiazepines, neuroleptic agents, and psychotropic medications in combination (Olazarán et al., 2013). A recent study found a significant relationship between hip fracture and the use of nonbenzodiazepine hypnotic drugs (Zolpidem tartrate, Eszopiclone, or Zaleplon) (Berry et al., 2013). Cognitive impairment and dementia are important risk factors for falls, and these conditions frequently coexist with other risk factors. The most common risk factors for falls that occur in patients with cognitive impairment and dementia are postural instability, hazardous medications, and neurocardiovascular instability (Tinetti et al., 1988).

Because NH residents with dementia fall more often than their nondemented counterparts, such patients are important candidates for NH fall prevention programs. However, dementia patients are particularly challenging because they typically forget to follow prevention protocols or other directions, are often still ambulatory, and usually require more supervision for safety than nondemented patients (Montero-Odasso et al., 2012; Van Doorn et al., 2003).

Sarcopenia is a syndrome characterized by progressive and generalized loss of skeletal muscle mass and strength with a risk of adverse outcomes such as physical disability, poor quality of life, falls, and death (Hartman et al., 2007; Delmonico et al., 2007). The European Working Group on Sarcopenia in Older People recommends using the presence of both low muscle mass and low muscle function (strength or performance) for the diagnosis of sarcopenia (Cruz-Jentoft et al., 2010).

Frailty is a geriatric syndrome resulting from age-related cumulative declines across multiple physiologic systems, with impaired homeostatic reserve and a reduced capacity of the organism to withstand stress. This increases vulnerability to adverse health outcomes including falls, hospitalization, institutionalization, and mortality. Frailty and sarcopenia overlap; most frail older people exhibit sarcopenia, and many older people with sarcopenia are also frail. Both syndromes are very common in NH patients (Bauer and Sieber, 2008; Fried et al., 2001; Cruz-Jentoft et al., 2010). Studies have evaluated the relation between sarcopenia and falls. One found that sarcopenic participants were over three times as likely to fall during a follow-up period of two years relative to nonsarcopenic individuals, regardless of age, gender, and other confounding factors over the two-year follow-up ($p < .001$, HR 3.23). Another study concluded that, among subjects living in a NH, sarcopenia is highly prevalent and is associated with a significantly increased risk of all-cause death. The current findings support the possibility that sarcopenia has an independent effect on survival among NH residents (Landi et al., 2012).

Muscle weakness, related to sarcopenia and frailty as well as simple inactivity, is another highly predictive risk factor for falls. It is also very common in the NH population, and its presence should be specifically looked for (Moreland et al., 2004).

3.4 Therapy and Prevention Programs

Prevention of falls in the NH setting is challenging, since the risk factors associated with these patients are multiple and often hard to alter. The reason that a person is admitted to long-term NH care is usually multifactorial and is often directly and indirectly related to falls and instability.

One study showed that the main chronic medical conditions associated with NH admission were dementia and stroke. Mental disorders represent 48% of all admissions, somatic disorders 43%, and social/emotional problems 8%. Of the somatic disorders, most frequently mentioned are diseases of the circulatory system (35%) (2/3 sequellae of stroke and 1/5 heart failure), followed by diseases of the nervous system (15%) (largely Parkinson's disease) and the musculoskeletal system (14%) (largely osteoarthritis). The most striking evolution from 1993 to 2005 was an increased prevalence of complicated diabetes mellitus (from 4.3% to 11.4%; $p < .0001$), especially with amputations and blindness. Symptoms such as dizziness, impaired vision, mobility problems, functional impairment, and frailty are also important contributory reasons for NH admission (Van Rensbergen et al., 2010).

The 2011 clinical practice guidelines of the American and British Geriatrics Societies recommend a multifactorial fall risk assessment for all older adults who present with a fall, who report more than one prior fall, or who have gait and balance problems. A fall risk assessment is not considered necessary for older persons reporting only a single fall without reported or demonstrated difficulty or unsteadiness. While these guidelines were intended primarily for community-living elders, virtually all NH residents would be in the category of individuals for whom a full multifactorial fall risk assessment would be recommended (Panel on Prevention of Falls in Older Persons, American Geriatrics Society and British Geriatrics Society, 2011).

While not found in all studies, the preponderance of evidence from controlled trials, confirmed in meta-analyses, is that that fall prevention programs are effective in the overall reduction of falls. While most of this evidence is from community-based trials, a growing number of NH trials are showing positive results. In general, the evidence is less conclusive for single interventions in LTC facilities than for multifactorial and interdisciplinary interventions (Choi et al., 2012; Neyens et al., 2011). A cluster randomized controlled trial found that a multifactorial falls prevention program that included a 3-month gait and balance training program, a medication review, and podiatry and optometry components showed a substantial reduction in fall risk factors, which translated to a modest reduction in actual falls rates (Dyer et al., 2004).

Fall prevention planning for individual NH patients begins with a careful fall risk assessment, usually using a specific assessment tool. A systematic literature search on fall risk assessment tools found that many such tools are readily available and assess similar patient characteristics. Although their diagnostic accuracy and overall usefulness showed wide variability, there are several scales that can be used with confidence as part of an effective fall prevention program, and the authors make some specific recommendations. Consequently, there should be little need for facilities to develop their own scales. Moreover, to continue to develop fall risk assessments unique to individual facilities may be counterproductive because scores will not be comparable across facilities (Perell et al., 2001; Scott et al., 2007).

More challenging than fall risk assessment is taking the next step: coming up with effective treatments and interventions to prevent future falls. There is no standard approach for treatment and prevention for all people because the etiology of falls is multifactorial. Each patient must have an individualized plan that includes intrinsic and extrinsic risk factors and functional levels. When the fall is caused by a single acute event, the treatment is usually simple and effective; however, most patients fall because of multiple chronic and interacting conditions, and treatment will require a combination of medical, rehabilitative, environmental, and behavioral intervention strategies.

Patient compliance with recommendations and cooperation with staff interventions, especially among frail and cognitively impaired patients, is also problematic. Physical activity is and should be encouraged as a positive goal that can lead to higher function and quality of life; however, activity also facilitates the opportunity for falling and injuries. Although not well studied, active persons may have more falls overall but may also have fewer falls per unit of activity. These interactions among falls, activity levels, frailty, and injury need to be studied much more carefully (Rubenstein et al., 2002).

A recent review examined published studies as to whether sensor technologies could prevent falls and fall-related injuries in institutionalized elderly. While their review did not find definitive benefit, the authors concluded that further research should focus more comprehensively on user requirements and effective ways of using intelligent alarms. In general, alarms should be considered as part of a larger fall prevention program and should not be relied on alone (Kosse et al., 2013).

A Cochrane review of fall prevention trials in institutional settings (43 trials in care facilities such as NHs and 17 in hospitals) concluded that in NHs, vitamin D supplementation is effective in reducing the rate of falls but not the risk of falling. Exercise programs in subacute hospital settings appear to be effective, but their effectiveness in NHs remains uncertain due to conflicting results, possibly associated with differences in interventions and levels of dependency. There is evidence that multifactorial interventions reduce fall rates in hospitals, but the evidence for the risk of falling was inconclusive. Evidence for multifactorial interventions in NHs suggests possible benefits, but this was inconclusive (Cameron et al., 2012).

Studies finished after the Cochrane report have been more positive in support of NH exercise and rehabilitation programs. A more recent meta-analysis study that combined studies of frequent and long-term exercise programs showed effectiveness in preventing falls in LTC facilities (Silva et al., 2013).

3.4.1 Gait and Balance Impairments

Residents with gait and balance disturbances should be evaluated for the underlying process. After examination, this can usually be categorized into problems with strength, sensation, pain, joint mobility, spasticity, or central processing or, commonly, a combination of these (Trueblood et al., 1991). Alterations in gait in older adults are associated with falls, dementia, and disability; at the same time, emerging evidence indicates that early disturbances in cognitive processes such as attention, executive function, and working memory are associated with slower gait and gait instability during single- and dual-task testing and that these cognitive disturbances assist in the prediction of future mobility loss, falls, and progression to dementia (Montero-Odasso et al., 2012).

Treatment approaches should be individually tailored but generally involve programs of gait training, specific exercises, and prescription of assistive devices. Gait training, usually under the supervision of a physical therapist, can be particularly helpful for persons with stroke, hip fracture, arthritis, or parkinsonism. Exercise interventions for weakness have been discussed in the previous section. Residents should be referred to a podiatrist for foot problems such as toe deformities and calluses (Rubenstein et al., 2002).

3.4.2 Exercise

In 2010, the American and British Geriatrics Societies Clinical Practice Panel on Fall Prevention concluded that there was no conclusive evidence for the effectiveness of exercise for fall prevention in NHs, even though there were some promising studies. The reasons for their conclusion included small sample sizes, heterogeneity, and absence of well-designed controlled trials. Since then, the Cochrane Collaboration concluded in 2013 that physical rehabilitation for LTC residents may be effective. Finally, a 2013 meta-analysis concluded that exercise programs are effective in preventing falls in LTC facilities. By then, a critical number of published studies had accumulated to reach this new and more optimistic conclusion (Panel on Prevention of Falls in Older Persons, American Geriatrics Society and British Geriatrics Society, 2011; Cameron et al., 2012; Silva et al., 2013) (Figure 3.1).

A Cochrane meta-analysis concluded that physical rehabilitation for LTC residents may be effective, reducing disability with few adverse events, although effects appear small and may not be applicable to all residents. The researchers felt that there is insufficient evidence to reach conclusions about improvement sustainability, cost-effectiveness, or which interventions are most appropriate. They also felt that future large-scale trials are justified (Crocker et al., 2013).

Studies finished after the Cochrane report have continued to solidify the evidence in support of NH exercise and rehabilitation programs. A more recent meta-analysis study that combined studies of frequent and long-term exercise programs showed effectiveness in preventing falls in LTC facilities (Silva et al., 2013).

3.4.3 Cognitive Impairment

As noted previously, patients with cognitive impairment represent one of the biggest challenges for fall prevention in LTC, due to their poor memory and impaired judgment together with their preserved ability to mobilize and put themselves at risk. At this time, there is insufficient evidence to recommend, for or against, single or multifactorial interventions in older adults with known cognitive impairment (Panel on Prevention of Falls in Older Persons, American Geriatrics Society and British Geriatrics Society, 2011).

The only trial that investigated the effectiveness of multifactorial intervention after a fall in cognitively impaired older patients was done in a community hospital emergency

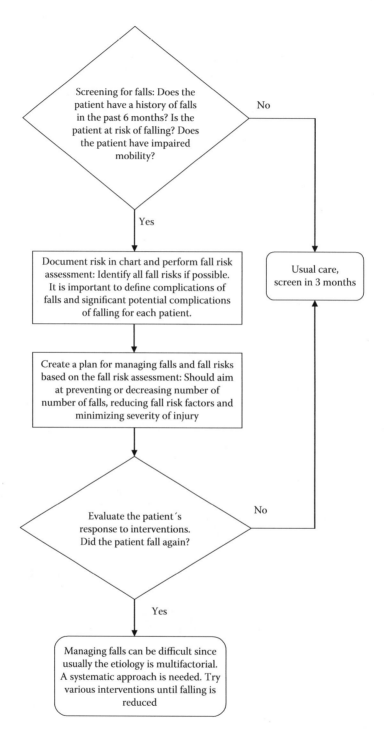

FIGURE 3.1
Falls and fall risk in the long-term care setting.

department, and this trial demonstrated lack of efficacy (Shaw et al., 2003). Thus, this remains an area greatly in need of further study. From a practical standpoint, in the absence of hard evidence, most LTC clinicians would recommend a combination of preventive interventions for cognitively impaired patients that include increased staffing ratios; closer observation; frequent toileting routines; frequent reminders to ask for help; avoidance of any activity known or suspected to be associated with falls; and the use of bed or chair alarms, wheelchair safety belts, low beds, short (not full length) bedrails, impact-absorbing flooring, and hip protectors, to name but afew.

3.4.4 Fear of Falling

Fear of falling and post-fall anxiety are very common symptoms associated with poor confidence in mobility secondary to a previous fall, altered gait or balance, or other physical problem. This fear has a great impact on the patient's lifestyle by decreasing participation in social and physical activities, contributing to functional decline and isolation, and contributing to a higher risk of falling. One analysis that reviewed 26 studies on the epidemiology of fear of falling in NHs and assisted-living facilities, as well as intervention studies in these settings, found that fear of falling is common, affecting more than 50% of LTC elders, and is associated with negative outcomes, including falls, functional impairments, depression, and poor quality of life (Lach and Parsons, 2013).

Another study determined the prevalence of fear of falling in patients after a hip fracture and concluded that in these patients fear of falling is common and correlates with anxiety and falls-related impaired self-efficacy (Visschedijk et al., 2013).

3.5 Summary

Although considerable evidence has shown that falls can be reduced, there is a marked difference between falls in NHs and in the community. While published NH studies are somewhat inconsistent due to differences in NHs and NH policies in different countries and regions, in general a multifactorial NH fall prevention plan has the most well-documented efficacy and is the most well-accepted approach. Such a plan begins with a fall risk assessment on admission to the facility tied to an individualized intervention program linked to the identified risk factors. Other components of effective NH fall prevention include regular staff training and updates, continuous monitoring of at-risk patients for falls and presence of additional risk factors, maintaining an adequate and safe environment for residents, participating in a regular exercise routine, having appropriate nutritional support, performing frequent reconciliations of medications to avoid unnecessary polypharmacy, and monitoring of chronic diseases so as to detect exacerbations early.

References

Agashivala, N., and Wu, W. K., Effects of potentially inappropriate psychoactive medications on falls in US nursing home residents: Analysis of the 2004 National Nursing Home Survey database. *Drugs Aging*, 2009;26:853–860.

Bauer, J. M. and Sieber, C. C., Sarcopenia and frailty: A clinician's controversial point of view. *Exp Gerontol*, 2008;43:674–678.

Becker C. and Rap, K., Fall prevention in nursing homes. *Clin Geriatr Med*, 2010;26(4):693–704.

Berry, S. D., Lee. Y., Cai. S., Dore. D. D., Non-benzodiazepine sleep medication use and hip fractures in nursing home residents. *JAMA Intern Med*, 2013;173:754–761.

Cameron, I. D., Gillespie, L. D., Robertson, M. C., et al., Interventions for preventing falls in older people in care facilities and hospitals. *Cochrane Database Syst Rev*, 2012;12:CD005465.

Choi, M. and Hector, M., Effectiveness of intervention programs in preventing falls: A systematic review of recent 10 years and meta-analysis. *J Am Dir Assoc*, 2012;13(2):188.e13–188.e21.

Consensus Committee of the American Autonomic Society and the American Academy of Neurology. Consensus statement on the definition of orthostatic hypotension, pure autonomic failure, and multiple system atrophy. *Neurology*, 1996;46:1470.

Crocker, T., Forster, A., Young, J., et al., Physical rehabilitation for older people in long-term care. *Cochrane Database Syst Rev*, 2013;CD004294.

Cruz-Jentoft, A. J., Baeyens, J. P., Bauer, J. M., Boirie, Y., Cederholm, T., Landi, F., et al., Sarcopenia: European consensus on definition and diagnosis. Report of the European working group on sarcopenia in older people. *Age Ageing*, 2010;39:412–423.

Damian, J., Pastor-Barriuso, R., Valderrama-Gama, E., de Pedro-Cuesta, J. Factors associated with falls among older adults living in institutions. *BMC Geriatr*, 2013;13:6.

Deandrea, S., Bravi, F., Turati, F., et al., Risk factors for falls in older people in nursing homes and hospitals. *Arch Gerontol Geriatr*, 2013;56(3):407–415.

Delmonico M. J., Harris, T. B., Lee, J. S. et al., Alternative definitions of sarcopenia, lower extremity performance, and functional impairment with aging in older men and women. *J Am Geriatr Soc*. 2007;55:769–774.

Dyer, C., Taylor, G., Reed, M., et al., Falls prevention in residential care homes: A randomised controlled trial. *Age Ageing*, 2004;33:596–602.

Freeman, R., Wieling, W., Axelrod, F. B., et al., Consensus statement on the definition of orthostatic hypotension, neurally mediated syncope and the postural tachycardia syndrome. Clin Auton Res 2011;21:69–72.

Fried L. P., Tangen, C. M., Walston, J., et al., Frailty in older adults: Evidence for a phenotype. *J Gerontol A BiolSci Med Sci*, 2001;56:M146–56.

Frith, J., Newton, J. L., Parry, S. W. Measuring and defining orthostatic hypotension in the older person. *Age Ageing*, 2014;43:168–170.

Gangavati, A., Hajjar, I., Quach, L., Jones, R. N., Kiely, D. K., Gagnon, P., Lipsitz, L. A., Hypertension, orthostatic hypotension, and the risk of falls in a community-dwelling elderly population: The maintenance of balance, independent living, intellect, and zest in the elderly of Boston study. *J Am Geriatr Soc*, 2011;59:383–389.

Hartman, M. J., Fields, D. A., Byrne, N. M., et al., Resistance training improves metabolic economy during functional tasks in older adults. *J Strength Cond Res*, 2007;21:91–95.

Heitterachi, E., Lord, S. R., Meyerkort, P., McCloskey, I., Fitzpatrick, R. Blood pressure changes on upright tilting predict falls in older people. *Age Ageing*, 2002;31:181–186.

Kim, D. H., Brown, R. T., Ding, E. L., et al., Dementia and medications and risk of falls, syncope, and related adverse events: Meta-analysis of randomized controlled trials. *J Am Geriatr Soc*, 2011;59:1019–1031.

Kosse, N. M., Brands, K., Bauer, J. M., et al., Sensor technologies aiming at fall prevention in institutionalized old adults: A synthesis of current knowledge. *Int J Med Inform*, 2013;82(9):743–752.

Lach, H. and Parsons, J., Impact of fear of falling in long term care: An integrative review. *J Am Med Dir Assoc*, 2013;14(8):573–577.

Landi, F., Liperoti, R., Russo, A., Giovannini, S., Tosato, M., Capoluongo, E., Bernabei, R., Onder, G., Sarcopenia as a risk factor for falls in elderly individuals: results from the ilSIRENTE study. *Clin Nutr*, 2012;13(5):652–658.

Lipsitz, L. A., Wei, N., Rowe, J. W., Syncope in an elderly, institutionalized population: Prevalence, incidence, and associated risk. *QJ Med*, 1985;55:45–55.

Luciano, G. L., Brennan, M. J., Rothberg, M. B., Postprandial hypotension. *Am J Med,* 2010;123:281.

Montero-Odasso, M., Levinson, P., Gore, B., et al., A flowchart system to improve fall data documentation in a long-term care institution: A pilot study. *J Am Med Dir Assoc,* 2007;8(5):300–306.

Montero-Odasso, M., Verghese, J., Beauthet, O., et al., Gait and cognition. A complementary approach to understanding brain function and the risk of falling. *J Am Geriatr Soc,* 2012;60:2127–2136.

Moreland, J. D., Richardson, J. A., Goldsmith, C. H., Clase, C. M., Muscle weakness and falls in older adults: A systematic review and meta-analysis. *J Am Geriatr Soc,* 2004;52:1121–1129.

National Center for Health Statistics. Health, United States, 2005, with: Chartbook on Trends in the Health of Americans. National Center for Health Statistics. Hyattsville, MD, 2005.

Neyens, J. C., van Haastregt, J. C., Dijcks, B. P., Martens, M., van den Heuvel, W. J., et al., Effectiveness and implementation aspects of interventions for preventing falls in elderly people in long-term care facilities: a systematic review of RCTs. *J Am Med Dir Assoc,* 2011;12:410–425.

Olazarán, J., Valle, D., Serra, J. A., et al., Psychotropic medications and falls in nursing homes: a cross-sectional study. *J Am Med Dir Assoc,* 2013;14(3):213–217.

Ooi, W. L., Hossain, M., and Lipsitz, L. A., The association between orthostatic hypotension and recurrent falls in nursing home residents. *Am J Med,* 2000;108:106–111.

Panel on Prevention of Falls in Older Persons, American Geriatrics Society and British Geriatrics Society. Summary of the Updated American Geriatrics Society/British Geriatrics Society Clinical Practice Guideline for Prevention of Falls in Older Persons. *J Am Geriat Soc,* 2011;59:148–157.

Perell, K. L., Nelson, A., Goldman, R. L., et al., Fall risk assessment measures: An analytic review. *J Gerontol A Biol Sci Med Sci,* 2001;56:M761–766.

Raj, S., Coffin, S., Medical therapy and physical maneuvers in the treatment of the vasovagal syncope and the orthostatic hypotension. *Prog Cardiovasc Dis,* 2013;55:425–433.

Rapp, K., Becker, C., Cameron, I., Konig, H., Buchele, G. Epidemiology of falls in residential aged care: Analysis of more than 70,000 falls from residents of Bavarian nursing homes. *J Am Med Dir Assoc,* 2012;13:187.e1–187.e6.

Robinovitch, S., Feldman, F., Yang, Y., et al., Video capture of the circumstances of falls in elderly people residing in long-term care. *Lancet,* 2013;381(9860):47–54.

Rubenstein, L. Z., Preventing falls in the nursing home. *J Am Med Ass,* 1997;278(7):595–596.

Rubenstein, L. Z., Falls in older people: Epidemiology, risk factors and strategies for prevention. *Age Ageing,* 2006,35:ii37–ii41.

Rubenstein, L. Z., Josephson, K. R., The epidemiology of falls and syncope. *Clin Geriatr Med,* 2002,18:141–158.

Rubenstein, L. Z., Josephson, K. R., Robbins, A. S., Falls in the nursing home. *Ann Int Med,* 1994;121:442–451.

Rubenstein, L. Z., Robbins, A. S., Schulman, B. L., Rosado, J., Osterweil, D., Josephson, K. R., Falls and instability in the elderly. *J Am Geriatr Soc,* 1988;36:266–278.

Sahyoun, N. R., Pratt, L. A., Lentzner, H., Dey, A., Robinson, K. N., The changing profile of nursing home residents: 1985–1997. *Aging Trends,* No.4, Hyattsville (MD): National Center for Health Statistics; 2001.

Scott, V., Votova, K., Scanlan, A., et al., Multifactorial and functional mobility assessment tools for fall risk among older adults in community, home-support, long-term and acute care settings. *Age Ageing,* 2007;36(2):130–139.

Shaw, F. E., Bond, J., Richardson, D. A., et al., Multifactorial intervention after a fall in older people with cognitive impairment and dementia presenting to the accident and emergency department: Randomized controlled trial. *BMJ,* 2003;326:73.

Silva, R., Eslick, G., Duque, G., et al., Exercise for falls and fracture prevention in long term care facilities: A systematic review and meta-analysis. *J Am Med Dir Assoc,* 2013;14:685–689.

Son, J. T., Lee, E., Postprandial hypotension among older residents of a nursing home in Korea. *J Clin Nursing,* 2012;21: 3565–3573.

Soteriades, E. S., Evans, J. C., Larson, M. G., et al., Incidence and prognosis of syncope. *N Engl J Med,* 2002;347:878–885.

Thapa, P. B., Brockman, K. G., Gideon, P., Fought, R. L., Ray, W. A., Injurious falls in non-ambulatory nursing home residents: A comparative study of circumstances, incidence and risk factors. *J Am Geriatr Soc*, 1996;44:273–278.

Tinetti, M. E., Baker, D. I., McAvay, G., et al., A multifactorial intervention to reduce the risk of falling among elderly people living in the community. *N Engl J Med*, 1994;331:821–827.

Tinetti, M. E., Han, L., Lee, D. S. H., McAvay, G. J., Peduzzi, P., Gross, C. P., Zhou, B., Lin, H., Antihypertensive medications and serious fall injuries in a nationally representative sample of older adults. *JAMA Intern Med*, 2014;174(4):588–595.

Tinetti, M. E., Speechley, M., Ginter, S. F., Risk factors for falls among elderly persons living in the community. *N Engl J Med*, 1988;319:1701–1707.

Trueblood, P. R. and Rubenstein, L. Z., Assessment of instability and gait in elderly persons. *Compr Ther*, 1991;17:20–29.

Van Doorn, C., Gruber-Baldini, A. L., Zimmerman, S., et al., Dementia as a risk factor for falls and fall injuries among nursing home residents. *J Am Geriatr Soc*, 2003;13:1213–1218.

Van Rensbergen, G., and Nawrot, T., Medical conditions of nursing home admissions. *BMC Geriatr*, 2010;10:46.

Visschedijk, J., van Balen, R., Hertogh, C., Achterberg, W., Fear of falling in patients with hip fractures: Prevalence and related psychological factors. *J Am Med Dir Ass*, 2013;14:218–220.

4

Fall Risk Characteristics in the Construction Industry

Xiuwen Sue Dong, Xuanwen Wang, Julie A. Largay, Bruce Lippy,
Chris Trahan Cain, Erich Pete Stafford, and James W. Platner

CONTENTS

ABSTRACT This chapter profiles the U.S. construction industry and its workers, describes the fall hazards on construction worksites, and analyzes the trends and patterns in fatal and nonfatal falls among U.S. construction workers in the last decades. The statistics reported in this chapter were obtained from several large, nationally representative datasets collected by the U.S. Census Bureau and the Bureau of Labor Statistics. In addition to injury statistics, this chapter discusses how the characteristics of the construction industry and changing demographics, such as small establishments, self-employment, increasing use of temporary workers and temporary agencies, the aging construction workforce, and increasing immigrant employment affect fall injuries. Fall prevention efforts and resources in construction, including the national campaign launched by the Occupational Safety and Health Administration (OSHA) and the National Institute for Occupational

Safety and Health (NIOSH), and the CPWR—The Center for Construction Research and Training (CPWR) website are also introduced.

KEY WORDS: *construction industry, fall hazard, fall injury, injury trend and pattern, older worker, Hispanic worker, foreign-born worker, roofer, small establishment, self-employed, fall prevention.*

4.1 Profile of the U.S. Construction Industry

4.1.1 Construction Industry

Construction is a large, dynamic, and complex industry sector in the United States. This industry has nearly three million establishments, about 78% (2.35 million) of which have no payroll employees (U.S. Census Bureau, 2012). Among payroll construction establishments, more than 80% have fewer than 10 employees (Table 4.1). In residential building construction (North American Industry Classification System [NAICS] 2361), about 94% of establishments had fewer than 10 employees in 2012, and 82% of establishments had four or fewer employees. Smaller construction establishments lag far behind their larger counterparts with regard to safety practices (McGraw-Hill, 2013), and are also less likely to be targeted by Occupational Safety and Health Administration (OSHA) inspections (Weil, 2001). Consequently, existing safety and health regulations and solutions may not be applied to, or adopted by, small construction companies and independent contractors.

Over the last decades, the construction industry has experienced a vast amount of expansion and contraction in terms of employment. Between 2003 and 2007, construction employment, especially among Hispanics, benefited from a strong and sustained growth in the U.S. housing market, in which employment grew by nearly two million (Figure 4.1). The number of Hispanic workers in construction peaked at three million in 2007, 43% higher than in 2003 and four times the number in 1990 (705,000; CPWR, 2009). It was estimated that Hispanic workers occupied about 78% of new construction jobs in production when the industry was expanding (CPWR, 2013). Starting at the end of 2007, construction employment was significantly impacted by the "great recession" (National Bureau of Economic Research, 2010). Following the recession, about three million construction workers lost their jobs, of which nearly one million were Hispanic.

The changes in employment varied greatly across construction subsectors. For example, residential building construction (NAICS 2361) showed more volatility than nonresidential building construction (NAICS 2362) over time. In residential building construction, employment grew 20% between 2003 and 2006 and dropped 32% below the 2003 level in 2011 (Figure 4.2), reflecting the boom and collapse of the U.S. housing market. In contrast, employment in nonresidential building construction remained relatively stable, at 8% above the 2003 level in 2006 and 11% below the 2003 level in 2011.

4.1.2 Construction Workforce

The construction workforce is diverse and composed of distinctive demographic subgroups. Disparities are striking when the workforce is stratified by Hispanic ethnicity. The average age of Hispanic construction workers was 37.7 in 2012, 6.3 years younger than

TABLE 4.1

Number and Percentage of Construction Establishments, Residential versus Nonresidential, by Establishment Size, 2012 (with Payroll)

Establishment Size (Number of Employees)	Residential Building Construction				Nonresidential Building Construction				All Construction			
	Establishments		Employees		Establishments		Employees		Establishments		Employees	
	Number	%	Number	%	Number	%	Number	%	Number	%	Number	%
1–4	124,508	82.4	176,524	34.0	20,866	50.9	35,812	6.9	443,145	67.9	694,399	13.2%
5–9	16,822	11.1	107,675	20.7	8,185	20.0	54,437	10.4	101,002	15.5	660,473	12.6%
10–19	6,275	4.2	82,141	15.8	6,221	15.2	84,026	16.1	57,657	8.8	773,444	14.7%
20–49	2,666	1.8	77,091	14.9	4,057	9.9	120,991	23.2	35,209	5.4	1,050,136	20.0%
50–99	581	0.4	38,280	7.4	1,039	2.5	70,231	13.5	10,123	1.6	685,643	13.0%
100–249	150	0.1	21,434	4.1	492	1.2	73,272	14.1	4,444	0.7	658,017	12.5%
250–499	24	0.0	8,431	1.6	109	0.3	35,504	6.8	932	0.1	310,840	5.9%
500–999	5	0.0	—	—	32	0.1	21,171	4.1	263	0.0	176,333	3.4%
1,000+	3	0.0	—	—	17	0.0	25,668	4.9	127	0.0	251,657	4.8%
Total	151,034	100	519,070	100	41,018	100	521,112	100	652,902	100	5,260,942	100

Source: U.S. Census Bureau, 2012 County Business Patterns.

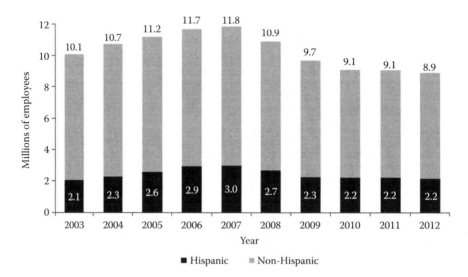

FIGURE 4.1
Construction employment in the United States, 2003–2012 (all employment). (From U.S. Bureau of Labor Statistics, 2003–2012 Current Population Survey. Calculations by the authors.)

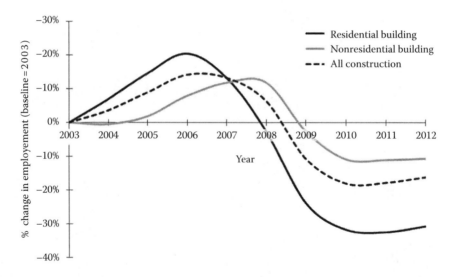

FIGURE 4.2
Percentage change in construction employment from 2003 through 2012 (private wage-and-salary workers). (From U.S. Bureau of Labor Statistics, 2003–2012 Current Employment Statistics. Calculations by the authors.)

white, non-Hispanic workers. Only 7% of Hispanic workers were aged 55 or older, while 23% of white, non-Hispanic construction workers were in this age group (Table 4.2). But overall, the construction workforce is aging. The average age of construction workers was 42.3 in 2012, a jump from 36.0 in 1985 (CPWR, 2013).

With regard to education, Hispanic construction workers have a much lower educational attainment than their white, non-Hispanic counterparts. About half of Hispanic construction workers had less than a high-school education, compared with just 9% of

TABLE 4.2

Characteristics of Construction Workers, Hispanic versus White, Non-Hispanic, 2012

Characteristics	Hispanic (%)	White, Non-Hispanic (%)	All (%)
Age (average years)	37.7	44.0	42.3
16–24	10.2	7.7	8.2
25–34	33.5	20.1	23.5
35–44	30.1	21.3	23.8
45–54	18.8	27.9	25.7
55–64	6.1	18.6	15.3
65+	1.2	4.5	3.5
Gender			
Male	96.5	89.3	91.1
Education			
Less than high school	48.5	9.2	19.0
High-school graduate	33.7	43.2	40.8
Some college and above	17.9	47.5	40.2
Foreign born	73.9	4.3	22.8
Region			
Northeast	10.4	19.9	17.4
Midwest	6.1	25.3	19.4
South	47.4	36.6	40.1
West	36.2	18.2	23.1
Type of Employment			
Self-employed	18.0	28.9	25.9
Private employees	80.7	65.9	69.6
Public employees	1.3	5.1	4.4
Occupation			
Blue-collar	89.4	65.9	72.3
Construction laborer	25.0	10.2	14.8
Carpenter	15.0	11.7	12.4
Painter	8.0	3.3	4.5
Roofer	4.0	1.5	2.0
Plumber	3.8	4.6	4.4
Drywall installer	3.8	0.8	1.5
Electrician	3.2	6.0	5.1
White-collar	10.6	34.1	27.7
Foreman	4.0	6.9	6.0
Construction manager	3.9	12.8	10.3
Union member	8.2	16.9	14.4
Total (weighted)	**2.2 million**	**6.0 million**	**8.9 million**

Source: 2012 Current Population Survey. Calculations by the authors.

white, non-Hispanic workers. In addition, the share of women in the construction industry has remained low—less than one in ten construction workers was female in 2012, despite women constituting almost half of the workforce in the United States (U.S. BLS, 2014a). The proportion of females was even smaller among Hispanic construction workers at less than 4%.

Almost 75% of Hispanic construction workers are immigrants (Table 4.2). Among foreign-born construction workers, more than 80% reported they spoke only Spanish at home (CPWR, 2013), therefore it is not surprising that many immigrant workers do not speak English very well. More than 80% of the Hispanic immigrants were from Mexico and other Latin-American countries (CPWR, 2013) and reside predominantly in the southern and western regions of the United States (47% and 36% of Hispanic construction workers, respectively).

In terms of construction occupations, almost 90% of Hispanics worked blue-collar jobs compared with 66% of their white, non-Hispanic counterparts (Table 4.2). About one in four Hispanic workers were employed as construction laborers, compared with just one in ten white, non-Hispanic workers. Hispanic workers are also less likely to be unionized. Only 8% of Hispanic construction workers were union members in 2012, less than half the percentage of white, non-Hispanic workers (17%). Nonunion jobs paid lower wages, had smaller benefit packages (e.g., health insurance coverage), and were less likely to provide job-related training for workers (CPWR, 2013). As a result, these demographic and employment factors have made Hispanic construction workers more vulnerable to work-related injuries (Dong et al., 2009; Anderson et al., 2000).

Self-employment is common in construction. In 2012, 2.3 million construction workers were self-employed, accounting for 26% of the construction workforce (Table 4.2). Among white, non-Hispanic workers, the proportion was as high as 29%. However, Hispanic workers were less likely to be self-employed (18%). Self-employed workers are not subject to federal or state labor laws or OSHA regulations, meaning they are not required to complete safety trainings, use personal protective equipment (including fall protection), or conduct workplace hazard inspections (Mirabelli et al., 2003). Self-employed workers are also more likely to be older and work longer hours, both of which increase the risk of fatigue, muscular pain, and ultimately falls (Dong et al., 2014a).

4.1.3 Fall Hazards in Construction

The construction industry is one of the most hazardous industries in the United States. Among the numerous dangers and risks faced by construction workers, falls are a common hazard and a leading cause of fatality in construction. According to the Occupational Information Network (O*NET), many construction occupations require working in high places and climbing ladders or scaffolds more than once a week (Table 4.3). Elevator installers, roofers, drywall installers, power-line installers, mechanical insulation workers, and ironworkers are exposed to heights on the job almost every day. Mechanical insulation workers, drywall installers, roofers, and painters spend more time climbing ladders, scaffolds, or poles than other occupations. It is estimated that nearly 60% of workers in construction production occupations work at heights at least once a month and climb ladders or scaffolds during half of their work time (CPWR, 2013). Working outdoors or exposed to severe weather can also increase the risk of falls. Several factors, such as ice, rain, and wind, can affect the likelihood of a fall. Roofers and cement masons are predominantly exposed to weather while working, followed closely by brickmasons.

TABLE 4.3

Fall Hazards and Other Exposures in Construction, Selected Occupations

Exposure Scores

Occupations	Exposed to High Places[a]	Climbing Ladders, Scaffolds, or Poles[b]	Outdoors, Exposed to Weather[a]
Elevator installers and repairers	100	45	62
Roofers	97	76	100
Drywall installers	92	79	56
Power-line installers	90	32	95
Insulation workers, mechanical	88	83	65
Ironworkers	88	51	97
Plasterers	84	58	75
Brickmasons	84	45	99
Solar photovoltaic installers	81	59	82
Electricians	72	63	63
Construction and building inspectors	72	28	93
Telecommunications line installers and repairers	71	37	94
Insulation workers	70	63	87
Pipe fitters and steamfitters	70	46	69
Reinforcing iron and rebar workers	68	51	94
Heat A/C mechanic	68	47	84
Painters	66	74	64
Weatherization installers and technicians	61	35	88
Sheet-metal workers	60	49	64
Carpenters	58	45	78
Construction laborers	58	44	87
Boilermakers	56	40	53
Hazardous materials removal workers	53	32	70
Plumbers	50	37	74
Construction managers	43	23	57
Welders	31	24	33
Cement masons	26	24	100
Operating engineers	21	13	96
Carpet installers	13	7	27
Pipe layers	9	27	97
Solderers and brazers	4	6	7

Source: O*NET OnLine, Work context: Physical work conditions. Retrieved May 2014 from http://www.onetonline.org/find/descriptor/browse/Work_Context/4.C.2/.

[a] Exposure scores: 0 = Never; 25 = Once a year or more, but not every month; 50 = Once a month or more, but not every week; 75 = Once a week or more, but not every day; and 100 = Every day.

[b] Exposure scores: 0 = Never; 25 = Less than half the time; 50 = About half the time; 75 = More than half the time; and 100 = Continually or almost continually.

4.2 Occupational Injuries in Construction

4.2.1 Overall Fatal and Nonfatal Injury Trends

The injury rates in construction declined considerably in the last two decades, regardless of year-to-year fluctuations. In 1992, the annual fatality rate was 14.3 per 100,000 full-time equivalent workers (FTEs; Figure 4.3). By 2012, the rate was down 31% to 9.8 per 100,000 FTEs. Nonfatal injuries and illnesses trended downward as well. The nonfatal injury rate dropped from 529.5 to 143.4 per 10,000 FTEs during the same time period. However, estimates for nonfatal occupational injuries and illnesses before and after 2002 may not be comparable since OSHA revised the record-keeping requirements in 2002. Even so, the nonfatal injury rate dropped 48% between 2002 and 2012—more than the 20-year drop for the fatality rate.

4.2.2 Leading Causes

Although fatal and nonfatal injury rates in construction have dropped over time, the construction industry still remains one of the most dangerous industries in the United States. The construction industry had the highest number of annual fatalities when compared with other industries—849 in 2012 (U.S. BLS, 2014b). Leading causes, such as falls to a lower level, contact with electrical current, highway incidents, and being struck by objects are still a major concern for the industry (CPWR, 2013). However, leading causes of fatal and nonfatal injuries differ. In 2012, falls caused more than one-third of fatalities in construction and also accounted for about 26% of nonfatal injuries resulting in days away from work (Figure 4.4).

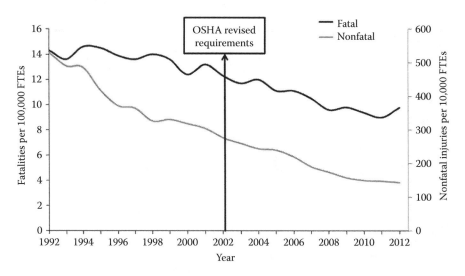

FIGURE 4.3

Fatal and nonfatal injury trends in construction, 1992–2012. FTE = Full-time equivalent worker, defined as 2000 h worked per year. *Note*: Effective January 1, 2002, OSHA revised its requirements for recording occupational injuries and illnesses. Due to the revised record keeping rule, the estimates since the 2002 survey are not comparable with those from previous years for nonfatal injuries. (From U.S. Bureau of Labor Statistics, 1992–2012 Census of Fatal Occupational Injuries, Survey of Occupational Injuries and Illnesses, and Current Population Survey.)

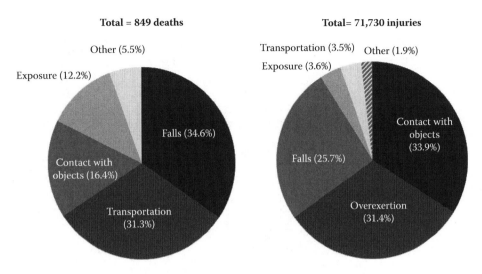

FIGURE 4.4
Distribution of leading causes of work-related fatal and nonfatal injuries in construction, 2012. (From U.S. Bureau of Labor Statistics, 2012 Census of Fatal Occupational Injuries and Survey of Occupational Injuries and Illnesses. Numbers are from the online CFOI database.)

4.3 Fall Injuries in Construction

4.3.1 Trends of Fall Injuries

Falls consistently cause a large number of fatalities in construction. Between 1992 and 2012, 7421 construction workers died as a result of falls—an average of 353 deaths per year or one death per day (Figure 4.5). During the economic boom in 2007, annual fall fatalities in construction peaked at 450. Despite the finding that overall fatal injuries had declined, the proportion of fatal falls in construction increased from 28% in 1992 to 33% in 2010. The number of fatalities from falls in 2011 and 2012 cannot be compared with data from previous years due to coding/classification system changes. In 2011, the Census of Fatal Occupational Injuries (CFOI) switched to the Occupational Injury and Illness Classification System (OIICS) version 2.01. In the new version, slips, trips, and falls are categorized together, whereas slips and trips were classified as *bodily action* in the previous version. Between 2011 and 2012, the number of fall fatalities increased 9% from 269 to 294. The overall proportion of fatalities from falls increased modestly as well—from 34% to 35% between these two years.

4.3.2 Fall Injuries by Demographics

Fatal and nonfatal fall injuries were distributed differently among demographic groups. In general, younger workers were more likely to suffer nonfatal injuries from falls, while more fatal falls were found among older workers. About 11% of fatal falls were among workers aged 65 years and older, but less than 1% of the nonfatal falls were in this age group (Table 4.4). On the other hand, 32% of nonfatal fall injuries were among workers under 35 years old, while this age group shared less than 20% of fatal falls. The largest proportion

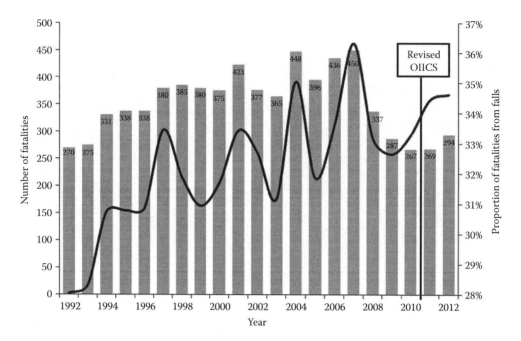

FIGURE 4.5

Trends of fatal falls in construction, 1992–2012. *Note*: In 2011, the CFOI switched to OIICS version categorizes slips, trips, and falls together. In previous years, slips and trips were categorized elsewhere. (From U.S. Bureau of Labor Statistics, 1992–2012 Census of Fatal Occupational Injuries. Numbers are from the online CFOI database.)

of fall injuries, both fatal and nonfatal, occurred among workers aged 45–54 years (29.6% and 26.6%, respectively), exceeding the share of construction employment (25.7%; see Table 4.2) by this age cohort. The percentage of nonfatal falls for this age group could be higher if self-employed workers were included, since self-employed workers tend to be older (Dong et al., 2012).

Hispanics accounted for about 25% of the construction workforce; however, 31% of fall fatalities occurred among this group. Contradictory to fatal injuries, the proportion of nonfatal fall injuries among Hispanic workers was 15%—slightly lower than the proportion of nonfall injuries. The nonfatal injury data show little variation between ethnicities. However, previous research has suggested significant injury underreporting (Rosenman et al., 2006), specifically among Hispanics (Dong et al., 2011). Foreign-born workers were also at an elevated risk of fatal falls, accounting for nearly one-third of falls. This is likely a reflection of the disparities faced by Hispanics and foreign-born workers, which are widely overlapping worker groups. With regard to nonfatal injuries, information on foreign-born workers is unavailable.

4.3.3 Fall Injuries by Employment Status

Almost all fatal and nonfatal falls occurred among blue-collar workers in construction, accounting for 96.6% and 95.2% of the overall injuries in this industry, respectively (Table 4.5). In 2012, about 22% of all fatal injuries were among self-employed construction workers, but 28% of fall fatalities were among this group.

Fatal falls are more likely to occur among small construction establishments. Nearly half (49.3%) of fall fatalities in construction were among establishments with 10 or fewer

TABLE 4.4

Demographic Characteristics of Construction Injuries, Fatal versus Nonfatal Injuries, 2012

	Fatal Injuries[a]			Nonfatal Injuries[b]		
Demographic Characteristics	Falls (*n* = 294) (%)	Nonfalls (*n* = 555) (%)	All (*n* = 849) (%)	Falls (*n* = 18,400) (%)	Nonfalls (*n* = 53,330) (%)	All (*n* = 71,730) (%)
Age						
16–24 years	4.8	9.6	7.9	9.8	9.7	9.7
25–34 years	15.0	18.2	17.1	22.2	29.8	27.9
35–44 years	20.4	19.5	19.8	21.6	26.1	25.0
45–54 years	29.6	27.6	28.3	26.6	24.7	25.1
55–64 years	19.4	18.4	18.7	15.0	8.5	10.1
65+ years	10.9	6.9	8.2	0.9	0.7	0.7
Not reported	—	—	—	3.9	0.6	1.3
Gender						
Male	99.3	98.9	99.1	95.7	98.7	98.0
Race/Ethnicity						
Hispanic	31.0	23.6	26.2	15.1	15.8	15.6
White, non-Hispanic	62.2	67.4	65.6	53.9	57.0	56.2
Black, non-Hispanic	3.7	7.0	5.9	4.0	3.5	3.6
Other	3.1	2.0	2.4	0.5	2.5	2.1
Not reported	—	—	—	26.6	21.2	22.5
Foreign born	32.7	18.9	23.7	—	—	—
Hispanic	25.5	15.5	19.0	—	—	—
Region						
Northeast	18.4	11.4	13.8	—	—	—
Midwest	21.8	24.5	23.6	—	—	—
South	41.5	49.0	46.4	—	—	—
West	18.4	15.1	16.3	—	—	—

Source: Fatal-injury data were generated by the authors with restricted access to the BLS CFOI microdata. Nonfatal-injury data were from the BLS SOII through a special request.

[a] All types of employment.

[b] Private wage-and-salary workers.

employees, compared with 32.5% of nonfall fatalities. Excluding those without establishment size information, the proportion of fatal falls among these small establishments was as high as 66%. Smaller establishments may have many disadvantages in terms of fall protection availability (Dong et al., 2014a; McGraw-Hill Construction, 2013; Choi, 2006), which is a considerable challenge for improving construction safety and health.

4.3.4 Fall Injuries among Construction Subsectors

In 2012, roofing contractors (NAICS 23816) accounted for more than one in five fatal falls in construction (Table 4.6), reflecting the high exposure to fall hazards for roofers (see Table 4.3). However, roofing contractors accounted for a much smaller proportion of non-fatal falls (4.7%), which is indicative of the severity of falls among roofing contractors. Residential building construction (NAICS 23611) ranked the second highest in percentage

TABLE 4.5

Employment Characteristics of Construction Injuries, Fatal versus Nonfatal Injuries, 2012

Employment Characteristics	Fatal Injuries[a]			Nonfatal Injuries[b]		
	Falls (*n* = 294) (%)	Nonfalls (*n* = 555) (%)	All (*n* = 849) (%)	Falls (*n* = 18,400) (%)	Nonfalls (*n* = 53,330) (%)	All (*n* = 71,730) (%)
Occupation						
Blue-collar	96.6	93.5	94.6	95.2	96.6	96.2
White-collar	3.4	6.5	5.4	4.8	3.4	3.8
Employee Status						
Self-employed	28.2	18.2	21.7	—	—	—
Wage-and-salary	70.4	81.6	77.7	—	—	—
Establishment size[c]						
1–10 employees	49.3	32.5	37.7	—	—	—
11–19 employees	8.2	8.2	8.2	—	—	—
20–49 employees	6.8	13.5	11.4	—	—	—
50–99 employees	2.4	8.8	6.8	—	—	—
100 + employees	7.7	15.9	13.3	—	—	—
Not Reported	25.6	21.2	22.6	—	—	—

Source: Fatal-injury data were generated by the authors with restricted access to the BLS CFOI microdata. Nonfatal-injury data were from the BLS SOII through a special request.

[a] All types of employment.
[b] Private wage-and-salary workers.
[c] Self-employed workers were excluded from this tabulation.

TABLE 4.6

Fatal and Nonfatal Fall Injuries, Selected Construction Subsectors, 2012

Construction Subsectors	NAICS Code	Fatal Falls[a] (*n* = 294)		Nonfatal Falls[b] (*n* = 18,400)	
		Number	(%)	Number	(%)
Roofing contractors	23816	65	22.1	860	4.7
Residential building construction	23610	49	16.7	2,510	13.6
Painting and wall covering	23832	25	8.5	380	2.1
Nonresidential building construction	23620	23	7.8	1,990	10.8
Electrical contractors	23821	19	6.5	2,520	13.7
Framing contractors	23813	12	4.1	160	0.9
Highway, street, and bridge construction	23730	12	4.1	820	4.5
Masonry contractors	23814	11	3.7	270	1.5
Structural steel and precast concrete	23812	10	3.4	370	2.0
Plumbing, heating, and air conditioning	23822	9	3.1	2,460	13.4
Finish carpentry	23835	7	2.4	230	1.3
Drywall and insulation	23831	6	2.0	1,110	6.0
Poured concrete foundation and structure	23811	6	2.0	630	3.4

Source: Fatal-injury data were generated by the authors with restricted access to the BLS CFOI microdata. Nonfatal-injury data were from the BLS SOII, http://www.bls.gov/iif/oshwc/osh/case/ostb3596.pdf.

[a] All types of employment.
[b] Private wage-and-salary workers.

of fatal falls, with 49 fatal falls in 2012—an 82% increase from 2011 (Dong et al., 2014b). Electrical contractors (NAICS 23821) experienced about 2500 nonfatal falls in 2012, the largest proportion of any construction subsector (13.7%). This suggests that work on live circuits may be the proximal cause of some falls, possibly related to weak OSHA lock-out tag-out requirements in construction relative to general industry. A similar proportion of nonfatal falls occurred in residential building construction (13.6%) as well as the specialty trade of plumbing, heating, and air-conditioning (NAICS 23822; 13.4%).

4.3.5 Fall Injuries among Construction Occupations

Between 2011 and 2012, there were 563 fatal falls in construction, with an annual injury rate of 3.2 per 100,000 FTEs (Table 4.7). The rate of fatal falls varied significantly among construction occupations. While construction laborers accounted for 22% of fall fatalities in this industry, roofers had the highest fall fatality rate (31.0 per 100,000 FTEs)—about 10 times the average for all construction. Power-line installers had a fall fatality rate of 21.1, corresponding to their elevated exposure to high places (exposure score = 90; see Table 4.3). Ironworkers ranked third in terms of risk of fatal falls with a rate of 20.5 per 100,000 FTEs.

TABLE 4.7

Number and Rate of Fatal Falls, Selected Construction Occupations, 2011 and 2012

| | Fatal Falls[a] | | | | Nonfatal Falls[b] | | | |
| | | Rate[c] | | | | Rate[d] | | |
Occupations	Number	Point Estimate	95% CI		Number	Point Estimate	95% CI	
Roofer	101	31.0	27.9	34.9	1,260	48.1	42.9	54.9
Power-line installer	9	21.1	15.9	31.4	350	87.0	65.1	131.1
Ironworker	22	20.5	17.1	25.7	420	44.2	36.4	56.2
Helper	10	9.8	8.1	12.6	1,400	151.2	123.4	195.2
Welder	12	7.7	6.6	9.3	330	22.5	19.1	27.4
Foreman	70	6.3	5.9	6.7	1,610	21.1	19.6	22.8
Painter	42	5.7	5.3	6.1	930	20.0	18.3	22.0
Construction laborer	122	5.3	5.1	5.6	7,270	40.6	38.8	42.6
Brickmason	12	5.0	4.4	5.8	550	28.5	24.8	33.5
Drywall installer	8	3.0	2.7	3.5	790	38.4	33.5	44.9
Carpenter	57	2.7	2.6	2.9	4,820	37.8	35.8	40.0
Electrician	24	2.5	2.4	2.7	3,580	47.2	44.1	50.8
Heat A/C mechanic	10	2.2	2.0	2.4	1,810	46.8	42.5	52.2
Truck driver	5	1.5	1.3	1.6	1,210	42.6	38.0	48.4
Plumber	6	0.8	0.7	0.8	1,710	27.6	25.5	30.0
Construction manager	11	0.6	0.6	0.6	1,040	10.5	9.9	11.3
All construction	**563**	**3.2**	**3.2**	**3.3**	**37,300**	**30.1**	**29.9**	**30.4**

Source: Fatal-injury data were generated by the authors with restricted access to the BLS CFOI microdata. Nonfatal-injury data were from the BLS SOII through a special request. Rates were calculated by the authors using FTEs from the CPS.

[a] All types of employment.

[b] Private wage-and-salary workers.

[c] Rate = Number of fatal fall injuries per 100,000 FTEs.

[d] Rate = Number of nonfatal fall injuries per 10,000 FTEs.

4.3.6 Types of Fall Injuries

Information on the circumstances preceding fall injuries is important to prevent similar incidents from occurring in the future. In 2011, the CFOI began collecting information on the height of falls and providing more information on the circumstances preceding fall injuries. Between 2011 and 2012, nearly 20% of construction fall decedents fell from 31 ft or higher (Table 4.8). Within these two years, half of the fatal falls were from 11 to 30 ft, resulting in 285 deaths. In addition, the number of fall fatalities in construction increased by 7% for falls from 30 ft or below, and dropped by 7% for falls from over 30 ft (Dong et al., 2014b). This may reflect the rise in fatalities in residential construction, as heights of more than 30 ft may be less common in this subsector. Most of these construction fall fatalities were due to falls to a lower level. Between 2011 and 2012, 77 construction workers died from falling through a surface or existing opening, such as an elevator or skylight; another 40 were killed when falling from a collapsing structure or equipment, such as scaffolding or a building. Nearly 75% of fatal falls were categorized as *other fall to a lower level.*

In addition to height of falls, data on where falls occur are also important for fall prevention activities. Previous research has shown that roof falls have accounted for the largest proportion of construction fall fatalities over the past decades (Dong et al., 2013). From 2011 to 2012, roofs were the source of one-third of all fall fatalities in construction, or 191 deaths (Table 4.8). Ladders were the second leading source with 22% of fatal falls, followed by scaffolds and staging (14%). By location, 242 fatal falls occurred at residential construction sites (28%) and homes (15%); another 231 falls or 41% occurred at industrial places or premises. Activities when fatal falls occurred were various, but one-fourth occurred while workers were constructing, assembling, dismantling, or removing. Another 18% of workers were installing (e.g., skylights or guardrails), and 12% were repairing or performing maintenance work. Despite having detailed descriptions of these activities, more specific data on working environments, safety-and-health training, personal protective equipment, implementation of prevention through design (PtD) recommendations, work organization, and safety culture are needed for enhancing fall prevention.

4.4 Fall Preventions in Construction

4.4.1 Fall Hazard Training Materials and Other Products Developed

To prevent fall injuries, the CPWR—The Center for Construction Research and Training a leading organization in construction safety and health, and others have developed a wealth of training materials to help contractors and workers prevent falls. However, training must be viewed in the correct perspective. Effective worker training is considered by OSHA, the National Institute for Occupational Safety and Health (NIOSH), and the American National Standards Institute (ANSI) to be a key element of any health and safety management program, but when viewed in the hierarchy of controls that has underpinned occupational safety and health management for decades, training is an administrative control and low in the hierarchy (Figure 4.6). Consequently, employers should try to eliminate all fall hazards or apply engineering controls to reduce the risk before relying on training as a control strategy. PtD interventions, such as parapet walls and nonfragile skylights, can cheaply eliminate fall hazards. Passive restraints such as guard rails and personnel nets are more likely to be effective. NIOSH has published several PtD fall prevention fact sheets,

TABLE 4.8

Types of Fatal Falls in Construction, 2011and 2012

Fatal Falls		
Types	**Number**	**%**
Height of Falls		
0 ft	16	2.8
1–5 ft	24	4.3
6–10 ft	55	9.8
11–15 ft	90	16.0
16–20 ft	84	14.9
21–25 ft	59	10.5
26–30 ft	52	9.2
31+ ft	105	18.7
Unspecified	78	13.9
Event		
Falls on same level	15	2.7
Falls through surface or existing opening	77	13.7
Falls from collapsing structure or equipment	40	7.1
Other falls to a lower level	413	73.4
Falls to a lower level, unspecified	11	2.0
Other	7	1.3
Source		
Roofs	191	33.9
Ladders	126	22.4
Scaffolds, staging	77	13.7
Vehicles	27	4.8
Floors, walkways, ground surfaces	24	4.3
Machinery	19	3.4
Other structural elements	15	2.7
Trusses, girders, beams	13	2.3
Bridges, dams, locks	10	1.8
Towers, poles	9	1.6
Confined spaces	8	1.4
Other	44	7.8
Location		
Industrial place and premises	231	41.0
Residential construction sites	158	28.1
Homes (i.e., apartment, farm house, home unspecified, home n.e.c.[a])	84	14.9
Public buildings	36	6.4
Streets and highways	20	3.6
Other places	34	6.1
Activity		
Installing	99	17.6
Repair, maintenance	70	12.4

(Continued)

TABLE 4.8 (CONTINUED)

Types of Fatal Falls in Construction, 2011and 2012

Fatal Falls

Types	Number	%
Constructing, assembling	59	10.5
Climbing, descending	52	9.2
Constructing, assembling, dismantling, n.e.c.	50	8.9
Painting, etc.	50	8.9
Constructing, repairing, cleaning, n.e.c.	42	7.5
Dismantling, removing	33	5.9
Inspecting or checking	20	3.6
Materials handling operations	15	2.7
Body position	14	2.5
Operating heavy equipment/machinery	11	2.0
Cleaning, washing	7	1.2
Using power tools	7	1.2
Vehicular and transportation operations	7	1.2
Other	27	4.8
Total	**563**	**100**

Source: Fatal-injury data were generated by the authors with restricted access to the BLS CFOI microdata.

[a] n.e.c. = not elsewhere classified.

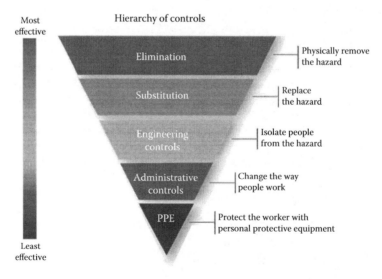

FIGURE 4.6

Hierarchy of controls. (From NIOSH, https://www.cdc.gov/niosh/topics/hierarchy/.)

and CPWR's Construction Solutions Database (http://CPWRConstructionSolutions.org) includes information on a variety of fall hazard reduction options.

As part of its construction research efforts, in 2006 CPWR developed a fall-protection training program targeting fall hazards when using ladders, titled "Don't Fall for It." This program includes an 11-min DVD that features first-person accounts of workers who have fallen from ladders, emotional testimony from the family of a fatal-fall victim, and information about how to work safely with ladders. There are four one-page fact sheets that accompany this training program and reinforce the DVD's systematic instructions on choosing, inspecting, setting up, and safely climbing ladders. Within a few months of the DVD's release, 450 construction workers had seen the DVD and responded to pre- and posttest questions about their ladder use. Posttests showed the proportion of workers who intended to inspect ladders before using them went from 44% to 83%. Follow-up telephone surveys conducted three months later found that workers had changed their actual work-site behavior. Over 50,000 people have seen the DVD, and 5,000 copies have been distributed. The DVD and supplemental materials are available in English and Spanish.

CPWR maintains the Electronic Library of Construction Occupational Safety and Health (eLCOSH) as a repository for a broad array of construction-related materials, but one of its primary target audiences is trainers. A search of eLCOSH using the term *falls* revealed 15 PowerPoint presentations and 331 images (which trainers can include in their training materials), and 52 toolbox talks. Toolbox talks (or tailgate talks) have been a primary mechanism for training on construction sites; these are short presentations that are given in the morning before starting work and focus on a particular safety topic generally related to the upcoming tasks and delivered by the foreman to his or her crew.

Incredibly, there has been almost no research on what makes for an effective toolbox talk. NIOSH researchers have suggested that an effective toolbox talk should (1) involve the crew with discussion questions, (2) include relevant case studies that have sufficient details to be seen as credible by the crew, (3) include details from the current jobsite, and (4) seek commitments from the crew to apply what was presented (Carol Stephenson, personal communication, 2011). These principles have been employed in several toolbox talks on fall protection that are currently housed on eLCOSH. The International Union of Operating Engineers developed six talks on falls under a larger program called the Focus Four—a reference to the four main killers on construction jobs, of which falls is the leading cause. In 2013, CPWR worked with NIOSH to develop a series of 52 talks (one for each week of the year) that cover falls, along with other hazards on construction sites. This innovative series contains a compelling graphic with three main bullet points on the back of the page so the crew has something to look at while the foreman delivers the talk. After the talk, the graphic side can be posted in the trailer to continue to reinforce the weekly message.

CPWR has developed a series of hazard alert cards that are available on paper and electronically. The card provided on ladders makes three strong points on how to avoid a fall: (1) Inspect the ladder before every use, (2) position the ladder properly, and (3) use the ladder safely. The card has been extremely popular, going through an initial printing of 5000 within months (Figure 4.7).

Training materials, no matter how well crafted, are only as effective as the underlying research they represent. To that end, CPWR has provided small study grants to university and nonprofit organizations to conduct research into the cause and prevention of falls in construction, particularly in residential construction. An example is the development of the St. Louis Audit of Fall Risks (SAFR) by researchers at the Washington School of Medicine (Kaskutas et al., 2008). The researchers found that the audit was a "reliable instrument for measuring fall safety risks at residential construction sites." Its ease of use makes it a "potentially useful instrument for safety monitoring by foremen and crew."

A more recent small study resulted in the creation of a compendium of available fall protection devices suitable for use in residential construction. The inventory contains more

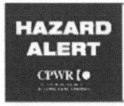
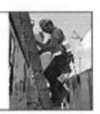

LADDERS

Am I in danger?

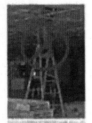

If you use a ladder on a construction site, then the answer is YES.

Falls are the leading cause of deaths and injuries in the construction industry

• Each year, more than 4,000 construction workers are injured so seriously by ladder falls that they miss work.

• Each year, about 70 construction workers DIE in falls from ladders.

Electrocution Hazard

Falls aren't the only way to get hurt on a ladder!

Contact with overhead power lines is a common, and sometimes fatal, source of injury for those working with ladders. Make sure your ladder is positioned **at least 10 feet from power lines.**

Aluminum is an excellent conductor of electricity. Working around wiring? Fiberglass is a better choice.

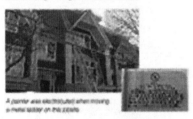

A painter was electrocuted when moving a metal ladder on this jobsite.

Find out more about construction hazards.

Get more of these Hazard Alert cards — and cards on other topics.

Call 301-578-8500

To avoid a fall ...

Not every defect is this obvious

1 Inspect the ladder before every use

Inspect the rails, rungs, feet, and spreaders or rung locks of your ladder for defects or damage **every time** you use it. If you see any damage, **tag it** "do not use" and request another ladder in proper working order. And check your ladder's duty rating – certain ladders may not support you and your toolbelt!

The minute you take to tie off could save your life

2 Position your ladder properly

For all ladders:

• Make sure you have level, solid footing for your ladder.

• Position the ladder near your work to avoid overreaching.

For extension ladders:

• Set the base one foot away from the building for every four feet of height.

• Tie off the ladder at the top – and bottom where possible!

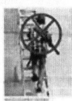

3 Use the ladder safely

• Maintain three-point contact with the ladder at all times.

• Do not stand on the top two rungs of a stepladder, or the top four rungs of an extension ladder.

• Have your partner hold the ladder to steady it as you ascend.

• **Don't carry tools and materials while climbing. Use a rope to haul or hoist materials to the upper level!**

Is a ladder the right tool for the job?

For **work at heights**, consider using a **scaffold** or **aerial lift.** The wider work platform and guard rails can substantially reduce your risk of falls.

If you think you are in danger: Contact your supervisor. Contact your union. Call OSHA 1-800-321-OSHA

FIGURE 4.7
Hazard alert.

than 150 products made by 23 different manufacturers (http://www.ot.wustl.edu/fptech/homepage.htm).

CPWR's Construction Solutions Database also provides information on a large number of effective controls for fall hazards. The website is directed toward construction employers who need information on available controls.

4.4.2 National Fall Prevention Campaign

To bring national awareness to the risk of fall hazards in the construction sector, CPWR joined with OSHA, NIOSH, and the National Occupational Research Agenda (NORA) Sector Council to launch a nationwide outreach campaign to raise awareness among workers and employers about the hazards of falls from roofs, ladders, and scaffolds. The fall prevention campaign provides abundant resources to construction employers and workers to assist with their fall protection plans and programs, including CPWR's website and the main campaign website, titled Stop Construction Falls website (www.stopconstructionfalls.com). The website provides information about the campaign, how to join, and a wealth of resources, including training programs, toolbox talks, videos, and other materials. There are also training tools for employers to use and posters to display at their worksites. Many of the new resources target vulnerable workers with limited English proficiency. New information and tools will be added to this page. As part of the campaign, a national weeklong stand-down was conducted during the week of June 2, 2014. OSHA documented participation through a voluntary website; employers could register stand-down activities and request a certificate of completion. OSHA asked CPWR to analyze the data collected. Feedback was submitted by almost 5000 participating stand-down sites and organizations and an estimated 1.5 million individuals in both construction and general industry were reached through the first national safety stand-down on falls. The event gave owners and contractors the opportunity and momentum needed to bring together large numbers of employees for training, toolbox talks, equipment inspections, and a variety of other activities in an organized manner, carrying the Campaign to Prevent Falls in Construction message further than initially conceived.

To support the national campaign, CPWR has also developed an online fatality map on the Stop Construction Falls website. Using a combination of OSHA inspection data and mass-media reporting, the map is a graphic representation of construction fatalities in the United States. This method of data collection has captured about 70% of the construction fall fatalities included in the CFOI from 2011 to 2013. By clicking on the pinpoints, users can locate where a construction worker lost his or her life on the job and learn how the incident happened and how the information was gathered. The map is updated regularly. Trainers have reported that the map is a valuable tool for reinforcing training efforts with information on local construction workers killed on the job.

4.5 Data Sources and Definitions

4.5.1 Data Sources

Fatal injury data were generated by the authors with restricted access to the U.S. Bureau of Labor Statistics's (BLS) Census of Fatal Occupational Injuries (CFOI), a federal-state cooperative program that has compiled fatal injury data annually since 1992. Nonfatal injury data are estimated from the BLS's Survey of Occupational Injuries and Illnesses (SOII), which collects information from a sample of employers each year. More information on work-related injuries, illnesses, and fatalities can be found online: http://www.bls.gov/iif/.

Information on fall hazards was estimated according to O*NET, a national program providing a wide variety of occupation-specific data. An O*NET exposure score is assigned from zero to 100, where zero represents no exposure to a given hazard and 100 represents continuous or daily exposure. Data are updated periodically to reflect changing work contexts. For more information, please visit http://www.onetonline.org/.

Demographic and employment data were from the *Current Population Survey*, the primary source for national labor force statistics in the United States. These data were also used for injury rate estimates. Please visit http://www.census.gov/cps/ for more information.

Data from the *County Business Patterns* were used for information on establishment size. This annual series provides economic data by industry across the nation and is available at http://www.census.gov/econ/cbp/.

4.5.2 Definitions

Full-time equivalent workers (FTEs): To make incidence rates comparable, researchers use the number of hours, or full-time workers (also known as person-years), to calculate such rates. Typically, it is assumed that a full-time worker works 2000 h per year (50 weeks of 40 h) in the United States. To determine the number of full-time equivalent workers in a population, divide the number of hours worked in the population by 2000.

Hispanic: Persons who identified themselves as being Spanish, Hispanic, or Latino. Persons of Hispanic or Latino ethnicity may be of any race.

References

Anderson JT, Hunting KL, Welch LS. 2000. Injury and employment patterns among Hispanic construction workers. *J Occup Environ Med*, 42(2):176–186.

Choi SD. 2006. A survey of the safety roles and costs of injuries in the roofing contracting industry. *J Safety Health Environ Res*, 3(1):1–20.

Dong X, Choi SD, Borchardt JG, Wang X, Largay JA. 2013. Fatal falls from roofs among U.S. construction workers. *J Safety Res*, 44:17–24.

Dong X, Fujimoto A, Ringen K, Men Y. 2009. Fatal falls among Hispanic construction workers. *Accid Anal Prev*, 41(5):1047–1052.

Dong X, Fujimoto A, Ringen K, Stafford E, Platner JW, Gittleman JL, Wang X. 2011. Injury underreporting among small establishments in the construction industry. *Am J Ind Med*, 54(5):339–349.

Dong X, Largay J, Wang X. 2014b. New trends in fatalities among construction workers. *CPWR Data Brief*, 3(2):1–10.

Dong X, Wang X, Daw C. 2012. Fatal falls among older construction workers. *Hum Factors*, 54(3):303–315.

Dong X, Wang X, Largay J, Choi S, Platner J, Trahan Cain C, Stafford E. 2014a. Fatal falls in the U.S. residential construction industry. *Am J Ind Med*, 57(9):992–1000.

Kaskutas VK, Dale AM, Lipscomb HJ, Evanoff BA. 2008. Development of the St. Louis audit of fall risks at residential construction sites. *Int J Occup Environ Health*, 14(4):243–249.

McGraw-Hill Construction. 2013. Safety management in the construction industry: Identifying risks and reducing accidents to improve site productivity and project ROI. *SmartMarket Report*, McGraw-Hill Construction.

Mirabelli MC, Loomis D, Richardson DB. 2003. Fatal occupational injuries among self-employed workers in North Carolina. *Am J Ind Med*, 44(2):182–190.

National Bureau of Economic Research. 2010. Business Cycle Dating Committee. Retrieved from http://www.nber.org/cycles/sept2010.pdf.

Rosenman K, Kalush A, Reilly M, Gardiner J, Reeves M, Luo Z. 2006. How much work-related injury and illness is missed by the current national surveillance system? *J Occup Environ Med*, 48(4): 357–365.

The Center for Construction Research and Training (CPWR). 2009. Hispanic employment in construction. *CPWR Data Brief,* 1(1):1–17.

The Center for Construction Research and Training (CPWR). 2013. *The Construction Chart Book: The U.S. Construction Industry and its Workers.* Silver Spring, MD: CPWR.

U.S. Bureau of Labor Statistics. 2014a. 2012 Current Population Survey. Retrieved from http://www.census.gov/programs-surveys/cps.html.

U.S. Bureau of Labor Statistics. 2014b. 2012 Census of Fatal Occupational Injury. Retrieved from online database, http://www.bls.gov/iif/#data.

U.S. Census Bureau. 2012. 2012 Nonemployer statistics. Retrieved from http://censtats.census.gov/cgi-bin/nonemployer/nondetl.pl.

Weil D. 2001. Assessing OSHA performance: New evidence from the construction industry. *J Pol Anal Manage,* 20(4): 651–674.

Section II

Sciences behind Human Falls and Injury Risk

5

Vision Impairment and Fall Risk in the Elderly

Philippe Lacherez and Stephen R. Lord

CONTENTS

ABSTRACT Vision is highly important for balance and gait, and visual impairments are significantly associated with locomotion problems and falls in older people. There is now a large body of research linking falls and fall-related injuries with visual problems, some of which are easily remedied by surgery or refractive correction. However, there is also evidence that the kind of refractive correction provided (in terms of single-vision or multifocal correction) can have an effect on fall risk. This chapter provides an overview of the major findings in this area.

KEY WORDS: *accidental falls, aged, balance, fractures, vision.*

5.1 The Problem of Falls in Older Adults: The Role of Vision

Falls are common in old age, and can have severe consequences in that they can lead to fractures, internal injuries, and even death. Most estimates suggest that approximately one-third of adults over 65 experience at least one fall in a year, and this figure increases to over 60% in those aged over 90 years (Black and Wood, 2005; Elliott, 2012). Age-related changes in visual function have been highlighted as a risk factor for falls that is amenable to intervention and, therefore, remediation.

Moving around in complex environments requires coordination of information from sensory inputs as well as coordinated motor control. Even in static postures (standing or sitting upright), visual information is important for maintaining posture. Sensory information for balance control is provided by the vestibular, proprioceptive (or somatosensory), and visual systems. However, the visual system often predominates, in that information from the visual system can override information from the other systems. For instance, postural sway typically increases by up to 70% when participants stand with eyes closed (Lord et al., 1991; Magnusson et al., 1990; Paulus et al., 1984), and exposure to moving visual stimuli produces a strong illusion of self-motion in a stationary stance (Berthoz et al., 1975). Studies have also shown that among people with somatosensory impairments, visual cues become even more important for balance control (Paulus et al., 1987). As a result, older adults (who often experience some loss of somatosensory function) demonstrate greater postural sway with eyes closed than their younger counterparts (Pyykko et al., 1990).

It is difficult to quantify precisely the contribution of visual function to the overall incidence of falls, due to the variety of measures and definitions employed in the literature. While not all epidemiological studies have found significant associations between visual function and falls, on the whole, vision has been shown to play a key role (Black and Wood, 2005; Dhital et al., 2010; Salonen and Kivelä, 2012). In one study (Jack et al., 1995), 76% of older adults admitted to a geriatric unit with a fall-related injury were visually impaired, and 79% of these visual impairments were correctable by refractive correction or cataract surgery. The following sections outline some key visual risk factors for falls.

5.2 Eye Disease

Several common eye diseases have been investigated as factors that may predispose older people to falls. These include cataracts, age-related macular degeneration (AMD), and glaucoma.

5.2.1 Cataracts

Cataracts greatly impair contrast sensitivity, and most studies examining objective measures of cataract severity as predictors of falls have found significant associations (Ivers et al., 1998, 2003; McCarty et al., 2002), the exception being one study by Felson et al. (1989). Cataract is a common visual problem (affecting up to 30% of older people) (Rochtchina et al., 2003), but in most cases can be readily corrected. Thus, early intervention for cataract is strongly recommended.

5.2.2 Age-Related Macular Degeneration

There is currently mixed evidence for the precise risk of falls associated with AMD. Three early studies failed to find any association between AMD and falls (Felson et al., 1989; Ivers et al., 1998, 2003), while two more recent studies have reported some association (Szabo et al., 2008; Wood et al., 2011). Szabo et al. (2008) observed that the fall risk of older women with AMD (as measured by an established predictor battery) was elevated, but they did not examine fall incidence. Wood et al. (2011) observed that within a group of AMD patients, higher fall incidence was associated with greater disease severity, as indexed by measures of visual function. Wood et al. (2009) also demonstrated, in an earlier analysis using the same cohort, that AMD patients with greater visual function loss also exhibited poorer balance and gait.

5.2.3 Glaucoma

Whether fall risk is increased in glaucoma remains uncertain. While some studies have reported an increased risk (Dolinis et al., 1997; Guse and Porinsky, 2003; Ivers et al., 2003), several others have found no significant associations (Coleman et al., 2004; Ivers et al., 1998; McCarty et al., 2002). Additionally, it appears that certain medications for glaucoma (particularly β-blockers) may themselves be associated with a higher fall risk (Glynn et al., 1991; Graafmans et al., 1996), so it is difficult to establish whether the associations reported are a result of the eye disease or the treatments prescribed.

5.3 Specific Functional Aspects of Vision

There are a number of ways in which visual function can change with age or disease processes, including changes in visual acuity, contrast sensitivity, and visual field loss. Additionally, each eye may be impaired to a different extent, leading to changes in binocular depth perception (stereoacuity). In the following sections, we summarize the findings about the contribution of each of these visual functions to fall risk.

5.3.1 Visual Acuity

Although visual acuity is a common measure employed in functional assessment, the impact of loss of acuity on fall risk is unclear. Distance visual acuity has been shown to be related to fall risk among people living in assisted care accommodation (Tinetti et al., 1986) as well as among those living independently in the community (Ivers et al., 1998; Klein et al., 2003; Lord and Menz, 2000; Nevitt et al., 1989; Patino et al., 2010; Yip et al., 2014). Some studies have reported an increased fall risk among those with visual acuity loss coupled with balance or hearing impairments (Kulmala et al., 2009). On the other hand, several studies have failed to find an association between reduced visual acuity and falls, particularly when adjusting for age (Brocklehurst et al., 1982; Campbell et al., 1989; Coleman et al., 2007; Freeman et al., 2007; Ivers et al., 2000; Lord et al., 1991; Robbins et al., 1989; Tinetti et al., 1988). One early study by Koski et al. (1998) may help to partly explain this discrepancy. They found that while visual acuity related strongly to the risk of falls among those in assisted living, there was no significant relationship among those living independently in the community. Thus, visual acuity may interact with other functional domains among those who are already otherwise impaired. Visual acuity loss has also been shown to be an independent predictor of fall-related injuries in two of three prospective studies (Cummings et al., 1995; Dargent-Molina et al., 1996; Felson et al., 1989), as well as one large case–control study (Ivers et al., 2000). In the Blue Mountains Eye Study (which involved 3299 people aged over 49 years), hip fractures were 8.4 times more likely among those with visual acuity worse than 6/18 (Ivers et al., 2003).

Uncorrected refractive error is common in older people, leading to unnecessary visual acuity loss (Thiagalingam et al., 2002). Therefore, an assessment of visual acuity and the regular provision of correct spectacles are advisable, given the possibility of increased fall risk indicated by the literature (although the kind of prescription, e.g., single-vision or multifocal, should also be considered—see Section 5.4).

5.3.2 Contrast Sensitivity

Contrast sensitivity is the ability to detect low-contrast stimuli in the environment. Contrast sensitivity, therefore, aids in detecting low-contrast contours and graduations in terrain (steps, street curbs, pavement cracks, and misalignments) over which people may trip. As with visual acuity, the data have been mixed with regard to the role that contrast sensitivity plays in relation to falls. Some studies have not found that reduced contrast sensitivity is a predictor of falls after adjustment for age and confounding factors such as cognition (Coleman et al., 2007; Freeman et al., 2007; Klein et al., 1998; Nevitt et al., 1989). However, several studies have found that poor edge-contrast sensitivity significantly increases fall risk in older people (Lord and Dayhew, 2001; Lord and Ward, 1994), as well as the risk of multiple falls and fractures (de Boer et al., 2004), suggesting, indeed, that it may be a better predictor than either visual acuity or visual field loss (Ivers et al., 1998). In the Beaver Dam Eye study, there was a nonsignificant association between retrospective falls and contrast sensitivity as measured by the Pelli–Robson test; however, their 5 year follow-up study revealed a significant association (Klein et al., 2003). One issue with this diverse literature is the inconsistency of measures, with few of the studies examining contrast sensitivity across a range of spatial frequencies (mostly using the Melbourne Edge Test and the Pelli–Robson test, which test contrast sensitivity at only a single spatial frequency) (Black and Wood, 2005). Since hazards that may lead to trips or falls in everyday life comprise a variety of spatial frequencies, it is important that future research should examine the predictive power of tests incorporating a range of spatial frequencies.

5.3.3 Stereopsis and Depth Perception

Binocular depth perception (stereopsis) affects the ability to accurately judge distances and to correctly perceive spatial relationships among objects, which suggests that it should be important for visually guided locomotion in the environment. Reductions in binocular depth perception have been found to increase the risk of multiple falls (Lord and Dayhew, 2001; Nevitt et al., 1989) as well as fall-related injuries (Felson et al., 1989; Ivers et al., 2000). Those exhibiting good vision in both eyes also have a lower rate of falls compared with those who have good vision in one eye but moderate or poor vision in the other (Lord and Dayhew, 2001). Similarly, older people with good vision in one eye, but only moderately good vision in the other, have been shown to have an elevated hip fracture risk (Felson et al., 1989). Only one study (Freeman et al., 2007) has reported a nonsignificant association between binocular depth perception and falls.

5.3.4 Visual Field Loss

Visual field loss has been less extensively examined than either visual acuity or contrast sensitivity; however, the results available indicate a strong association. Although two early studies reported weak associations between visual fields and falls (Glynn et al., 1991; Nevitt et al., 1989), more recent studies have found visual field loss to be a significant risk factor for falls (Black et al., 2011; Ivers et al., 1998; Patino et al., 2010; Ramrattan et al., 2001), multiple falls (Coleman et al., 2007; Klein et al., 2003), and fractures (Klein et al., 2003). It has also been reported that this risk remains significant when adjusting for demographic and health measures (Coleman et al., 2007; Freeman et al., 2007), with one exception (Friedman et al., 2002). Notably, the Beaver Dam Eye Study found that visual field loss almost doubled the risk of falls and fractures (Klein et al., 1998, 2003). Again, different measures of visual field loss have been used across the studies (Black and Wood, 2005), but the overall findings suggest that screening for visual field loss is a useful component of visual fall risk assessments in older people.

5.4 Spectacle Correction

Although, as noted in the previous section, appropriate refractive correction is an inexpensive and effective treatment for reduced visual acuity in the vast majority of cases, the kind of prescription dispensed may also have a direct impact on fall risk. Current literature suggests that multifocal (bifocal, trifocal or progressive lens) glasses also pose a significant risk of falling for older people. Multifocals are widely prescribed, as they reduce the need to change spectacles while undertaking daily activities (reading, using the computer, cooking, etc.). However, multifocal glasses may also predispose older people to falls, because viewing the environment through their lower lenses creates blur when viewing the ground while standing and walking. It has been documented that people generally look two steps ahead (approximately 1.5–2 m) when walking (Patla and Vickers, 1997). Without downward pitch head movement, multifocal glasses wearers view their forward path through their lower lens segments (typically set to a focal point around 60 cm), resulting in blurred vision and impaired ability to detect and discriminate floor-level hazards.

In one epidemiological survey (Davies et al., 2001), it was found, among older persons who had experienced "underfoot accidents" (including falls, trips on stairs, etc.), that habitual multifocal users reported significantly more incidents involving missing the edge of a step. Johnson et al. (2007, 2008) also investigated the accuracy of foot placement when stepping onto a step, in older people wearing single-lens glasses versus multifocal glasses (progressive and bifocal lenses). Older people wearing multifocal glasses showed more variable vertical toe clearance when stepping up (Johnson et al., 2007) and more variable foot placement when negotiating the step (Johnson et al., 2008). Contacts with the step edge (12 out of 875 trials) (Johnson et al., 2008) and trips (Johnson et al., 2007) occurred only in the multifocal glasses conditions, and participants tripped more often with multifocal than with single-distance glasses (Johnson et al., 2007).

Multifocal glasses have also been shown to impair older people's ability to divide their attention while walking (when the task is to negotiate multiple obstacles). In one study (Menant et al., 2009), 30 older adults who habitually wore multifocal glasses negotiated an obstacle course. In some conditions, the participants wore their multifocal spectacles; in the others, they wore a matched pair of single-lens distance glasses. Additionally, in half the trials, the participants were also required to read a series of letters presented in front of them at eye level as a secondary task. The participants contacted significantly more obstacles in the condition that combined the dual-task and multifocal correction. Eye and head positioning were also measured, and analysis of these data suggested that in the dual-task condition, participants did not incline their head sufficiently when wearing multifocal glasses, resulting in increased blur at floor level (seen through the lower lens).

In one prospective cohort study of 156 participants aged 63–90 years (Lord et al., 2002), participants who were regular wearers of multifocal glasses showed significantly poorer distant depth perception and edge-contrast sensitivity when viewing test stimuli through the lower segments of their glasses. Multifocal glasses wearers also fell significantly more often in the 1 year follow-up period than nonmultifocal glasses wearers (adjusting for age and known physical risk factors for falls) and experienced more falls when outside their homes and when walking up or down stairs.

5.5 Visual Interventions for Preventing Falls

A small number of randomized controlled trials (RCTs) have been undertaken to investigate one or more visual interventions in terms of their ability to prevent falls. One RCT evaluated a targeted home-safety assessment and modification intervention program for older adults with severe visual impairment (Campbell et al., 2005; La Grow et al., 2006). Three hundred and ninety-one visually impaired people aged 75 years and over living in the community were randomized to either a home-safety program (n = 100), an exercise program with vitamin D supplementation (n = 97), both interventions (n = 98), or a social visit control group (n = 96). Falls were reduced by 41% in the group randomized to the home-safety program (Campbell et al., 2005). The authors attributed the success of this intervention to (i) the effectiveness of the reduction of home hazards (for hazard-related falls); (ii) participants' increased awareness regarding home hazards; and (iii) possible increased fear of falling, leading to activity restriction and in turn, reduced exposure to risk (La Grow et al., 2006).

The effect of cataract surgery in reducing fall incidence has been investigated in two prospective RCTs. The first, involving 306 women aged 70 years and over, examined the efficacy of cataract surgery on the first eye (Harwood et al., 2005). Participants were randomly allocated to receive either expedited (approximately 4 weeks' wait) or routine (12 months' wait) surgery, and it was found that the fall rate in the expedited group was reduced significantly, by 34%, compared with the controls. A follow-on study by the same authors evaluated whether surgery on the second eye led to further reductions in falls (Foss et al., 2006). Again, participants (239 women aged over 70) were randomized to either expedited (approximately 4 weeks' wait) or routine (12 months' wait) surgery. The 1 year prospective rate of falls was again reduced by 32% in the operated group, although this was a nonsignificant reduction in this sample, likely due to reduced power from the smaller sample size. In one nonrandomized study, McGwin et al. (2006) observed no difference in the 1 year prospective rate of falls among participants who elected to have cataract surgery and patients who did not. The patients were matched in terms of selection criteria (visual acuity worse than 20/40 and cataract in at least one eye) and age; however, the patients electing to have surgery did have worse vision at baseline. One recent longitudinal population study examining over 28,000 hospital records for participants who had received cataract surgery found that the rate of hospital admissions for fall-related injuries *increased* in the 2 years following surgery to each eye (Meuleners et al., 2014). It is worth noting, however, that this is in comparison with their fall rate before surgery and not in comparison with a control group. In stark contrast, a population study conducted in the United

States that examined over 1 million records, including those who did and those who did not receive cataract surgery, found that cataract surgery effectively reduced the rate of falls (Tseng et al., 2012).

Two RCTs have evaluated the efficacy of visual assessment and provision of new glasses as an intervention to prevent falls. Day et al. (2002) used a factorial design to assess the separate and combined effects of interventions aimed at vision improvement, home hazard reduction, and group exercise among 1090 participants aged 70 years and over. In the visual-improvement intervention, participants with impaired vision were provided with a referral to their usual eye-care provider (if they exhibited poor visual acuity, decreased stereopsis, and/or reduced field of view). The 12 month prospective falls rate was reduced by 4.4% for those in the visual intervention group, a nonsignificant reduction. It is worth noting, however, that of the 547 participants randomly assigned to receive the vision intervention, only 26 received a treatment they would not otherwise have had.

In the second study (Cumming et al., 2007), 616 older people aged 70 years and over were randomized to either an intervention group (n = 309) or a control group (n = 307). Of the intervention group, 44% (n = 92) received vision-related treatments (most often a new pair of glasses). During the 12 month follow-up period, participants in the intervention group reported significantly *more* falls than those in the control group. This was a highly unexpected finding given the hypotheses of the study. The authors conjectured that since the participants in the intervention group often received prescriptions quite different from their current glasses, they might have needed more time to adapt to their new glasses (Elliott and Chapman, 2010); alternatively, they might have become overconfident, adopting more risk-taking activities (thus increasing the exposure to falls) as a result of experiencing better vision. As evidence of the former, the authors observed that fall risk was higher among those who had a larger change in prescription than those who had a smaller change. Thus, some period of adaptation is needed, and it is recommended that optometrists gradually change prescriptions and counsel patients as to the likely short-term risks of a new prescription (Elliott, 2014).

Another RCT, which imbedded visual functional assessment into a broader intervention (Close et al., 1999), produced a significant reduction in falls, but with this multifactorial study design, it is not possible to determine whether the vision-intervention component was a key aspect of the overall efficacious intervention.

A recent RCT (Haran et al., 2009), involving 606 older people and 13 months of follow-up, assessed whether fall rates among habitual multifocal users could be reduced by facilitating participants to wear single-vision correction when active outdoors or in unfamiliar indoor settings. The intervention was aimed at older habitual multifocal wearers at increased risk of falls (i.e., who had suffered one or more falls in the past year or had a Timed Up and Go test >15 s). Participants were provided with an additional pair of single-vision spectacles and counseled to wear these for walking or outdoor activities (participants were counseled to restrict their use of their multifocal glasses to activities that require changes in focal length, including everyday tasks such as driving, shopping, and cooking, which pose little risk for falls). Overall, there was a nonsignificant 8% reduction in all falls as a result of the intervention and a significant 40% reduction in the subgroup who more regularly undertook outside activities. However, outside falls *increased* in the intervention group in those who habitually undertook less outside activity. The authors suggest that single lenses may be beneficial for those who take part in regular outdoor activities but may increase risk for those with low levels of outdoor activity.

5.6 Summary

In summary, the visual system provides important information for balance and gait, and visual impairment can have direct and measurable impacts on postural stability, falls, and fall-related injuries in older people. Eye diseases such as AMD, glaucoma, and cataracts and suboptimal refractive correction may predispose older people to falls. Cataract surgery and home-safety interventions can significantly reduce falls in visually impaired older people. With respect to glasses prescription, the kind of refractive correction dispensed appears to be important, with single-vision correction generally being preferable to multifocal correction for outdoor walking.

References

Berthoz, A., Pavard, B. and Young, L. R. (1975). Perception of linear horizontal self-motion induced by peripheral vision (linearvection): Basic characteristics and visual-vestibular interactions. *Experimental Brain Research*, 23(5), 471–489.

Black, A. A. and Wood, J. M. (2005). Vision and falls. *Clinical and Experimental Optometry*, 88(4), 212–222.

Black, A. A., Wood, J. M. and Lovie-Kitchin, J. E. (2011). Inferior field loss increases rate of falls in older adults with glaucoma. *Optometry and Vision Science*, 88(11), 1275–1282.

Brocklehurst, J. C., Robertson, D. and Jamesgroom, P. (1982). Clinical correlates of sway in old-age: Sensory modalities. *Age and Ageing*, 11(1), 1–10.

Campbell, A. J., Borrie, M. J. and Spears, G. F. (1989). Risk-factors for falls in a community-based prospective-study of people 70 years and older. *Journals of Gerontology*, 44(4), M112–M117.

Campbell, A. J., Robertson, M. C., La Grow, S. J. et al. (2005). Randomised controlled trial of prevention of falls in people aged >=75 with severe visual impairment: The VIP trial. *British Medical Journal*, 331(7520), 817–820A.

Close, J., Ellis, M., Hooper, R., Glucksman, E., Jackson, S. and Swift, C. (1999). Prevention of falls in the elderly trial (PROFET): A randomised controlled trial. *Lancet*, 353(9147), 93–97.

Coleman, A. L., Cummings, S. R., Yu, F. et al. (2007). Binocular visual-field loss increases the risk of future falls in older white women. *Journal of the American Geriatrics Society*, 55(3), 357–364.

Coleman, A. L., Stone, K., Ewing, S. K., et al. (2004). Higher risk of multiple falls among elderly women who lose visual acuity. *Ophthalmology*, 111(5), 857–862.

Cumming, R. G., Ivers, R., Clemson, L. et al. (2007). Improving vision to prevent falls in frail older people: A randomized trial. *Journal of the American Geriatrics Society*, 55(2), 175–181.

Cummings, S. R., Nevitt, M. C., Browner, W. S. et al. (1995). Risk-factors for hip fracture in white women. *New England Journal of Medicine*, 332(12), 767–773.

Dargent-Molina, P., Favier, F., Grandjean, H. et al. (1996). Fall-related factors and risk of hip fracture: The EPIDOS prospective study. *Lancet*, 348(9021), 145–149.

Davies, J. C., Kemp, G. J., Stevens, G., Frostick, S. P. and Manning, D. P. (2001). Bifocal/varifocal spectacles, lighting and missed-step accidents. *Safety Science*, 38(3), 211–226.

Day, L., Fildes, B., Gordon, I., Fitzharris, M., Flamer, H. and Lord, S. (2002). Randomised factorial trial of falls prevention among older people living in their own homes. *British Medical Journal*, 325(7356), 128–131.

de Boer, M. R., Pluijm, S. M., Lips, P. et al. (2004). Different aspects of visual impairment as risk factors for falls and fractures in older men and women. *Journal of Bone and Mineral Research*, 19(9), 1539–1547.

Dhital, A., Pey, T. and Stanford, M. R. (2010). Visual loss and falls: A review. *Eye*, 24(9), 1437–1446.

Dolinis, J., Harrison, J. E. and Andrews, G. R. (1997). Factors associated with falling in older Adelaide residents. *Australian and New Zealand Journal of Public Health*, 21(5), 462–468.

Elliott, D. B. (2012). Falls and vision impairment: Guidance for the optometrist. *Optometry in Practice*, 13(2), 65–76.

Elliott, D. B. (2014). The Glenn A. Fry award lecture 2013: Blurred vision, spectacle correction, and falls in older adults. *Optometry and Vision Science*, 91(6), 593–601.

Elliott, D. B. and Chapman, G. J. (2010). Adaptive gait changes due to spectacle magnification and dioptric blur in older people. *Investigative Ophthalmology and Visual Science*, 51(2), 718–722.

Felson, D. T., Anderson, J. J., Hannan, M. T., Milton, R. C., Wilson, P. W. F. and Kiel, D. P. (1989). Impaired vision and hip fracture: The Framingham study. *Journal of the American Geriatrics Society*, 37(6), 495–500.

Foss, A. J. E., Harwood, R. H., Osborn, F., Gregson, R. M., Zaman, A. and Masud, T. (2006). Falls and health status in elderly women following second eye cataract surgery: A randomised controlled trial. *Age and Ageing*, 35(1), 66–71.

Freeman, E. E., Munoz, B., Rubin, G. and West, S. K. (2007). Visual field loss increases the risk of falls in older adults: The Salisbury eye evaluation. *Investigative Ophthalmology and Visual Science*, 48(10), 4445–4450.

Friedman, S. M., Munoz, B., West, S. K., Rubin, G. S. and Fried, L. P. (2002). Falls and fear of falling: Which comes first? A longitudinal prediction model suggests strategies for primary and secondary prevention. *Journal of the American Geriatrics Society*, 50(8), 1329–1335.

Glynn, R. J., Seddon, J. M., Krug, J. H., Sahagian, C. R., Chiavelli, M. E. and Campion, E. W. (1991). Falls in elderly patients with glaucoma. *Archives of Ophthalmology*, 109(2), 205–210.

Graafmans, W., Ooms, M., Hofstee, H., Bezemer, P., Bouter, L. and Lips, P. (1996). Falls in the elderly: A prospective study of risk factors and risk profiles. *American Journal of Epidemiology*, 143(11), 1129–1136.

Guse, C. E. and Porinsky, R. (2003). Risk factors associated with hospitalization for unintentional falls: Wisconsin hospital discharge data for patients aged 65 and over. *Wisconsin Medical Journal*, 102(4), 37–42.

Haran, M. J., Lord, S. R., Cameron, I. D. et al. (2009). Preventing falls in older multifocal glasses wearers by providing single-lens distance glasses: The protocol for the VISIBLE randomised controlled trial. *BMC Geriatrics*, 9(1), 10.

Harwood, R. H., Foss, J. E., Osborn, F., Gregson, R. M., Zaman, A. and Masud, T. (2005). Falls and health status in elderly women following first eye cataract surgery: A randomised controlled trial. *British Journal of Ophthalmology*, 89(1), 53–59.

Ivers, R. Q., Cumming, R. G., Mitchell, P. and Attebo, K. (1998). Visual impairment and falls in older adults: The Blue Mountains eye study. *Journal of the American Geriatrics Society*, 46(1), 58–64.

Ivers, R. Q., Cumming, R. G., Mitchell, P., Simpson, J. M. and Peduto, A. J. (2003). Visual risk factors for hip fracture in older people. *Journal of the American Geriatrics Society*, 51(3), 356–363.

Ivers, R. Q., Norton, R., Cumming, R. G., Butler, M., and Campbell, A. J. (2000). Visual impairment and risk of hip fracture. *American Journal of Epidemiology*, 152(7), 633–639.

Jack, C. I. A., Smith, T., Neoh, C., Lye, M. and Mcgalliard, J. N. (1995). Prevalence of low vision in elderly patients admitted to an acute geriatric unit in Liverpool: Elderly people who fall are more likely to have low vision. *Gerontology*, 41(5), 280–285.

Johnson, L., Buckley, J. G., Harley, C. and Elliott, D. B. (2008). Use of single-vision eyeglasses improves stepping precision and safety when elderly habitual multifocal wearers negotiate a raised surface. *Journal of the American Geriatrics Society*, 56(1), 178–180.

Johnson, L., Buckley, J. G., Scally, A. J. and Elliott, D. B. (2007). Multifocal spectacles increase variability in toe clearance and risk of tripping in the elderly. *Investigative Ophthalmology and Visual Science*, 48(4), 1466–1471.

Klein, B. E. K., Klein, R., Lee, K. E. and Cruickshanks, K. J. (1998). Performance-based and self-assessed measures of visual function as related to history of falls, hip fractures, and measured gait time: The Beaver Dam Eye Study. *Ophthalmology*, 105(1), 160–164.

Klein, B. E. K., Moss, S. E., Klein, R., Lee, K. E. and Cruickshanks, K. J. (2003). Associations of visual function with physical outcomes and limitations 5 years later in an older population: The Beaver Dam eye study. *Ophthalmology*, 110(4), 644–650.

Koski, K., Luukinen, H., Laippala, P. and Kivela, S. L. (1998). Risk factors for major injurious falls among the home-dwelling elderly by functional abilities. A prospective population-based study. *Gerontology*, 44, 232–238.

Kulmala, J., Viljanen, A., Sipila, S. et al. (2009). Poor vision accompanied with other sensory impairments as a predictor of falls in older women. *Age and Ageing*, 38(2), 162–167.

La Grow, S., Robertson, M. C., Campbell, A. J., Clarke, G. and Kerse, N. M. (2006). Reducing hazard related falls in people 75 years and older with significant visual impairment: How did a successful program work? *Injury Prevention*, 12(5), 296–301.

Lord, S. R., Clark, R. D. and Webster, I. W. (1991). Postural stability and associated physiological factors in a population of aged persons. *Journals of Gerontology*, 46(3), M69–M76.

Lord, S. R. and Dayhew, J. (2001). Visual risk factors for falls in older people. *Journal of the American Geriatrics Society*, 49(5), 508–515.

Lord, S. R., Dayhew, J. and Howland, A. (2002). Multifocal glasses impair edge-contrast sensitivity and depth perception and increase the risk of falls in older people. *Journal of the American Geriatrics Society*, 50(11), 1760–1766.

Lord, S. R. and Menz, H. B. (2000). Visual contributions to postural stability in older adults. *Gerontology*, 46(6), 306–310.

Lord, S. R. and Ward, J. A. (1994). Age-associated differences in sensorimotor function and balance in community-dwelling women. *Age and Ageing*, 23(6), 452–460.

McCarty, C. A., Fu, L., and Taylor, R. (2002). The risks of everyday life: Predictors of falls in the Melbourne visual impairment project. *Australian and New Zealand Journal of Public Health*, 26(2), 116–119.

McGwin G., Jr., Gewant, H. D., Modjarrad, K., Hall, T. A. and Owsley, C. (2006). Effect of cataract surgery on falls and mobility in independently living older adults. *Journal of the American Geriatrics Society*, 54(7), 1089–1094.

Magnusson, M., Enbom, H., Johansson, R. and Wiklund, J. (1990). Significance of pressor input from the human feet in lateral postural control: The effect of hypothermia on galvanically induced body-sway. *Acta Oto-Laryngologica*, 110(5–6), 321–327.

Menant, J. C., St George, R. J., Sandery, B., Fitzpatrick, R. C. and Lord, S. R. (2009). Older people contact more obstacles when wearing multifocal glasses and performing a secondary visual task. *Journal of the American Geriatrics Society*, 57(10), 1833–1838.

Meuleners, L. B., Fraser, M. L., Ng, J. and Morlet, N. (2014). The impact of first- and second-eye cataract surgery on injurious falls that require hospitalisation: A whole-population study. *Age and Ageing*, 43(3), 341–346.

Nevitt, M. C., Cummings, S. R., Kidd, S. and Black, D. (1989). Risk-factors for recurrent nonsyncopal falls: A prospective study. *Journal of the American Medical Association*, 261(18), 2663–2668.

Patino, C. M., McKean-Cowdin, R., Azen, S. P., Allison, J. C., Choudhury, F. and Varma, R. (2010). Central and peripheral visual impairment and the risk of falls and falls with injury. *Ophthalmology*, 117(2), 199–206.

Patla, A. E. and Vickers, J. N. (1997). Where and when do we look as we approach and step over an obstacle in the travel path? *Neuroreport*, 8(17), 3661–3665.

Paulus, W. M., Straube, A. and Brandt, T. (1984). Visual stabilization of posture: Physiological stimulus characteristics and clinical aspects. *Brain*, 107(Dec), 1143–1163.

Paulus, W. M., Straube, A. and Brandt, T. H. (1987). Visual postural performance after loss of somatosensory and vestibular function. *Journal of Neurology, Neurosurgery and Psychiatry*, 50(11), 1542–1545.

Pyykko, I., Jantti, P. and Aalto, H. (1990). Postural control in elderly subjects. *Age and Ageing*, 19(3), 215–221.

Ramrattan, R. S., Wolfs, R. C., Panda-Jonas, S. et al. (2001). Prevalence and causes of visual field loss in the elderly and associations with impairment in daily functioning: The Rotterdam Study. *Archives of Ophthalmology*, 119(12), 1788–1794.

Robbins, A. S., Rubenstein, L. Z., Josephson, K. R., Schulman, B. L., Osterweil, D. and Fine, G. (1989). Predictors of falls among elderly people: Results of 2 population-based studies. *Archives of Internal Medicine*, 149(7), 1628–1633.

Rochtchina, E., Mukesh, B. N., Wang, J. J., McCarty, C. A., Taylor, H. R. and Mitchell, P. (2003). Projected prevalence of age-related cataract and cataract surgery in Australia for the years 2001 and 2021: Pooled data from two population-based surveys. *Clinical and Experimental Ophthalmology*, 31(3), 233–236.

Salonen, L. and Kivelä, S. L. (2012). Eye diseases and impaired vision as possible risk factors for recurrent falls in the aged: A systematic review. *Current Gerontology and Geriatrics Research*, Article ID 271481.

Szabo, S. M., Janssen, P. A., Khan, K., Potter, M. J. and Lord, S. R. (2008). Older women with age-related macular degeneration have a greater risk of falls: A physiological profile assessment study. *Journal of the American Geriatrics Society*, 56(5), 800–807.

Thiagalingam, S., Cumming, R. and Mitchell, P. (2002). Factors associated with undercorrected refractive errors in an older population: The Blue Mountains Eye Study. *British Journal of Ophthalmology*, 86(9), 1041–1045.

Tinetti, M. E., Speechley, M. and Ginter, S. F. (1988). Risk-factors for falls among elderly persons living in the community. *New England Journal of Medicine*, 319(26), 1701–1707.

Tinetti, M. E., Williams, T. F. and Mayewski, R. (1986). Fall risk index for elderly patients based on number of chronic disabilities. *American Journal of Medicine*, 80(3), 429–434.

Tseng, V. L., Yu, F., Lum, F. and Coleman, A. L. (2012). Risk of fractures following cataract surgery in Medicare beneficiaries. *Journal of the American Medical Association*, 308(5), 493–501.

Wood, J. M., Lacherez, P. F., Black, A. A., Cole, M. H., Boon, M. Y. and Kerr, G. K. (2009). Postural stability and gait among older adults with age-related maculopathy. *Investigative Ophthalmology and Visual Science*, 50(1), 482–487.

Wood, J. M., Lacherez, P. F., Black, A. A., Cole, M. H., Boon, M. Y. and Kerr, G. K. (2011). Risk of falls, injurious falls, and other injuries resulting from visual impairment among older adults with age-related macular degeneration. *Investigative Ophthalmology and Visual Science*, 52(8), 5088–5092.

Yip, J. L. Y., Khawaja, A. P., Broadway, D. et al. (2014). Visual acuity, self-reported vision and falls in the EPIC-Norfolk Eye study. *British Journal of Ophthalmology*, 98(3), 377–382.

6

Influence of Personal Protective Equipment Use on Fall Risk

Sharon S. Chiou and Paul R. Keane

CONTENTS

Personal protective equipment (PPE) is apparatus that is designed to prevent or limit the exposure of wearers to physical hazards as well as to chemical, biological, radiological, or nuclear (CBRN) hazards. The apparatus may include respirators, garments, head protection, hearing protection, eyewear, footwear, gloves, protective vests or ensembles, or other devices that provide a barrier between the wearer and the environment. PPE ranks last on the hierarchy of hazard controls, following elimination and substitution of hazards, engineering controls, and administrative measures. As such, it constitutes the final line of defense for worker exposure to hazardous substances, and it should be used in cases when other means of protecting the worker cannot be implemented.

According to Occupational Safety and Health Administration (OSHA) standards (29 CFR 1910.134), when effective engineering controls are not feasible or while they are being instituted, appropriate respirators shall be used. Approximately 20 million workers use PPE regularly in occupational settings to protect them from exposure to hazards [1]. Workers across all industry sectors, including agriculture, forestry, fishing, construction, health care, manufacturing, services, transportation, the wholesale and retail trade, and mining, regularly use PPE [2]. Proper use of PPE can result in effective reduction in exposure to inhalation hazards and also to hazards to skin, hearing, and traumatic injury, which often correlates directly to reduced injury, disease, and fatality rates [3].

Since 2001, there has been growing concern about CBRN agents, because of the danger of both deliberate attacks and industrial accidents [4]. First responders (e.g., firefighters, law enforcement, HAZMAT workers, and emergency medical teams) are frequently the first personnel at the scenes of mass-casualty incidents, and they are required, as a condition of compliance with existing OSHA standards (OSHA 1910.95, 120, 132–138, 156; 1926.56–106), to wear significant amounts of PPE to protect them against a wide range of hazards [5].

The 2014 Ebola outbreak in West Africa highlighted the importance of PPE in protecting health-care workers from the deadly Ebola virus. It also emphasized the urgent need for improved protection of health-care workers so that they could respond safely and efficiently to infectious disease epidemics in adverse environments. It is known that the use of PPE may prevent the worker from direct contact with an environmental hazard, but it does impose additional hazards: reduced visibility, increased weight and bulk, increased propensity to fall as a function of gait and proprioception effects, and other human factors hazards [6–8]. All of these factors may affect the ability of the workers to function effectively and safely in performing designated tasks, and since these tasks frequently involve public safety and health, the design and manufacture of PPEs that are safe, comfortable, and designed with the task and user in mind are pressing concerns for researchers, government agencies that are concerned with public safety and health, hospital administrators, and first-responder incident commanders.

PPE has limitations in that it does not eliminate the hazard at its source and may result in employees being exposed to the hazard if the equipment fails; damage to PPE may subject workers to traumatic injuries, pulmonary diseases, dermal exposures, and, under extreme circumstances, may cause immediate danger to their lives and health. Since physical damage is known to occur in dynamic situations, the ability of PPE to resist damage and to impose minimal constraints while maintaining a barrier against exposure becomes significant.

The current chapter addresses the effects of additional constraining factors or limitations imposed by PPE in terms of additional weight, reduced visibility, confinement, and impacts on workers' postural balance. The National Institute for Occupational Safety and Health (NIOSH) has devoted considerable effort to understanding this issue and has conducted various research projects aimed at understanding the contribution of PPE to postural balance and subsequent fall-related injury risk. This chapter starts with a background review of motor control, balance control, and gait control as they are related to fall injuries. Intrinsic and extrinsic factors that are related to postural balance and that may increase the propensity to loss of balance are described herein. The chapter further discusses the effects of PPE on postural instability and the slip-trip-fall (STF) injury potential of two groups of first responders—firefighters and hospital first receivers who treat contaminated patients—while wearing PPE. A full complement of firefighting turnout gear conforming to National Fire Protection Association (NFPA) standards and a set of first-receiver PPE that met the requirements of OSHA are used as examples to examine fall risks associated with PPE.

This chapter identifies the restrictive nature of PPE and its relationship with fall risk and presents previous and current findings. It promotes the recognition of the fall injury hazards associated with PPE and the current leading research for injury prevention and hazard evaluation to better understand the stresses PPE may impose on workers and to provide scientific information for future recommendations for improved work practices and PPE design.

6.1 Background

6.1.1 Slips, Trips, and Falls

A fall is an event that results in a person unintentionally coming to rest on the floor or on lower levels. Prior to the moment in which a fall incident occurs, a person first experiences postural instability or loss of balance. The duration between the sense of loss of balance and the event of fall is usually very short. When a person is not able to recover from loss of balance, a fall incident occurs. A slip is a type of fall causing loss of balance and commonly causing a subsequent fall; slips are often caused by environmental factors, such as contaminated floors. Falls are commonly categorized by the location where the incidents occur: falls on the same level, falls from elevation, and stair falls. Slips and trips are the main contributors to falls on the same level. Examples of falls from elevations are falls from roofs, scaffolds, or ladders. Stair falls may include slips or trips while descending or ascending.

Trips are also loss-of-balance events, frequently leading to a subsequent fall. OSHA defines trips as events involving loss of balance caused by striking an object with the foot or lower leg while the upper body continues its trajectory, or an event causing loss of balance involved with stepping down to a lower level [9].

In 2014, there were approximately 316,650 injuries attributable to work-related STF involving days away from work in private industry [10]. STF is one of the leading causes of workplace injuries in the United States with an estimated cost of $5.7 billion each year [11]. In many industries, falls are the key cause of injuries in the workplace. Falls frequently result in severe bodily injury, permanent disability, and even fatality. Take the health-care industry as an example; the Bureau of Labor Statistics (BLS) reported that health-care workers suffered a greater than average rate of injuries due to falls on the same level (BLS 2014). In 2014, the BLS incidence rate of lost-workday injuries from STF on the same level in hospitals was 31.3 per 10,000 FTEs [10], which was 52% greater than the average rate for all private industries combined. Epidemiological, biomechanical, psychological, and tribological studies have been conducted to reduce slips and falls, and it has been found that the causes of STF are complex and multidimensional [12–16]. Previous studies examined causes of STF in workplaces and have shown that STF can result from personal, environmental, and job-task factors [12]. Understanding the causes of STF enables the development of intervention strategies to reduce the incidence of STF. The three factors related to STF will be discussed further in later sections of the chapter.

6.1.2 Control of Postural Balance

Control and maintenance of postural balance is essential in daily life as well as in the workplace. Postural control is the ability of the body to maintain its center of gravity over the base of support during standing or dynamic movement. The maintenance of postural balance is a complex process involving the coordination among musculoskeletal, sensory, motor, and CNSs. In daily life or in an occupational setting, postural balance is constantly challenged by perturbations arising from environmental changes, sudden movement of body segments, or task demands, such as working at heights or the use of PPE. These perturbations could be visual, vestibular, or proprioceptive input changes resulting in conditions that challenge the body's equilibrium. Functionally, postural control can be divided into different activities, including maintenance of posture during standing or sitting, controlling the movement of the body's center of mass, and response to external perturbations [13].

Several physiological systems provide afferent information for maintaining postural balance. Afferents—that is, vision, proprioception, the vestibular system, and the cutaneous apparatus—elicit postural reflexes when they are individually or collectively challenged. Visual inputs are essential in the maintenance of postural equilibrium, and the characteristics of the base of support determine the extent to which the vestibular system is involved [14]. The role of the proprioceptive system and the vestibular system becomes critical when the base of support on which the subject stands becomes uneven and the visual input is excluded. Despite the availability of multiple sensory inputs for healthy adults, the preferred sensory input for balance control is the proprioceptors at the feet [15]. Although the CNS generally relies on one sense at a time for balance, when one source is reduced, alternative sensory inputs are used for balance [16]. Postural balance is widely used as an indicator of susceptibility to loss of balance or fall. The control of postural stability plays an important role in fall prevention among the elderly as well as among individuals performing workplace activities.

When the body's center of mass is shifted near the outer perimeter of the basal support due to perturbations, the instability is detected via afferent inputs from muscles, joints, the vestibular system, and vision. Subsequently, motor processes coordinate the muscle actions into discrete synergies to minimize postural sway and keep the body's center of mass within the base of support [17,18]. This entire process is controlled by the central nervous system (CNS). If static balance cannot be maintained, a rapid step or additional external support such as holding onto a guard rail is needed to reestablish the base of support. Motor control is a dynamic process that coordinates human movements and regulates the ability of the human body to move, to carry out daily activities, and to perform industrial tasks. It is a continuous and complex process that involves processing sensory information including body segment (e.g., position, force magnitude and directions) and environmental changes (e.g., floor slipperiness and lighting) and initiates the commands to regulate the movement of the human body.

6.1.3 Control and Maintenance of Dynamic Balance

A variety of tasks performed in a standing position can place the human body's ability to maintain balance at risk; however, task performance during walking places even more demands on the body's ability to maintain balance. In human gait, the body's equilibrium is lost and gained from one step to another. During gait, the center of gravity of the body ventures out of the basal support momentarily. An unexpected perturbation or an external loading may be enough to cause the center of gravity to travel outside the basal support area and cause a fall. Gait requires an integration of a complex neuromuscular–skeletal system as well as the coordination of muscles acting across many joints. This dynamic balance could be disturbed by traumatic injury, neurological damage and deterioration, and even fatigue [19]. It can also be challenged by perturbations arising from environmental changes, that is, floor slipperiness and clutter, or job-task requirements, such as working at heights and/or the use of PPE [20–23].

Previous studies have indicated that, to achieve safe and efficient locomotion, major motor functional requirements needed to be met. Upright posture and total body balance must be maintained [24], and the upper body should be fully supported against the force of gravity during locomotion. Foot trajectory needs to be well controlled to achieve safe ground clearance [25]. In addition, sufficient mechanical energy needs to be generated by the body to maintain forward velocity during progression [26]. Moreover, the motor patterns at the hips, knees, and ankles have the major function of absorbing and generating energy [26], and the CNS must integrate and coordinate efferent commands with proprioceptive feedback and vestibular and visual inputs to generate the correct patterns of moment of force at each joint.

Previous studies on gait [21,27,28] have documented that people changed their gait as they approached and encountered slippery surfaces. Humans can adjust their gait to perceived changes indicated by sensory feedback and can safely negotiate many different friction-surface levels. The typical protective gait strategy adopted in response to increased slipperiness includes shorter steps and increased knee flexion to reduce vertical acceleration and forward velocity [29]. Gait changes are also observed in poorly lit environments. Subjects experiencing these conditions walked significantly more slowly and exhibited decreased incoming velocity and heel contact angle [21]. It is the sudden and unanticipated changes in surface slipperiness or other environmental factors (e.g., changes in floor/surface pitch and elevation) that often cause most slips and falls [30].

6.1.4 Factors Affecting Postural Stability

6.1.4.1 Personal Factors

There are many personal risk factors that are related to STF, such as gender, age, fatigue, obesity, physical inactivity, poor muscle strength, and poor fitness levels [31–38]. Other personal factors associated with an increased risk of falls include vision impairment, hearing problems, functional limitations, history of falls, and one's ability to perceive an impending fall [31–41].

Postural stability undergoes maturation from birth to about 10 years of age. After 25–30 years of age, body balance begins to deteriorate gradually [31]. A major determinant of postural instability in old age is the reduced attentional capacity and inability in the allocation of available resources to dampen sway. Reduced sensation, muscle weakness in the legs, and increased reaction time are important factors associated with aging and postural instability. The effects of age on postural control have been studied by previous researchers, and postural stability during upright standing has been shown to decrease with age [31]. When compared with younger adults (20–35 years old), older adults (60–75 years old) showed greater postural sway regardless of conditions, that is, with or without visual inputs [32]. No gender differences were found in several studies of postural stability during standing or mild perturbations [19,20]; however, when more challenging tasks are involved—such as those with visual and somatosensory inputs that are reduced or eliminated—the results indicated that elderly women showed greater impairments compared with elderly men [31]. Healthy elderly adults with no musculoskeletal or neurological disorders differ from healthy young adults in their responses to modest perturbations of upright stance; they tend to be unable to reduce small random perturbations as easily [34].

An analysis of the percentage increases in sway under conditions where visual and peripheral sensation systems are removed or diminished, compared with sway under optimal conditions, indicated that peripheral sensation is the most important sensory system in the maintenance of static postural stability [42]. A thorough understanding of falls requires the study of personal factors—such as the effect of age on a person's ability to maintain balance, postural adjustment capability due to sudden movement of body segments, and the perception of an impending fall—under various workloads, surface conditions, environmental lighting, and lack of availability of peripheral vision. Previous studies have shown an association between blocked peripheral vision and fall potential [32].

6.1.4.2 Environmental Factors

Loss of balance can also arise from various environmental hazards. Major environmental factors associated with an increased risk of workplace STF are those related to lighting, walking surface conditions [30], and the shoe–floor interfaces [21,27,29]. Examples of environmental factors are surface evenness, surface firmness, contaminants and/or obstacles on the floor, type of floor, shoe-sole material and tread, and shoe wear conditions.

Previous studies have shown that poor lighting along with obstruction of peripheral vision, which can be due to poor workplace layout, oversized material, or the use of PPE, can place the worker at the risk of a fall incident [35]. A clear view of the walkway and of any potential hazard is a necessity. Any lack of visual acuity due to poor lighting or poor contrast can lead to slips and falls [43]. Poor lighting detrimentally influences postural balance, especially in more demanding tasks, such as tasks involving reaching or bending [22].

Visual cues play an important role in postural stabilization. They are used in a feedback mode to control balance during standing and walking, or in an anticipatory mode to guide locomotion [44]. When working at heights without close visual references, the destabilizing effect is similar to that of eyes closed at ground level [13]. Other environmental factors are exposure to noise and organic solvents [45] and the surface conditions. Tasks being performed on conformable, narrow, sloped, or slippery surfaces challenge workers' balance control system, and workers often need to adopt different strategies to maintain postural balance [27]. An increase in the slope and height of the working surface increases postural sway synergistically [46].

6.1.4.3 Job-Task Factors

Job-task factors related to falls are those that involve tasks placing the human body's ability to maintain upright balance at risk. Examples are tasks that are physically demanding and tasks requiring the use of elevated devices such as ladders, scaffolds, or aerial lifts. Additional tasks/activities that may place workers at risk for falls include lifting a load, bending down to pick up an object from floor level, excessive arm reach, handling sudden loadings, and the use of PPE.

Physically demanding tasks cause perturbations to the body and trigger anticipatory postural adjustments [47] that actively initiate muscle adjustments when possible disturbances of balance are anticipated by the CNS [48]. When there is a discrepancy between the anticipation and perturbation, such as an overestimation of the weight to be lifted or the handling of sudden loadings, an unnecessarily high momentum of the body may disturb balance and lead to a fall [49]. Tasks performed on ladders are extremely challenging as the workers standing on the rung of a ladder have a limited base of support. Any perturbations may easily shift the body's center of mass outside the base of support, thus causing a fall incident. Manual material lifting such as lifting a sheet of drywall places great demands on the workers' postural control, especially when the drywall is lifted vertically [50]. Tasks involving excessive arm reach shift the body's center of mass forward and may require the body to take a step to reestablish balance. When the center of mass moves outside the base of support and workers are not able to take a step, such as on a ladder, a fall will occur. The use of bulky tools and PPE increases the demand for highly developed and flexible balance skills [12]. Specific items of protective equipment, such as footwear, clothing, eyewear, and respirators, can affect workers' postural balance [12].

6.1.5 Effect of PPE on Postural Stability and Dynamic Balance

6.1.5.1 Full-Face Respirator and Eyewear

While protective eyewear, respirators, masks, and head protectors can function as protective devices, they can affect workers' postural stability due to the restrictions they place on the wearers' peripheral vision. More importantly, the limitation in vision may further interact with other work conditions, such as workload and shift work. In a study of effects of respirators and workload, subjects wearing a respirator showed increases in postural sway length during demanding physical work, which were attributable to the work load-induced proprioceptive fatigue effect [51]. Self-contained breathing apparatus (SCBA) is the most significant piece of PPE negatively affecting functional balance [52].

Protective eyewear can cause deleterious effects on sensory input from the visual system, and compensatory strategies are usually enacted to maintain or regain postural stability [53]. Full-face respirators affected human cognitive performance negatively in an experiment conducted to compare three respirators—dust, mist, fume respirators, powered air-purifying respirators, and full-face respirators [53]. There is a potential for full-face, negative-pressure respirators to negatively affect jobs demanding high cognitive skills such as problem-solving and decision-making [54]. Workers who employ respirators, protective eyewear, and other face/head protection on a daily basis need to be aware of the effect of altered visual input resulting from PPE use on their postural stability, especially during sensory-challenging tasks, such as navigating ladders, roofs, uneven surfaces, scaffolding, and the elevated surfaces found in most construction work.

6.1.5.2 Protective Clothing and Ensemble

It has been well documented that personal protective clothing affects mobility in terms of the range of body motions defined by the maximum angular changes available at joints [55,56]. Such negative effects often impede work performance and may prolong the time required to perform hazardous tasks [55]. Furthermore, the reduction in lower extremity range of motions, such as knee and hip flexion/extension, may affect workers' abilities to negotiate obstacles or handle an impending fall/slip [57].

A previous study on military load carriage indicated that load bearing increased the stance time and step width used to provide stability to the body [58]. The impact of PPE weight on body movement is an issue that may affect workers' efficiency and create detrimental impacts on postural balance. In a study investigating the impact of body armor on lower body mobility, wearing an 18 lb ballistic outer tactical vest significantly increased knee flexion, foot plantar flexion, anterior pelvic tilt, stance phase, and the time required to establish stability during gait [59]. These changes reflect the increased demand of postural balance and energy expenditure, which can negatively affect soldiers' performance and increase injury risk. Subjects who wore heavier protective equipment contacted tall floor obstacles more frequently during locomotion, suggesting a greater risk of tripping [59]. Heavier equipment also resulted in greater forces by the trailing leg in both the anterior–posterior and vertical directions, suggesting greater risk of slipping [59].

Besides the reduction in mobility and increase in load bearing, the effect of PPE may interact with other task, environmental, or personal factors to create additional adverse impact on users. In a study of firefighters' postural stability, it was shown that prolonged work shifts may be an important contributor to the high prevalence of slips and falls among firefighters [60]. Postural sway variables showed negative/impaired differences in postural stability in workers wearing different levels of PPE required by the U.S. Environmental Protection Agency (EPA) while having fatigued muscle [35]. Level A protection is required when the greatest potential for exposure to hazards exists and when the greatest level of skin, respiratory, and eye protection is necessary [61]. Level B protection is required under circumstances demanding the highest level of respiratory protection, with a lesser level of skin protection [61]. The PPE Level B produced greater instability than PPE Level A when subjects were tested with eyes closed and standing on a four-inch foam. This result indicated that postural stability may be altered with PPE use and with fatigued postural muscles [35]. Wearing PPE negatively affects postural and functional balance, and the effects were more pronounced among older subjects (43–56 years old) than younger subjects (33–38 years old) [52].

6.1.5.3 Protective Footwear

Footwear can affect postural stability from many perspectives. Shoes act as a sensory interface between the foot and surface of support, and the modification of this interface may affect postural stability [62,63]. A number of shoe-design aspects have been shown to impact balance, including heel height, heel-collar height, sole hardness, heel, and the midsole geometry and slip resistance of the outer sole [64,65]. Studies have shown that shoes with thin hard soles provided better stability for men, while shoes with thick soft midsoles destabilized walking stability due to a decreased awareness of foot position [66,67]. An evaluation of midsole hardness on dynamic balance control during response to gait termination suggested that variations in midsole material impaired the dynamic balance control system [66]. Enhancing rear foot motion control and improving ankle proprioception were identified as two major shoe-design pathways for improving walking ability at elevations in a study of roofer footwear [62]. For public and outdoor workers, such as construction and service workers, studies have shown that slip-resistance properties were the top requirements by the users [68].

There have been numerous studies conducted to examine the impact of sports shoes on joint loadings, postures, performance, balance, and slip resistance [69–71]. A few articles on biomechanical evaluation of military boots were found [72,73]. Most of them emphasized the climatic comfort, flexibility, and energy absorption quality of shoes. Research specifically focused on protective footwear, especially properties or designs that are related to slips and trips, were scarce. Studies on sports footwear may not be generalizable to protective footwear for workers due to the inherent differences in the activities the wearers were involved in and the different design characteristics of protective footwear. A few studies were found to have examined the biomechanical and physiological effects of firefighter boots specifically [74,75]. The heavy weight of firefighter boots has been shown to significantly increase the physiological stresses of firefighters [76]. Significant differences were found in sway velocity between the pre- and posttest measures and among two different firefighter boots, suggesting that rubber firefighter boots elicit greater postural instability [77]. The slip resistance of firefighter boots for the different boot–surface interfaces firefighters may be exposed to, however, have not been studied in detail.

6.2 NIOSH Case Studies

6.2.1 Firefighter PPE

Firefighting is one of the most dangerous jobs in the United States, with the work-related injury rate exceeding those of most occupations [78]. In 2007, an estimated 80,100 firefighter injuries occurred in the line of duty, and fall-related injuries were the leading cause, accounting for 27.3% of total fire ground injuries [79]. In firefighting and rescuing operations, firefighters are exposed to varied, complex, and unpredictable conditions as well as a rapidly changing environment. They are constantly exposed to chemical and physical hazards, such as carbon monoxide, heat, and noise. They also frequently work on roofs, stairs, and ladders, and the walking surfaces are often cluttered or slippery due to the existence of debris, building materials, or contaminants.

6.2.1.1 Effect of Firefighter PPE on Risk of Tripping

In 2010, NIOSH conducted a study to evaluate the effect of firefighters' ensemble on their physiological and biomechanical responses during simulated firefighting tasks. One important objective for the study was to examine workers' mobility and their ability to negotiate obstacles while wearing a full turnout gear and different types of fire boots. Firefighters have traditionally worn heavily insulated rubberized boots as protective footwear, which can add 10 lb (4.4 kg) of extra weight to the body, significantly increasing energy expenditure and biomechanical stress such as joint loadings. There are two general types of certified (UL/SEI) structural firefighting boots in use today: 13″–16″ rubber bunker boots and 8″–16″ leather boots. Rubber boots are generally approximately 3lb (1.7 kg) heavier than leather boots, while leather boots are lighter but generally are more expensive than rubber boots. A 5%–12% increase in oxygen consumption per kilogram of weight added to the foot has been observed [80,81]; however, the increase may depend on gender, task, ankle-fit, and whether or not subjects are wearing additional protective clothing or equipment.

The objective of the NIOSH study was to investigate the effect of firefighter boot weight on firefighters' gait characteristics and risk of fall injuries while negotiating obstacles. Twelve healthy men (28.9 ± 5.0 years) and nine healthy women (35.3 ± 3.1 years), employed as professional firefighters and aged between 23 and 39 years, participated in the study. Four models of firefighter boots conforming to NFPA 1971 Standards for structural firefighting were selected for the study [82]. These boots were pull-up bunker boots that were commercially available. The four models of boots represented two models of leather boots, one model of leather/fabric hybrid boots, and one model of rubber boots. The boot characteristics are shown in Table 6.1. The sole flexibility was determined by the longitudinal stiffness of footwear testing based on the TM 194 procedures of the UK SATRA Technology Center [83].

The test protocol involved subjects walking along a 6.3m path and stepping over two 15 cm and two 30 cm obstacles. The participants, while wearing full turnout gear and randomly assigned boots, walked from one end of the walkway, stepping over four obstacles to travel to the other end. They then turned around and continued walking and crossing obstacles for five minutes at a mean speed of 0.57 m/s. The walking speed was paced using a metronome. A six-camera motion analysis system (Peak Motion Analysis System™, Vicon Inc., Centennial, CO) was used to collect 3-D marker trajectory data at 60 Hz and was low-pass filtered using a fourth-order Butterworth filter with a cutoff frequency of 6 Hz. Two 10 s sequences of kinematic data were collected during the 5-min walk, one in the beginning after 30 s of walking and the other during the last 30 s of walking. Each

TABLE 6.1

Boot Characteristics by Model

Boot Model	A	B	C	D
Upper material	Leather	Leather	Leather/fabric	Rubber
Sole flexibility[a]	More flexible	Less flexible	Less flexible	More flexible
Boot weight (men)	3.1 (0.1)	2.9 (0.1)	2.5 (0.1)	3.8 (0.1)
Boot weight (women)	2.5 (0.1)	2.4 (0.1)	2.0 (0.1)	3.3 (0.04)
Boot length (men)	31.2 (0.9)	31.2 (0.8)	30.9 (0.9)	30.7 (1.0)
Boot length (women)	27.1 (0.9)	27.0 (0.8)	26.5 (1.0)	26.8 (0.6)
Boot width (men)	10.8 (0.2)	10.1 (0.2)	10.6 (0.2)	11.1 (0.3)
Boot width (women)	9.6 (0.2)	9.0 (0.2)	9.6 (0.2)	10.1 (0.2)

Note: Standard deviations are shown in parenthesis. Boot weights are in kilograms and boot length and width are in centimeters.

[a] SATRA TM 194 Testing performed.

subject was allowed to select his or her preferred limb for leading over the obstacle. A total of eight reflective markers were placed on the subjects at the toe, heel, fifth metatarsal joint, and the ankle to monitor gait patterns and rear foot motions for both leading and trailing feet. Two markers were placed on the two ends of each obstacle to define its position in 3-D space. The obstacles were made of lightweight PVC pipes measuring 3.5 cm in diameter and one meter in length. They posed little to no risks of falls if contacted.

The motion data were analyzed from the toe-off of the trailing foot before stepping over the first obstacle to the heel strike of the trailing foot after crossing the second obstacle. Swing foot trajectories were assessed through the examination of crossing step length, toe–obstacle clearance, lead foot heel-strike distance, and trail foot approach distance. The cross step length was the distance from the trailing toe-off to the leading heel contact. Toe–obstacle clearance was defined as the vertical distance between the toe and the top of the obstacle at the instant when the toe was directly above the obstacle. The heel-strike distance was the distance from the lead heel to the obstacle, while the trailing foot approach distance was the distance from the trailing toe to the obstacle. During testing, it was observed that subjects tended to displace their crossing limb laterally when clearing the obstacle. Therefore, the lateral position of the lead foot was quantified, which is the horizontal position of the lead toe from the stance foot at the time it crossed over the obstacle.

Data from successful trials for which the subjects stepped over the obstacle without contacting the obstacle was included in the analysis. Of all 168 trials collected, 19 (11.3%) tripping incidents occurred. All tripping over obstacles occurred with the trailing foot. Repeated-measure analyses of variance (ANOVAs) were performed to test the effect of gender, boot weight, boot-sole flexibility, and time period (beginning vs. end of 5-min walk) on the temporal–distance variables. The effect of boot weight and time period was found to be significant on trailing foot toe–obstacle clearances for both high and low obstacles ($p < .02$). As the boot weight increased, the toe–obstacle clearances decreased. For each 1 kg increase in boot weight, there was a 2.8 cm decrease in toe–obstacle clearance for the taller obstacle. Subjects were able to maintain a toe–obstacle clearance of 23.5 cm in the beginning of the walk (Figure 6.1); however, the clearance was decreased to 21.9 cm near the end of the 5-min walk over the high obstacle ($p < .05$). In addition, significant differences were observed for lateral toe position by gender ($p < .01$) and time period ($p < .03$). On average, the lead toe was initially 42 cm to the right of the stance foot when crossing the high obstacle, but it was increased to 46 cm near the end of the walk. Women firefighters were found to displace the toe farther away from the stance foot than the men firefighters (Figure 6.1).

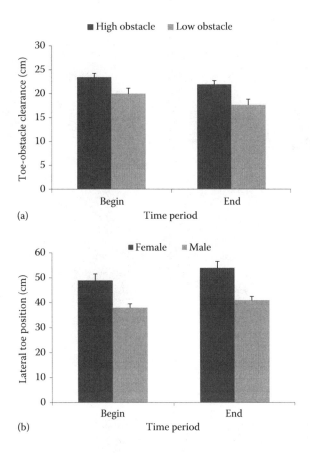

FIGURE 6.1
(a) Mean toe-obstacle clearance for two obstacles by time period and (b) mean lateral toe position by gender and time period.

In summary, successful navigation through the fire ground necessitates the effective avoidance of obstacles and securing adequate footing. In this study, the toe–obstacle clearances significantly decreased as boot weight and task time period increased. Insufficient toe–obstacle clearances often result in unsuccessful obstacle avoidance at the job site and may lead to tripping [84]. Results from this study indicated that boot weight and task time period affected firefighters' gait characteristics in negotiating obstacles. Subjects were more likely to trip over obstacles when wearing heavier boots and after walking for a period of time. Men and women firefighters adopted different kinematic strategies in negotiating obstacles. By swinging the foot outward, female subjects increased the toe height to help maintain toe clearance above the obstacle. Findings from this study may provide scientific evidence for firefighters and manufacturers in boot selection and design for preventing falls on the fire ground.

6.2.1.2 Slip Resistance Properties of Firefighter Boots

Previous studies have documented the evidence on the effect of PPE on firefighters' postural balance [85]. Firefighters are at an increased risk for STF injuries since they are exposed to extreme conditions such as high temperatures, wet surfaces, and strenuous tasks. Their working conditions are often varied and fast-changing. In many firefighting

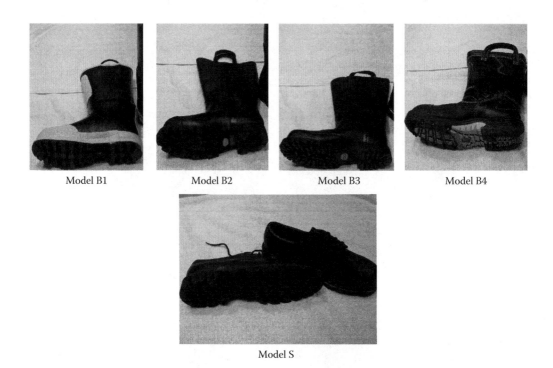

Model B1   Model B2   Model B3   Model B4

Model S

FIGURE 6.2
Four types of firefighter boots (B1–B4) and one type of safety shoe (S) tested in the study.

tasks, they are required to hastily ingress and egress from the fire truck while they are on the fire ground. Footwear plays an important in role in slip-and-fall prevention. Loss of foot traction between footwear and the work surface is considered as a major source of slip injuries [30]. In addition to the slip-resistant properties of the shoe sole itself, characteristics of shoe wear and tear can also affect the available coefficient of friction (COF) of the shoes [86].

In an NIOSH study of the slip resistant properties of firefighter boots, four pairs of NFPA certified firefighter boots and one pair of safety shoes (Figure 6.2) were tested using a Brungraber Mark II Slip Meter. The shoe soles were conditioned with fresh P400-grit abrasive paper prior to slip testing. The characteristics of the firefighter boots and safety shoes are provided in Table 6.2.

The slip resistance of firefighter boots as indicated by COF values on a wet surface ranged from 0.15 to 0.53. Boot model B1 was a pair of rubber boots with the lowest COF values. Boot model B3 exhibits the best slip resistance of all. The shoe sole samples were maintained in a controlled environment with a constant temperature of 21°C and relative humidity of 17% RH.

Figure 6.3 shows the COF results between each heel sample of footwear and stainless-steel plate abraded with 36-grit abrasive paper as a function of the number of trials. In general, the COF values of all tested footwear decreased as more trials were performed. This trend was consistent for both testing days. The decrease in COF values can be attributed to wear and tear due to repeated trials and/or a possible hydration phenomenon, in that shoe-sole material gradually saturated with fluid under wet conditions. Since firefighters consistently walk on wet surfaces, further research is needed to examine the changes in slip resistance due to wear and tear and surface contaminations.

TABLE 6.2

Shoe Sole Properties and Tread Characteristics

| Model | Hardness[a] | Surface[b] Roughness (Rz) | Tread Configuration (mm) | | | | COF[c] |
			Max. Width	Min. Width	Max. Depth	Min. Depth	
S	76.17	14.650	9.8	0.9	5.5	0.6	0.42
	(1.47)	(1.470)					
B1	69.25	15.795	8.6	3.4	5.7	2.2	0.15
	(0.97)	(2.885)					
B2	83.83	11.718	27.6	1.4	9	1.2	0.36
	(1.11)	(2.217)					
B3	75.58	19.270	10.1	3.3	7.1	1.6	0.53
	(2.78)	(3.374)					
B4	68.75	40.192	4.1	0.8	5.3	0.8	0.40
	(1.48)	(3.798)					

[a] Mean and (SD) of Shore A hardness measured by HPSA-M durometer (mm).
[b] Mean and (SD) of Surface Roughness Parameter Rz (μm) measured by Mitutoyo Surftest SJ301P.
[c] COF (Coefficient of Friction) measured by Brungraber Mark II on a wet stainless steel plate.

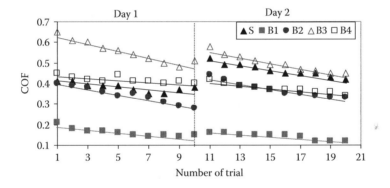

FIGURE 6.3
COF values between footwear sole samples and a wet stainless steel plate abraded with 36-grit abrasive paper measured on two different days.

6.3 First-Receiver PPE

According to OSHA's best-practices document for hospital-based first receivers, the minimum PPE needed to provide protection from a wide range of unknown hazards includes a powered air-purifying respirator (PAPR) (Figure 6.4), a double layer of protective gloves, chemical-protective boots, and a chemical-resistant suit (e.g., Tychem® or Tyvek®) with its openings sealed with tape [87]. A PAPR is a respirator composed of a headpiece or hood, breathing tube, filter, and battery-powered blower. The user wears the battery and the pump while it draws ambient air in through a filter and supplies it to the loose-fitting hood. The design of protective ensembles often focuses on the physical and mechanical properties of protective materials, with few considerations of usability [88]. The weight, the

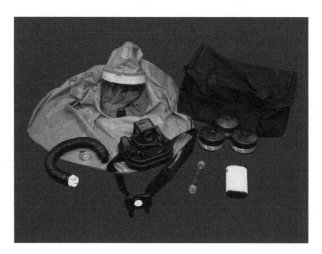

FIGURE 6.4
Example of first-receiver PAPR system.

bulk, and the corrugated breathing tube of the PAPR and the restrictive nature of the protective suit and gloves may immobilize first receivers to some extent, thus encumbering dexterity and limiting first receivers' effective emergency response. In addition, especially under mass-emergency conditions, triage, decontamination, and treatment operations could take place at outdoor facilities or outside hospitals in order to handle a large patient volume and to keep contaminated patients away from emergency departments [89]. Under those conditions, there is an ongoing concern about inclement weather, especially the thermal environment, which can affect operational tasks as well as affecting the ensemble conditions itself; physiological constraints can be magnified under these circumstances.

To date, quantified data on biomechanical, ergonomic, and physiological stresses imposed by the first-receiver ensemble have been limited. Performance criteria and test methods specific to the biomechanical and ergonomic stresses of wearing first-receiver gear have not been established. Little to no research has been conducted to evaluate the injury potential for overexertion and slips/trips/falls associated with the first-receiver protective ensemble among health-care workers performing job-specific tasks. Furthermore, scientific data for the effects of first-receiver PPE on performance for both male and female workers in a hot environment remains lacking.

Beginning in 2014, NIOSH undertook a study to evaluate the ergonomic and physiologic burden imposed on first receivers, wearing OSHA-recommended PPE, performing simulated decontamination and treatment tasks in the environmentally controlled Human Factors Laboratory. The test ensemble included a 3M Breathe Easy PAPR system, Ansell Sol-Vex gloves, Bata Hazmax boots, and a DuPont Tychem® CPF3 suit (model C3125T). The 3M Breathe Easy PAPR system is a motorized unit powered by a battery pack, which filters air surrounding the wearer through cartridges to provide respiratory protection. This system consists of a loose-fitting butyl rubber hood, a blower, a battery pack, a breathing tube, and cartridges. The system weighs approximately 4.0 kg, and it protects the wearer against CBRN hazards. The DuPont Tychem® CPF3 protective garment is composed of a multi-layer barrier that protects against a broad range of chemicals. The Bata Hazmax boots are 16in high with steel toes and slip-resistant soles; to assure an air-tight seal, boots are taped to the suit legs. The Ansell Sol-Vex gloves are made of chemical-resistant nitrile compound. They are worn over vinyl exam gloves and are taped to the Tychem® suit sleeves.

PPE enables workers to perform tasks in environments that are potentially hazardous, but it can negatively affect work productivity and expose those working in hazardous environments for a long period of time to hazardous substances. The bulky PPE ensemble can restrict mobility, limit effective emergency response, and increase risks for overexertion and STF injuries. The objective of this study was to quantify the barriers to the use of first-receiver ensembles by evaluating ergonomic and biomechanical stresses imposed on the wearers.

The restriction of body motions caused by the use of PPE may affect workers' ability to respond to perturbations arising from the work environment or job tasks. It may also affect workers' ability to react to an impending fall. Range of motion (ROM) is an important measure for workers wearing PPE as it is a way to assess worker mobility. In the NIOSH study of first receivers, ROM measurements were collected from 24 health-care workers (mean age: 31.2 ± 8.1 years) with at least 12 months of experience wearing surgical masks or N-95 (particulate-filtering facepiece) respirators. Measurements of ROM at the shoulders, elbows, trunks, hips, and knees in both sagittal and frontal planes were taken for each subject while wearing PPE or regular clothing (T-shirt and shorts) using a universal goniometer (Model 01135, Lafayette Instrument, Lafayette, IN). All measurements were taken using a universal goniometer by the same researcher to avoid any possible intertester reliability concerns.

Repeated-measure ANOVAs were performed to determine the effects of PPE and gender on 14 ROM variables. The effects of PPE and gender were significant on all ROM variables ($p < .01$) except for hip abduction and elbow flexion.

Figure 6.5 shows the percentage decrease in ROM due to the effect of PPE. The use of PPE had a significant effect on all movements. Subjects' ROM capabilities decreased consistently across all joints with PPE use. The most restricted areas were shoulders with more than 30% reduction in extension and 40% reduction in adduction. Frontal plane motions were more restricted than sagittal plane motions as indicated by more than 20% ROM reduction in hip abduction and trunk lateral flexion and more than 40% reduction in shoulder adduction.

To assess first receivers' dynamic stability, gait tests were conducted, which include normal walking and obstacle negotiation. The normal walking task required subjects to walk across a 12 m (40 ft) walkway with two embedded force plates. The subjects walked at a self-selected speed (e.g., natural cadence). They were required to step on the first force plate with their right foot (right foot heel strike), and take the subsequent step (left foot heel strike) on the second force plate. The gait starting position from the force plate was adjusted for each subject to achieve a right heel strike approximately at the center of the first force platform.

For obstacle negotiation trials, subjects walked at a self-selected pace along the same walkway used for the normal walk task, also stepping over an obstacle. The obstacle was placed in the middle of the walkway between two force plates. Prior to the experiment, the participants were given time to familiarize themselves with the walkway and the obstacle. A total of eight reflective markers were placed on the boots at the toe, heel, fifth metatarsal joint, and ankle for the monitoring of foot trajectories. The obstacle was either 15 cm or 30 cm in height. The obstacles were made of PVC pipes measuring 2.5 cm diameter and 1 m in length. The pipes were rigid but light, posing little to no risks of falls if contacted.

Of all 96 obstacle-crossing trials for which data was collected, 18 (18.8%) involved contacting or knocking down the obstacle, which were considered to constitute tripping incidents. Of all 18 tripping incidents, 16 (89%) occurred while negotiating a high obstacle, and 83% occurred when subjects were wearing PPE, possibly due to reduced

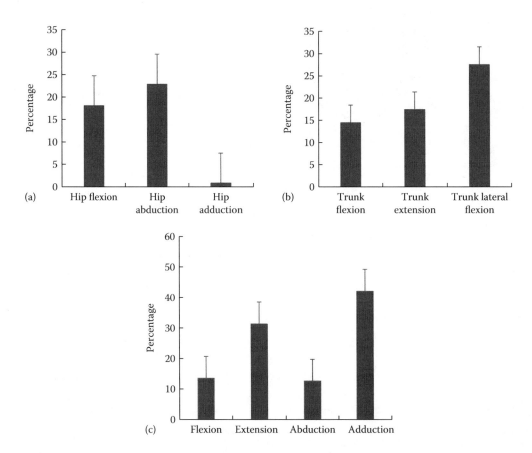

FIGURE 6.5
Percentage decrease in range of motion due to PPE at (a) hip, (b) trunk, and (c) shoulder joints.

hip and knee range of motion. All tripping over obstacles occurred with the trailing foot. This phenomenon can be attributed to the fact that neither the trailing foot nor the obstacle was within the subject's field of vision when the trailing foot was clearing the obstacle. In addition, the trailing foot was one step length closer to the obstacle than the toe of the leading limb. Thus, workers need to be advised that their trailing foot is more likely to trip on obstacles when wearing PPE. Subjects were able to negotiate a 6″ obstacle, but it was shown that they may trip over a 12″ obstacle while wearing first-receiver PPE.

With regard to gait characteristics, the effect of PPE was significant on step width ($p < .002$) and double stance time ($p < .001$) (Figure 6.6). First-receiver PPE affected health-care workers' gait stability as reflected in significant increases in step width and double stance time. While wearing PPE, the demand on postural stability was increased; therefore, workers needed to maintain a wider step width to increase their base of support. In addition, their foot contacted the ground for a longer period of time in each gait cycle to maintain balance from one step to another. Wearing first-receiver PPE significantly changed subjects' walking patterns and reduced ROMs at trunk, hips, and shoulders, which can negatively affect the free movement of the lower body, introduce more rapid fatigue, increase ankle injuries, and limit workers' ability to negotiate obstacles [90].

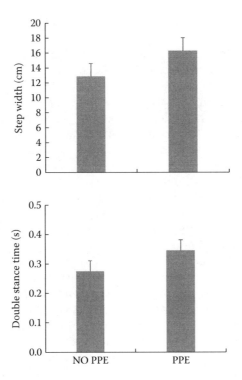

FIGURE 6.6
Effect of PPE on double stance time and step width.

6.4 Future Directions

In this chapter, basic aspects of PPE, postural stability, and motor control were presented, along with more comprehensive discussions of factors affecting postural balance and how PPE affects postural stability and dynamic balance. There are many directions in which research on effects of PPE on postural instability and fall risks described in the chapter could be extended.

A primary concern is the wide range in COF among the acceptable boots worn for firefighting tasks, as observed in the NIOSH case study. Research should focus on standardization of a slip tester and establish minimum required footwear COF criteria, so that firefighters are able to don firefighter boots with well-established characteristics and an acceptable safety profile. Firefighters may be required to adjust gait and stance according to environmental conditions on the fire ground, but footwear friction criteria would eliminate or reduce an additional variable. At a minimum, the establishment of a minimum COF and a standardized slip tester should be pursued, so that available boots should be roughly comparable in terms of the ability of footwear to produce comparable performance.

Similarly, safety-boot manufacturers should focus on weight reduction of their products, in the context of research that indicates a decrement in firefighters' ability to negotiate obstacles as a function of increases in time on the fire ground and the overall weight of boots.

It should also be recognized that heat stress and physiologic stress of various kinds can be increased among users of PPE. This is especially the case with first receivers within hospitals, who may be forced to perform critical tasks while subject to environmental stresses; and firefighters, who face increased dynamic, orientation, and communication tasks while on the fire ground.

Further, it should be recognized that the use of respirators carries a performance decrement, and this can be significant for certain types of industrial tasks. Currently, respirator use and selection is guided by NIOSH and OSHA requirements; however, it is not widely recognized that the use of certain items of protective equipment reduces the ability of the user to perform specific tasks, and further research could be undertaken to determine the manner in which ROM and limitations in perceptual ability and cognitive function, as well as related variables, can function to decrement task-specific performance. Future research should focus on performance speed and efficiency and the effect of time wearing PPE, time to complete tasks, or other measures on the performance decrement that is to be expected when a respirator is required.

Future research should also explore the impact of PPE bulkiness, peripheral field of view, weight, and weight distribution on both upper and lower extremity mobility and task performance. This is especially important for firefighters and first receivers who heavily reply on PPE for protection against hazards in unpredictable outdoor environments. Depending on the results of such studies, criteria and recommendations could be developed to improve the design of PPE. Evaluation of the slip resistance of protective footwear with the considerations of the walking surfaces for occupation-specific environments and tasks would provide important information for preventing falls due to loss of foot traction.

Causes of slips and falls are multidimensional, involving personal, environmental, and job-task factors. The prevention of fall injury due to PPE requires the evaluation of the contribution of individual PPE components (e.g., google, respirator, gown, footwear) to postural instability, as well as the impact of the ensemble as a whole. The contribution of PPE individually or collectively to common injury risks for traumatic injuries is intuitively apparent but not substantiated by sufficient research efforts. Efforts to incorporate biomechanical, tribological, anthropometric, and psychological findings into a systematic approach should be pursued to establish a better understanding of the pathways of fall injury and the resultant preventive strategies. Testing methods and performance criteria for various classes of protection defined by OSHA, ranging from maximal protection, Level A, to minimal protection, Level D, are needed. Further in-depth understanding in these areas will provide insights to improve PPE design and to develop intervention strategies to reduce STF.

6.5 Disclaimer

The findings and conclusions presented in the report are those of the authors and do not necessarily represent the views of National Institute for Occupational Safety and Health (NIOSH). Mention of any company names or products does not constitute endorsement by NIOSH.

In addition, citations to websites external to NIOSH do not constitute NIOSH endorsement of the sponsoring organizations or their programs or products. Furthermore, NIOSH is not responsible for the content of these websites. All web addresses referenced in this document were accessible as of the publication date.

References

1. OSHA 29 CFR 1926.134 Respiratory Protection. https://www.osha.gov/pls/oshaweb/owadisp. show_document?p_table=STANDARDS&p_id=12716.
2. National Institute for Occupational Safety and Health. *Worker Health Chartbook*. DHHS (NIOSH) publication no. 2004-146. Washington, DC: NIOSH, 2004.
3. National Institute for Occupational Safety and Health, Personal Protective Technology Program Portfolio. http://www.cdc.gov/niosh/programs/ppt/.
4. Tan, G. A. and Fitzgerald, M. C. Chemical-biological-radiological (CBR) response: A template for hospital emergency departments. *The Medical Journal of Australia*, 177, no. 4 (2002): 196–199.
5. OSHA Safety and Health Topic. https://www.osha.gov/SLTC/personalprotectiveequipment/
6. Adams, P. S. and Keyserling, W. M. The effect of size and fabric weight of protective coveralls on range of gross body motions. *American Industrial Hygiene Association* 56, no. 4 (1995): 333–340.
7. Krausman, A. S. and Nussbaum, N. A. Effects of wearing chemical protective clothing on text entry when using wearable input devices. *International Journal of Industrial Ergonomics*, 37, no. 6 (2007): 525–530.
8. Chiou, S. S., Turner, N., Zwiener, J., Weaver, D. L., and Haskell W. E. Effect of boot weight and sole flexibility on gait and physiological responses of firefighters in stepping over obstacles. *Human Factors: The Journal of the Human Factors and Ergonomics Society*, 54, no. 3 (2012): 373–386.
9. OSHA 29 CFR 1910 Subpart D, Walking-working surfaces. https://www.osha.gov/SLTC/walkingworkingsurfaces/standards.html.
10. Bureau of Labor Statistics. Nonfatal occupational injuries and illnesses requiring days away from work, 2014. http://www.bls.gov/news.release/pdf/osh2.pdf.
11. Kong, P. W., Suyama, J., and Hostler, D. A review of risk factors of accidental slips, trips, and falls among firefighters. *Safety Science*, 60 (2013): 203–209.
12. Hsiao, H. and Simeonov, P. Preventing falls from roofs: A critical review. *Ergonomics*, 44, no. 5 (2001): 537–561.
13. Kim, I., Hsiao, H., and Simeonov, P. Functional levels of floor surface roughness for the prevention of slips and falls: Clean-and-dry and soapsuds-covered wet surfaces. *Applied Ergonomics*, 44, no. 1 (2013): 58–64.
14. Simeonov, P. and Hsiao, H. Height, surface firmness, and visual reference effects on balance control. *Injury Prevention*, 7, no. suppl 1 (2001): i50–i53.
15. Rubenstein, L. Z. Falls in older people: Epidemiology, risk factors and strategies for prevention. *Age and Ageing*, 35, no. suppl 2 (2006): ii37–ii41.
16. Leamon, T. B. and Murphy, P. L. Occupational slips and falls: More than a trivial problem. *Ergonomics*, 38, no. 3 (1995): 487–498.
17. Sainburg, R. L., Poizner, H., and Ghez, C. Loss of proprioception produces deficits in interjoint coordination. *Journal of Neurophysiology*, 70, no. 5 (1993): 2136–2147.
18. Nashner, L. M. Adapting reflexes controlling the human posture. *Experimental Brain Research*, 26, no. 1 (1976): 59–72.
19. Winter, D. A. *Biomechanics and Motor Control of Human Movement*. Waterloo, Ontario, Canada: University of Waterloo Press, 1991.
20. Bhatt, T., Wening, J. D., and Pai, Y. C. Adaptive control of gait stability in reducing slip-related backward loss of balance. *Experimental Brain Research*, 170 (2006): 61–73.
21. Chiou, S., Bhattacharya, A., and Succop, P. A. Evaluation of workers' perceived sense of slip and effect of prior knowledge of slipperiness during task performance on slippery surfaces. *American Industrial Hygiene Association Journal*, 61 (2000): 492–500.
22. Redfern, M. S., Cham, R., Gielo-Perczak, K., Gronqvist, R., Hirvonen, M., Lanshammar, H., Marpet, M., Pai, C. Y., and Powers, C. Biomechanics of slips. *Ergonomics*, 44 (2001): 1138–1166.

23. Nasher, L. M. Balance adjustments of human perturbed while walking. *Neurophysiology*, 44 (1980): 650–664.

24. Nasher, L. M. Adaptation of human movement to altered environments. *Trends in Neurosciences*, 5 (1982): 358–361.

25. Winter, D. A. Energy generation and absorption at the ankle and knee during fast, natural, and slow cadences. *Clinical Orthopaedics and Related Research*, 175 (1983): 147–154.

26. Winter, D. A. Foot trajectory in human gait: A precise and multifactorial motor control task. *Physical Therapy*, 72 (1992): 45–53.

27. Cham, R. and Redfern, M. S. Heel contact dynamics during slip events on level and inclined surfaces. *Safety Science*, 40, no. 7–8 (2002): 559–576.

28. Tang, P. F., Woollacott, M. H., and Chong, R. K. Control of reactive balance adjustments in perturbed human walking: Roles of proximal and distal postural muscle activity. *Experimental Brain Research*, 119 (1998): 141–152.

29. Llewellyn, M. G. A., and Nevola, V. R. Strategies for walking on low-friction surfaces. In Lotens, W. A., and Havenith, G. (Eds.), *Proceedings of the Fifth International Conference on Environmental Ergonomics*. Masstricht, The Netherlands, pp. 156–157, 1992.

30. Grönqvist, R., Abeysekera, J., Gard, G., Hsiang, S. M., Leamon, T. B., Newman, D. J., and Pai IV, C. Y. C. Human-centred approaches in slipperiness measurement. *Ergonomics*, 44, no. 13 (2001): 1167–1199.

31. Wolfson, L., Whipple, R., Derby, C. A., Amerman, P., and Nashner, L. Gender differences in the balance of healthy elderly as demonstrated by dynamic posturography. *Journal of Gerontology*, 49, no. 4 (1994): M160–M167.

32. Hageman, P. A., Leibowitz, J. M., and Blanke, D. Age and gender effects on postural control measures. *Archives of Physical Medicine and Rehabilitation*, 76, no. 10 (1995): 961–965.

33. Maki, B. E. Aging and postural control: A comparison of spontaneous and induced sway tests. *Journal of the American Geriatrics Society*, 38 (1991): 1–9.

34. Gu, M. J., Schultz, A. B., Shepard, N. T., and Alexander, N. B. Postural control in young and elderly adults when stance is perturbed: Dynamics. *Journal of Biomechanics*, 29, no. 3 (1996): 319–329.

35. Kincl, L. D., Bhattacharya, A., Succop, P. A., and Clark, C. S. Postural sway measurements: A potential safety monitoring technique for workers wearing personal protective equipment. *Applied Occupational and Environmental Hygiene*, 17, no. 4 (2002): 256–266.

36. Hue, O., Simoneau, M., Marcotte, J., Berrigan, F., Doré, J., Marceau, P., Marceau, S., Tremblay, A., and Teasdale, N. Body weight is a strong predictor of postural stability. *Gait and Posture*, 26, no. 1 (2007): 32–38.

37. Skelton, D. A. Effects of physical activity on postural stability. *Age and Ageing*, 30 (2001): 33–40.

38. Lord, S. R., Clark, R. D., and Webster, I. W. Postural stability and associated physiological factors in a population of aged persons. *Journal of Gerontology*, 46, no. 3 (1991): M69–M76.

39. Juntunen, J., Ylikoski, J., Ojala, M., Matikainen, E., Ylikoski, M., and Vaheri, E. Postural body sway and exposure to high-energy impulse noise. *The Lancet*, 330, no. 8553 (1987): 261–264.

40. Chiou, S., Bhattacharya, B., Lai, C., and Succop, P. A. Effects of environmental and task risk factors on workers' perceived sense of postural sway and instability. *Occupational Ergonomics*, 1, no. 2 (1998): 81–93.

41. Lord, S. R. and Menz, H. B. Visual contributions to postural stability in older adults. *Gerontology* 46, no. 6 (2000): 306–310.

42. Bhattacharya, A., Morgan, R., Shukla, R., Ramakrishanan, H. K., and Wang, L. Non-invasive estimation of afferent inputs for postural stability under low levels of alcohol. *Annals of Biomedical Engineering*, 15, no. 6 (1987): 533–550.

43. Brooke-Wavell, K., Perrett, L. K., Howarth, P. A., and Haslam, R. A. Influence of the visual environment on the postural stability in healthy older women. *Gerontology*, 48, no. 5 (2002): 293–297.

44. Patla, A. E. Understanding the roles of vision in the control of human locomotion. *Gait and Posture*, 5, no. 1 (1997): 54–69.

45. Smith, L. B., Bhattacharya, A., Lemasters, G., Succop, P., Puhala, I. I. E., Medvedovic, M., and Joyce, J. Effect of chronic low-level exposure to jet fuel on postural balance of US Air Force personnel. *Journal of Occupational and Environmental Medicine,* 39, no. 7 (1997): 623–632.

46. Bhattacharya, A., Succop, P., Kincl, L., Lu, M. L., and Bagchee, A. Postural stability during task performance on elevated and/or inclined surfaces. *Occupational Ergonomics,* 3, no. 2 (2003): 83–97.

47. Patla, A. E., Ishac, M. G., and Winter, D. A. Anticipatory control of center of mass and joint stability during voluntary arm movement from a standing posture: Interplay between active and passive control. *Experimental Brain Research,* 143, no. 3 (2002): 318–327.

48. Zettel, J. L., McIlroy, W. E., and Maki, B. E. Environmental constraints on foot trajectory reveal the capacity for modulation of anticipatory postural adjustments during rapid triggered stepping reactions. *Experimental Brain Research,* 146, no. 1 (2002): 38–47.

49. Commissaris, D., ACM, and Toussaint, H. M. Anticipatory postural adjustments in a bimanual, whole body lifting task with an object of known weight. *Human Movement Science,* 16, no. 4 (1997): 407–431.

50. Pan, C. S., Chiou, S., and Hendricks, S. The effect of drywall lifting method on workers' balance in a laboratory-based simulation. *Occupational Ergonomics,* 3, no. 4 (2003): 235–249.

51. Seliga, R., Bhattacharya, A., Succop, P., Wickstrom, R., Smith, D., and Willeke, K. Effect of work loan and respirator wear on postural stability, heart rate, and perceived exertion. *The American Industrial Hygiene Association Journal,* 52, no. 10 (1991): 417–422.

52. Punakallio, A., Lusa, S., and Luukkonen, R. Protective equipment affects balance abilities differently in younger and older firefighters. *Aviation, Space, and Environmental Medicine,* 74, no. 11 (2003): 1151–1156.

53. Wade, L., Weimar, W., and Davis, J. Effect of personal protective eyewear on postural stability. *Ergonomics,* 47, no. 15 (2004): 1614–1623.

54. AlGhamri, A. A., Murray, S. L., and Samaranayake, V. A. The effects of wearing respirators on human fine motor, visual, and cognitive performance. *Ergonomics,* 56, no. 5 (2013): 791–802.

55. Adams, P. S. and Keyserling, W. M. The effect of size and fabric weight of protective coveralls on range of gross body motions. *American Industrial Hygiene Association,* 56, no. 4 (1995): 333–340.

56. Huck, J. Protective clothing systems: A technique for evaluating restriction of wearer mobility. *Applied Ergonomics,* 19, no. 3 (1988): 185–190.

57. Chiou, S. S., Turner, N., Zwiener, J., Weaver, D. L., and Haskell, W. E. Effect of boot weight and sole flexibility on gait and physiological responses of firefighters in stepping over obstacles. *Human Factors: The Journal of the Human Factors and Ergonomics Society,* 54, no. 3 (2012): 373–386.

58. Birrell, S. A. and Haslam, R. A. The effect of load distribution within military load carriage systems on the kinetics of human gait. *Applied Ergonomics,* 41, no. 4 (2010): 585–590.

59. Park, H., Nolli, G., Branson, D., Peksoz, S., Petrova, A., and Goad, C. Impact of wearing body armor on lower body mobility. *Clothing and Textiles Research Journal,* 29, no. 3 (2011): 232–247.

60. Sobeih, T. M., Davis, K. G., Succop, P. A., Jetter, W. A., and Bhattacharya, B. Postural balance changes in on-duty firefighters: Effect of gear and long work shifts. *Journal of Occupational and Environmental Medicine,* 48, no. 1 (2006): 68–75.

61. U.S. EPA [2016]. Personal protective equipment. www.epa.gov/emergency-response/personal-protective-equipment.

62. Simeonov, P., Hsiao, H., Powers, J., Ammons, D., Amendola, A., Kau, T., and Cantis, D. Footwear effects on walking balance at elevation. *Ergonomics,* 51, no. 12 (2008): 1885–1905.

63. Menz, H. B. and Lord, S. R. Footwear and postural stability in older people. *Journal of the American Podiatric Medical Association,* 89, no. 7 (1999): 346–357.

64. Menant, J. C., Steele, J. R., Menz, H. B., Munro, B. J., and Lord, S. R. Optimizing footwear for older people at risk of falls. *Journal of Rehabilitation Research and Development,* 45, no. 8 (2008): 1167–1181.

65. Lord, S. R., Bashford, G. M., Howland, A., and Munro, B. J. Effects of shoe collar height and sole hardness on balance in older women. *Journal of the American Geriatrics Society*, 47, no. 6 (1999): 681–684.

66. Robbins, S., Waked, E., Gouw, G. J., and McClaran, J. Athletic footwear affects balance in men. *British Journal of Sports Medicine*, 28, no. 2 (1994): 117–122.

67. Robbins, S. and McClaran, J. Effect of footwear midsole hardness and thickness on proprioception and stability in older men. In *Biomedical Engineering Conference, 1995: Proceedings of the 1995 Fourteenth Southern*, Shreveport, LA. p. 166. IEEE, 1995.

68. Gao, C., Holmér, I., and Abeysekera, J. Slips and falls in a cold climate: Underfoot surface, footwear design and worker preferences for preventive measures. *Applied Ergonomics*, 39, no. 3 (2008): 385–391.

69. Frederick, E. C. Optimal frictional properties for sport shoes and sport surfaces. *ISBS-Conference Proceedings Archive* 1, no. 1 (1993).

70. Majid, F. and Bader, D. L. A biomechanical analysis of the plantar surface of soccer shoes. *Proceedings of the Institution of Mechanical Engineers, Part H: Journal of Engineering in Medicine*, 207, no. 2 (1993): 93–101.

71. Bergmann, G., Kniggendorf, H., Graichen, F., and Rohlmann, A. Influence of shoes and heel strike on the loading of the hip joint. *Journal of Biomechanics*, 28, no. 7 (1995): 817–827.

72. DeMoya, R. G. A biomechanical comparison of the running shoe and the combat boot. *Military Medicine*, 147, no. 5 (1982): 380.

73. Rosenblad-Wallin, E., FS. The design and evaluation of military footwear based upon the concept of healthy feet and user requirement studies. *Ergonomics*, 31, no. 9 (1988): 1245–1263.

74. Neeves, R., Barlow, D., Richards, J., Provost-Craig, M., and Castagno, P. *Physiological and Biomechanical Changes in Firefighters due to Boot Design Modifications. Final Report*. International Association of Firefighters and the Federal Emergency Management Association, August, 1989.

75. Smolander, J., Louhevaara, V., Hakola, T., Ahonen, E., and Klen, T. Cardiorespiratory strain during walking in snow with boots of differing weights. *Ergonomics*, 32, no. 1 (1989): 3–13.

76. Turner, N. L., Chiou, S., Zwiener, J., Weaver, D., and Spahr, J. Physiological effects of boot weight and design on men and women firefighters. *Journal of Occupational and Environmental Hygiene*, 7, no. 8 (2010): 477–482.

77. Garner, J. C., Wade, C., Garten, R., Chander, H., and Acevedo, E. The influence of firefighter boot type on balance. *International Journal of Industrial Ergonomics*, 43, no. 1 (2013): 77–81.

78. Walton, S. M., Conrad, K. M., Furner, S. E., and Samo, D. G. Cause, type, and workers' compensation costs of injury to fire fighters. *American Journal of Industrial Medicine*, 43, no. 4 (2003): 454–458.

79. Karter, M. J. and Molis, J. L. *US Firefighter Injuries 2008*. Quincy, MA: National Fire Protection Association, 2009.

80. Jones, B. H., Toner, M. M., Daniels, W. L., and Knapik, J. J. The energy cost and heart-rate response of trained and untrained subjects walking and running in shoes and boots. *Ergonomics*, 27, no. 8 (1984): 895–902.

81. Knapik, J. J., Reynolds, K. L., and Harman, E. Soldier load carriage: Historical, physiological, biomechanical, and medical aspects. *Military Medicine*, 169, no. 1 (2004): 45.

82. National Fire Protection Association. *NFPA 1971 Standard on Protective Ensemble for Structural Fire Fighting*, 2000 Edition. Quincy, MA: National Fire Protection Association, 2000.

83. SATRA Technology, SATRA's Dynamic Footwear Stiffness Test machine. https://www.satra.co.uk/bulletin/article_view.php?id=754.

84. Krell, J. and Patla, A. E. The influence of multiple obstacles in the travel path on avoidance strategy. *Gait and Posture*, 16 (2002): 15–19.

85. Punakallio, A., Lusa, S., and Luukkonen, R. Functional, postural and perceived balance for predicting the work ability of firefighters. *International Archives of Occupational and Environmental Health*, 77, no. 7 (2004): 482–490.

86. Chiou, S., Bhattacharya, A., and Succop, P. A. Effect of workers' shoe wear on objective and subjective assessment of slipperiness. *American Industrial Hygiene Association Journal*, 57, no. 9 (1996): 825–831.
87. Occupational Safety and Health Administration. *OSHA Best Practices for Hospital-Based First Receivers of Victims from Mass Casualty Incidents Involving the Release of Hazardous Substances.* Washington, DC: The Administration, 2005.
88. Ziegler, J. P. FAQs & fables about protective clothing. *Occupational Health and Safety (Waco, Tex.),* 69, no. 7 (2000): 42.
89. Schultz, C. H., Mothershead, J. L., and Field, M. Bioterrorism preparedness: I: The emergency department and hospital. *Emergency Medicine Clinics of North America*, 20, no. 2 (2002): 437–455.
90. Chiou, S., Zwiener, J., Powers, J., Hause, M., Ronaghi, M., and Weaver, D. Effect of first receiver protective ensemble on range of motion and postural balance. National Occupational Injury Research Symposium, May 19–21, 2015, Kingwood, WV.

7

Suspension Tolerance Time and Risk after a Fall

Anil Adisesh

CONTENTS

ABSTRACT   A fall into harness suspension has been considered a life-threatening emergency due to the risk of loss of consciousness in harness suspension. This chapter introduces the history of these concerns and reviews the experimental evidence from human studies. It moves on to look at the pathophysiologic mechanisms that operate, appropriate management by first responders, and preventive measures.

KEY WORDS: *motionless, orthostasis, pathophysiology, presyncope, suspension, syncope.*

7.1 Introduction

Falls into suspension may occur in work, leisure, or home activities at height above ground or when below ground from one level to another lower level. To become suspended, the victim will have either purposefully worn a protective harness, tied themselves into a rope, or become entangled in some material that is preventing a completed fall. In considering the possible effects of a fall resulting in suspension, it is first necessary to understand the context, the antecedent events, and the personal factors of the individual suspended.

In a work situation, it may be reasonable to expect that some planning has gone into the conduct of the work task, involving selection of appropriate access equipment, personal protective equipment including a harness, and trained personnel. In a leisure or home activity, for example, rock climbing or home roof repairs, there may be more variability in any of these factors. In addition, there are environmental circumstances, such as the weather conditions for outdoor activities that may affect both the likelihood of a fall and the medical outcome.

A fall into harness suspension has been noted as a potentially serious hazard by the United States Occupational Safety & Health Administration in a bulletin on suspension trauma/orthostatic intolerance.[1] The term *orthostatic intolerance* refers to the ability of a person to maintain an upright posture (orthostasis) and the period for which this can be endured. The classical example of an inability to tolerate prolonged standing is that of soldiers standing to attention, particularly on a warm day, and then fainting. This uncontrollable fainting is the result of the pooling of blood in the legs while relatively motionless. In an effort to avoid this somewhat embarrassing eventuality, soldiers are often advised to gently rock forward and backward, since rising on the toes will activate the calf muscles, assisting blood return to the heart. *Suspension trauma* is an unfortunate term that is best avoided. Despite its common use, trauma does not have to occur, although suspension, usually in a harness, is a required feature. This term appears to have been first introduced by Petermeyer and Unterhalt in their 1997 publication entitled *Das Hängetrauma* (suspension trauma).[2] In this report, they note that "simply being suspended from a rope without even suffering a fall or trauma" may be sufficient cause for syncope. They then go on to attribute certain pathophysiologic changes to this situation, which they maintain to be specific to suspension. This author prefers the term *suspension syncope*, with *syncope* meaning a sudden loss of consciousness and postural tone, which is typically reversible if the horizontal posture follows, as happens in the example given of a soldier on parade.

7.2 Historical Aspects

The history of suspension syncope includes crucifixion, in which victims may endure the torture for several hours to days.[3] It was considered a kindness to perform "crurifragium" or fracturing of the lower legs just below the knees. This practice would prevent the victim from supporting themselves upright and cause a slumping posture, thereby hampering breathing, and with blood loss at the fracture site contributing to syncope and death.[3] However, the problem of syncope and death in rope and harness suspension was brought to wider attention following the 1972 Second International Conference of Mountain Rescue Doctors,[4,5] in which one section dealt with "Falls into the rope." It is clear from these reports that head-up suspension in mountaineering or caving has led to fatalities; however, the causality was not always well defined due to the nature of the circumstances, often in remote locations and sometimes with lone individuals. The types of harness varied, but most of the injuries and fatalities occurred while using a simple rope-tied chest harness. Factors such as exhaustion, hypothermia, injuries from falling, injuries from ill-fitting harnesses, and restriction of respiration by the chest harness would have contributed to death by making motionless suspension more likely, with suspension syncope then supervening. Once syncope has occurred, the victim will succumb either to airway obstruction or to profound loss of blood pressure, leading to death if not rescued. Such self-tied rope harnesses are now perhaps only to be encountered in nonwork situations, and then under improvisation.

The type of harness and its fit for the individual user are also factors affecting tolerance when in suspension, either motionless or not. Simple tied rope harnesses around the thorax are not well tolerated and are associated with pain, paralysis, and swelling of the arms from compression of the upper chest and axillae.[5] From the post-injury and postmortem findings described by Flora and Holzl as well as others, it appears that the venous blood return from the upper torso is impaired, causing facial suffusion, swelling, and likely respiratory difficulty from direct mechanical compression.[5]

7.3 Experimental Evidence

French studies in the early 1980s arose from some incidents of falls into harness suspension by stuntmen, particularly when using a light thoracic harness.[6] A series of investigations used five subjects, each testing three full body harnesses in motionless suspension: a parachute harness, a thoracic belt, and a waist belt with shoulder straps were also tested by some subjects. The thoracic and waist belts were not tolerated by any of the three tested subjects for more than 2 min due to pain and nausea with compression. The full body harnesses were better tolerated; however, even then, the shortest suspension duration for each harness was less than half of the longest period endured. The reasons for termination included pain in the arms, legs, and chest; numbness of the arms; abdominal compression; chest compression; nausea; dizziness; and in one case, heart rhythm changes. Perhaps notably, this was in the subject suspended for the longest time: 43 min.

Orzech et al.[7] describe studies from their laboratory in 1968 with five subjects suspended in a parachute harness. While four subjects tolerated the protocol, one subject lost consciousness at 28 min, but recovered 2 min after being lowered down. Studies by Orzech et al. in 1987[7] evaluated three types of fall-protection harnesses. They tested a body belt, a chest harness, and a full body harness with 13 subjects undergoing motionless suspension. There was a clear order of preference for the harness types, with the full body harness, then the chest harness, being better tolerated than the body belt. However, there was one case of syncope, and this occurred during use of the full body harness after only 6 min of suspension, emphasizing the importance of individual factors as well as harness type. This subject recovered by lying supine and had an unconscious period of 30 sec. It was noted that this subject had bradycardia prior to the collapse, and that this normalized after 20 sec. Among their conclusions were the concerns that a body belt is likely to cause internal injury during fall arrest, and the chest harness restricts breathing and causes pressure on the axillae, while the full body harness is superior, as it tends to distribute the load over the body.

A study of harness suspension[8] was commissioned by the German Federal Post Office following a fatal accident, although the details of this event are not reported, so harness suspension can only be supposed to have been a possible contributory factor. Fifteen subjects participated in two scenarios of motionless suspension, one free hanging from a platform and the other hanging from a ladder. The subjects completed a number of maneuvers to simulate working in the harnesses prior to being placed in motionless suspension. Three full body harnesses were tested and appear to have had both front and rear attachment points for suspension, the rear point being used for the platform hang test and the front for the ladder hang test. Monitoring of electrocardiogram, breathing, blood pressure, and thigh circumference was performed using instrumentation. There was no difference between the three types of harness, but the ladder hang was tolerated for a median of 9 min and 47 sec, compared with 26 min and 3 sec for the free hang from a platform. The criteria for stopping the test were unbearable pain, orthostasis symptoms or signs, and orthostasis indicated by physiological measurements. The numbers stopping by indication for test termination are not given in the available data; however, the authors performed multinomial regression analyses to derive prediction equations (Equations 7.1 and 7.2):

Front suspension duration (TL) hanging from a ladder[8]

$$TL = (2.97 \times \text{body weight}) + (-0.86 \times \text{body height}) + (-1.47 \times \text{shoulder width})$$
$$+ (-0.22 \times \text{body depth}) + (0.49 \times \text{hip width}) + (-0.40 \times \text{upper thigh circumference})$$
$$+ (-1.86 \times \text{stomach girth}) + (0.46 \times \text{torso length})$$

$$(7.1)$$

Rear suspension duration (TF) free hanging from a platform[8]

$$TF = (3.55 \times \text{body weight}) + (-1.44 \times \text{body height}) + (-1.74 \times \text{shoulder width})$$
$$+ (-0.61 \times \text{body depth}) + (0.57 \times \text{hip width}) + (-0.54 \times \text{upper thigh circumference})$$
$$+ (-0.96 \times \text{stomach girth}) + (0.55 \times \text{torso length})$$

$$(7.2)$$

This approach seems useful, although the data set is limited and only included three females, so the influence of gender difference is uncertain, despite no significant findings being reported. Body weight, body height, shoulder width, and stomach girth are the most influential factors on suspension tolerance from these findings. Figure 7.1 shows the important factors. Other authors do not seem to have employed similar anthropometric analysis, and it should probably be encouraged to assist harness design. Body fat composition might be easily included in future studies with the advent of electrical impedance devices. It might also be considered that any change in blood pressure from supine to standing may be a useful baseline measure, although not mentioned in previous papers.

Roeggla and colleagues[9] were interested in looking at the effects of suspension in a chest harness and a sit harness, such as may be used in rock climbing. They had six subjects use both harness types in a random order with motionless suspension for 3 min and took

> Constriction of the chest and respiratory movements
> Head-up tilt angle
> Vertical dependency of lower limbs
> Motionless suspension
> Duration of suspension
> Discomfort from harness compression
> Harness fit
> Harness attachment point position
> Body weight
> Body height
> Shoulder width
> Abdominal girth
> Environmental conditions
> Medication/drugs
> Alcohol
> Co-morbid medical conditions

FIGURE 7.1
Factors known or likely to be associated with suspension syncope.

measurements of blood pressure, cardiac output, respiratory function, oxygen saturation, and carbon dioxide retention prior to and during testing. They found that the chest harness caused impairment of all measured variables other than oxygenation, but there were no changes with the sit harness. These findings would be compatible with mechanical embarrassment of respiration caused by the chest harness. This would reduce carbon dioxide clearance, as was evidenced by the reduced lung volumes measured in suspension; also, reduced chest expansion and increased intrathoracic pressure would impair blood return to the right ventricle, contributing to the lower cardiac output. The heart rate in chest harness suspension decreased, which is in contrast to other reports of an initial tachycardia, although the latter finding was present for the sit harness.

A case of death apparently from suspension in a chest strop was described in a paper by Madsen et al.[10] They described a 25-year-old otherwise fit soldier who was asked to simulate hanging in a chest strop suspended from a wall. He became unconscious after 6 min of not being observed, and despite initial successful cardiac resuscitation, he remained unconscious and died. The authors go on to describe their studies to define the limits of normal tolerance of head-up tilt. They used a cardiac tilt table, which can be tipped upright to a varying angle and allows body weight to be supported on a bicycle seat leaving the legs dependent, with 79 subjects, of whom 15 were female. Invasive and noninvasive cardiovascular measurements were made during tilt testing. With tilt to 50°, 69 of 79 subjects (87%) experienced presyncope in head-up tilt. However, three of the 79 subjects withdrew due to discomfort, meaning that 91% of the subjects remaining had presyncope. Notably, six subjects (8%) had presyncope within 5 min, 17 (22%) within 10 min, and 50% within 27 min. Only seven subjects (9%) completed the planned 1 h of tilting without presyncope. The Kaplan–Meier survival curve for head-up tilt showed an almost linear decrease with time, emphasizing the dependence on duration of motionless suspension. The heart rate changes observed were consistent with other reports showing an initial tachycardia with normal blood pressure and, with the onset of presyncope, a bradycardia associated with low blood pressure. In a further experiment, the same authors went on to examine the effect of being suspended in a double strop: one chest strop and one under the knees to raise the legs. Nine subjects, one female, undertook the study with the same monitoring as for the tilt test. The eight male subjects completed the 1 h suspension without presyncope. The female subject tolerated 50 min in the double strop but had only managed 5 min in the head-up tilt test. These maneuvers allowed the investigators to conclude that the main effect of head-up suspension is a depletion of central blood volume, resulting in bradycardia and low blood pressure. The cosine of the head-up tilt angle relates to the orthostatic stress experienced, which is maximal at the vertical.

A study conducted by the National Institute for Occupational Safety and Health (NIOSH)[11] set out to investigate whether a self-deploying harness accessory to elevate the subjects' legs after fall arrest would improve suspension tolerance. The device was used with a back attachment point harness and elevated the legs into much the same posture as Madsen's study had employed with a double strop. The comparison was against each of a front and back attachment point harness alone. The study included 22 men and 18 women, allowing gender differences to be assessed. Prior to suspension, it was noted that the harnesses did not fit women as well as they did men. Forty percent of women studied had a poor harness fit and the remainder a fair fit, whereas 48% of men had a fair fit, with the remainder having a good fit. Perhaps significantly, all the male subjects and 14 women had construction experience, therefore being authentic subjects. The authors performed Kaplan–Meier survival analysis, which showed that 5% of subjects had reached their tolerance by 7 min for the front attachment point and by 11 min for the back attachment point.

This short time period has implications for the rescue of workers who are, or become, motionless in harness suspension.

7.4 Mechanism of Onset

Motionless suspension leads to syncope because of loss of cerebral perfusion, meaning that the conscious state can no longer be maintained. The precipitating event is a fall in blood pressure. Since blood pressure is the product of cardiac output and the total peripheral resistance of the peripheral blood vessels, anything that reduces either factor can lead to reduced blood pressure. The underlying pathophysiology of suspension syncope principally relates to the gravitational dependence of the lower limbs and torso in the absence of the return of blood from the legs by the muscle pump effect. Blood pools in the leg veins, as it does on a normal rise from sitting, when 500–800 mL of blood moves towards the abdomen and legs under gravity. However, with a normal postural change, the cardiac output will increase, and the resistance to blood flow of the blood vessels also increases to maintain blood pressure. Then, during movement, the leg muscle pump assists venous return. However, the lack of this mechanism in motionless suspension tends to sequester blood volume in the lower limbs, reducing the cardiac output, which can then result in a spiral of reduced cardiac filling with consequent reduced stroke volume, increased heart rate as a compensatory mechanism, and decreased blood pressure due to reduced circulating blood volume.[12–14] Reflex mechanisms associated with low ventricular volume, the Bezold–Jarisch reflex, can trigger bradycardia and vasodilation, which in this situation might be responsible for precipitating syncope.[14] The onset of syncope may be influenced by other factors that contribute to these mechanisms. Anxiety and pain may lead to an increased heart rate; pain may also cause a vasovagal response. Alcohol and some drugs can act as vasodilators as well as affecting heart rate and level of consciousness. Physical exertion during or prior to suspension may also lead to vasodilation and dehydration, as might a hot environment. Preexisting medical conditions that are themselves associated with syncopal events may make an individual more susceptible to adverse responses from motionless suspension.

The onset of syncope may be associated with symptoms that are termed indicative of presyncope (see Figure 7.2). The presence of these symptoms in someone who is in a state of suspension may herald imminent collapse into an unconscious state followed by death.

> Light headedness
> Nausea
> Sensation of flushing
> Tingling of peripheries
> Numbness of peripheries
> Tremulousness
> Palpitations
> Drowsiness
> Visual disturbance
> Anxiety

FIGURE 7.2
Symptoms indicative of presyncope in a suspended subject.

Presyncope has been used as an indication for termination of experimental motionless suspension followed by placing the subject in a supine position.

7.5 Management

It can be appreciated from the pathophysiologic mechanism described, as well as from experimental evidence, that motionless suspension will be better tolerated with reduced head-up tilt angle and with the lower limbs less dependent. That is to say, the closer the subject is to the horizontal position, the less likely they are to experience symptoms. It is, therefore, unsurprising that when cardiac tilt table tests are conducted and symptoms are provoked, the maneuver is terminated by laying the subject horizontally, usually in a supine position with face looking upwards. In a medically supervised situation, the subject can be monitored, and even if an unconscious state ensues, the person's airway can be maintained. In a field setting, whether at leisure or in the workplace, any subject who is unconscious but spontaneously breathing should be managed according to standard first aid guidelines, which would typically mean laying the subject in a recovery position, with a lateral recumbent posture.[12,13,15] Similarly, subjects who are thought to be presyncopal would be expected to recover more quickly on lying down. First responders would, from their training, be expected to consider the presence of any other complicating factors such as head injury, other trauma, or medical conditions and prioritize treatment appropriately. Failure to place an unconscious spontaneously breathing victim in a recovery position by supporting the person in an erect or semirecumbent position can only be expected to exacerbate the clinical situation.[12–14,16] Unconscious victims will require medical advice and treatment, usually from emergency services. Persons experiencing presyncope may only require being allowed to recover by suitable positioning, depending on the circumstances and the presence or absence of any other medical conditions.

7.6 Prevention

The principles of risk management should be applied to ensure the use of the most appropriate means of access for work at heights. Where harnesses with fall-arrest systems are used, planning and training can minimize the risks from falls into suspension. Consideration needs to be given to rescuing anyone who may fall into suspension, bearing in mind the potentially very brief tolerance for individuals who are motionless. Motionless suspension immediately after a fall is most likely due to consequences of the fall, such as head injury, or the reason for the fall, perhaps a sudden cardiac event. In such circumstances, the victim may succumb within a matter of a few minutes if the airway cannot be maintained, and thereafter from the underlying medical condition or suspension syncope. A conscious victim may be able to self-rescue or use foot strops to raise the body and actuate their calf muscles, thereby maintaining venous blood return. Elevation of the lower limbs in a strop beneath the knees will place the victim in a more horizontal posture and encourage venous return while limiting gravitational dependency.[11] It therefore follows that using a harness and fall-arrest system while lone working is an unsafe practice, as there is by necessity reliance on either self-rescue or passers-by.

References

1. "Suspension Trauma/Orthostatic Intolerance" SHIB 03-24-2004, updated 2011. https://www.osha.gov/dts/shib/shib032404.html. Last accessed: 19 April 2015.

2. Petermeyer M, Unterhalt M. *Das Hängetrauma (Suspension trauma)*. German to English translation by HSE Language Services. Transl. No. 16367(A) *Der Notarzt* 1997;13:12–15.

3. Edwards WD, Gabel WJ, Hosmer FE. On the Physical Death of Jesus Christ. *JAMA* 1986;255:1455–1463.

4. Seddon P. *Harness Suspension: Review and Evaluation of Existing Information. CRR* 451/2002, HSE Books, Norwich: HMSO; 2002.

5. Various. Falls into the rope: Skull injuries in alpine regions. *Papers of the Second International Conference of Mountain Rescue Doctors (Austria)*; 1972. German to English translation by HSE Language Services Transl. No. 16372(I).

6. Noel G, Ardouin M G, Archer P, Amphoux M, Sevin A. Some aspects of fall protection equipment employed in construction and public works industries. In: Sulowski A C, ed. *Fundamentals of Fall Protection*. Toronto, Canada: International Society for Fall Protection; 1991:1–32.

7. Orzech M A, Goodwin M D, Brinkley J W, Salerno M D, Seaworth J. *Test Program to Evaluate Human Response to Prolonged Motionless Suspension in Three Types of Fall Protection Harnesses*. Wright-Patterson Air Force Base, OH: Harry G. Armstrong Aerospace Medical Research Laboratory; 1987.

8. Weber P, Michels-Brendel G. *Physiologie beanspruchungen beim hägen in Auffanggurten (Physiological Limits of Suspension in Harnesses)*. German to English translation by Johann Wolfgang Goethe University, Frankfurt, Germany, 1990.

9. Roeggla M, Brunner M, Michalek A, et al. Cardiorespiratory response to free suspension simulating the situation between fall and rescue in a rock climbing accident. *Wilderness Environ. Med.* 1996;7:109–114.

10. Madsen P, Svendsen L B, Jorgensen L G, et al. Tolerance to head-up tilt and suspension with elevated legs. *Aviat. Space Environ. Med.* 1998;69:781–784.

11. Turner N L, Wassell J T, Whisler R, Zwiener J. Suspension tolerance in a full-body safety harness, and a prototype harness accessory. *J. Occup. Env. Hygiene* 2008;5:227–231.

12. Adisesh A, Lee C, Porter K. Harness suspension and first aid management: Development of an evidence-based guideline. *Emerg. Med. J.* 2011;28:265–268.

13. Adisesh A, Robinson L, Codling A, Harris-Roberts J, Lee C, Porter K. 2009. *Evidence-Based Review of the Current Guidance on First Aid Measures for Suspension Trauma*. HSE Research Report RR708. HSE Books, Norwich, UK.

14. Mortimer R B. Risks and management of prolonged suspension in an alpine harness. *Wilderness Env. Med.* 2011;22:77–86.

15. International First Aid and Resuscitation Guidelines 2011. International Federation of Red Cross and Red Crescent Societies, Geneva, 2011. https://www.ifrc.org/PageFiles/53459/IFRC%20-International%20first%20aid%20and%20resuscitation%20guideline%202011.pdf. Last accessed: 19 April 2015.

16. Pasquier M, Yersin B, Vallotton L, Carron P-N. Clinical update: Suspension trauma. *Wilderness Env. Med.* 2011; 22:167–171.

8

Suspension Trauma and Fall-Arrest Harness Design

Hongwei Hsiao

CONTENTS

ABSTRACT After a successfully arrested fall, fall victims may develop suspension trauma, a potentially fatal reduction of return blood flow from legs to the heart and brain, if they are not rescued quickly or the harness does not fit them well. This chapter describes human suspension tolerance time while wearing full-body harnesses, the factors that affect suspension tolerance, current suspension injury control measures, and rescue procedures.

KEY WORDS: *body weight, body shape, harness fit, suspension, anthropometry, fall arrest, rescue.*

8.1 Introduction

In 1995, the Occupational Safety and Health Administration (OSHA) mandated a construction standard that specified that full-body harnesses replace waist belts for fall arrest in a personal fall-arrest system, effective in 1998 (U.S. Department of Labor, 2011a). The requirement has resulted in an increase in the use of full-body harnesses for fall protection. Along with the OSHA mandate, safety professionals and scientists have furthered our knowledge about fall protection over the past decades, including the fall-arrest harness fit assessment, post-fall suspension control, and post-fall rescue issues.

Once a worker's fall has been successfully arrested by a full-body harness, the suspended worker needs to be rescued promptly. A prolonged suspension can cause the pooling of blood in the legs and the reduction of the return blood flow to the heart. The motionless posture after a traumatic shock and restrictions of the femoral arteries and veins caused by the harness straps can worsen venous pooling. Other factors such as heat, dehydration, immobilization due to injury, neurological disorders, aging, or norepinephrine-transporter deficiency can further speed the detrimental effects, which may damage vital organs such as the kidneys (Seddon, 2002; Robertson, 2008; Shannon et al., 2000). This phenomenon of venous pooling is known as suspension trauma.

This chapter describes human suspension tolerance time while wearing full-body harnesses, the factors that affect suspension tolerance, current suspension trauma prevention practice, and rescue procedures. Suspension tolerance was defined by Streeten (1987) as the duration of motionless suspended time until any sign of medical orthostatic intolerance (a temporary loss of consciousness). The signs of orthostatic intolerance included (1) a systolic blood pressure (BP) decrease of more than 20 mm Hg below the pretest value; (2) a diastolic BP decrease of more than 10 mm Hg below the pretest value; (3) a heart rate (HR) increase of more than 28 bpm over the pretest value; (4) a HR decrease of more than 10 bpm from baseline; (5) a pulse pressure decrease to less than 18 mm Hg; or (6) an observed shortness of breath, nausea, dizziness, or diastolic BP greater than 100 mm Hg (Streeten, 1987).

8.2 Suspension Tolerance Time

Some laboratory studies have investigated the tolerance of participants to motionless suspension, mainly for men while wearing fall-arrest harnesses (Brinkley, 1988; Weber and Michels-Brendel, 1990). With small sample sizes, suspension tolerance, as measured, ranged from 3.5 to 60 min. Specifically, the literature has shown some variant results regarding tolerance time for the use of similar full-body harnesses: from 8 to 45 min ($N=5$) (Noel et al., 1978), 6 to 37 min ($N=2$) (Bariod and Théry, 1997), and 5.1 to 30.1 min (mean $= 14.38$, $N=13$) (Brinkley, 1988). The literature has also reported differences in suspension tolerance time for different styles of full-body harness, with an average of 17.1 min (minimum to maximum of 3.5–32) to 28.4 min (minimum to maximum of 10.2– 49.8) for four harness types ($N=10$) (Brinkley, 1988), as well as median suspension durations of 20–27 min for five styles of harness ($N=15$) (Weber and Michels-Brendel, 1990). In any case, suspension tolerance varies considerably from person to person. Scientists have speculated about the harness fit effect on suspension tolerance time because about half the trials in the mentioned studies terminated voluntarily by the participants, possibly due to discomfort caused by poor harness design or fit (Noel et al., 1978). In a recent controlled laboratory study, Hsiao et al. (2012) reported that the suspension tolerance time was measured to be an average of 29.1 min and that the harness fit to the human body played a role. The study also evidenced large variability ($s=12.1$ min, $N=37$) with a minimum to maximum of 5–56 min (Figure 8.1). With a comparatively larger sample size ($N=37$), the study provided

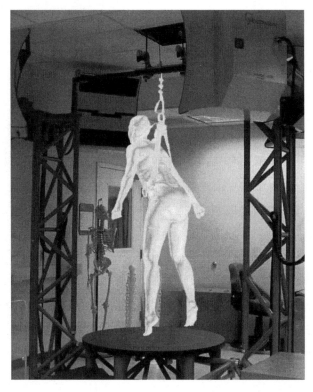

FIGURE 8.1
A custom-made suspension system was used to suspend the participant for a suspension-tolerance capability test and for registering the interface between the harness and participant.

the most updated data for estimating the time constraints in rescuing a worker suspended after a fall. It is worth noting that the range of the participants' body weight in this study was 50–107.6 kg, although the harnesses have been designed to accommodate 50–141 kg. Given that body weight has a negative correlation with suspension tolerance time, harness users with a body weight above 107.6 kg may experience an even shorter suspension tolerance time than that reported in this study.

8.3 Factors That Affect Full-Body Harness Suspension Tolerance

8.3.1 Body Weight and Stature Effects

Researchers have reported that body weight (Turner et al., 2008) and stature (Seddon, 2002) were predictors for suspension tolerance. Specifically, the Pearson correlation coefficient showed significant negative correlations between suspension tolerance time and body weight ($r = -.45$, $p = .005$) and stature ($r = -.43$, $p = .007$) (Hsiao et al., 2012). In practical harness–torso interface design applications, greater upper-torso depth ($r = -.37$, $p = .02$) and lower-torso depth ($r = -.36$, $p = .03$) are associated with shorter suspension tolerance time

(Hsiao et al., 2012), which is understandable since greater upper- and lower-torso depths generally correspond to heavier body weights.

8.3.2 Gender Effect

An absence of gender difference in the ability to tolerate harness suspension has been reported elsewhere (Weber and Michels-Brendel, 1990). However, the true effect cannot be determined in that there were only three and four women in the two tests of the Weber and Michels-Brendel study. In a recent study, a mean suspension tolerance time comparison by gender also revealed no significant difference ($p = .261$). The mean suspension tolerance time was 27.1 min for men (95% CI: 21.2–33.0; $N = 20$) and 31.6 min for women (95% CI: 25.7–37.6; $N = 17$) (Hsiao et al., 2012). While the larger sample size (17 women) in that study offered a good prospect for examining the gender effect, an obstacle remained. The study was not a matched-pairs study; 71% of the female participants weighed less than 70 kg, while 80% of the male participants weighed above 70 kg. With the confounding between gender and body weight, the insignificant effect of gender (anatomical and physiological characteristics) ($p = .26$) cannot be confidently confirmed.

8.3.3 Effect of Harness Fit to Human Body

Harness fit can be attributed to four key parameters: harness ring location (static fit to body), torso angle of suspension, strap configuration, and human body characteristics (i.e., size and shape) (Hsiao et al., 2009a).

8.3.3.1 Static Fit (Harness Ring Location)

There is a general understanding that the harness dorsal D-ring should be positioned between the inferior and superior borders of the scapula while the harness user is standing. Also, the chest ring is to be placed at the sternum area. Harness manufacturers have more detailed ring-location specifications, which are generally included in product manuals. In the past, fall-arrest harnesses were designed based on the body dimensions of male workers; static harness fit was in general worse for women than for men (Hsiao et al., 2003). However, harness users need to be aware that a static fit does not guarantee that a person suspended motionless in such a harness will be exempt from suspension trauma (Hsiao et al., 2012).

8.3.3.2 Torso Angle of Suspension and Suspension Fit

The second element of harness fit to the user's body is the torso angle of suspension (Hsiao et al., 2009a). The angle of suspension is measured between the torso center line and the harness vertical suspension line (Figure 8.2a). Using a rigid torso dummy for drop testing, the American National Standards Institute (ANSI) Z359.1 standard specifies that the suspension angle at rest shall not exceed 30° (ASSE, 2015). The Canadian CAN/CSA-Z259.10-06 standard also allows a maximum angle of 30° (CSA, 2006). The International Organization of Standards (ISO) 10333-1 and European EN 361standards allow maximum angles of 45° and 50°, respectively (ISO, 2002; CEN, 1992). These standards, however, do not elaborate on why these angle limits were specified and how they affect suspension tolerance (Seddon, 2002). A recent study showed that participants with a suspension angle >35° had shorter suspension tolerance time than those with smaller suspension angles ($p < .001$). Respective

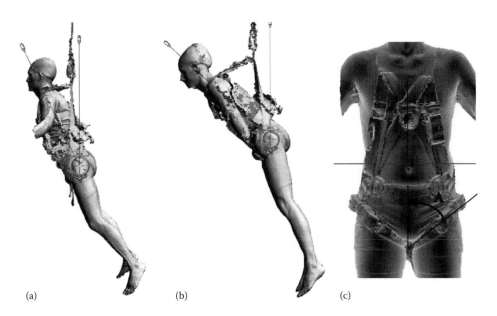

(a)   (b)   (c)

FIGURE 8.2
The angle of suspension is measured between the torso center line and the harness vertical suspension line. (a) The suspension fit rating is a pass (angle of suspension=26°); (b) the suspension fit rating is a fail (angle of suspension=48°). The thigh-strap angle A in (c) is defined by the line that connects the highest point and the lowest point of the thigh strap and in reference to the body sagittal plan.

suspension times were 34.9 min (95% CI: 30.1–39.6; $N=22$) for the group with the smaller angle of suspension (angle of suspension ≤35°) and 20.9 min (95% CI: 15.9–25.8; $N=15$) for the group with the greater angle of suspension (angle of suspension >35°) (Hsiao et al., 2012; Figure 8.2b).

In a critical review, Seddon (2002) was puzzled as to why the maximum angle requirements were set differently in different standards. From the perspective of biomechanics, an increased torso suspension angle results in a larger moment arm at the low back, which, in turn, can cause lower-back discomfort and increased consumption of oxygen, thus posing an increased risk of suspension trauma. When the torso suspension angle is more than 30°, the force imposed by the weight of the upper body will increase dramatically, based on the basic trigonometric concept. The harness industry and fall protection professional community can consider testing body-harness designs using a series of anthropometric manikins in suspension and checking on suspension angles, in lieu of relying on traditional static-fit testing criteria to provide an increased protection against suspension trauma.

8.3.3.3 Thigh-Strap Angle

The third element for harness fit is thigh-strap configuration fit (thigh-strap angle). The thigh-strap angle is defined as the angle between the thigh strap and the sagittal plane (Figure 8.2c). A study of 216 participants using an overhead-style harness revealed that a greater thigh-strap angle from the sagittal plan was correlated with an increase in torso suspension angle and hence in harness-fit failure (Hsiao et al., 2007). The thigh-strap angle may be considered as a fit criterion to possibly minimize the need for a suspension test to predict the angle of suspension and suspension tolerance.

8.3.3.4 Body Size and Shape and Effect of Harness Match Level

The last element for harness fit is human body size and shape. Past studies have shown that body weight is a fair predictor for suspension tolerance (Turner et al., 2008; Seddon, 2002) and that a relatively bulky chest combined with a short torso is associated with a poor harness-fit rating (Hsiao et al., 2009b). A previous study has also shown that individuals who used a size of harness that was different from the best-fit size had shorter suspension tolerance times (Hsiao et al., 2012). Individuals with disparity of body dimensions often are "forced" to choose a harness size that does not fit their body, thereby increasing their risk of suspension trauma.

Large changes have taken place over the last decades in body dimensions among the U.S. civilian population (U.S. Department of Health and Human Services, 2001), and the harness industry has updated harness sizing systems based on government research suggestions (Hsiao et al., 2009a,b). Workers whose combination of body weight and stature is at the proximity of the size boundaries of the sizing scheme continue to need to try on more than one size to select the best-fit size because the overall combination of their body dimensions (i.e., body shape) governs the size; some of their body dimensions may fall on different sides of the boundaries. When purchasing a safety harness, clearly, the harness should be tested so that an individual can find a model that best fits the shape of his or her body, thus delaying the onset of suspension trauma (Bariod and Théry, 1997).

8.4 Current Prevention and Protection Practice

8.4.1 Rescue Time

Past studies have reported a wide range of suspension tolerance times among individuals, from 3.5 to 60 min. With small sample sizes, typically 2–13 participants, most studies in the literature did not or were unable to suggest a required critical time frame in which to rescue a victim. Hsiao et al. (2012) suggested that a rescue action be accomplished in 9 min. This was proposed based on the fact that the mean and standard deviation of suspension tolerance time were 29.2 and 12.1 min, respectively, from 37 participants and that the data are normally distributed: $T_{0.05} = \text{mean} - (1.645 * s) = 29.2 - 1.645 * 12.1 = 9.26$ min. This is to ensure that no more than 5% of suspended workers would experience suspension trauma. The explanatory information in ANSI Z359.2 recommends a goal of establishing contact with the fall victim within 6 min after a fall incident (Feldstein, 2007).

8.5 Rescue Procedure

Under 29 CFR 1926.502 (d) (Fall Protection Systems Criteria and Practices), OSHA requires that employers provide for "prompt rescue of employees in the event of a fall or shall assure that employees are able to rescue themselves" (U.S. Department of Labor, 2011b). To fulfill this requirement, three topics must be understood: signs and symptoms of suspension trauma, suspension trauma control, and post-rescue treatment.

8.5.1 Signs and Symptoms of Suspension Trauma

Workers should be trained to be aware of factors that can increase the risk of suspension trauma and the symptoms of trauma. In general, body characteristics (i.e., weight, stature, upper- and lower-torso depths), and poor harness fit are associated with decreased suspension tolerance time. The signs of developing suspension trauma include a systolic BP decrease of more than 20 mm Hg below the individual's normal value, a diastolic BP decrease of more than 10 mm Hg, a HR increase of more than 28 bpm, a HR decrease of more than 10 bpm, a pulse pressure decrease to less than 18 mm Hg, shortness of breath, nausea, dizziness, and a diastolic BP greater than 100 mm Hg (Streeten, 1987).

8.5.2 Suspension Trauma Control

To reduce suspension trauma risk, workers are to be trained to use fall-arrest systems correctly while performing their jobs. They also need to know that they can move their legs during a suspension to reduce the risk of venous pooling. Many fall-arrest harnesses have a pair of "built-in" footholds. Harness users need to be familiar with the use of footholds to alleviate pressure and delay symptoms. In addition, efforts should be made to rescue suspended workers as quickly as possible. Moreover, everybody who is suspended in a safety harness runs the risk of shock and unconsciousness due to trauma incident consequence; a prototype self-deployable suspension trauma-relief accessory that converts a suspension posture to a seated posture at the moment of a fall was proposed, which can significantly delay the onset of suspension trauma (Turner et al., 2008).

8.5.3 Post-Rescue Treatment

The best method to recover harness suspension victims has not been clear over the past 20 years, with some authors advising against standard first-aid practices (i.e., placing victims in a horizontal position), while others have contended that there is no evidence to support the safety or efficacy of positioning a victim in a semi-seated position. Some safety training materials published in the early 2000s have emphasized that the victim should be positioned with the upper body raised, that is, in a seated or possibly squatting or crouched posture. The rationale was that laying the victim down horizontally can be life threatening because blood that has accumulated in the legs can flow abruptly into the heart, creating a risk of heart failure due to overstrain. The concept can be traced back to a harness suspension information report (Seddon, 2002) that cited a German report on first aid following suspension in a fall-arrest harness (Lieblich and Rensing, 1997). This positioning recommendation was also supported by an earlier conference proceeding paper, which contended that rescued suspension victims may experience adverse effects if laid horizontally (Flora et al., 1972).

Through a systematic review of 29 papers relevant to the subject, Adisesh et al. (2011) identified nine articles as a basis for guideline recommendations and concluded that no evidence indicates the efficacy or safety of positioning a victim in a semiseated position. They suggested that the standard first-aid guidance for recovery of a semiconscious or unconscious person in a horizontal position be followed. OSHA has updated its suspension trauma/orthostatic intolerance information bulletin (U.S. Department of Labor, 2011b) by removing the statement that "Some authorities recommend that the patient be transported with the upper body raised" from the earlier version (U.S. Department of Labor, 2004). Other first-aid practices include unfastening all restrictive belts and clothing, calling a doctor, and continuously monitoring respiration and circulation as necessary.

8.6 Summary

Body weight, stature, and upper- and lower-torso depths were negatively correlated with suspension tolerance time. Harness suspension angle, thigh-strap angle, and harness-size match level were also precursors for suspension tolerance. Selecting well-fitting harnesses and establishing a 9-min rescue plan are suggested to ensure that no more than 5% of suspended workers would experience suspension trauma. This short rescue time is challenging. A self-deployable suspension trauma relief accessory or mechanism that can be integrated into harness design to further harness-user protection would be useful. To avoid any post-rescue injuries, the current practice is that the victim be positioned in a horizontal posture, per the standard guidelines for the recovery of an unconscious or semiconscious person after a rescue.

8.7 Disclaimer

The findings and conclusions in this article are those of the author and do not necessarily represent the views of the National Institute for Occupational Safety and Health (NIOSH). Mention of company names or products does not constitute endorsement by NIOSH.

References

Adisesh, A., Lee, C., and Porter, K. (2011). Harness suspension and first aid management: Development of an evidence-based guideline. *Emergency Medicine Journal*, 28: 265–268.

American Society of Safety Engineers (ASSE). (2015). American National Standards Institute ANSI Z359.1-1992, *Safety Requirements for Personal Fall Arrest Systems, Subsystems and Components*. Des Plaines, IL: American Society of Safety Engineers (Secretariat).

Bariod, J. and Théry, B. (1997). *Medizinische Auswirkungen des Hängens in Sicherheitsgurten (The Medical Effects of Being Suspended in Safety Harnesses)*. Cited from Seddon, P. (2002). Harness suspension: Review and evaluation of existing information. *Health and Safety Executive Contract Research Report 451/2002*. Norwich, England: Her Majesty's Stationery Office.

Brinkley, J.W. (1988). Experimental studies of fall protection equipment. *Proceedings of the 1st International Fall Protection Symposium*. Toronto, Canada: International Society for Fall Protection, 51–65.

Canadian Standards Association (CSA). (2006). Canadian Standard CAN/CSA-Z259.10-06 *Full Body Harnesses*, Etobicoke, Ontario, Canada: Canadian Standards Association.

European Committee for Standardization (CEN). (1992). European Standard EN 361:1992. *Personal Protective Equipment against Falls from a Height—Full Body Harnesses*. Brussels, Belgium: European Committee for Standardization.

Feldstein, J. (2007). ANSI/ASSE Z359 Fall Protection Code: Revisions Strengthen Benchmark Consensus Standard. In *By Design—A Technical Publication of ASSE's Engineering Practice Specialty*. Des Plaines, IL: American Society of Safety Engineers.

Flora, G., Margreiter, R., Dittrich, P., et al. (1972). Hanging tests—Conclusions for the mountaineer. The Second International Conference of Mountain Rescue Doctors, Austria. German to English translation by HSE Language Services Translation No. 16372(I), cited from Adisesh et al., 2011.

Hsiao, H., Bradtmiller, B., and Whitestone, J. (2003). Sizing and fit of fall-protection harnesses. *Ergonomics*, 46(12), 1233–1258.

Hsiao, H., Friess, M., Bradtmiller, B., and Rohlf, J. (2009b). Development of sizing structure for fall arrest harness design. *Ergonomics*, 52(9), 1128–1143.

Hsiao, H., Turner, N., Whisler, R., and Zwiener, J. (2012). Impact of harness fit on suspension tolerance. *Human Factors*, 54(3), 346–357.

Hsiao, H., Whitestone, J., and Kau, T. (2007). Evaluation of fall-arrest harness sizing schemes. *Human Factors*, 49(3), 447–464.

Hsiao, H., Whitestone, J., Taylor, S., Godby, M., and Guan, J. (2009a). Harness sizing and strap adjustment configurations. *Human Factors*, 51(4), 497–518.

International Standards Organization (ISO). (2002). ISO 10333-1: 2000 + AMD 1: 2002 *Personal Fall-Arrest Systems—Part 1: Full-Body Harnesses*. Geneva, Switzerland: International Standards Organization.

Lieblich, M. and Rensing, M. (1997). Rescuing people who have fallen and first aid following suspension in a safety harness, German to English translation by HSE Language Service. *ASvorORT*, 1997, 12, cited from Seddon, P., 2002.

Noel, G., Ardouin, M.G., Archer, P., Amphoux, M., and Sevin, A. (1978). Some aspects of fall protection equipment employed in construction and public works industries, French to English translation. In Sulowski, A.C., ed. *Fundamentals of Fall Protection* (1991), Chapter 1. Toronto, Ontario, Canada: International Society for Fall Protection, ISBN 0-921952-01-5.

Robertson, D. (2008). The pathophysiology and diagnosis of orthostatic hypotension. *Clinical Autonomic Research*, 18[Supply 1], 2–7.

Seddon, P. (2002). Harness suspension: Review and evaluation of existing information. *Health and Safety Executive Contract Research Report 451/2002*. Norwich, England: Her Majesty's Stationery Office.

Shannon, J., Flattem, N., Jordan, J., Jacob, G., Black, B., Biaggioni, I., Blakely, R., and Robertson, D. (2000). Orthostatic intolerance and tachycardia associated with norepinephrine-transporter deficiency. *New England Journal of Medicine*, 342, 541–549.

Streeten, D. (1987). Orthostatic disorders of blood pressure control: Definitions and classification. In: *Orthostatic Disorders of the Circulation: Mechanisms, Manifestations, and Treatment*, pp. 111–125. New York: Plenum Medical Book Company.

Turner, N., Wassell, J., Whisler, R., and Zwiener, J. (2008). Suspension tolerance in a full-body safety harness, and a prototype harness accessory. *Journal of Occupational and Environmental Hygiene*, 5, 227–231.

U.S. Department of Health and Human Services. (2001). *The Surgeon General's Call to Action to Prevent and Decrease Overweight and Obesity*. Washington, DC: U.S. Government Printing Office.

U.S. Department of Labor. (2004). *Suspension Trauma/Orthostatic Intolerance*. Safety and Health Information Bulletin SHIB 03-24-2004, Washington, DC: Author. Retrieved June 10, 2010.

U.S. Department of Labor. (2011a). *Safety and Health Regulations for Construction*. Subpart M—Fall Protection, 1926.502(d). Washington, DC: Author. Retrieved June 1, 2011, from http://www.osha.gov/pls/oshaweb/owadisp.show_document?p_table=STANDARDS&p_id=10758.

U.S. Department of Labor. (2011b). *Suspension Trauma/Orthostatic Intolerance*. Safety and Health Information Bulletin SHIB 03-24-2004, updated 2011, Washington, DC: Author. Retrieved April 4, 2015, from https://www.osha.gov/dts/shib/shib032404.pdf.

Weber, P. and Michels-Brendel, G. (1990). *Physiologie beanspruchungen beim hägen in Auffanggurten (Physiological Limits of Suspension in Harnesses)*. Frankfurt, Germany: Johann Wolfgang Goethe University.

9

Fall Risk Associated with Restricted and Elevated Support Surfaces

Peter Simeonov

CONTENTS

ABSTRACT This chapter addresses the effects of restricted and elevated support surfaces on balance control as related to the risk of occupational falls from elevation. The chapter presents a summary of the pioneering research studies conducted at the National Institute for Occupational Safety and Health (NIOSH) to evaluate and apply virtual reality technology for fall prevention research. The described research outcomes include practical strategies and solutions to improve workers' balance control in challenging construction work environments. Also included is a brief review of related research on balance control, in which exposures to restricted and elevated surfaces are used to understand and prevent falls in the elderly. The chapter concludes with a brief summary of suggested measures to control falls from restricted and elevated surfaces.

9.1 Problem of Falls from Elevation

Falls remain a leading cause of fatal injury in the workplace. In 2012, there were approximately 704 fatal work-related falls in the United States. More than 80% (570) of these fatal fall injuries were due to falls from elevation, and nearly 50% (279) of the falls from elevation occurred in the construction industry (BLS, 2013). In addition, in 2012, there were 56,890 nonfatal injuries with days away from work due to falls from elevation in the United States (BLS, 2014). According to the 2013 Liberty Mutual Workplace Safety Index, the cost of injury resulting in falls from elevation in 2011 in the United States was $4.9 billion (Liberty Mutual, 2013). These staggering statistics reveal the persistent nature of fall hazards in the workplace and, specifically, the fall prevention challenges that remain within the construction industry.

Work at elevation, especially in construction, is associated with frequent standing and walking on restricted surfaces, such as temporary work platforms (scaffolding planks), structural components and elements (trusses, rafters, and steel beams in metal construction), and unfinished work surfaces (wall top plates), which are not designed for but are frequently used as support surfaces. Temporary support surfaces at elevation are frequently compliant (they can bend, yield, and move when loaded). Restricted and elevated surfaces can also be sloped (e.g., in residential roofing).

Developing a good understanding of the fall risks associated with exposure to restricted and elevated surfaces may help in selecting effective fall prevention strategies. An important first step in this process is the adequate characterization of the components of this exposure.

9.2 Restricted and Elevated Support Surfaces

Restricted and elevated support surfaces are characterized by open unprotected edges and are therefore associated with a fall-from-height hazard; they may be characterized by visual exposure to elevation (open space with distant visual references) and therefore associated with reduced visual feedback for balance control and increased risk of losing balance; and they also may be limited in at least one dimension that can reduce the base of support (BOS) during standing or restrict stepping control strategies during walking, and therefore they may be associated with an increased risk of losing balance.

How high must a support surface be to be considered elevated? For practical purposes, the Occupational Safety and Health Association (OSHA) General Industry Standard (29 CFR 1910) "Walking-working surfaces"—1910.23(c)(1) has defined a lower limit of dangerous surface height by requiring guarding of open-sided floors or platforms 1.22 m (4 ft) or more above adjacent floor or ground level (OSHA, 1984), while the OSHA Safety and Health Regulations for Construction (29 CFR 1926) Subpart M "Fall Protection"—1926.501(b)(1) sets the height limit for fall protection at 1.83 m (6 ft) (OSHA, 1995). However, in steel erection

(OSHA Safety Standards for Steel Erection)—1926.760(a)(1), fall protection is required for all work above 4.5 m (15 ft) and, for some tasks, above 9 m (30 ft) (OSHA, 2001). An increase in fall height has been positively correlated with higher injury severity (Lau et al. 1998) and increased risk of fatal injury (Warner and Demling, 1986); however, even falls from very low heights can be fatal.

What are the dimensions that define a support surface as restricted? There is practically no lower limit for the width of a surface used as support while standing and performing tasks at elevation—examples include the rungs or steps of a ladder, scaffolding frames, roof trusses, and other structural components. However, balance on such narrow support surfaces is usually maintained by using the hands or body for extra support. Walking and balancing tasks for short distances are frequently performed by construction workers without any protection on elevated surfaces as narrow as 10–15 cm (4–6 in.), such as wall top plates, rafters, and beams.

Some practical determinations for the dimensions of restricted support surfaces can be found in the safety standards and regulations. For example, the OSHA Safety and Health Regulations for Construction (29 CFR 1926) Subpart L "Scaffolds" sets the minimum width for a scaffolding plank at 30 cm (12 in.); however, this requirement is not enforced for roofing planks (1926.451(b)(2)(i)), and the common roofing practice is to use 25 cm (10 in.) and even 15 cm (6 in.)-wide planks (OSHA, 1996). The OSHA General Industry Standard (29 CFR 1910) Subpart D "Walking-working surfaces"—1910.23(c)(2) sets a minimum width requirement of 46 cm (18 in.) for a runway that is unguarded on one side (OSHA, 1984). The OSHA Safety and Health Regulations for Construction (29 CFR 1926) Subpart M "Fall Protection"—1926.502(g)(1)(i) defines the distance of 183 cm (6 ft) from an unprotected edge as critical for workers' safety in setting the requirements for controlled access zones (OSHA, 1995).

9.3 Fall Risk Associated with Restricted and Elevated Support Surfaces

9.3.1 Theoretical Considerations for Fall Causation

From the perspective of mechanics, biomechanics, and human factors, a fall can be defined as uncontrolled descent under the influence of gravity, and the causes of falls can be regarded as failures or disruptions in the control of dynamic postural stability during human interaction with the environment. Control of balance is a complex process in which the central nervous system integrates sensory information from visual, vestibular, and somatosensory inputs and uses knowledge acquired through past experience to select and implement postural control strategies (Horak, 2006). The postural control goal is to maintain the body's center of mass (COM) within its stability limits, considering the instant position and velocity of the COM with relation to its BOS defined by the position of the feet.

Loss of balance incidents (falls) occur when one or several modes of the proactive and reactive mechanisms of balance control are disrupted during human–environment interactions (Patla, 1997b; Woollacott and Tang, 1997). The proactive mechanism of balance control, modulated mainly by visual information (Patla, 1997a), involves the activation of postural adjustments prior to the occurrence of destabilizing forces and acts to minimize balance disturbances. The reactive mechanism of balance control, triggered by somatosensory and vestibular inputs, involves the activation of postural adjustments after an external distur-bance is encountered, thus enacting balance recovery (Patla, 1993). Restricted and elevated support surfaces can affect the control-of-balance process, and thus the risk of falls, by one or more of the following mechanisms: inducing fearful perceptions and triggering protec-tive behavior; reducing and modifying the adequate sensory information; and restricting the performance of some of the available balance-control strategies.

9.3.2 Psychophysiological Effects of Exposure to Elevation

Exposure to close-by unguarded edges on elevated support surfaces can affect workers' balance through fear-related behavioral and physiological responses (Brown and Frank, 1997). The feeling of anxiety or fear of falling in some cases can lead to overreaction in controlling posture and cause instability. Increased postural threat has been associ-ated with enforced tight control over COM kinematics (Brown and Frank, 1997), selec-tion of a wider BOS (Maki et al., 1994), reduced stride length and velocity (Maki, 1997), and enhanced gain of the vestibular–ocular reflex (Yardley et al., 1995). Furthermore, the increased postural threat does not have to be directly visually induced—any awareness of an existing immediate danger is sufficient to trigger protective responses (Tersteeg et al., 2012).

The level of anxiety experienced from a perceived postural threat is associated with the worker's perceptions of danger, which are a function of the perceived risk for fall and the perceived severity of the expected injury (Menzies and Clarke, 1995). The risk parameters for a fall from elevation may include the worker's task and posture, distance to the edge of the restricted and elevated support surface, availability of fall protec-tive devices and barriers, and stability of the structure (Cloe, 1979; Suruda et al., 1995; Janicak, 1998). The physical factors that determine the severity of injury from a free fall are the height of the fall, properties of the surface of impact, body orientation at impact, and body mass (Warner and Demling, 1986). On the other hand, habituation to a spe-cific dangerous environment can significantly diminish workers' danger perceptions—experienced roofers have been found to underestimate the risk associated with their job (Zimolong, 1985).

9.3.3 Physiological Effects of Exposure to Elevation

A visual environment of elevation is characterized by a lack of close visual references, which can influence balance control through the mechanism of visual stabilization (Bles et al., 1980; Brandt et al., 1980). Bles et al. (1980) reported that when at elevation, human body sway gradually increases both in lateral and fore–aft directions with increasing dis-tance between the eye and the closest object within a person' s visual field. This correla-tion is stronger when a higher proprioceptive interference is involved (e.g., standing on unstable surface). The sway reaches its maximum at eye–object distances of 5 m and over. Postural instability associated with eye–object distance is not significant at ground level because cues from nearby stationary contrasts (provided by peripheral vision) prevent the instigating sensory mismatch (Brandt et al., 1980). Paulus et al. (1984) reported that pos-tural instability due to height effect begins at 3–4 m eye height.

While on an elevated and restricted surface, workers may direct their eyes to a tree moving in the wind or look at swinging objects such as materials moved by a crane. Given the absence of other stable visual references, these actions might degrade a worker's balance. Research has demonstrated that exposure to moving visual scenes can affect a person's postural stability (Lee and Lishman, 1975; Berthoz et al., 1979; Stoffregen, 1985). Peterka and Benolken (1995) found that, in conditions with inaccurate somatosensory cues, the visually induced postural sway increased significantly (with amplitude almost three times greater than the stimulus) and caused occasional falls in their test subjects.

9.3.4 Biomechanical Effects of Restricted Support Surfaces

Depending on the level of restriction, a support surface can affect balance control in several ways: by directly reducing the BOS determined by feet/shoes dimensions and position; by limiting the availability of a stepping control strategy for balance recovery; and by limiting the affordance of some of the walking balance-control strategies.

Narrow surfaces, supporting only part of the foot, may diminish or eliminate the somatosensory input, subserving the normal mode of postural control, and they may also reduce the effectiveness of the "ankle" postural control strategy (Horak and Nashner, 1986). Perturbation studies in standing (Maki et al., 1996) have shown that a sudden displacement of the BOS is frequently compensated for with stepping responses within a radius of 60 cm, and sometimes several steps are required to restore equilibrium. Restricted support surfaces reduce the potential for effective emergency-reactive control; the worker has a reduced ability to use stepping strategies to recover from occasional instability.

Lateral stability during walking on unrestricted surfaces is most efficiently controlled by the "mediolateral foot placement" (MacKinnon and Winter, 1993; Bauby and Kuo, 2000; Patla, 2003). On narrow walking surfaces (e.g., 15 cm), which enforce suboptimal step width (Donelan et al., 2001), the "mediolateral foot placement" strategy is not available, and the only remaining effective way to control balance in the frontal plane is the individual or combined use of "ankle" and "hip" strategies, applied by lateral tilting movements at the foot and the trunk. During walking, a tripping perturbation is usually compensated for with an increase in the subsequent step length or with several small steps. The magnitude of the movement responses and the distance required for recovery of balance depend on many factors, including the walking velocity, perturbation characteristics, timing, and perceived threat of the task (Eng et al., 1994). If the reactive control fails after a perturbation, and a fall occurs, a restricted support surface may not afford the possibility of arresting the falling body, and a fall to a lower level will follow.

The standing/walking distance from the edge of elevated surfaces has been reported to be associated with the risk of fall incidents. Based on his own observations of people's behavior in the vicinity of elevated edges, Davis (1983) defined a "biomechanically safe distance." It is equal to the subject's own height (at the eyes), which, for the average male, was a little less than 183 cm. He related this distance to the fear of falling and defined a "45° rule." People stopped approaching elevated edges when the edge was seen as being 45° below the horizontal at a distance equal to their eyes' height, a distance they perceived to be biomechanically safe. Workers can fall from a standing position over an edge within 183 cm by tripping, slipping, stubbing their toes, or experiencing other loss-of-balance events (Ellis, 2001).

Generally speaking, there is sufficient experimental evidence in the literature that standing or walking on narrow supports degrades the control of balance. Furthermore, the standing/walking distance to an edge of a restricted surface is recognized as a factor associated with the risk of falling. However, studying the dose-response relations between the parameters of the restricted and elevated support surfaces and their effects on balance control, and the risk of fall remains a challenging research area.

9.4 Fall Prevention Research with Virtual Reality Simulations of Height

In contrast to the considerable number of experimental studies on the causes and prevention of slips and falls on the same level (Grönqvist et al., 2001), very little experimental research has been conducted to systematically investigate the contributing factors leading to falls from elevation. A serious barrier to such research is the high risk of injury, for both human participants and researchers, associated with the unprotected exposure to elevation, for example, in an experimental setup such as a roof or a scaffold.

The virtual reality (VR) technology that emerged and was developed during the last two decades provided an opportunity for conducting research at simulated elevated workplaces without the risk of injury. However, a systematic preliminary research project was needed to develop and validate this approach before it could be used for practical applications. The efforts to develop and use the VR technology for fall prevention research included the following logically interconnected activities: preliminary studies at real height and development of the VR laboratory; validation studies of virtual models of height and elevated workplaces; and evaluation studies of new fall prevention strategies with the application of virtual models of elevated workplaces.

9.4.1 Efforts to Develop Adequate Models of Elevation

9.4.1.1 Preliminary Studies at Real Height

The development of adequate models of elevation and elevated workplaces could benefit from preliminary information on workers' perceptions and performance at height. Since an adequate balance control at elevation was critical to avoid a fall, a study was initiated to evaluate the effects of height exposure on workers' balance performance and perceptions under various support conditions. Earlier research had suggested that the open space at elevation may lead to postural instability and height vertigo (Bles et al., 1980). The height exposure was per se exposure to distant visual scenes in conditions deficient in close visual references (Lee and Lishman, 1975). One of the study hypotheses was that a close visual structure may serve as a frame of reference and act as a countermeasure to the height-induced instability.

The first stage of the study investigated the effects of deformable/unstable work surfaces, height, and visual references—two vertical bars and the balcony edges in the visual field periphery—on the standing balance of construction workers. The participants were tested in a laboratory setting under two surface conditions (firm and deformable), at three heights (0, 3, and 9 m), and under two visual conditions (with and without visual references). The second stage of the study investigated the effects of the roof work environment characteristics of surface slope, height, and visual reference on standing balance in construction workers. The participants were tested in a laboratory setting at four slopes (0°, 18°, 26°, and 34°), at two heights (0, 3 m), and under two visual conditions (with and without visual references). Postural sway characteristics were calculated using center-of-pressure recordings from a force platform. Workers' perceptions of postural sway and instability were also evaluated.

The results of the study indicated that height exposure without close visual references significantly increased all sway parameters. The destabilizing effects of height increased dramatically on deformable surfaces, while the presence of close visual references resulted in improved postural stability (Simeonov and Hsiao, 2001). Slope surface and height synergistically increased workers' standing postural instability. While workers recognized the individual destabilizing effects of slope and height, they did not recognize the synergistic effect of the two. Visual references significantly reduced the destabilizing effects of height and slope (Simeonov et al., 2003).

This preliminary study had two main implications. First, it provided supporting evidence for the effectiveness of some simple practical measures and strategies for improving workers' balance at elevation, such as the use of temporary level work surfaces and the proximal vertical reference structures as postural instability control measures during roofing work. Second, it provided a basis for the comparative evaluation of virtual models of elevated workplaces. In this respect, one limitation of this study was that it addressed only the physiological effects of height on balance during protected exposure to elevation. Conducting experiments with unprotected exposure to simulate existing work practices in a construction workplace would be ethically acceptable only in a model of elevation within a VR system.

9.4.1.2 The NIOSH Virtual Reality Laboratory

The NIOSH fully immersive VR laboratory was designed and built in 1996 and was upgraded to a digital format in 2010—it is among the largest in scale of its kind and is one of very few being utilized for occupational safety research applications in the country. At present, this laboratory, measuring 8.5 m (28 ft) × 10.7 m (35 ft) × 4.3 m (14 ft), is being utilized to better understand human behavior, physical responses, and decision-making skills under simulated conditions of elevated work, such as scaffolding, roofing, and ladder-use tasks.

The VR laboratory is equipped with a projection-based CAVE-type surround-screen virtual reality (SSVR) system (MechDyne Corporation, Marshalltown, Iowa), with three 4.0 (13 ft)×3.0 m (10 ft) rear-projection screens for the walls and a 4.0 (13 ft)×4.0 m (13 ft) front-projection screen for the floor (Figure 9.1). The projected images are generated and controlled by a PC with four graphic cards. The participants wear a pair of liquid-crystal shutter glasses that separate the left- and right-eye images that are being projected, making the images appear three-dimensional. A position tracking system tracks the head

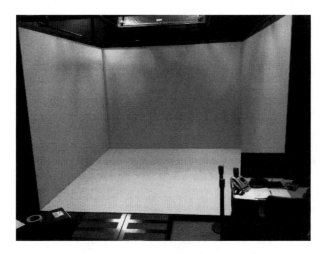

FIGURE 9.1
The NIOSH surround-screen virtual reality (SSVR) system.

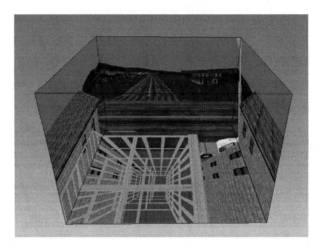

FIGURE 9.2
A SSVR model of a construction environment featuring restricted and elevated surfaces.

movements of the participants, and the image generator continuously updates the VR environment to give the subjects the right perspective. The fully immersive SSVR system, which has an active floor-projection screen and head-tracking functionality, is an excellent tool for the simulation of construction environments featuring restricted and elevated support surfaces (Figure 9.2).

Other equipment used in the VR laboratory include a portable force platform (Accusway, Advanced Mechanical Technologies, Inc., Watertown, MA), an Optotrak-3020 motion measurement system (Northern Digital Inc., Waterloo, Ontario), and since 2010, a six-camera VICON motion measurement system (VICON, Oxford Metrics Group, Oxford, United Kingdom), as well as a Biolog Data Recorder (Biolog 3992, UFI, Morro Bay, CA) capturing users' physiological responses.

9.4.2 Validation Studies of Virtual Models of Elevated Workplaces

9.4.2.1 Comparative Evaluation of Real and Virtual Height Effects

Humans detect and recognize elevation and exposure to elevation exclusively by the available visual information. Elevation in the environment is perceived by the observer as a vertical distance from the surface of support to a lower surface, in other words, height perception is a special case of depth perception (Gibson and Walk, 1960). Exposure to elevation may induce a psychological effect of fear of falling, leading to physiological and behavioral protective responses, and it can also affect human balance control due to degraded visual stabilization. The visual nature of the height effects suggested that they could be successfully induced by computer-generated models in a VR system.

To test this idea, a study was designed to compare the human responses with height exposure in real and similar virtual environments of elevation. The NIOSH high-bay laboratory, with the 3 m and 9 m high balconies, used in the preliminary studies was selected as the real height environment, and a virtual model of the laboratory was created with reasonable detail in the NIOSH VR laboratory. The study compared human perceptions of height, danger, and anxiety, as well as skin conductance and heart-rate responses and postural instability effects, in real and virtual height environments. The study hypothesis

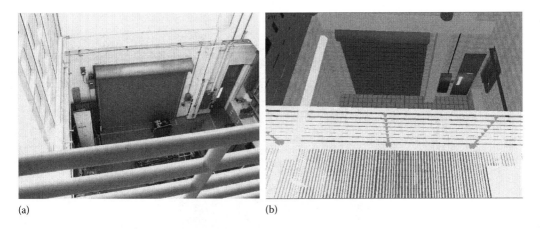

(a)   (b)

FIGURE 9.3
Exposure to elevation effects—validation study. View over the railing of a 9 m-high balcony: (a) Real height environment in the High-bay laboratory. (b) Virtual height environment in the SSVR system.

was that virtual and real height can induce similar perceptions, physiological responses, and postural instability effects.

The participants performed "lean-over-the-railing" and standing tasks on real and comparable virtual balconies, using the SSVR system (Figure 9.3). The results indicated that the virtual display of elevation provided realistic perceptual experience and induced some physiological responses and postural instability effects comparable with those found in a real environment (Simeonov et al., 2005). The study demonstrated that the simulation of elevated work environment in a SSVR system, although with reduced visual fidelity, is a valid tool for safety research. A direct follow-up from this study was the design of virtual models of scaffolding and a roof on a construction site for the safe evaluation of human performance and the assessment of new fall prevention strategies.

9.4.2.2 Augmenting Virtual Scaffolding Models with Real Planks

A scaffolding structure on a construction site is one of the most challenging work environments, involving the use of narrow and deformable or unstable planks as walking and working surfaces at height. Designing an adequate virtual model of a scaffold required careful consideration and representation of the properties of the supporting surfaces. A key question was whether a visual representation of a plank on the floor of the SSVR system was sufficiently realistic. The strong interactions between the destabilizing visual conditions at elevation and the properties of the support surface in the preliminary studies suggested that including a real plank in the virtual scaffolding model may provide a more realistic experience and improve the overall fidelity of the model.

To test this hypothesis, a study was designed to investigate the effect of adding real planks to virtual scaffolding models of elevation on human performance in the SSVR system. Construction workers and inexperienced controls performed walking tasks on real and virtual planks at three virtual heights (0, 6, 12 m) and under two scaffolding platform–width conditions (30 and 60 cm) (Figure 9.4). Gait patterns, walking instability measurements, and cardiovascular reactivity were assessed. The results showed differences in human responses to real and virtual planks in walking patterns, instability score, and heart rate interbeat intervals, and they supported the hypothesis that real planks in the virtual scaffolding models enhanced its realism (Hsiao et al., 2005).

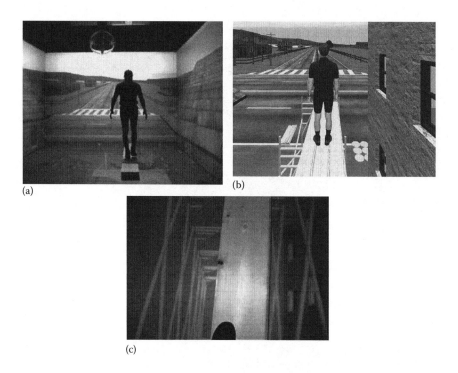

FIGURE 9.4
Virtual model of elevated and restricted surface (scaffolding)—validation study. (a) A participant on a virtual scaffold with a real wood plank. (b) A participant on a virtual scaffold with virtual planks. (c) A view over the edge of a real scaffolding plank at virtual height.

This study had two main implications: First, it suggested a new element of a comprehensive fall prevention strategy—the significant differences in performance between construction workers and the control group implied that inexperienced construction workers may benefit from a program of balance-control training in simulated environments before entering a construction job at elevation; second, it provided supporting experimental evidence for the adoption of augmented virtual models of elevated construction environments for the purpose of injury-prevention research.

9.4.3 Evaluation Studies Using Virtual Models of Elevated Workplace

9.4.3.1 Footwear Effects on Balance at Restricted and Elevated Surfaces

Simple measures to improve workers' balance at elevation can serve as efficient interventions for the reduction of fall incidents and injuries. As already mentioned, appropriate use of visual references is one of the very effective strategies for balance control at elevation. Although inexpensive, such an approach still requires some environment and behavioral modifications and thus the involvement of the worker. A strategy of using passive controls, which minimize worker involvement, is more promising since it guarantees automatic compliance. For example, appropriate design modification of personal protective equipment, including work apparel and shoes, may improve balance control by enhancing critical aspects of the available sensory information (Hsiao and Simeonov, 2001).

Due to the visually induced instability at elevation, a worker's postural control system relies heavily on proprioceptive inputs from the feet. Shoes act as a sensory interface between the worker's feet and the support surface, and their design can modify balance control (Menz and Lord, 1999). To evaluate the importance of shoe type and style as a potential balance-control intervention in an elevated construction environment, a study was designed using a virtual model of a sloped residential roof in the SSVR system (Figure 9.5). To enhance the realism of the simulation, the virtual model was augmented with real roofing planks (15 and 25 cm wide), which were used as walking surfaces. The study hypothesis was that shoe design may be essential for adequate control of balance on a narrow walking surface at elevation.

Construction workers were tested while walking on the narrow planks at a virtual residential roof in the SSVR system (Figure 9.6). Dependent variables included three athletic and three work shoe styles (Figure 9.7) and walking surfaces with different widths and lateral slopes. The angular velocities of the trunk and the foot in the medial–lateral direction

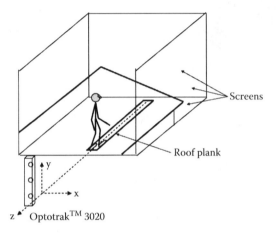

FIGURE 9.5
Footwear effects on walking stability at restricted and elevated surface—evaluation study. Schematic diagram of the virtual roof setup with a real wood roofing plank in the SSVR system.

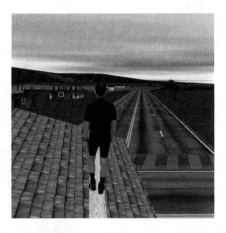

FIGURE 9.6
Footwear effects on walking stability at restricted and elevated surface—evaluation study. Virtual roof environment with a participant on a roofing plank.

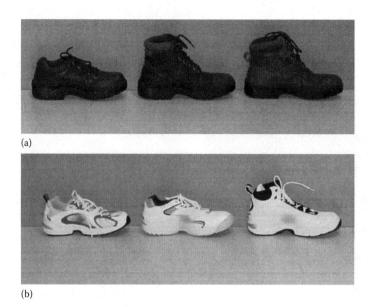

(a)

(b)

FIGURE 9.7
Footwear effects on walking stability at restricted and elevated surface—evaluation study. The test shoes: (a) work shoe styles, from left to right: low-cut work shoe; work boot; safety boot; (b) athletic shoe styles, from left to right: running shoe; tennis shoe; basketball shoe.

were calculated from data recorded with a motion measurement system. Workers' perceptions of instability were assessed with a computerized visual analogue scales.

The results demonstrated that shoe style significantly affected workers' walking instability at elevated work environments and highlighted two major shoe-design pathways for improving walking balance at elevation: enhancing rear foot motion control; and improving ankle proprioception (Simeonov et al., 2008). The study adds to the knowledge in the area of balance control by emphasizing the role of footwear as a critical human–support surface interface during work on narrow surfaces at height. The results can be used for footwear selection and footwear design improvements to reduce the risk of falls from elevation.

9.4.3.2 Vibration Effects on Balance at Restricted and Elevated Surfaces

The risk of falls from height on a construction site increases under conditions that degrade workers' postural control. At elevation, workers depend heavily on sensory information from their feet to maintain balance. Prior research suggested that imperceptible random vibrations applied to the feet can improve the feedback from the pressure receptors and lead to a more stable posture, especially in conditions with reduced visual input (Priplata et al., 2003). A study was designed to test the "sensory enhancement" hypothesis that subsensory (undetectable) random mechanical vibrations at the plantar surface of the feet can improve a worker's balance at elevation; and an alternative "sensory suppression" hypothesis that suprasensory (detectable) random mechanical vibrations can have a degrading effect on balance in the same experimental settings.

Workers were tested while standing in standard and semitandem postures on instrumented gel insoles, which applied sub- or suprasensory levels of random mechanical vibrations to the feet (Figure 9.8). The tests were conducted in a SSVR system, which

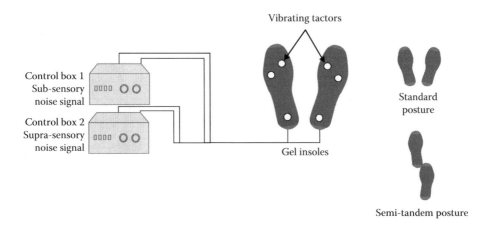

FIGURE 9.8
Vibration effects on balance at restricted and elevated surface—evaluation study. The instrumented gel insoles experimental setup.

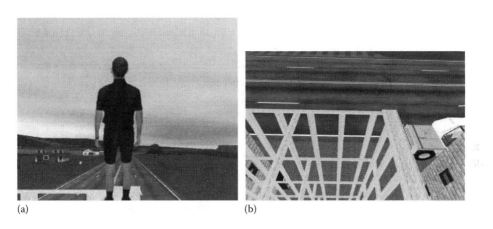

FIGURE 9.9
Vibration effects on balance at restricted and elevated surface—evaluation study. Experimental setup in the SSVR system. (a) A participant on a restricted surface at simulated elevation. (b) A view over the edge of a restricted surface at virtual height.

simulated a narrow plank at elevation on a construction site (Figure 9.9). Upper-body kinematics was assessed with a motion measurement system. Postural stability effects were evaluated by conventional and statistical mechanics sway measures as well as trunk angular displacement parameters. The results did not confirm the "sensory enhancement" hypothesis but provided evidence for the "sensory suppression" hypothesis. The suprasensory vibration had a destabilizing effect, which was considerably stronger in the semitandem posture and affected most of the sway variables (Simeonov et al., 2011).

There are several practical implications from this study. Sensory suppression associated with vibration in a supporting structure at a construction site may increase the risk of losing balance. Construction workers at height might be at elevated risk of falling if they can detect vibrations under their feet. This risk may be significantly increased when they are in a more unstable posture (on a beam or narrow plank). To reduce the possibility of losing balance, mechanical vibration to the supporting structures used as walking/working surfaces should be minimized when performing tasks at elevation.

9.4.4 Methodological Limitations and Future Research

The reviewed VR validation research addressed the following major issues related to the virtual modeling of elevated workplaces: postural stability and fearful responses during elevation exposure, and responses to tactile augmentation with real walking surfaces. The level of understanding of these key aspects and the associated limitations in virtual modeling development and evaluation will determine, to a great extent, the validity of any future research applications.

The similarly increased postural instability at both real and virtual elevation as compared with that at ground level is related to deficient visual information; however, the underlying causation mechanisms in both environments are different. While postural instability at real heights is the result of exposure to distant visual scenes and references, instability in the virtual height simulation is related to a different set of visual information deficiencies in addition to the distant references, including image resolution, contrast, and refresh rate or, in other words, reduced visual fidelity. In this respect, for certain tasks, the destabilizing effects of a virtual height model may be overrepresented. Overall, virtual elevation modeling still remains a very safe and efficient research methodology for the evaluation of instability control measures in dangerous workplaces. The fast progress in digital technology and the constant improvements in the visual fidelity of digital imaging will improve this aspect of the virtual height models.

The comparable anxiety and skin conductance responses to height exposures at real and virtual environments demonstrate the viability of the modeling approach. The reduced danger perceptions at virtual height, however, and especially the lack of heart rate response, indicated some deficiencies in the models. A defining factor is the lower level of visual fidelity of the simulation, which is also reflected in the reduced height/distance perceptions in the virtual model. The low danger levels of the simulated protected exposure in the validation study may have also contributed to the absence of heart rate response. Another powerful factor in VR is the associated level of presence—awareness of the laboratory setup and the simulated exposure can significantly reduce danger perceptions. Overall, it is reasonable to consider that the levels of induced postural threat and the corresponding fearful responses from exposure to virtual height models will be generally underrepresented. Further improvements in VR technology will lead to an increased sense of presence and ultimately more realistic danger perceptions.

The augmented virtual models with real walking surfaces enhanced both the visual and the somatosensory feedback and thus improved the overall sensory fidelity of the virtual model. However, the presence of a real object in the virtual world could be a distraction and thus reduce the sense of presence in the participants. The cost/benefit balance between distraction and enhancement effects from adding a real object in a virtual environment depends exclusively on the specific application. For the walking tasks during height exposure on a scaffold, the presence of real planks with visible edges and unstable/deformable walking surfaces provided improved fidelity both for walking instability and fearful responses.

The success and validity of future studies using VR models of elevated workplaces will depend on many factors, defined by the specific research goals and objectives of the investigation. Careful consideration of the benefits and limitations of this methodology is needed to design a study with optimal outcomes. Some of the future projects at virtual height may address ladder design modification effects on transitioning tasks at elevation; work–rest cycles and task-related fatigue interactions with height; and specially designed exercise programs as potential balance control enhancing interventions. Other potential research applications may include the development and evaluation of balance control screening procedures to detect and warn of dangerous personal conditions before work at elevation is initiated.

9.5 Other Related Research Using Real Models of Height

In recent years, exposure to height has become a well-established research paradigm for inducing postural threat. A growing number of research studies have used experimental setups of restricted and elevated surfaces to study postural behavior under conditions of increased postural threat (Adkin et al., 2000, 2002; Brown et al., 2002; Caetano et al., 2009; Carpenter et al., 1999, 2001; Davis et al., 2009; Delbaere et al., 2009; Sibley et al., 2007; Tersteeg et al., 2012). Most of these studies have been directed to identify postural control mechanisms, aiming toward an understanding how fear of falling, especially among the elderly, might influence postural control. Overall, the studies have suggested that postural control is modulated according to the degree of the impending postural threat and that the postural accommodations that occur would serve well to reduce the risk of falling (Brown et al., 2002).

The experimental methods in these studies have included setups with relatively low threat levels, for example, standing 50 cm away from the edge of a 160 cm-high platform (Adkin et al., 2000); or walking on restricted surfaces at elevations of less than 60 cm (Caetano et al., 2009; Delbaere et al., 2009; Brown et al., 2002). In setups with higher threat levels, such as standing at the edge of a platform with heights of up to 3.2 m (Davis et al., 2009) or walking on a 22 cm-wide surface at height of 3.5 m (Tersteeg et al., 2012), the participants have been protected by fall-arrest equipment. Along with young and healthy individuals (Adkin et al., 2000; Davis et al., 2009; Brown et al., 2002; Tersteeg et al., 2012), the test participants have included elderly subjects (Brown et al., 2002; Caetano et al., 2009; Delbaere et al., 2009), height-fearful subjects (Delbaere et al., 2009), and participants with pathological conditions (Caetano et al., 2009).

The findings of these studies indicate that postural threat triggers protective responses. Such responses for standing trials have been characterized with tighter postural control, described by smaller amplitude and higher frequency of COP displacements as compared with standing on the ground (Adkin et al., 2000). In walking trials, responses include an increase in the double-support phase, reduced velocity, reduced step length, and reduced cadence (Brown et al., 2002; Caetano et al., 2009; Delbaere et al., 2009). Overall, the reviewed research suggests that the postural control responses and the mechanisms associated with danger perceptions serve as a very powerful and effective fall prevention strategy. However, the direct applicability of the results from these studies for the prevention of falls from elevation may be limited—it is known that experienced workers in construction are well adapted to working at elevation, and as a consequence their danger perceptions are generally low.

Some of the limitations of the studies with real height models are that they use either conditions with low danger exposure or conditions with protected exposures. Exposing participants to lower heights may not be sufficiently dangerous and thus may induce some anxiety but not real fearful perceptions—it has been suggested that fear and anxiety are associated with two different postural behaviors (Davis et al., 2009). Harnessing the participants in studies with exposure to higher elevations affects their knowledge of the consequences of a potential fall and therefore reduces their danger perceptions and consequently affects their postural behavior. Furthermore, the full body harness and the attached lanyard might also affect their movement strategies to some extent.

Another limitation of the real height models is that, in laboratory conditions, they cannot recreate the visual exposure of an elevated workplace, characterized by open space and distant visual references, and therefore they cannot account well for some of the visual effects of height. Since these studies were not directed to understand and prevent falls from elevation, their experimental setups did not try to simulate all aspects of a dangerous workplace at elevation, include the use of experienced construction workers as test subjects, or to test appropriate fall prevention strategies.

9.6 Measures to Control Falls from Restricted and Elevated Surfaces

9.6.1 Fall Protection Measures

Applying fall protection measures remains the required practice for controlling the risk of fall injury during construction work on restricted and elevated surfaces (OSHA, 1995). However, short-term construction work on restricted and elevated surfaces usually associated with temporary and unfinished structures, presents a number of challenges for the effective application of fall protection systems. Some of these challenges and the available solutions are discussed in the OSHA's Fall Protection Directive STD 03-11-002 "Compliance Guidance for Residential Construction" (OSHA, 2011) and the related preceding documents.

Fall protection measures are directed and designed to reduce the dangerous consequences of a fall after it has initiated, to reduce the risk of impact injury by controlled transfer of the kinetic energy of the falling body to a supporting structure. A broader view is to recognize that a fall event can be characterized by three phases: initiation, descent, and landing (Hayes et al., 1993). With this classification, the initiation phase uses protective barriers and fall restraint systems. The descent phase uses fall-arrest systems, catch platforms, and safety nets; and the impact phase uses soft landing systems.

Fall protection systems have also been classified as collective and individual, passive and active by their protective range and the need for user action in achieving their protective function (Sulowski, 1993). Collective fall protection systems (protective barriers, catch platforms, nets, and soft landing systems) are generally passive, while individual fall protection systems (fall-arrest and restraint systems) are mostly active. From a design perspective, collective fall protection systems can also be described as environment-oriented interfaces, while individual fall protection systems can be considered as human-oriented interfaces. The environment-oriented interfaces are engineering control systems designed to guard or modify the hazard, while the human-oriented interfaces are personal protective equipment systems guarding the human.

All these classes of fall protection system have their advantages and disadvantages and their optimal application areas as related to controlling the fall injury risk on restricted and elevated surfaces. Furthermore, numerous products are available and new products are continuously being introduced to the market, providing flexibility in the selection and implementation of an effective fall protection approach. Collective and passive systems controlling the fall initiation are preferred but are not always practical for use on restricted and elevated surfaces. Simplicity of operation, reliability, cost-effectiveness, efficiency, requiring minimal time for installation and removal, and having minimal interference with the work task, would be among the desired features of an optimal fall protection system.

The most common fall protection measure used to control the fall risk on restricted and elevated surfaces remains the fall-arrest system. The fall-arrest system is an active, individual fall protection system consisting of a full body harness, a lanyard, and an anchor point. The anchor point remains the most critical element in the system because its installation has to be customized for the specific environment. Selecting or designing an appropriate anchor point is not a trivial task, and usually requires careful work-task analysis and environment-specific engineering design solutions. Adequate preplanning is a key requirement for the proper selection and installation of anchor points and the safe application of a fall-arrest system (NAHB, 2007). Many light temporary structures may not be sufficiently strong and stable to support a fall-arrest anchor—in such cases a structure-independent fall-arrest anchoring system may be needed.

An effective alternative solution to the use of fall protection for controlling the fall risk on restricted and elevated surfaces is the application of strategies to reduce or eliminate the fall hazard by using equipment for work at elevation and by modifying the construction work process.

9.6.2 Hazard Elimination Measures

Aerial lifts have become the equipment of choice for work at elevation in construction, maintenance, and repair jobs. Aerial lifts eliminate the need for work on restricted and elevated surfaces by providing convenient and flexible access to elevated locations with a controllable and protected platform. Scissor lifts, telescoping and articulating boom lifts, and a variety of other personnel aerial lifts have been suggested as a safer alternative measure to working at elevation (OSHA, 2011). Aerial lifts are designed for safe operation; however, proper training is an important safety requirement for lift operators. One limitation of the aerial lifts is that they are heavy equipment that requires road access around a structure, which may not always be available on small construction sites with light structures. In addition, some contractors may not be able to afford such equipment, and renting it for small construction projects may be economically infeasible (OSHA, 2011).

The best fall risk control solution would be to reduce or eliminate the need to work at elevation altogether by preplanning the construction process and applying constructability and safety-in-design principles. Constructability analyses can be applied to identify tasks that can be finished on the ground. Furthermore, implementing safety-in-design principles may reduce the need for work at elevation both in the short term during the construction process and in the long term during maintenance (Toole and Gambatese, 2008). For example, roof truss assembly on the ground has been suggested as a construction practice that can eliminate or reduce the need for standing and working on restricted and elevated surfaces such as wall top plates and trusses (NHAB, 2007).

9.7 Conclusions

Falls from elevation remain a persistent occupational injury problem, mainly associated with construction activities. On construction projects, workers are frequently exposed to restricted and elevated surfaces without any protection. Furthermore, these conditions present a considerable challenge for the workers' postural control systems and therefore increase their risk of falls. Conducting research on falls from elevation to identify risk factors and test fall prevention strategies remains a challenging research area due to the associated injury risk for both researchers and test participants.

The NIOSH fall prevention research program established a cornerstone in VR technology applications. The reviewed research studies provide a theoretical and methodological background for using VR as an adequate tool for simulating elevated construction workplaces. Furthermore, the studies deliver direct results of practical significance in fall prevention. Future VR applications will benefit from the enhanced fidelity of the subsequent generations of displays, improved computer graphics, and increased computing power.

Workers do not always correctly perceive the increased instability associated with height exposure on restricted and unstable support surfaces, which may increase their risk of loss-of-balance and fall incidents. Taking advantage of existing or enhanced visual references may be an effective approach to improving workers' balance at elevation. Other effective strategies to improve workers' balance at elevation may be the adequate selection of shoes, which act as sensory interfaces between the foot and the support surface; and avoiding or eliminating conditions such as detectable vibration in the support surface, which can degrade sensory inputs.

Fall protection remains the required practice for controlling the risk of fall injury during construction work on restricted and elevated surfaces; however, the short-term work on temporary or unfinished structures presents a number of challenges for the effective application of these systems. The best strategy to control falls from restricted and elevated surfaces is to modify and reduce the hazard by using safer equipment for work at elevation, or to completely eliminate the hazard by preplanning the construction process and applying constructability and safety-in-design principles.

9.8 Disclaimers

The findings and conclusions in this report are those of the author and do not necessarily represent the views of the National Institute for Occupational Safety and Health (NIOSH). Mention of any company or product does not constitute endorsement by NIOSH. In addition, citations to websites external to NIOSH do not constitute NIOSH endorsement of the sponsoring organizations or their programs or products. Furthermore, NIOSH is not responsible for the content of these websites. All web addresses referenced in this document were accessible as of the publication date.

References

Adkin, A. L., Frank, J. S., Carpenter, M. G., and Peysar, G. W., Postural control is scaled to level of postural threat. *Gait Posture*, 12, no. 2, (2000): 87–93.

Adkin, A. L., Frank, J. S., Carpenter, M. G., and Peysar, G. W., Fear of falling modifies anticipatory postural control. *Exp Brain Res*, 143, no. 2, (2002): 160–170.

Bauby, C. E., and Kuo, A. D., Active control of lateral balance in human walking. *J Biomech*, 33, no. 11, (2000): 1433–1440.

Berthoz, A., Lacour, M., Soechting, J. F., and Vidal, P.-P., The role of vision in the control of posture during linear motion. In *Progress in Brain Research: Reflex Control of Posture and Movement* (New York: Elsevier, 1979), 197–209.

Bles, W., Kapteyn, T. C., Brandt, T., and Arnold, F., The mechanism of physiological height vertigo: II. Posturography. *Acta Oto-Laryngol*, 89, no. 3–6, (1980): 534–540.

BLS [Bureau of Labor Statistics], 2013. Census of Fatal Occupational Injuries in 2012. http://www.bls.gov/iif/oshwc/cfoi/cftb0276.pdf

BLS [Bureau of Labor Statistics], 2014. Nonfatal cases involving days away from work in 2012. http://www.bls.gov/iif/data.htm

Brandt, T., Arnold, F., Bles, W., and Kapteyn, T. C., The mechanism of physiological height vertigo, I. Theoretical approach and psychophysics. *Acta Oto-Laryngol*, 89, (1980): 513–523.

Brown, L. A., and Frank, J. S., Postural compensations to the potential consequences of instability: Kinematics. *Gait and Posture*, 6, no. 2, (1997): 89–97.

Brown, L. A., Gage, W. H., Polych, M. A., Sleik, R. J., and Winder, T. R., Central set influences on gait. *Exp Brain Res*, 145, (2002): 286–296.

Caetano, M. J. D., Gobbi, L. T. B., Del Rosario Sánchez-Arias, M., Stella, F., and Gobbi, S., Effects of postural threat on walking features of Parkinson's disease patients. *Neurosci Lett*, 452, (2009): 136–140.

Carpenter, M. G., Frank, J. S., and Silcher, C. P., Surface height effects on postural control: A hypothesis for a stiffness strategy for stance. *J Vestib Res*, 9, (1999): 277–286.

Carpenter, M. G., Frank, J. S., Silcher, C. P., and Peysar, G. W., The influence of postural threat on the control of upright stance. *Exp Brain Res*, 138, (2001): 210–218.

Cloe, W. W., *Occupational Fatalities Related to Roofs, Ceilings and Floors as Found in Reports of OSHA Fatality/Catastrophe Investigations*. (Washington, DC: Occupational Safety and Health Administration, US Department of Labor, 1979).

Davis, P. R., Human factors contributing to slips, trips, and falls. *Ergonomics*, 26, (1983): 51–59.

Davis, J.R., Campbell, A.D., Adkin, A.L., and Carpenter, M.G., The relationship between fear of falling and human postural control. *Gait & Posture*, 29, no. 2 (2009): 275–279.

Delbaere, K., Diana, L. S., Geert, C., and Stephen, R. L., Concern about falls elicits changes in gait parameters in conditions of postural threat in older people. *J Gerontol A Biol Sci Med Sci*, 64, (2009): 237–242.

Donelan, J. M., Kram, R., and Kuo, A., Mechanical and metabolic determinants of the preferred step width in human walking. *Proc Royal Soc London, Series B*, 268, (2001): 1985–1991.

Ellis, J. N., Walking and working surface hazards. In *Introduction to Fall Protection*, 3rd edn, Chapter 4, pp. 77–114. (Des Plaines, IL: American Society of Safety Engineers, 1994).

Eng, J. J., Winter, D. A., and Patla, A. E., Strategies for recovery from a trip in early and late swing during human walking. *Exp Brain Res*, 102, (1994): 339–349.

Gibson, E. J., and Walk, R. D., The "visual cliff." *Scientific Amer*, 202, (1960): 64–71.

Grönqvist, R., Abeysekera, J., Gard, G., Hsiang, S. M., Leamon, T. B., Newman, D. J., Gielo-Perczak, K., Lockhart, T. E., and Clive, Y.-C. Pai IV. Human-centered approaches in slipperiness measurement. *Ergonomics*, 44, no. 13, (2001): 1167–1199.

Hayes, W. C., Myers, E. R., Morris, J. N., Gerhart, T. N., Yett, H. S., Lipsitz, L. A., Impact near the hip dominates fracture risk in elderly nursing home residents who fall. *Calc Tiss Int*, 52, (1993): 192–198.

Horak, F. B., Postural orientation and equilibrium: What do we need to know about neural control of balance to prevent falls? *Age Ageing* 35–S2, (2006): ii7–ii11.

Horak, F. B., and Nashner, L. M., Central programming of postural movements: Adaptation to altered support-surface configurations. *J Neurophysiol*, 55, (1986): 1369–1381.

Hsiao, H., and Simeonov, P., Preventing falls from roofs: A critical review. *Ergonomics*, 44, no. 5, (2001): 537–561.

Hsiao, H., Simeonov, P., Dotson, B., Ammons, D., Kau, T-Y., and Chiou, S., Human responses to augmented virtual scaffolding models. *Ergonomics*, 48, no. 10, (2005): 1223–1242.

Janicak, C. A., Fall-related deaths in the construction industry. *J Safety Res*, 29, no. 1, (1998): 35–42.

Lau, G., Ooi, P. L., and Phoon, B., Fatal falls from a height: The use of mathematical models to estimate the height of fall from the injuries sustained. *Forensic Sci Int*, 93, (1998): 33–44.

Lee, D. N., and Lishman, R. L., Visual proprioceptive control of stance. *J Human Mov Studies*, 1, no. 2, (1975): 87–95.

Liberty Mutual (Liberty Mutual Research Institute for Safety). *2013 Liberty Mutual Workplace Safety Index*. (Hopkinton, MA: Liberty Mutual Research Institute for Safety, 2013).

Maki, B. E., Gait changes in older adults: Predictors of falls or indicators of fear? *J Am Geriat Soc*, 45, (1997): 313–320.

Maki, B. E., Holliday, P. J., and Topper, A. K., A prospective study of postural balance and risk of falling in an ambulatory and independent elderly population. *J Gerontol: Med Sci*, 49, (1994): M72–M84.

Maki, B. E., McIlroy, W. E., and Perry, S. Influence of lateral destabilization on compensatory stepping responses. *J Biomech*, 29, no. 2, (1996): 343–353.

MacKinnon, C. D., and Winter, D. A., Control of whole body balance in the frontal plane during human walking. *J Biomech*, 26, no. 6, (1993): 633–644.

Menz, H. B., and Lord, S. R., Footwear and postural stability in older people. *J Am Podiatric Med Assoc*, 89, no. 7, (1999): 346–357.

Menzies, R. G., and Clarke, J. C., Danger expectancies and insight in acrophobia. *Behav Res Ther*, 33, no. 2, (1995): 215–221.

NAHB (National Association of Home Builders). *NAHB-OSHA Fall Protection Handbook*. (Washington, DC: National Association of Home Builders, 2007).

OSHA (Occupational Safety and Health Administration). General Industry Standard (29 CFR 1910). Subpart D: "Walking-working surfaces." (Washington, DC: US Department of Labor, 1984). https://www.osha.gov/pls/oshaweb/owadisp.show_document?p_table=standards&p_id=9715

OSHA (Occupational Safety and Health Administration). Safety and Health Regulations for Construction (29 CFR 1926). Subpart M: Fall Protection. (Washington, DC: US Department of Labor, 1995). https://www.osha.gov/pls/oshaweb/owadisp.show_document?p_table=STANDARDS&p_id=10757.

OSHA (Occupational Safety and Health Administration). Safety and Health Regulations for Construction (29 CFR 1926). Subpart L "Scaffolds." (Washington, DC: US Department of Labor, 1996). https://www.osha.gov/pls/oshaweb/owadisp.show_document?p_table=standards&p_id=10752.

OSHA (Occupational Safety and Health Administration). Safety and Health Regulations for Construction (29 CFR 1926). "Safety Standards for Steel Erection"—Final Rules 66:5317–5325. (Washington, DC: US Department of Labor, 2001). https://www.osha.gov/pls/oshaweb/owadisp.show_document?p_id=16290&p_table=FEDERAL_REGISTER.

OSHA (Occupational Safety and Health Administration). Safety and Health Regulations for Construction (29 CFR 1926). Subpart M: Fall Protection, Directive STD 03-11-002 "Compliance Guidance for Residential Construction." (Washington, DC: US Department of Labor, 2011). https://www.osha.gov/pls/oshaweb/owadisp.show_document?p_table=DIRECTIVES&p_id=4755.

Patla, A. E., Age-related changes in visually guided locomotion over different terrains: Major issues. In *Sensorimotor Impairment in the Elderly* (Dordrecht: Kluwer, 1993), 231–252.

Patla, A. E., Understanding the role of vision in the control of human locomotion. *Gait & Posture*, 5, (1997a): 54–69.

Patla, A. E., Slips, trips and falls: Implications for rehabilitation and ergonomics. In *Perspectives in Rehabilitation Ergonomics* (London: Taylor & Francis, 1997b), 196–209.

Patla, A. E., Strategies for dynamic stability during adaptive human locomotion. *IEEE Eng Med Biol Mag*, 22, no. 2, (2003): 48–52.

Paulus, W. M., Straube, A., and Brandt, T. H., Visual stabilization of posture. Physiological stimulus characteristics and clinical aspects. *Brain*, 107, no. 4, (1984): 1143–1163.

Peterka, R. J., and Benolken, M. S., Role of somatosensory and vestibular cues in attenuating visually induced human postural sway. *Exp Brain Res*, 105, (1995): 101–110.

Priplata, A. A., Niemi, J. B., Harry, J. D., Lipsitz, L. A., and Collins, J. J., Vibrating insoles and balance control in elderly people. *Lancet*, 362, no. 9390, (2003): 1123–1124.

Sibley, K. M., Carpenter, M. G., Perry, J. C., and Frank, J. S., Effects of postural anxiety on the soleus H-reflex. *Hum Mov Sci*, 26, no. 1, (2007): 103–112.

Simeonov, P., and Hsiao, H., Height, surface firmness and visual reference effects on balance control. *Inj Prev*, 7(Suppl I), (2001): i50–53.

Simeonov, P., Hsiao, H., Dotson, B., and Ammons, D., Control and perception of balance at elevated and sloped surfaces. *Human Factors*, 45, (2003): 136–147.

Simeonov, P., Hsiao, H., Dotson, B., and Ammons, D., Height effects in real and virtual environments. *Human Factors* 47, no. 2, (2005): 430–438.

Simeonov, P., Hsiao, H., Powers, J., Ammons, D., Amendola, A., Kau, T.-Y., and Cantis, D., Footwear effects on walking balance at elevation. *Ergonomics*, 51, no. 12, (2008): 1885–1905.

Simeonov, P., Hsiao, H., Powers, J., Ammons, D., Kau, T.-Y., and Amendola, A., Postural stability effects of random vibration at the feet of construction workers in simulated elevation. *Appl Ergonomics*, 42, (2011): 672–681.

Stoffregen, T. A., Flow structure versus retinal location in the optical control of stance. *J Exp Psychol: Human Percept Perform*, 11, (1985): 554–565.

Sulowski, A. C., *Fundamentals of Fall Protection*. (Toronto: International Society for Fall Protection, 1993).

Suruda, A., Fosbroke, D., and Braddee, R., Fatal work-related falls from roofs. *J Safety Res*, 26, no. 1, (1995): 1–8.

Tersteeg, M. C. A., Marple-Horvat, D. E., and Loram, L. D., Cautious gait in relation to knowledge and vision of height: Is altered visual information the dominant influence? *J Neurophysiol*, 107, (2012): 2686–2691.

Toole, M. T., and John, G. The trajectories of prevention through design in construction. *J Safety Res* 39, (2008): 225–230.

Warner, K. G., and Demling, R. H., The pathophysiology of free-fall injury. *Annals Emerg Med*, 15, no. 9, (1986): 1088–1093.

Woollacott, M. H., and Tang, P.-F., Balance control during walking in the older adult: Research and its implications. *Phys Therapy*, 77, no. 6, (1997): 646–660.

Yardley, L., Watson, S., Britton, J., Lear, S., and Bird, J. Effect of anxiety arousal and mental stress on the vestibulo-ocular reflex. *Acta Oto-Laryngol*, 115, no. 5, (1995): 597–602.

Zimolong, B. Hazard perception and risk estimation in accident causation. In *Trends in Ergonomics/ Human Factors II* (Amsterdam: Elsevier, 1985), 463–470.

10

Role of Support Surfaces in Preventing Slip, Trip, and Fall Injuries

Kurt E. Beschorner and Mark S. Redfern

CONTENTS

ABSTRACT   The properties of support surfaces such as flooring, ramps, sidewalks, and outdoor ground have a dramatic impact on a person's fall risk. For example, floor surface properties that can lead to falls are insufficient friction with shoes, resulting in a slip; uneven surfaces causing the toe to collide with the ground during the swing phase of gait and leading to a trip; and the compliance of a floor surface impacting an individual's balance. This chapter specifically focuses on current research to describe the effects of walkway surfaces on slip and trip risk as well as injury risk after a fall.

10.1 Design for Preventing Slips

The coefficient of friction (COF) between a shoe and the floor is a key parameter that impacts the risk for slips and falls. The introduction of a contaminant, such as water, oils, or powders, can also dramatically affect the COF. The probability of a slip occurrence is largely dependent on the difference between the amount of friction required for walking, typically termed the *required coefficient of friction* (RCOF), and the amount of friction at the shoe–floor interface, typically termed the *available coefficient of friction* (ACOF) [1,2]. The probability of a slip is described using a logistic regression equation (Equation 10.1) where β_0 and β_1 are constants (Figure 10.1) [2]. Therefore, the probability of a slip can be reduced either by increasing the ACOF [1] or by reducing the RCOF. Flooring characteristics have a dramatic impact on the ACOF and therefore have a substantial impact on slipping risk.

$$p_{slip} = \frac{e^{(\beta_0 + \beta_1{}^*(ACOF-RCOF))}}{1 + e^{(\beta_0 + \beta_1{}^*(ACOF-RCOF))}} \tag{10.1}$$

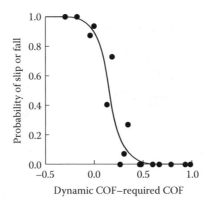

FIGURE 10.1
Logistic regression fit to actual data points relating the difference between ACOF and RCOF to the probability of a slip or fall. (Reproduced with permission from Hanson, J.P. et al., *Ergonomics*, 42(12), 1619–1633, 1999.)

The use of slip-resistant flooring has been epidemiologically demonstrated to have significant potential for reducing slip and fall accidents. For example, a prospective study demonstrated that the number of occupational slip and fall accidents in limited-service restaurant workers decreased by 21% for each 0.1 increase in the ACOF throughout the restaurant kitchen [3]. Comprehensive slip and fall prevention programs that included the new installation of slip-resistant flooring have been demonstrated to be effective in preventing slips in the retail [4] and health-care industries [5]. Slip-resistant flooring clearly is an effective component of a slip and fall prevention strategy. Identifying the appropriate flooring for a specific environment can be enhanced through testing of various flooring surfaces and understanding the underlying tribological mechanisms that are relevant to shoe–floor COF.

Several devices and standardized methods are available for testing shoe–floor contaminant COF. The most commonly used devices can be broadly categorized into whole-shoe testers, impact testers, and steady-state drag testers (Figure 10.2, Table 10.1). Whole-shoe testers, which include the SATRA STM 603 [6] and the portable slip simulator [7], typically move an entire shoe across a floor surface while applying normal forces, shoe–floor angles, and sliding speeds approximating those that occur during actual walking and recording the forces between the shoe and the floor (Figure 10.2a). In whole-shoe testing, COF is calculated as the average ratio of friction forces to normal forces over a period of time when the shoe is sliding relative to the floor. The American Society for Testing and Materials (ASTM) International (ASTM F2913) [8] and the International Standards Organization offer testing standards for whole-shoe testers (EN ISO 13287) [9]. Impact devices can be categorized into two subcategories: pendulum tribometers (Figure 10.2b) and variable angle tribometers (Figure 10.2c). Pendulum tribometers measure COF by swinging a shoe material that is attached to the end of a pendulum against a floor sample. COF is determined from the energy that is lost in the collision, which is measured by recording the maximum height that the pendulum reaches after the collision. Europe, Australia, and New Zealand maintain standard methods for measuring COF with pendulum testers [10–12]. Variable angle devices measure COF based on an iterative process of changing the angle of contact between the shoe material and the flooring. The COF is determined based on the angle at which the shoe material transitions from sticking to the floor surface to slipping. The shoe material can either be accelerated to the floor surface using gravity (as with the portable inclinable articulated strut tribometer) or pneumatically (as with the variable incidence tribometer) [13]. ASTM International formerly maintained standards for these devices, but the

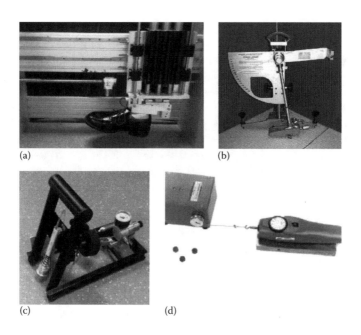

(a)   (b)

(c)   (d)

FIGURE 10.2
Different devices are available to measure COF between shoes and floor surfaces, including whole-shoe testers (a), pendulum skid testers (b), variable angle testers (c), and drag testers (d). More detailed information for these slip-testers is found in Table 10.1. (Figures 10.2b and 10.2d reproduced with permission from Chang, W.-R., et al., *Ergonomics*, 44(13), 1233–1261, 2001.)

TABLE 10.1

Overview of Common Slip-Testers

Name	Category	Manufacturer/Model[a]	Related Standards	Figure
Portable slip simulator	Whole-shoe tester	(None)	ASTM F2913, EN ISO 13287	Figure 10.2a
Slip resistance testing machine	Whole-shoe tester	SATRA STM 603	ASTM F2913, EN ISO 13287	None
British portable skid tester	Impact (pendulum) tester	Munro Stanley 89100/ABS/BSI	DIN EN 14231; AS/NZS 4663:2013; AS/NZS 4586:2013	Figure 10.2b
Portable inclinable articulated strut tribometer	Impact (variable angle) tester	Brungraber Mark II	ASTM F1677-05 (withdrawn)	None
Variable incidence tribometer	Impact (variable angle) tester	English XL	ASTM F1679-04 (withdrawn)	Figure 10.2c
Horizontal pull slipmeter	Drag tester	American slip meter ASM 725	ASTM F609-05 (2013)	Figure 10.2d

[a] Other manufacturers and models may be available that comply with a specific standard.

standards were withdrawn in 2004 and 2005 [14,15]. Drag slip-testers are devices by which a shoe sample is dragged across a floor surface at a constant speed. These devices allow the determination of the static COF (the force required to move the shoe material from a static position) and the dynamic COF (the force required to maintain relative motion between two surfaces). Typically, the static COF is determined as the ratio of peak shear force to the vertical force as the shoe material starts sliding, and the dynamic COF is the average force once the object is in motion. Numerous standard methods are available for drag testers, including from ASTM International, the American National Standards Institute/National Floor Safety Institute (ANSI/NFSI), and the Japanese Institute of Standards [16–18]. This chapter only covers some common tribometers. A more comprehensive review of slip-resistance testing methods is available in [19].

Ultimately, shoe-floor COF is created by the interaction between the shoe and the floor material at a microscopic level. A visually flat floor surface is actually made up of many microscopic peaks and valleys, termed *asperities*. During typical contact during standing or walking, softer shoe materials viscoelastically form around the hard asperities of flooring (Figure 10.3). The contact between these surfaces results in two types of COF, which are described in the tribology literature as adhesion and hysteresis. Adhesion friction refers to the adhesive or bonding force that occurs at the surface between two contacting surfaces that resists sliding motion [20]. Hysteresis friction is caused by energy loss as flooring asperities deform viscoelastic shoe asperities [20]. Adhesion COF is largely dependent on the contact area formed between the two surfaces, while hysteresis COF is dependent on the level of viscoelastic deformation in the shoe material [21,22]. Adhesion COF tends to be large for conforming surfaces (i.e., two smooth and flat surfaces), since these surfaces allow higher contact area. Thus, smooth and polished floor surfaces tend to have high adhesion COF [23,24]. Hysteresis COF, however, is larger for support surfaces that cause significant deformation in the shoe surface. Increased deformation can be caused by rough flooring surfaces, because these surfaces have larger asperities, which will dig into the shoe material. The positive correlation between floor roughness and hysteresis COF and the negative correlation between floor roughness and adhesion COF have been demonstrated experimentally [23,24] and verified using finite element models [25,26] (Figure 10.4 demonstrates these concepts). The effect of roughness on COF with a dry surface may be subtle and inconsistent, since higher-roughness floors increase hysteresis COF but reduce adhesion COF. With fluid-contaminated surfaces, however, the total COF is likely to be more dependent on the hysteresis COF than the adhesion COF, since adhesion COF is more sensitive to fluid contaminants. Specifically, fluid contaminants with higher viscosity tend to cause larger reductions in adhesion COF [24]. Hysteresis COF, on the other hand, is

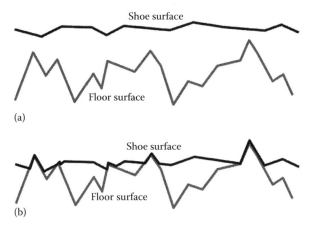

FIGURE 10.3
During contact, the shoe surface (original geometry shown in (a)) conforms around the asperities of the harder floor (b).

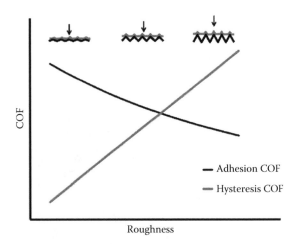

FIGURE 10.4
Conceptual model for how adhesion COF (black line) and hysteresis COF (gray line) vary with roughness. As surface roughness increases, a reduction in contact area reduces the adhesion COF, whereas an increase in shoe material deformation increases the hysteresis COF. The pictures above the figure represent a low-roughness (left), moderate-roughness (center), and high-roughness (right) flooring against a deformable shoe surface (gray lines).

largely independent of fluid contaminant in the boundary lubrication regime [24]. Thus, floor surfaces with high hysteresis COF and low adhesion COF are minimally affected by fluid contaminants. This point is demonstrated by data from Chang, who found that the correlations between roughness and COF were higher in the presence of higher-viscosity fluids [27]. Designing and selecting flooring that increases hysteresis COF (i.e., rough and textured surfaces), therefore, provides protection against slips in the presence of high-viscosity fluids that minimize adhesion.

Floor roughness is a characteristic that can be measured using a profilometer and characterized with roughness parameters. Profilometers can be broadly categorized as two-dimensional (2-D) contact profilometers and three-dimensional (3-D) optical profilometers. The 2-D profilometers yield an array of asperity heights (Equation 10.2a and Figure 10.5a), whereas the 3-D profilometers yield a surface of asperity heights (Equation 10.2b and Figure 10.5b). The measured asperity height data from a 2-D contact profilometer is typically processed by high-pass frequency filtering (removing large wavelength asperities from the arrays) with cutoff lengths between 0.8 and 8.0 mm to characterize the roughness of the surface. After profilometer data have been collected and processed, several roughness parameters can be calculated, including the average roughness (R_a), the root mean square roughness (R_q), the average peak asperity height over five equal sections (R_{pm}) (see Figure 10.5a for example of five equal sections), the average distance between the most extreme valley and the most extreme asperity across five equal sections (R_{tm}) and the average slope (Δ_a). These parameters tend to be correlated with each other and are good predictors of lubricated COF [28,29]. Stronger correlations have been observed between floor roughness parameters and COF in the presence of high-viscosity fluid contaminants [29,30], indicating that roughness may be more critical in conditions where adhesion COF is low. Data processing methods can have an impact on the correlations. Chang et al. found that the highest correlation between roughness parameters and COF is observed when the data are processed with a high-pass filter using a cutoff frequency of 8.0 mm [29].

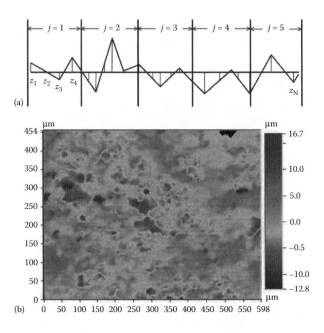

FIGURE 10.5
Example of a 2-D profile discretized into n points and five equally sized sections (a) and a 3-D profile surface (b). The color scale in the 3-D profile represents height of asperities, with the highest points represented by red colors and the lowest points represented by blue colors.

$$z_{2D\_Profilometer} = \left[z_1, z_2, z_3, ..., z_n \right] \tag{10.2a}$$

$$z_{3D\_Profilometer} = \begin{bmatrix} z_{11} & z_{12} & \cdots & z_{1n} \\ z_{21} & z_{22} & \cdots & z_{2n} \\ \vdots & \vdots & \ddots & \vdots \\ z_{n1} & z_{n2} & \cdots & z_{nn} \end{bmatrix} \tag{10.2b}$$

$$R_a = \frac{\sum_{i=1}^{n} |z_i|}{n}$$

$$R_q = \frac{1}{n} \sum_{i=1}^{n} \sqrt{z_i^2}$$

$$R_{pm} = \frac{1}{5} \sum_{j=1}^{5} z_{max,j}$$

$$R_{tm} = \frac{1}{5} \sum_{j=1}^{5} \left(z_{max,j} - z_{min,j} \right)$$

$$\Delta_a = \frac{1}{n} \sum_{i=1}^{n} \left| \frac{dz_i}{dx} \right| \tag{10.3}$$

Another tribological mechanism relevant to shoe–floor–contaminant COF is hydrodynamic pressures. Hydrodynamic pressures occur when shoes without tread slide over a floor surface in the presence of a fluid contaminant [31,32]. Hydrodynamic pressures are more prevalent in the presence of high-viscosity fluids [32,33]. Floor surfaces with macroscopic features (i.e., surfaces with wavelengths on the order of 1 mm) can take the form of waviness or raised edges and have an impact on the slip resistance through fluid pressure dispersion. The waviness of a floor surface can be characterized by including millimeter-scale wavelength features in the roughness calculations. This is performed by altering the processing parameters used on the profilometer data, specifically, the cutoff frequency of the filters, or by using a low-pass filter instead of a high-pass filter [29]. Waviness parameters (W_a, W_q, W_{pm}, W_{tm}, and $W_{\Delta a}$) are then calculated using the same roughness equations (Equation 10.3) but with the low-pass filtered data. Chang et al. found that the COF of a nontreaded shoe against different floor surfaces had a better correlation with waviness parameters than roughness parameters as the viscosity of the fluid increased [29], while COF had a better correlation with roughness in the presence of lower-viscosity fluids (Figure 10.6). The results of this study can be explained by the fact that fluid drainage capacity (related to the floor waviness) was more important for high-viscosity fluids, while hysteresis COF (related to the floor roughness) was more important for low-viscosity fluids. Therefore, in certain environments where high-viscosity fluids are expected, designing or selecting flooring with macroscopic features and high waviness may be appropriate to minimize hydrodynamic effects.

Few studies have considered the impact that the floor material properties, independent of roughness or waviness, have on shoe–floor COF. However, tribological theory provides some insights into how flooring material properties impact shoe–floor COF. Generally, the material from which the floor is made has a smaller impact on COF than the topography of the flooring. Most flooring materials (concrete, ceramic, and vinyl composition tile [VCT]) are significantly stiffer than shoe materials, which causes the shoe material to conform around the floor asperities. In certain cases, when the floor material is not substantially more rigid than the shoe material (i.e., carpet or compliant surfaces), increased COF values have been observed [2]. One interesting animal study that has implications for human slip prevention found fewer slips in cattle with soft flooring [34]. The explanation of this effect is that increased COF occurs due to the ability of the floor to deform around the shoe geometry, allowing more contact area and lower contact pressures, which could increase hysteresis and adhesion COF [25]. Clearly, research into flooring material characteristics and their potential for affecting slips could lead to new approaches to fall prevention.

Selecting or designing the appropriate flooring for the prevention of slipping accidents depends on the expected use of the floor. Increasing floor roughness is critical for floors that are expected to be exposed to liquid contaminants. In the presence of high-viscosity fluids, increased surface waviness may also be important to allow drainage channels.

10.2 Design for Preventing Trips

Tripping is a major source of falling accidents occupationally and among elderly adults. A review article by Courtney et al. found that trips accounted for between 17% and 22% of occupational falling accidents [35]. Tripping is also prevalent among older adults: previous studies have reported that 53% of falls by elderly adults in their home are initiated

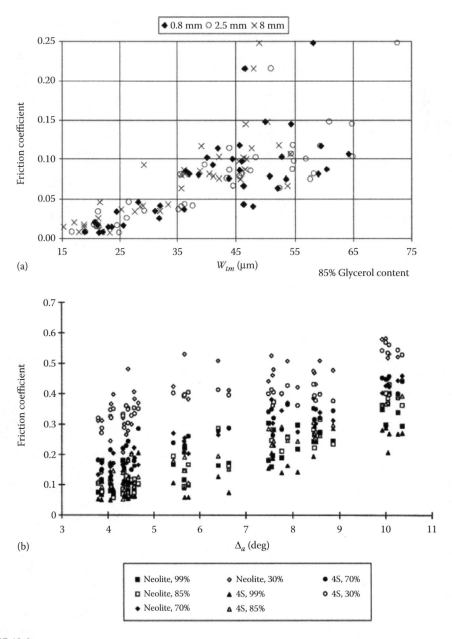

FIGURE 10.6
Correlation between waviness and COF (a) and correlation between roughness and COF (b). (Figure 10.6a reproduced with permission from Chang, W.-R. et al., *Ergonomics*, 47(8), 890–906, 2004; Figure 10.6b reprinted from *Applied Ergonomics*, 32(2), Chang, W.-R., The effect of surface roughness and contaminant on the dynamic friction of porcelain tile, 173–184, Copyright (2001), with permission from Elsevier.)

by a trip [36], and 21% of falls in long-term care facilities are initiated by a trip [37]. Thus, reducing tripping accidents is a priority for preventing fall-related injuries across multiple environments.

Tripping and stumbling accidents typically occur when a part of the foot collides with the floor surface during the swing phase or due to improper foot placement at the heel contact phase of gait. Laboratory studies on tripping have revealed that a sudden obstruction of the swing leg causes an impulse force, which introduces angular momentum that rotates the trunk forward toward the ground [38]. A person's strength, coordination, and reaction time directly affect recovery from a trip. Older adults, who are known to have reduced strength and reaction time, are at increased risk of falling from a trip compared with younger adults [39,40]. Thus, walkway surfaces that minimize tripping events are an important fall prevention strategy in general, and particularly for aging adults.

The trajectory of the foot during the swing phase is the key factor in tripping and is controlled to avoid a collision with the floor. The kinematics of the foot during swing include an initial elevation of the foot soon after toe-off, followed by a local minimum during mid-swing, and then a local maximum just before heel contact (Figure 10.7). Minimum foot clearance (MFC) has been quantified using a marker attached to the toe [41,42], a virtual marker at the most anterior and inferior location of the toe (reproduced using a geometric model based on two other markers) [43,44], the fifth metatarsal–phalangeal joint [42], and a point cloud representing the geometry of the shoe outsole (tracked relative to a local coordinate system) [45]. The local minimum during mid-swing is particularly relevant to tripping risk, since the foot is moving at about three times the gait speed during this part of swing [46]. The MFC during the swing phase is somewhat variable both within subjects and across environmental conditions. MFC has a mean of 13–20 mm [42,46] and a standard deviation of 4 mm [46]. Begg et al. noted a positive skewness in the distribution [43]. This positive skewness indicates that more variability occurs above the mean than below the mean, which suggests that foot control prioritizes minimizing small MFC values as opposed to the overall variability [43]. Mean MFC values increase, however, during circumstances where the floor is perceived as possibly uneven. For example, Schulz reported that MFC values increased from 11.1 to 22.2 mm when subjects walked on an uneven surface [45]. The increase in MFC (11.1 mm) between even and uneven floors was similar to the height of the obstacles on the uneven floors. Thus, circumstances where ground-level obstacles occur *unexpectedly* are most likely to cause a trip event.

Tripping hazards are relatively frequent, particularly for outdoor walking surfaces. For example, a survey of uneven flooring found between 12 and 50 points of abrupt changes in elevation exceeding 13 mm over a mile of outdoor sidewalks in different California cities, whereas no abrupt changes in curb height were identified in an indoor mall [47]. To reduce hazards related to unexpected ground-level obstacles, the ASTM F1637-13 standard recommends beveling transitions between 6 and 12 mm and using marked transitions (stairs or ramps) to connect surfaces with an elevation change of greater than 12 mm [48]. Several intervention studies have included controls to reduce sudden floor-elevation changes as part of a comprehensive program [5,49,50]. Future research, however, is needed to quantify trip and fall risk based on the frequency or distribution of walkway trip hazards.

10.3 Design for Impact Attenuation and Postural Balance

One countermeasure to prevent falling injuries is to reduce the impact force on the hip or pelvis experienced during a fall by using low-stiffness flooring. Specifically, low-stiffness flooring can reduce the impact forces and reduce the risk of a fracture. Low-stiffness flooring can take the form of a portable mat (commonly referred to as a bedside mat) or

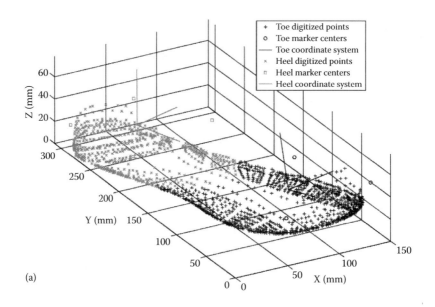

(a)

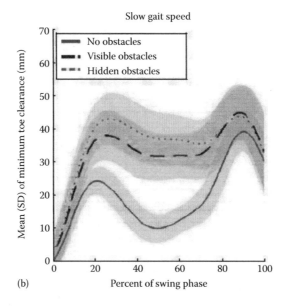

(b)

FIGURE 10.7
(a) Digitized point cloud of a shoe heel (gray data points) and toe (black data points); (b) time series of foot clearance in the absence of floor obstacles, in the presence of visible obstacles (dashed line), and in the presence of hidden obstacles (dotted line). (Reprinted from *Journal of Biomechanics*, 44(7), Schulz, B.W., Minimum toe clearance adaptations to floor surface irregularity and gait speed, 1277–1284, Copyright (2011), with permission from Elsevier.)

a soft material that is installed beneath another walkway surface (also known as safety, low-stiffness, or compliant floor). However, low floor stiffness can also negatively affect balance, which could increase the probability of a fall. Therefore, the use of this counter-measure should reduce impact forces experienced during a fall without having a substantial negative impact on balance, which would increase the risk of a fall.

Previous research has consistently demonstrated through both human-based and mechanical testing that lower-stiffness flooring reduces impact during a fall. Mechanical testing has been conducted using impact tests in which a model of the hip (i.e., the proximal femur region) collides against the floor surface. The ability of the flooring to attenuate impact forces is assessed based on the energy absorption [51] or the peak force [52,53] measured using a load cell or force plate (Figure 10.8a). Human testing has been conducted using a technique referred to as *pelvis release experiments* [54] (Figure 10.8b). In these experiments, a person is released from a sling above a force plate, and the impact force is measured as his or her pelvis strikes the floor. Both mechanical and human-based studies have demonstrated a reduction in peak forces for more compliant flooring. Force attenuation of between 20% and 80% has been observed with safety flooring [52,53]. Foam surfaces and bedside mats have been shown to attenuate forces and increase energy absorption more than other safety flooring or standard flooring [51–53]. For example, bedside mats were found to have 3.8–8 times better energy absorption, whereas safety floors had just 1.5–3.5 times better energy absorption than commercial-grade carpet [51]. Similarly, average force attenuation during impact testing was between 24% and 47% for safety flooring but was between 52% and 76% for different foam surfaces relative to rigid flooring [53]. Laing et al. found good agreement between the peak forces predicted by a simple linear mass spring model based on the material properties of the flooring and pelvis release experiments [54]. This finding suggests that there is a direct relationship between material properties and impact attenuation. However, when considering the effects of flooring on balance (i.e., fall risk), softer floor materials may not always be the best option.

Compliant flooring, while offering impact attenuation, can also negatively affect balance. This trade-off is demonstrated in a study by Simpson et al. which found that carpeted floors led to more frequent falls, yet a lower fracture rate, than uncarpeted wood or concrete flooring [55]. Compliant flooring negatively affects balance because it does not provide a firm and stable reference point, which negatively affects the quality of ankle proprioceptive information feedback [56]. Studies have demonstrated that safety flooring can increase sway during quiet standing [52,53], but that only the most compliant flooring reduces functional balance measures and the ability to respond to a backward translation perturbation [53]. Foam mats were found to be potentially too compliant for standing balance or gait [52,53]. To provide a combined measure of the impact of flooring on impact attenuation and balance, Glinka et al. reported the ratio of energy absorption during impact testing to vertical foot deflection under simulated walking [51] (Figure 10.9). This study found that safety flooring provided better energy absorption compared with rigid flooring and bedside mats when normalized to the deflection experienced during walking. Overall, the previous research has suggested that safety flooring can provide between 15% and 50% of force attenuation with minimal impacts on balance.

10.4 Conclusions

This chapter intends to offer insights into selecting an appropriate floor surface to minimize various slip, trip, and fall risks. Increasing COF through enhanced surface roughness and waviness is particularly relevant to preventing slipping accidents in the presence of a fluid-contaminated surface. Reducing unexpected floor transitions, particularly among outdoor surfaces where these transitions are most prevalent, may be an effective strategy

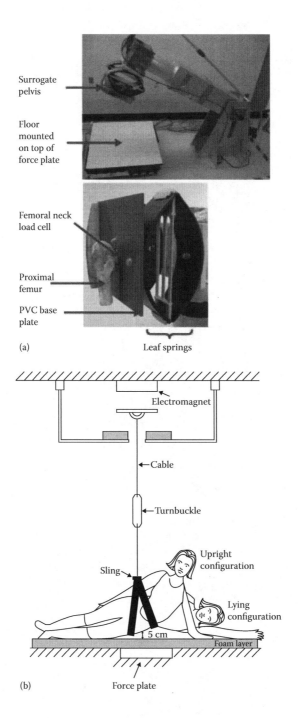

Surrogate pelvis

Floor mounted on top of force plate

Femoral neck load cell

Proximal femur

PVC base plate

(a)

Leaf springs

Electromagnet

Cable

Turnbuckle

Sling

Upright configuration

Lying configuration

5 cm

Foam layer

(b)

Force plate

FIGURE 10.8

Diagram of the hip impact simulator and the pelvis release experiment that are used to assess impact attenuation of safety flooring. (Figure 10.8a reprinted from *Accident Analysis and Prevention*, 41(3), Laing, A.C. and Robinovitch, S.N., Low stiffness floors can attenuate fall-related femoral impact forces by up to 50% without substantially impairing balance in older women, 642–650, Copyright (2009), with permission from Elsevier; Figure 10.8b reprinted from Laing, A.C., et al.: Effect of compliant flooring on impact force during falls on the hip. *Journal of Orthopaedic Research*. 2006. 24(7). 1405–1411. Copyright Wiley-VCH Verlag GmbH & Co. KGaA. Reproduced with permission.)

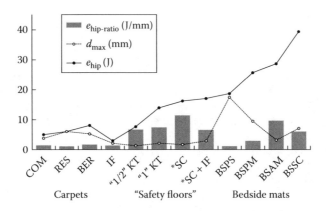

FIGURE 10.9
This graph shows the energy absorbed by different floor surfaces (solid line, e_{hip}), the surface deflection during a simulated step (dashed lines, d_{max}), and the ratio of energy absorption to surface deflection (gray bars, $e_{hip\text{-}ratio}$). The four carpet conditions (left four points) included commercial carpet (COM), residential carpet (RES), Berber carpet (BER), and a modular carpet (IF). The four safety floors (middle four points) included Kradal tile floors (Acma Industries Ltd., Wellington, New Zealand) at 13 mm thick (1/2"KT) and 25 mm thick (1"KT), SmartCell (SC, SATECH Inc., Chehalis, WA, SC) and a combination of SmartCell and modular carpet (SC + IF). The bedside mats (right four points) included soft (BSPS) and medium (BSPM) hardness products (Posey Company, Posey, Arcadia, CA), a high-density foam (BSAM) (Alimed Inc., Dedham, MA), and a medium-density foam (Skil-Care Corp., Yonkers, NY). (Reprinted from *Medical Engineering and Physics*, 35(1), Glinka, M.N., et al., Characterization of the protective capacity of flooring systems using force-deflection profiling, 108–115, Copyright (2013), with permission from Elsevier.)

for preventing trip and fall accidents. Lastly, safety flooring that reduces impact forces without reducing balance offers potential for reducing injuries that result from a fall.

No single walkway surface offers complete protection against different slip, trip, and fall accidents. The selection of an appropriate walkway surface should consider the hazards and likely fall-initiating events of a specific environment. For example, slip-resistant flooring should be prioritized in a kitchen environment where fluid contaminants are most likely to cause slipping accidents. However, falls may be caused by individual factors (poor balance, neurological events, etc.) in certain long-term care environments. In such environments, slip-resistant flooring may be less effective at preventing falls, and safety flooring, which protects the individual after a fall, may be needed to reduce fall-related injuries.

References

1. Burnfield, J. and C. Powers, Prediction of slip events during walking: An analysis of utilized coefficient of friction and available slip resistance. *Ergonomics*, 2006. 49(10): pp. 982–985.
2. Hanson, J.P., M.S. Redfern, and M. Mazumdar, Predicting slips and falls considering required and available friction. *Ergonomics*, 1999. 42(12): pp. 1619–1633.
3. Verma, S.K., Chang, W.R., Courtney, T.K., Lombardi, D.A., Huang, Y.H., Brennan, M.J., Mittleman, M.A., Ware, J.H., and Perry, M.J., A prospective study of floor surface, shoes, floor cleaning and slipping in US limited-service restaurant workers. *Occupational and Environmental Medicine*, 2011. 68(4): p. 279.
4. Lewis, R., Pier 1's slip-and-fall success. *Occupational Health and Safety*, 1997. 66(8): pp. 34–38.

5. Bell, J.L., Collins, J.W., Wolf, L., Grönqvist, R., Chiou, S., Chang, W.R., Sorock, G.S., Courtney, T.K., Lombardi, D.A., and Evanoff, B., Evaluation of a comprehensive slip, trip and fall prevention programme for hospital employees. *Ergonomics*, 2008. 51(12): pp. 1906–1925.

6. Wilson, M., Development of SATRA slip test and tread pattern design guidelines. Slips, Trips, and Falls: Pedestrian Footwear and Surfaces, ASTM STP 1103, 1990: pp. 113–123.

7. Aschan, C., Hirvonen, M., Mannelin, T., and Rajamäki, E, Development and validation of a novel portable slip simulator. *Applied Ergonomics*, 2005. 36(5): pp. 585–593.

8. ASTM International, *ASTM F2913–11: Standard Test Method for Measuring the Coefficient of Friction for Evaluation of Slip Performance of Footwear and Test Surfaces/Flooring Using a Whole Shoe Tester.* 2011, ASTM International: West Conshohocken, PA.

9. European Standards and International Standards Organization, *EN ISO 13287: Personal Protective Equipment—Footwear—Test Method for Slip Resistance.* 2012, Danish Standards: Charlottenlund, Denmark.

10. Deutsches Institut für Normung, *DIN EN 14231: Natural Stone Test Methods—Determination of the Slip Resistance by Means of the Pendulum Tester.* 2003, DIN Deutsches Institut für Normung: Berlin.

11. Standards Australia and Standards New Zealand, *AS/NZS 4663:2013: Slip Resistance Measurement of Existing Pedestrian Surfaces.* 2013, Standards Australia International: Sydney.

12. Standards Australia and Standards New Zealand, *AS/NZS 4586:2013: Slip Resistance Classification of New Pedestrian Surface Materials.* 2013, Standards Australia International: Sydney.

13. Chang, W.-R. and S. Matz, The slip resistance of common footwear materials measured with two slipmeters. *Applied Ergonomics*, 2001. 32(6): pp. 549–558.

14. ASTM International, *ASTM F1679–04: Standard Test Method for Using a Variable Incidence Tribometer (VIT).* 2004, ASTM International: West Conshohocken, PA.

15. ASTM International, *ASTM F1677–05: Standard Test Method for Using a Portable Inclineable Articulated Strut Slip Tester (PIAST).* 2005, ASTM International: West Conshohocken, PA.

16. American National Standards Institute and National Floor Safety Institute, *ANSI/NFSI B101.1: Test Method for Measuring Wet SCOF of Common Hard-Surface Floor Materials.* 2009, National Floor Safety Institute: Southlake, TX.

17. ASTM, *ASTM F609–05: Standard Test Method for Using a Horizontal Pull Slipmeter (HPS).* 2005, ASTM International: West Conshohocken, PA.

18. Japanese Industrial Standard, *JIS 1 1509-12:2008: Test Methods for Ceramic Tiles: Part 12—Determination of Slip Resistance.* 2008, Japanese Standards Association: Tokyo, Japan.

19. Chang, W.-R., Grönqvist, R., Leclercq, S., Brungraber, R.J., Mattke, U., Strandberg, L., Thorpe, S.C., Myung, R., Makkonen, L., and Courtney, T.K., The role of friction in the measurement of slipperiness, Part 2: Survey of friction measurement devices. *Ergonomics*, 2001. 44(13): pp. 1233–1261.

20. Bhushan, B., *Introduction to Tribology.* 2013, Wiley: New York.

21. Bowden, F.P. and D. Tabor, *The Friction and Lubrication of Solids-{Part I}.* 1950, Clarendon: Oxford.

22. Tabor, D., Friction, adhesion and boundary lubrication of polymers, in *Advances in Polymer Friction and Wear.* 1974, Springer. pp. 5–30.

23. Cowap, M.J.H., Moghaddam, S.R.M., Menezes, P.L., and Beschorner, K.E., Contributions of adhesion and hysteresis to coefficient of friction between shoe and floor surfaces: Effects of floor roughness and sliding speed. *Tribology-Materials, Surfaces & Interfaces*, 2015. 9(2): pp. 77–84.

24. Strobel, C.M., Strobel, C.M., Menezes, P.L., Lovell, M.R., and Beschorner, K.E., Analysis of the contribution of adhesion and hysteresis to shoe–floor lubricated friction in the boundary lubrication regime. *Tribology Letters*, 2012. 47(3): pp. 341–347.

25. Mirhassani Moghaddam, S.R., *Finite Element Analysis of Contribution of Adhesion and Hysteresis to Shoe-Floor Friction.* 2013, University of Wisconsin-Milwaukee: Milwaukee, WI.

26. Mirhassani Moghaddam, S.R. and K.E. Beschorner. Finite element model of shoe-floor hysteresis friction, in *STLE Tribology Frontiers.* 2014, Society of Tribologists and Lubrication Engineers: Chicago, IL.

27. Chang, W.-R., The effect of surface roughness and contaminant on the dynamic friction of porcelain tile. *Applied Ergonomics*, 2001. 32(2): pp. 173–184.
28. Chang, W.-R., The effect of surface roughness on dynamic friction between neolite and quarry tile. *Safety Science*, 1998. 29(2): pp. 89–105.
29. Chang, W.-R., Grönqvist, R., Hirvonen, M., and Matz, S., The effect of surface waviness on friction between Neolite and quarry tiles. *Ergonomics*, 2004. 47(8): pp. 890–906.
30. Chang, W.-R., The effect of surface roughness on the measurement of slip resistance. *International Journal of Industrial Ergonomics*, 1999. 24(3): pp. 299–313.
31. Beschorner, K.E., Albert, D.L., Chambers, A.J., and Redfern, M.S., Fluid pressures at the shoe–floor–contaminant interface during slips: Effects of tread & implications on slip severity. *Journal of Biomechanics*, 2014. 47(2): pp. 458–463.
32. Singh, G. and K.E. Beschorner, A method for measuring fluid pressures in the shoe-floor-fluid interface: Application to shoe tread evaluation. *IIE Transactions on Occupational Ergonomics and Human Factors*, 2014. 2(2): pp. 53–59.
33. Beschorner, K., Lovell, M., Higgs III, C.F., and Redfern, M.S., Modeling mixed-lubrication of a shoe-floor interface applied to a pin-on-disk apparatus. *Tribology Transactions*, 2009. 52(4): pp. 560–568.
34. Rushen, J. and A. De Passillé, Effects of roughness and compressibility of flooring on cow locomotion. *Journal of Dairy Science*, 2006. 89(8): pp. 2965–2972.
35. Courtney, T.K., Sorock, G.S., Manning, D.P., Collins, J.W., and Holbein-Jenny, M.A., Occupational slip, trip, and fall-related injuries—can the contribution of slipperiness be isolated? *Ergonomics*, 2001. 44(13): pp. 1118–1137.
36. Blake, A., Morgan, K., Bendall, M., Dallosso, H., Ebrahim, S., Arie, T., Fentem, P., and Bassey, E., Falls by elderly people at home: Prevalence and associated factors. *Age and Ageing*, 1988. 17(6): pp. 365–372.
37. Robinovitch, S.N., Feldman, F., Yang, Y., Schonnop, R., Leung, P.M., Sarraf, T., Sims-Gould, J., and Loughin, M., Video capture of the circumstances of falls in elderly people residing in long-term care: An observational study. *The Lancet*, 2013. 381(9860): pp. 47–54.
38. Pijnappels, M., M.F. Bobbert, and J.H. van Dieën, Contribution of the support limb in control of angular momentum after tripping. *Journal of Biomechanics*, 2004. 37(12): pp. 1811–1818.
39. Pavol, M.J., Owings, T.M., Foley, K.T., and Grabiner, M.D., The sex and age of older adults influence the outcome of induced trips. *The Journals of Gerontology Series A: Biological Sciences and Medical Sciences*, 1999. 54(2): pp. M103–M108.
40. Pijnappels, M., M.F. Bobbert, and J.H. van Dieën, Push-off reactions in recovery after tripping discriminate young subjects, older non-fallers and older fallers. *Gait and Posture*, 2005. 21(4): pp. 388–394.
41. Menant, J.C., Steele, J.R., Menz, H.B., Munro, B.J., and Lord, S.R., Effects of walking surfaces and footwear on temporo-spatial gait parameters in young and older people. *Gait and Posture*, 2009. 29(3): pp. 392–397.
42. Mills, P.M. and R.S. Barrett, Swing phase mechanics of healthy young and elderly men. *Human Movement Science*, 2001. 20(4): pp. 427–446.
43. Begg, R., Best, R., Dell'Oro, L., and Taylor, S., Minimum foot clearance during walking: Strategies for the minimisation of trip-related falls. *Gait and Posture*, 2007. 25(2): pp. 191–198.
44. Winter, D.A., Patla, A.E., Frank, J.S., and Walt, S.E., Biomechanical walking pattern changes in the fit and healthy elderly. *Physical Therapy*, 1990. 70(6): pp. 340–347.
45. Schulz, B.W., Minimum toe clearance adaptations to floor surface irregularity and gait speed. *Journal of Biomechanics*, 2011. 44(7): pp. 1277–1284.
46. Winter, D.A., Foot trajectory in human gait: A precise and multifactorial motor control task. *Physical Therapy*, 1992. 72(1): pp. 45–53.
47. Ayres, T. and R. Kelkar, Sidewalk potential trip points: A method for characterizing walkways. *International Journal of Industrial Ergonomics*, 2006. 36(12): pp. 1031–1035.
48. ASTM International, *ASTM F1637-13: Standard Practice for Safe Walking Surfaces*. 2013, ASTM International: West Conshohocken, PA.

49. Stevens, M., C.A.J. Holman, and N. Bennett, Preventing falls in older people: Impact of an intervention to reduce environmental hazards in the home. *Journal of the American Geriatrics Society*, 2001. 49(11): pp. 1442–1447.

50. Stevens, M., Holman, C.A.J., Bennett, N., and De Klerk, N., Preventing falls in older people: Outcome evaluation of a randomized controlled trial. *Journal of the American Geriatrics Society*, 2001. 49(11): pp. 1448–1455.

51. Glinka, M.N., Karakolis, T., Callaghan, J.P., and Laing, A.C., Characterization of the protective capacity of flooring systems using force-deflection profiling. *Medical Engineering and Physics*, 2013. 35(1): pp. 108–115.

52. Glinka, M.N., Cheema, K.P., Robinovitch, S.N., and Laing, A.C., Quantification of the trade-off between force attenuation and balance impairment in the design of compliant safety floors. *Journal of Applied Biomechanics*, 2013. 29(5): pp. 563–572.

53. Laing, A.C. and S.N. Robinovitch, Low stiffness floors can attenuate fall-related femoral impact forces by up to 50% without substantially impairing balance in older women. *Accident Analysis and Prevention*, 2009. 41(3): pp. 642–650.

54. Laing, A.C., Tootoonchi, I., Hulme, P.A., and Robinovitch, S.N., Effect of compliant flooring on impact force during falls on the hip. *Journal of Orthopaedic Research*, 2006. 24(7): pp. 1405–1411.

55. Simpson, A., Lamb, S., Roberts, P., Gardner, T., and Evans, J.G., Does the type of flooring affect the risk of hip fracture? *Age and Ageing*, 2004. 33(3): pp. 242–246.

56. Redfern, M.S., P.L. Moore, and C.M. Yarsky, The influence of flooring on standing balance among older persons. *Human Factors: The Journal of the Human Factors and Ergonomics Society*, 1997. 39(3): pp. 445–455.

Section III

Research on Slips, Trips, and Falls

11

Hazard Concept and Falls

Sylvie Leclercq

CONTENTS

ABSTRACT Many injuries and fatalities are the result of accidental falls and, more broadly, the result of movement disturbances. The accident process ends with an injury mechanism, which embodies the hazard concept involved in risk assessment and prevention strategies. If hazard taxonomy exists, it would seem that no category describes it precisely enough to represent the injury mechanism resulting from movement disturbance or loss of balance in particular. This chapter focuses on the injury mechanism and discusses the notion of "circumstantial hazard," which causes an injury, when combined with the energy of the victim's disturbed movement. The part played by the kinetic energy of the victim's movement in causing injury would imply that walking or moving is a hazard. Describing the injury mechanism in any accident triggered by movement disturbance enables us to highlight the difficulties or impossibilities of assessing the related risk and of setting up the most effective protective barriers against the injury. Widening the scope of analysis from falls to any accident triggered by movement disturbance is meaningful, and it increases the visibility of many accidents that are not specifically considered.

KEY WORDS: *hazard, fall, movement disturbance, energy.*

11.1 Introduction

Many injuries and fatalities are the result of accidental falls and, more broadly, the result of movement disturbances (e.g., colliding with an element in the environment, with an object when walking, or with a machine because a wrench slips when tightening a bolt). Such accidents are referred to in the literature by the acronym STFs (slips, trips, and falls) without being explicitly defined, and they represent a major issue. Among occupational accidents in particular, they represent a 25%–65% proportion of statistical database data depending on the injuries considered, based on data provided by the Communautés Européennes (CE [European communities]) (2008), the Caisse Nationale d'Assurance Maladie des Travailleurs Salariés (CNAMTS [the French national health insurance fund for salaried workers]) (2009), the Health and Safety Executive (HSE) (2011), and the Bureau of Labor Statistics (BLS) (2012). However, no in-depth study of the injury mechanism has been conducted in so-called STF cases, although accident prevention relies notably on this mechanism. The injury mechanism is not the entire sequence of events leading to injury but only its very final stage. It describes the process by which injury occurs, and it involves some form of energy (International Classification of External Causes of Injuries [ICECI], 2004). This mechanism develops when the contact/proximity between the victim and a form of energy is such that energy absorption by human tissue becomes injury-causing. The injury mechanism embodies the hazard concept usually involved in risk assessment and prevention strategies. Hazard is related to an exposed target and to the associated risk. There is no agreed definition of risk (Aven and Renn, 2009). In this chapter, the risk is the probability of an adverse outcome (Graham and Wiener, 1995) and, more precisely, the probability that a target will encounter a hazard. *Hazard* and *target* embrace different realities, depending on whether the accident is occupational or "major," yet all accidents are represented by the same general and theoretical models using these concepts (cf. e.g., Kjellen, 2000).

The term *hazard* takes on different meanings in the literature. Definitions are not systematically given: reference is therefore implicitly made to common sense or a general dictionary definition. However, professionals in the prevention field often give a meaning to the term *hazard* that is different to common meaning. ""Hazard concept" can also be specific to models used by researchers or experts who are either working on regulations or normative texts or performing company risk assessment. These general models do not take into account the specific characteristics of so-called STFs. To our knowledge, only Leclercq et al. (2009, 2010) have detailed the hazard involved when modeling STFs. In this chapter, we will therefore first discuss how the hazard concept is defined and used in the literature on accident prevention in general and on so-called STF prevention thereafter. The injury mechanism resulting from a loss of balance (leading to a fall), which is also relevant to any injury following a movement disturbance, will then be described by focusing on the hazard concept and its specific characteristics in any accident triggered by movement disturbance. Throughout the chapter, the diversity of these accidents and their associated hazards will be illustrated based on real occupational accident accounts taken from the Études de Prévention par l'Informatisation des Comptes rendus d'Enquêtes d'Accidents (EPICEA) database (Ho et al., 1986; EPICEA, 2011) or directly from companies. EPICEA is a French anonymous database consolidating more than 18,000 occupational accident cases that have occurred since 1990 at companies operating within the French general social security system. EPICEA lists nearly all fatal occupational accidents and some accidents that were serious or significant for prevention. Finally, the consequences of the specific characteristics of the injury mechanism in accidents triggered by movement disturbance will be discussed with reference to the field of protection and prevention.

11.2 Hazard Concept within the Scope of Accident Prevention

11.2.1 Multiple Definitions

Accident-related literature and regulations often focus on so-called major accidents (spills, toxic clouds, fires, or explosions). These are related to work within a process that is liable to suddenly release considerable energy (chemical, nuclear, etc.), thereby causing serious damage to people and the environment. The definition of a hazard is therefore specifically oriented toward this kind of process. The October 2005 glossary of technological risks defines a hazard as *"an intrinsic property* of a substance (butane, chlorine, etc.), a technical system (pressurizing gas, etc.), a provision (elevation of a load), a body (microbes), etc., *likely to cause damage* to a 'vulnerable target'."* In the same year, the International Risk Governance Council (IRGC, 2005) stated that "Hazards describe the *potential for harm* or other consequences of interest. They characterize the *inherent properties* of the *risk agent* and related processes." Kjellen (2000) adopts the following definition of hazard: "a source of possible injury to personnel or *damage to the environment or material assets."* This definition is close to the general one given in Webster (2002): "a thing that has potential to cause *harm, or a source of danger."* On the other hand, Rasmussen and Svedung (2000) refer to the "hazard sources" found in a system and suggest a pragmatic classification of sources as *"physical phenomena* that may lead to damage, if not adequately controlled."

Hazard is therefore frequently characterized by an intrinsic property of an element/agent likely to cause damage to a vulnerable target, which can be a human being and/or the environment. In most cases, these definitions refer, explicitly (see, e.g., the International Classification of External Causes of Injury [ICECI, 2004]) or not, to a hazard that is external to the target and recognizable as harmful when assessing a priori the risk. For example, when mapping hazards, Koehler and Volckens (2011) project the intensity or concentration of a chemical agent onto a two-dimensional floor plan or workplace layout. In this case, the hazard is a chemical agent (a chemical energy carrier) that is external to the target and identified a priori as a clear possible cause of damage if exposure occurs. The latter hazard characteristic is highlighted by Monteau (2010) in relation to occupational accidents, stating that hazards are "incompatible with human presence"; in other words, elements with which any contact would cause injury.

Other definitions of hazard are adopted in the specific context of occupational accidents, in which the target and the negative outcome are a *human being* and *an injury*, respectively. Unlike the previous definitions, these refer to the fact that *hazards can originate from humans or objects*, which are both energy carriers (kinetic, potential, thermal, chemical, or radiant) that can be harmful to humans (Hoyos, 1980). The kinetic energy involved in the injury mechanism associated with falling from a height, for example, is carried by humans. The expression *physical ergonomic hazard* is also used to qualify work activities and/or workplace conditions that create biomechanical stress for the workers (Tak and Calvert, 2011). This type of stress, applied when sitting in specific conditions, is therefore considered a hazard (Corlett, 2008). These wider definitions of a hazard blur the boundary between *risk factors* (each situation element which increases the risk of injury, even if it is not a direct cause of injury) and *hazard* regarded as the direct cause(s) of injury.

In this section, the injury mechanism involving direct causes of injury, that is, involving the hazard, will be described for accidents triggered by movement disturbance. In keeping with Gibson (1961), who deals with injuries in general, we will consider that injury to a human being resulting from a fall or a movement disturbance is caused by an accumulation of energy transferred excessively to a body.

11.2.2 Hazard Concept Usage

In the prevention field, the hazard concept is especially used for establishing hazard categories in order to

- Assess the risk corresponding to each category, that is, the risk that a target exposed to a hazard will encounter it and sustain damage
- Implement protection and prevention actions to prevent a target encountering a hazard

Hazard categorization using the accident energy model developed by Gibson (1961) is based on forms of energy that can harm people and can be "either mechanical, thermal, radiant, chemical or electrical." The International Classification of External Causes of Injury (ICECI, 2004) is another system of classification for describing how injuries occur and is also designed to assist injury prevention. Unlike accident-dedicated categorization based on forms of energy, the latter classification refers to all injuries (diseases or accidents).

Using the accident energy model, Haddon (1980) developed 10 countermeasures, also called *Haddon's strategies*, for reducing energy-related damage. These strategies are designed to set up barriers for protecting the human being when energy is transferring to the body, or for preventing energy transfer. Kjellen (2000) subsequently summarized these strategies as illustrated in Figure 11.1.

These strategies have been widely deployed in legislation (e.g., on harmful chemical products) or in standardization (e.g., on safety of machinery) when harmful energy is external to the victim and when it can be identified a priori as a clear possible cause of damage in the event of exposure. Hazard identification is often a first stage of accident risk assessment. This identification usually covers harmful energy, external to the victim, that is a clear possible cause of damage.

11.2.3 Hazard Concept and Slip, Trip, and Fall

Faced with the question "In what energy class belongs for cutting oneself in the hand?" Rasmussen and Svedung (2000) discard hazard taxonomy based on exclusive classification of energy forms that could harm people. They in fact adopt a more pragmatic classification of hazard sources based on a number of well-defined bounded sources (energy accumulation, accumulation of toxic substances, structural integrity, and stability) and a further category entitled "others, mixed." According to this pragmatic classification, the hazard is kinetic energy in the case of a fall from a height (the surface on which the victim falls is thus neglected); and sharp edges in the case of a fall on the level, on part of a machine with sharp edges, or in the case of cutting one's hand. Similarly, when considering injuries to children falling on playgrounds, Runyan (2003) identified explicitly playground equipment and devices (not the kinetic energy accumulated during the fall),

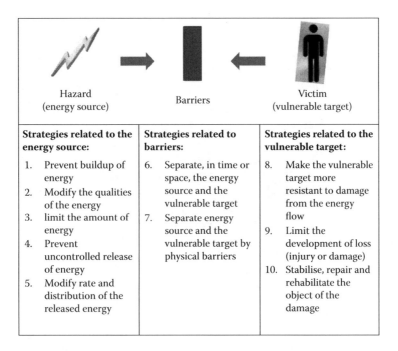

Strategies related to the energy source:	Strategies related to barriers:	Strategies related to the vulnerable target:
1. Prevent buildup of energy 2. Modify the qualities of the energy 3. limit the amount of energy 4. Prevent uncontrolled release of energy 5. Modify rate and distribution of the released energy	6. Separate, in time or space, the energy source and the vulnerable target 7. Separate energy source and the vulnerable target by physical barriers	8. Make the vulnerable target more resistant to damage from the energy flow 9. Limit the development of loss (injury or damage) 10. Stabilise, repair and rehabilitate the object of the damage

FIGURE 11.1
Haddon's 10 accident prevention strategies. (From Kjellén, U., *Prevention of Accidents through Experience Feedback*, Taylor & Francis, London, 2000. who adapted from Haddon [1980].)

as the accident-causing "agent/vehicle" (i.e., hazard). These studies prompt the following two observations. First, it would seem that, in cases of so-called STFs, the hazard is usually identified as the major direct cause of injury, obscuring the second cause, whose role in injury occurrence appears to be less. In cases of falls on a physical element in the environment, the identified hazard is either the kinetic energy or the physical element, depending on whether it is a fall from a height or a fall on the level. Secondly, the hazard in some loss-of-balance cases (e.g., a fall on the same level or on sharp edges) can be compared with the hazard in cases of a movement disturbance that does not lead to loss of balance (e.g., cutting one's hand). These observations will be questioned in the following part of the chapter when we accurately describe the injury mechanism in falls, and when we compare all accidents triggered by movement disturbance in terms of this mechanism.

11.3 Hazard and Injury Mechanism in Accidents Triggered by Movement Disturbance

11.3.1 Hazard and Injury Mechanism in Falls

This subsection is used to show that, in cases of falls (loss of balance), injury type and seriousness invariably result from a combination, at a given moment, of the energy accumulated during the fall and an element in the physical environment.

We consider the following three injury cases (the very end of the accident genesis):

- A person falling from a moderate height onto a very soft floor surface, resulting in bruises
- A person falling from a moderate height onto a curb, resulting in a fatal injury
- A person falling from his or her own height onto the corner of a table and suffering head injury

In all three cases, the kinetic energy of the victim's movement when falling is a direct cause of injury, regardless of the height of the fall. The greater the fall, the greater the accumulated energy when encountering an element in the physical environment (i.e., part of a floor, curb, or table). The injury mechanism is indeed developing when the person encounters such an element after his or her balance has been lost. Both the body and the physical element are assumed to absorb the kinetic energy accumulated at the moment of impact. The harder the physical element, the less its capacity for absorbing kinetic energy, which is then mainly absorbed by softer human tissue, thereby increasing the injury's seriousness. Soft floors in playgrounds therefore ensure greater absorption of kinetic energy by the floor than hard floors and decrease the seriousness of the injury if a fall occurs.

The contact area between the victim's body and the element in the physical environment, encountered during development of the injury mechanism, also determines the injury type and seriousness. The larger the contact area, the less injury-causing energy absorption by human tissue. Thus, the sharper the edges against which a person falls, the more serious his or her injury. Fall-related injury type and seriousness will thus depend not only on the accumulated energy when encountering an element in the physical environment, but also on the characteristics of this element (hardness, shape). Kinetic energy is therefore not the only direct cause of injury. Another element is involved in each of the three loss-of-balance cases referred to in the previous bulleted list: the soft floor surface, the curb, or the table. None of these elements alone causes the injury; every day, we interact with floor surfaces, curbs, furniture, and machines without suffering injury! Such an element of the physical environment can only be involved in an injury if it combines with sufficient kinetic energy accumulated when encountering it.

To sum up, the hazard is composite in injuries resulting from loss of balance. It combines the kinetic energy of the victim's movement and an element in the physical environment to create an injury. The same mechanism is encountered in any accident triggered by a movement disturbance that does not lead to a fall (loss of balance). The following subsection on the injury mechanism therefore applies not only to falls but also to all accidents triggered by movement disturbance.

11.3.2 Composite Hazard Involved in the Injury Mechanism

Occupational accidents occur in many different situations, and the great majority of them are triggered by movement disturbance (Leclercq et al., 2015). In these cases, the injury mechanism can result from a victim falling from a height or from his or her own height. It can also be part of a body colliding (without falling) with an element in the physical environment when walking or exerting forces on a resisting or supporting element that suddenly gives way. It can also be a person's hand slipping on a piece of ham, causing a hand injury. In all these accident cases, the injury is directly caused by the energy of the victim's disturbed movement and an element in the physical environment, which may or may not be characterized by sharp edges. For example, it may be a wall in case of an injury resulting from a person's arm striking a wall. Is the wall a hazard? It is, but only when combined with a sufficient amount of energy if there is movement disturbance. This is why Leclercq et al. (2009, 2010) have suggested calling this type of hazard a *circumstantial hazard*, that is, a physical element with which one interacts every day (a floor, furniture, a transported package, etc.) and which does not appear to be inherently harmful but can be a direct cause of injury under specific conditions. Instead of colliding with a wall, the victim could have collided with the moving parts of a machine. Moving parts appear to be inherently harmful if any contact with them causes injury. Such elements will be considered to be "*obvious hazards*" (Leclercq et al., 2009; 2010). The characteristics of an "obvious hazard" are compatible with most of the hazard definitions adopted in the accidentology field (cf. subsection 11.2.1 and Figure 11.1). The expressions *circumstantial hazard* and *obvious hazard* used in the remainder of the chapter refer to the related characteristics given in this paragraph. Furthermore, Table 11.1 provides three examples of injury mechanism in accidents triggered by movement disturbance that do not lead to a fall.

In these accidents, the victim's arm struck a duckboard when tightening a bolt, or his or her head struck a truck tailgate when climbing down, or his or her elbow struck a cupboard when transferring a patient. The victim's movement was disturbed and injury was caused by the conjunction of his or her energy of movement and a circumstantial hazard (duckboard, tailgate, or cupboard). The victim's balance was neither threatened nor lost. As in cases of falls, two components of hazard hence determine injury type and seriousness in accidents triggered by movement disturbance: the energy of the victim's disturbed movement and a physical element in the environment. The part played in the type and seriousness of injury by each of these components varies depending on both the accumulated kinetic energy at the moment of impact with the physical element and the characteristics of this physical element (shape, hardness). For example, the part played by kinetic energy in the case of a fall onto a floor from a height is greater than in the case of a fall from the victim's own height onto the same floor. Table 11.2 provides illustrations of this using five cases of injury mechanism resulting from a fall. In case "a," no physical element in the environment contributed to the injury. The energy of the victim's movement alone, in response to a slip on the floor, resulted in reactivating the knee pain. In most of the cases, however, a physical element is indeed involved in causing the injury, and this element may appear either inherently harmful, such as a rotating drum in accident case "e," or not inherently harmful, such as the lawn in accident case "b."

It should be noted that accidents caused by loss of balance and by movement disturbance, which does not lead to loss of balance do not necessarily follow the same time sequence,

TABLE 11.1

Three Cases of Accidents Triggered by Movement Disturbance That Do Not Lead to Loss of Balance

Extract from Occupational Accident Narrative Text Describing the Injury Mechanism
The wrench slipped when the victim wanted to tighten the bolt. He grazed his arm on duckboard.
When climbing down from the lorry, the employee's head struck the lowest point of the tailgate. He injured his scalp.
The employee struck his elbow against the cupboard when trying to transfer the patient from his bed to an armchair.

Source: Ho, M.T., et al., *Le Travail Humain*, 49(2), 137–146, 1986.

Note: Partial accounts of accidents are from EPICEA database or passed on by companies. EPICEA database is described by Ho, M.T. et al. (1986).

TABLE 11.2

Injury-Causing Contribution of Both Hazard Components in Five Cases ("a"–"e") of Falls

	Injury-Causing Contribution	
Extract of Accident Account Concerning Injury Mechanism	**Energy of Victim's Disturbed Movement**	**Physical Element External to the Victim (Shape, Hardness)**
Case a. The employee was in the consolidation phase following a sprained right knee. Her left foot slipped on the wet floor, provoking a reaction involving the right leg and reactivating her right-knee pain.	++++	0
Case b. Not having seen that the safety rail had been removed, the apprentice stepped back and fell 5 m onto the lawn of the house.	+++	+
Case c. The employee's feet caught in the forks (of the forklift truck) and he fell to the ground. He bruised his left thigh and left forearm.	++	++
Case d. The operator tripped on a batten lying on the ground and fell onto a concrete reinforcement starter bar....This bar entered his body at the chin.	+	+++
Case e. When servicing a cotton teasing machine...the assistant fitter slipped on the floor; he lost his balance and reached for support with his right hand, which was pulled into the rotating drum by its inertia; the hand injury required amputation.	0	++++

Source: Ho, M.T., et al., *Le Travail Humain*, 49(2), 137–146, 1986.

Note: Partial accounts of accidents are from EPICEA database or passed on by companies. EPICEA database is described by Ho, M.T. et al. (1986).

even if their injury mechanisms are of similar form. For example, Table 11.3 shows us that, in cases "a" and "b," the injuries develop shortly after movement disturbance and that movement disturbance and start of injury mechanism occur simultaneously in cases "c" and "d." The kinetic energy involved in the injury mechanism is the energy of the victim's movement when colliding with or striking an element in the environment. It can therefore be the energy accumulated before the movement disturbance (cases "c" and "d" in Table 11.3) or after movement disturbance and during the fall (cases "a" and "b" in Table 11.3).

An accurate description of the injury mechanism in a so-called STF in fact calls into question this acronym. STF associates "slip," "trip" (movement disturbances), and "fall" (one consequence of movement disturbance) without defining the set of targeted accidents. This leads to research into different groups of accidents without explicitly defining them. A definition of targeted accidents based on the concept of movement disturbance could offer a way forward from the injury prevention standpoint (cf. Leclercq et al., 2009; 2010).

11.3.3 Variety of Hazards Involved in Injury Mechanism

Subsections 11.3.1 and 11.3.2 include a wide variety of injury cases involving loss of balance and, more generally, movement disturbance. This concurs with the wide variety of occupational STF types, sites, and injury seriousness (Gaudez et al., 2006). This can be explained not only by the fact that a movement disturbance can occur a priori as soon as a worker performs a movement, but also by the fact that any physical element close to the person whose movement is disturbed can contribute to create an injury in a case involving movement

TABLE 11.3

Accidents Triggered by a Movement Disturbance with Different Time Sequences

Accident Case	Time Sequence of Events Close to Injury Mechanism
Case a. The employee's feet caught in the forks (of the forklift truck) and he fell to the ground. He bruised his left thigh and left forearm.	
Case b. When servicing a cotton teasing machine…the assistant fitter slipped on the floor; he lost his balance and reached for support with his right hand, which was pulled into the rotating drum by its inertia; the hand injury required amputation.	Movement disturbance leading to loss of balance: Impact with an element in the environment (ground, rotating drum) and start of the injury mechanism • Feet caught in the forks • Assistant fitter slipped
Case c. When climbing down from the lorry, the employee's head struck the lowest point of the tailgate. He injured his scalp.	Movement disturbance that does not lead to a loss of balance:
Case d. The employee struck his elbow against the cupboard when trying to transfer the patient from his bed to an armchair.	• Employee's head struck tailgate • Employee struck his elbow against the cupboard Impact with an element in the environment (tailgate, cupboard) and start of the injury mechanism

Source: Ho, M.T., et al., *Le Travail Humain*, 49(2), 137–146, 1986.

Note: Partial accounts of accidents are from EPICEA database or passed on by companies. EPICEA database is described by Ho, M.T. et al. (1986).

TABLE 11.4

Two Cases of Accidents Triggered by Movement Disturbances When a Manipulated Object Becomes a "Circumstantial Hazard"

Extract from Occupational Accident Narrative Text Describing Injury Mechanism
The employee pulls on the right-hand door leaf to open it. At that moment, the left-hand leaf swings toward him.
Two workers moved together a heavy item. When crossing the door window, one of the workers tripped against the window shutter stop. The worker didn't release the door in his fall and had the fingers of the right hand stuck between the door and the concrete floor.

Source: Ho, M.T., et al., *Le Travail Humain*, 49(2), 137–146, 1986.

Note: Partial accounts of accidents are from EPICEA database or passed on by companies. EPICEA database is described by Ho, M.T. et al. (1986).

disturbance. This is true even when this element does not appear as inherently harmful and whatever the element in the environment, if the kinetic energy is sufficient.

The injury mechanism representation in cases of accidents triggered by movement disturbance needs to cover at least the range of cases referred to in subsections 11.3.1 and 11.3.2. In addition, it needs to cover one more recurrent form of injury mechanism. This involves accident cases in which the object manipulated by the victim (if appropriate) can become a circumstantial hazard and thus contribute directly to the injury. For example, in the two partial accident accounts given in Table 11.4, the victim manipulated a swinging door or moved a heavy item with a colleague. When their movement was disturbed, the manipulated object was unexpectedly set into motion and contributed to injury. In such cases, the physical element manipulated by the victim becomes a circumstantial hazard when his or her movement is disturbed.

11.3.4 Representation of Injury Mechanism

Figure 11.2 illustrates the injury mechanism in any accident triggered by a movement disturbance. This is part of the model of accidents triggered by movement disturbance developed by Leclercq et al. (2009, 2010). Figure 11.2 includes elements necessary for directly causing the injury in any accident triggered by movement disturbance. These elements are combined on the basis of the range of combinations encountered in extracts of accident accounts referred to in the previous subsections.

It would appear that injury is caused by the combination of the energy of disturbed movement and an element in the physical environment. When present, this injury-causing element can be

- An obvious hazard: A physical element appearing inherently harmful and with which any contact would cause injury (e.g., moving parts of a machine)
- A negotiable hazard: A physical element with which contact would not cause injury but which appears potentially harmful if there is contact and if there is enough kinetic energy (e.g., reinforcement starter bar or object with sharp edges)

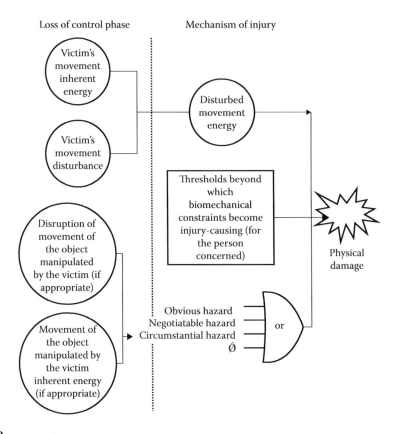

FIGURE 11.2
Mechanism of injury in case of accidents triggered by a movement disturbance. (Part of a model developed by Leclercq, S., et al., *Proceedings of the Conference of the International Ergonomics Association*, IEA, Beijing, China, 2009; Leclercq, S., et al., *PISTES*, 12(3), 16p, 2010.)

- A circumstantial hazard: A physical element with which one interacts every day, which does not appear inherently harmful but which can nevertheless be a direct cause of injury when combined with enough kinetic energy (e.g., a floor, furniture, transported package, etc.)

In Figure 11.2, the links between two elements indicate a necessity from a logical standpoint but not the progression of the final stage of the accident in time. These accidents in fact have different time sequences, depending on whether the movement disturbance and the start of injury mechanism occur simultaneously or not (cf. Section 11.3.2).

11.4 Impact on Prevention Strategies and Risk Assessment

Prevention actions are either related to a defended conception of health and safety (e.g., implementation of barriers) or to enhancing the system resilience (see Hollnagel [2010] for definition of resilience). Knowledge of the injury mechanism or hazard identification is an important step in the prevention field as explained in Section 11.2.2. Options for implementing barriers at a level close to the injury can be studied on the basis of this information. Barriers that can be implemented within the scope of prevention are described in detail by Hollnagel (2004, 2008). Barriers can be protective, such as a crankcase, a baluster, and so on, or they can embody any measure taken at any accident stage in order to curtail its genesis. Physical or functional barriers implemented close to the injury in the accident genesis are the most effective. Illustrated in Figure 11.1, *Haddon's strategies* are designed to establish such barriers. Options and potential problems relating to risk assessment and implementation of these strategies for accidents triggered by movement disturbances will be discussed in the following subsections.

11.4.1 Haddon's Strategies for Accidents Triggered by Movement Disturbance

Several, if not most, of Haddon's 10 strategies could be implemented when the element in the physical environment that directly causes an injury is an obvious hazard, or when a person is exposed to a fall from a height. While these strategies are widely deployed in legislation, regulations covering the risk of falling from a height need to be implemented as a priority. A wide variety of situations are subject to this kind of risk, so very many regulations specific to the situation are required. Even though the injury mechanism is similar for a fall from a height and for a fall on the level, it would therefore appear relevant to consider separately the management of the risk of falling from a height.

Let us now consider any accident triggered by a movement disturbance with the exception of a fall from a height. It appears from Figure 11.2 that most of Haddon's 10 strategies are impossible to implement for two reasons. First, the injury-causing energy is not external to the victim but is carried by him or her. Thus, strategy 6 in Figure 11.1, "Separate, in time or space, the energy source and the vulnerable target," is not applicable. Moreover, "separation in time or space of a vulnerable target and an element in the physical environment causing injury" is only possible for an obvious hazard or a negotiable hazard (cf. Section 11.3.3). Such actions are impossible in cases involving a circumstantial hazard (e.g., floor or wall).

Some personal protective devices (e.g., toe caps in safety shoes) protect one part of the body (e.g., the feet) from injury (e.g., when heavy objects can strike the feet in certain occupational situations). In cases of accidents triggered by movement disturbance, the injury site is unpredictable and the risk exposure time is nearly permanent if circumstantial hazards are considered. Thus, strategy 8 in Figure 11.1, "Make the vulnerable target more resistant to damage from the energy flow," for example, is unthinkable unless every part of a moving person's body is to be protected.

11.4.2 Risk Assessment for Accidents Triggered by Movement Disturbance

As far as occupational accidents are concerned, risk assessment is usually based first on identifying obvious (and negotiable) hazards or else work situations at height covered by regulations or instructions. Unlike these situations, when injury results from the energy of the victim's movement combined with a "circumstantial hazard," one needs to consider any worker movement or physical element in the environment as a potential hazard. Assessment of the risk of movement disturbance based on an identified hazard has therefore always been particularly difficult. It is just as difficult today since it cannot be based on relevant accident factors, as these accidents are only rarely analyzed in depth. When they are, a wide variety of accident factors emerges, related to equipment usage (Kines, 2003), access system configuration (Leclercq et al., 2007), work system design (Derosier et al., 2008), work organization (Leclercq and Thouy, 2004), or safety management (Bentley and Haslam, 2001).

11.5 Discussion and Conclusion

Today, a lack of interest in the accident injury mechanism is clearly apparent. According to Hovden et al. (2010), there would be little need in terms of new models for understanding the "direct causes" of occupational accidents, and Haddon's 10 strategies (cf. subsection 11.2.2) will remain significant for counteracting such accidents. While every single person, without exception, has sustained injuries caused by movement disturbance, the injury mechanism in such accidents has not been studied in detail using accidentology-developed concepts. This section reveals the constant significance of the accident sequence close to the injury by describing the injury mechanism involved in such accidents. This study shows that, although so-called STFs are perceived as "simple accidents" (Jorgensen, 2011), the hazard involved in the injury mechanism is in fact composite, being the conjunction of the energy of the victim's disturbed movement and an element in the physical environment. The injury mechanism representation of these accidents highlights that moving and walking can be viewed as hazards. The representation also introduces the notion of *circumstantial hazard* to account for the fact that any element in the physical environment can cause an injury if it combines with sufficient kinetic energy. The model therefore highlights the difficulty or even impossibility of implementing Haddon's strategies and assessing the risk for accidents triggered by movement disturbances that involve a circumstantial hazard but are not falls from a height (cf. subsection 11.3.1). A unified representation of the injury mechanism can be adopted for all accidents triggered by movement disturbance. This fact notwithstanding, does it really make sense to consider jointly all these accidents? Leclercq et al. (2009, 2010) have proposed a categorization of all such accidents occurring at work from a practical risk management standpoint. In particular, it is apparent that occupational falls from a height call for priority implementation of specific actions, which refer to extensive, complex regulations, to protect against falling. Falls from a height and other occupational accidents triggered by movement disturbance should therefore be considered independently.

Considering together accidents triggered by movement disturbance, leading or not leading to loss of balance, is meaningful if a systemic view of accidents is adopted. It would, moreover, ensure greater visibility of many accidents considered "simple" or caused by awkwardness and to which little attention is currently given.

Finally, falls at work or in the home are a major concern and would surely deserve greater attention. Although frequent and serious (CE, 2008; CNAMTS, 2009; HSE, 2011; BLS, 2012), these accidents do not receive consideration in keeping with the risk they pose, and their prevention encounters many obstacles and misconceptions frequently based on preconceived ideas (Leclercq, 2005).

A review of the available data on occupational accidents reveals that many are triggered by a movement disturbance that does not lead to loss of balance (an arm injury caused by a wrench slipping, a bruise on the head due to colliding with the tailgate when climbing down from a truck, colliding with furniture when walking, etc.). Accidents triggered by movement disturbances most often involve a circumstantial hazard; all activity sectors and work activities are concerned. Studies on these accidents in hospital settings were conducted by Saint Vincent (1995) and Leclercq et al. (2014). In these studies, the identified elements in the physical environment that directly caused the injury were only circumstantial hazards (an item of furniture or equipment generally present in a hospital room on a permanent basis, a mobile equipment item or a structural element [door, wall, window, floor]). The absence of an obvious hazard could explain why the individual is frequently called into question: if it is not an equipment-related problem, it can only be a human problem! However, movement disturbance may be explained by accident factors related to any component of the occupational situation, for example, work system design as well as work organization. Prevention actions to neutralize risk factors further upstream in the accident genesis are effectively the only actions possible when barriers cannot be set up at injury mechanism level.

Acknowledgments

The author gratefully acknowledges X. Cuny, honorary professor in Hygiene and Safety; and the late M. Monteau, head of the safety management laboratory at France's Institut National de Recherche et de Sécurité. They developed with the author the model for occupational accident with movement disturbance, which was first presented in its English version at the International Ergonomics Association Conference held in Beijing in 2009. This model covers the injury mechanism discussed in the present study. The author would also like to thank Corinne Grusenmeyer and Adriana Savescu for providing their constructive thinking in relation to writing this chapter.

References

Aven, T., and Renn, O. (2009). On risk defined as an event where the outcome is uncertain. *Journal of Risk Research*, 12(1), 1–11.

Bentley, T.A., and Haslam, R.A. (2001). Identification of risk factors and countermeasures for slip, trip and fall accidents during delivery of mail. *Applied Ergonomics*, 32, 127–134.

BLS (Bureau of Labor Statistics), Nonfatal occupational injuries and illnesses requiring days away from work, 2011. Available from http://www.bls.gov/iif/#tables/ (accessed 15 December 2012).

CE (Communautés Européennes), *Causes et circonstances des accidents du travail dans l'UE*. Office des publications officielles des communautés européennes, Luxembourg, 2008.

CNAMTS (French National Health Insurance Fund for Salaried Workers), *Statistiques Nationales des accidents du travail, des accidents de trajet et des maladies professionnelles*. CNAMTS, Paris, 2009.

Corlett, E.N. (2008). Sitting as a hazard. *Safety Science*, 46, 815–821.

Derosier, C., Leclercq, S., Rabardel, P., and Langa, P. (2008). Studying work practices: A key factor in understanding accident on the level. *Ergonomics*, 51(12), 1926–1943.

EPICEA (Études de Prévention par l'Informatisation des Comptes rendus d'Enquêtes d'Accidents), 2011. (Online). Available at: http://www.inrs.fr/accueil/produits/bdd/epicea.html (Accessed 1 October 2011).

Gaudez, C., Leclercq, S., et Derosier, C. National statistics of occupational accidents on the level in France. In Pikaar, P.N., Koningsveld, E.A.P., and Settels, P.J.M., eds, *Proceedings IEA2006 Congress*. P5. Elsevier, 2006, ISSN 0003-6870.

Gibson, J. The contribution of experimental psychology to the formulation of the problem of safety: A brief for basic research. In *Behavioral Approaches to Accident Research*. Association for the Aid of Crippled Children, New York, 1961, 77–89.

Graham, J.D., and Wiener, J.B., eds. *Risk versus Risk: Tradeoffs in Protecting Health and the Environment*. Cambridge: Harvard University Press, 1995.

Haddon, W., (1980). The basic strategies for reducing damage from hazards of all kinds. *Hazard Prevention*, September–October: 8–12.

Ho, M.T., Bastide, J.C., and Francois, C. (1986). Mise au point d'un système destiné à l'exploitation de comptes rendus d'analyse d'accidents du travail. *Le Travail Humain*, 49(2), 137–146.

Hollnagel, E. *Barriers and Accident Prevention*. Ashgate Publishing Limited, Aldershot, 2004.

Hollnagel, E. (2008). Risk + barriers = safety? *Safety Science*, 46, 221–229.

Hollnagel, E. How resilient is your organization? An introduction to the resilience analysis grid (RAG). In *Sustainable Transformation: Building a Resilient Organization*. Toronto, Canada, 2010. https://hal-mines-paristech.archives-ouvertes.fr/hal-00613986.

Hovden, J., Albrechtsen, E., and Herrera, I.A. (2010). Is there a need for new theories, models and approaches to occupational accident prevention? *Safety Science*, 48, 950–956.

Hoyos, C.G., *Psychologische Unfall und Sicherheitsforschung*. Kohlhammer, 1980.

HSE, The Health and Safety Executive Statistics 2009/2010. Available from http://www.hse.gov.uk/statistics/ (accessed June 18, 2011).

ICECI (International Classification of External Causes of Injuries), Consumer Safety Institute, Amsterdam and AIHW National Injury Surveillance Unit, Adelaide, 2004.

IRGC, White paper on risk governance. Towards an integrative approach. IRGC, Geneva, 2005.

Jorgensen, K. (2011). A tool for safety officers investigating "simple" accidents. *Safety Science*, 49, 32–38.

Kines, P. (2003). Case studies of occupational falls from heights: Cognition and behavior context. *Journal of Safety Research*, 34, 263–271.

Kjellén, U. *Prevention of Accidents through Experience Feedback*. Taylor and Francis, London, 2000, 423 p.

Koehler, K.A., and Volckens, J. (2011). Prospects and pitfalls of occupational hazards mapping: 'Between these lines there be dragons'. *Annals of Occupational Hygiene*, 55(8), 829–840.

Leclercq, S. (2005). Prevention of so-called "accidents on the level" in occupational situations: A research project. *Safety Science*, 43, 359–371.

Leclercq, S., Monteau, M., and Cuny, X. Occupational accidents with movement disturbance: In support of an operational definition. In *Proceedings of the Conference of the International Ergonomics Association*. IEA, Beijing, China, 2009.

Leclercq, S., Monteau, M., and Cuny, X. (2010). Avancée dans la prévention des « chutes de plain-pied » au travail. Proposition de édfinition opérationnelle d'une nouvelle classe: « les accidents avec perturbation du mouvement (APM) ». *PISTES*, 12(3), 16p.

Leclercq, S., and Thouy, S. (2004). Systemic analysis of so-called "accidents on the level" in a multi trade company. *Ergonomics*, 47(12), 1282–1300.

Leclercq, S., Thouy, S., and Rossignol, E. (2007). Progress in understanding processes underlying occupational accidents on the level based on case studies. *Ergonomics*, 1(15), 59–79.

Leclercq, S., Cuny-Guerrier, A., Gaudez, C., and Aublet-Cuvelier, A. (2015). Similarities between work related musculoskeletal disorders and slips, trips and falls. *Ergonomics*, 58(10), 1624–1636.

Leclercq, S., Saurel, D., Cuny, X., and Monteau, M. (2014). Research into cases of slips, collisions and other movement disturbances occurring in work situations in a hospital environment. *Safety Science*, 68, 204–211.

Monteau, M., *L'organisation délétère—La santé et la sécurité au travail au prisme de l'organisation*. L'Harmattan, Paris, 2010.

Rasmussen, J., and Svedung, I. *Proactive Risk Management in a Dynamic Society*. Swedish Rescue Services Agency, Karlstad, Sweden, 2000.

Runyan, C.W. (2003). Introduction: Back to the future—Revisiting Haddon's conceptualization of injury epidemiology and prevention. *Epidemiologic Reviews*, 25, 60–64.

Saint Vincent, M. *Analyse des accidents survenus durant une année dans trois centres hospitaliers*. Rapport IRSST, R-093, IRSST, Canada, 1995.

Tak, S., and Calvert, G.M. (2011). The estimated national burden of physical ergonomic hazards among US workers. *American Journal of Industrial Medicine*, 54, 395–404.

Webster, *Webster's Third New International Dictionary: Unabridged*. Merriam Webster, 2002.

12

Friction Measurement: Methods and Applications

Wen-Ruey Chang

CONTENTS

ABSTRACT Friction measurement has been widely used as an assessment of slipperiness at the shoe–floor interface. However, controversies around friction measurements remain. The purpose of this chapter is to summarize our understanding about friction measurement with mechanical measurement devices related to slipperiness assessment of the interface between shoe and floor. Commonly used devices for slipperiness measurement are summarized. Static friction measurement, using the traditional drag-type device, is only suitable for dry and clean surfaces due to its limitation in properly reflecting lubrication at the measurement interface. Dynamic and impact friction methods are needed to properly estimate the potential risk on contaminated surfaces. Friction assessment using the mechanical measurement devices described herein appears generally valid and reliable. However, the validity of most devices could be improved by bringing them within the range of human slipping conditions to compare the results with the required coefficient of friction measured in biomechanical studies. Future studies should focus on understanding the tribological phenomena at the shoe–floor interface. For portable devices, it is important to improve their tribo-fidelity.

KEY WORDS: *field based, laboratory based, slipperiness, slipmeter, tribometer.*

12.1 Introduction

Mechanical devices have been widely used to measure various types of friction at the shoe–floor interface. Controversies about friction measurements remain, however, including the question of which type of friction to measure (static, dynamic, etc.), the problems of inter-method and inter-device differences, and the bio-fidelity of the measurement (whether the movement and contact forces of the test foot used in these devices resemble those of shoes at the critical instants of slip events).

Despite these limitations, friction measurements remain one of the most common approaches for measuring slipperiness. Numerous friction measurement devices have been used to assess the slipperiness between footwear and walking surfaces. Although all these devices measure coefficient of friction (COF), they differ considerably in their characteristics. Different measurement principles have been used, including static drag-sled methods, constant velocity dynamic friction methods, and impact methods. Contact pressure, contact area, and sliding speed at the interface often differ substantially among devices within a given type. Due to diverse measurement characteristics, the results generated from different devices can be significantly different.

There are generally two categories of devices: laboratory based and field based. Detailed descriptions of these devices can be found in the literature (Chang et al. 2001a). Laboratory-based devices are usually stationary. Field-based devices, typically called *slipmeters* or *tribometers*, are portable. Although various laboratory- and field-based mechanical devices have been widely used around the world to measure friction at the shoe–floor interface, debates about the validity of their results continue.

12.2 Measurement Conditions

The biomechanical approach has been used to investigate human reaction to slips and falls. Although a slip can happen at any time during the stance phase, there appear to be two different directional slips that occur during a normal walking step: forward slip during landing phase of the leading foot and backward slip during take-off phase of the trailing foot (Perkins 1978). It is generally accepted in the literature that the forward slip at the landing phase is the most dangerous due to the body weight being progressively transferred onto the slipping foot (Chang et al. 2001b). The forward momentum of the body makes it difficult to remove the weight from that foot to regain balance, and a continued slip is likely to result in a completely irrecoverable situation.

When the friction required to support human walking exceeds the friction available at the shoe–floor interface, a slip occurs (Hanson et al. 1999, Chang 2004). The available COF for human locomotion is the maximum friction coefficient that can be supported without a slip at the shoe–floor interface and is measured with a mechanical device. The required COF is defined as the minimum friction coefficient needed at the shoe–floor interface to support human locomotion. The required COF is usually measured on dry surfaces with a force plate, and the human participants have full confidence while walking on the floor without any concern about a potential slip incident. Therefore, this criterion of comparing the required and available COF can be applied when a human unknowingly steps onto a contaminated surface from a dry surface. For the available COF measurement, a friction measurement device is intended to simulate a slip when measured on surfaces with or without contaminants to measure the maximum COF that could be supported at the shoe–floor interface. Although people are less likely to slip on dry surfaces, the devices are still intended to measure the breakaway force as the maximum COF that can be supported.

Perkins (1978) observed slip events on a slippery floor in a laboratory environment. The shoe lands normally, but begins to slip forward about 0.1 s after heel contact. The shoe and foot accelerate forward, leading to a loss of balance. Immediately prior to the slip, the heel is not quite flat on the floor; the forepart is still well clear, but touches down when the slip starts. In most of Perkins' observations, a slip started with only the back of the heel in contact with the floor. Any slip more than 10–15 cm resulted in a loss of balance. Based on a review of the literature, Chang et al. (2001b) concluded that measurement parameters and their range should reflect the biomechanics and tribophysics of actual slip incidents simulating the heel strike phase in walking. Chang et al. (2001b) recommended these test conditions: the normal force buildup rate should be at least 10 kN/s for the whole-shoe testing devices, the normal pressure at the interface should be between 0.2 and 1.0 MPa, sliding speed should be between 0 and 1.0 m/s, and the contact time prior to and during the COF computation should be between 0 and 600 ms.

Available features on portable slipmeters are limited due to constraints of weight and portability, and have limited fidelity to the actual shoe–floor interface. Although human movements during slip incidents have been reported in the literature (Perkins 1978, Lanshammar and Strandberg 1983, Cham and Redfern 2002), design and reproducibility issues necessitated some simplifications in shoe movements compared with the previous experimental observations in the construction of these devices. More drastic simplifications were made with portable slipmeters than with laboratory-based devices. These simplifications resulted in significant differences in the results measured with various devices. Moreover, there appear to be regional preferences around the world regarding which devices could best represent human gait involved in slip and fall incidents. Since conflicting results could be obtained from different devices when they are used to evaluate potential interventions, these problems further complicate efforts in the development of interventions.

12.3 Friction Mechanisms

The main contributors to friction of elastomers, such as shoe sole material, involved at a dry interface include adhesion, hysteresis, and tearing (Tabor 1974, Moore 1975). Adhesion is caused by a dissipative stick–slip process at a molecular level, while hysteresis is an irreversible and delayed response during an elastic contact stress cycle due to damping in materials that leads to energy dissipation and an increase in friction. On dry surfaces, the contribution of adhesion and hysteresis to the total COF of elastomers depends on contact pressure. Electrostatic and van der Waals forces are the main sources of adhesion for polymers, as pointed out by Tabor (1974). When an elastomer adheres to another surface, work must be expended to produce sliding, since the adhesion at the interface must be broken. The formation and rupture of adhesive bonds increase the hysteresis loss of the polymer, leading to an increase in friction. However, experimental results indicate that the strength of adhesion increases with contact duration (dwell time) (Barquins 1982). Kummer (1966) provided further explanations that both components of rubber and elastomer friction are manifestations of the same basic viscoelastic energy dissipation mechanism.

For liquid-contaminated surfaces, three major elements at the shoe–floor interface include the squeeze-film process for the drainage capability of the shoe–floor contact surface, the draping of the shoe heel and sole about the asperities of the underfoot surface (lubrication, hysteresis), and the true contact between the interacting surfaces (adhesion, hysteresis, tearing).

The hydrodynamic pressure and load support in liquid film are generated with the contributions of wedge, stretch, and squeeze effects. According to Strandberg (1985), the contribution of the squeeze effect can be formulated as

$$h^2 = \frac{K \cdot u \cdot A^2}{F_N \cdot t} \tag{12.1}$$

where:
- h is the liquid film thickness
- K is a shape constant
- u is the dynamic viscosity of the fluid
- A is the contact area between surfaces
- F_N is normal force
- t is descending time

For a given liquid viscosity, normal force, and liquid film thickness, the contaminant descending time for drainage and draping becomes four times longer when the contact area is doubled. A longer drainage and draping time may increase the actual risk of slipping, because the response time available to prevent a forward slip after heel contact is very short, only a few tenths of a second (Strandberg and Lanshammar 1981). According to Proctor and Coleman (1988), the contribution of the *wedge term* can be formulated as

$$h^2 = \frac{0.066ul^3v}{F_N} \tag{12.2}$$

where:
- h and u are film thickness and viscosity of the liquid, respectively
- l is length of contact area (a square contact area is assumed)
- v is sliding velocity
- F_N is normal force

Proctor and Coleman (1988) called this the *hydrodynamic squeeze-film model*. This model is related to the tapered wedge, and it shows that for a specific viscosity, vertical load, and slider dimensions, the film thickness varies as the square root of the sliding velocity. The contribution of the stretch term to the pressure generation was not discussed extensively in the literature. However, the stretch term could be critical for the elastomer, since it might undergo large deformation during contact with the floor surface.

For solid contamination, the friction mechanisms involved are still not well understood. Heshmat et al. (1995) hypothesized that the friction mechanisms for dry particulate could include rolling, shearing, normal fracture, elasticity, and slip. Kinetic and continuum models were developed for ideal rigid particles. In the kinetic model, it is assumed that all collisions occur in pairs and elastic collision occurs between particles, similarly to rarefied gases (Elrod 1988). The continuum model, in which the contaminant is treated as a continuous mass rather than as discrete particles, is basically a non-Newtonian quasi-hydrodynamic lubrication model derived from experimental observations (Heshmat et al. 1995). Good agreement between the continuum model and experimental results was obtained. More work is needed to expand the current understanding of friction mechanisms involved in solid contaminants.

The contribution of floor surfaces to friction has not been discussed extensively. Surface roughness on floor surfaces can play a significant role in determining friction at the interface through lubrication, adhesion, and hysteresis, as indicated by Chang (1999). In addition, the bulk deformation of floor surfaces, especially on resilient floor surfaces or carpet with padding, could potentially generate an interlocking effect similar to the one at the asperity level to increase friction.

12.4 Summary of Mechanical Devices

The measurement conditions of the laboratory-based methods and portable devices summarized in this section are listed in Tables 12.1 and 12.2, respectively. Detailed descriptions and discussions about these devices were given by Chang et al. (2001a).

12.4.1 Laboratory-Based Methods

These types of devices are usually not portable and cannot be used to measure floor surfaces under real operational and environmental conditions.

The James machine, shown in Figure 12.1 (James 1944, ASTM D2047-11 2015), is classified as a static device. A mass of approximately 34 kg placed on a shaft for a total mass of approximately 38 kg can move in a vertical direction only. An articulated strut is pinned to the bottom of the shaft and a test shoe material holder at each end. A 7.62 × 7.62 cm test shoe material (foot) is placed on top of the floor surface, which sits on a table that is moveable in a horizontal direction only. With the articulated strut in the vertical position when the test begins, the table starts to move at a constant speed, so the angle between the strut and the vertical increases. A slip at the interface between the foot and the floor surface occurs before the vertical shaft reaches the lowest allowable position. COF is determined from the angle between the strut and the vertical at which a drastic slip happens at the interface between the foot and the floor surface.

Dynamic devices include LabINRS, the programmable slip resistance tester (PSRT), the Stevenson et al. (1989) device, the Stevenson (1997) device, the STM603 slip tester, the step simulator, and the slip simulator. All these devices are capable of testing the whole shoe.

TABLE 12.1

Test Conditions of Laboratory-Based Friction Devices

Device/Developer	Contact Angle (°)	Normal Force (N)	Sliding Speed (m/s)
James Machine	—	161	—
LabINRS	0–20	600[a] (100–1000)[b]	0.2[a] (0–1.6)[b]
PSRT	0–15	40–80	0.01–0.2
Stevenson et al. (1989)	10	350	0.4[a] (0–0.6)[b]
Stevenson (1997)	5	490	0.25
STM603	5[a] (0–30)[b]	400[a] (up to 750)[b]	0.1[a] (0.015–0.5)[b]
Step simulator	0–10	350–750	0.1–0.4
Slip simulator	5[a] (±25)[b]	700[a] (100–1500)[b]	0.4[a] (0–1.0)[b]

[a] Typical value.
[b] Adjustable range.

TABLE 12.2

Test Conditions of Field-Based Friction Devices

Device	Average Normal Force (N)	Contact Area[a] (cm²)	Contact Pressure (kPa)	Horizontal Sliding Velocity (m/s)	Contact Duration for COF Computation	Mass (kg)	Dimension (L × W × H [cm])
HPS	2.7	3.8	71	—	—	2.8	26 × 8 × 7
PAST	52	58	9	—	—	70	50 × 20 × 50
PFT	112	2.8	400	0.3b (0–1)[c]	0.5–3.5 s	42	60 × 40 × 55
AFPV	360[b] (124, 196, 360)[c]	16	225[b] (77,123,225)[c]	0.83	—	—	230 × 72 × 45
Tortus	2	0.6	30	0.017	User specified	6.6	42 × 24 × 10
BOT3000	22.4	2.5	100	0.2	User specified	2.8	29 × 20 × 17
Schuster	40	26	15	—	User specified	4.1	16 × 10 × 3
BPST	22	2.2	100	2.8	—	130	63 × 50 × 70
PIAST	240[d]	58	41[d]	—	—	42	38 × 20 × 40
VIT	37[d]	7.9[d]	47[d]	—	—	2	30 × 14 × 25

[a] Plain surfaces.
[b] Typical value.
[c] Adjustable range.
[d] Generated with vertical impact.

For LabINRS, shown in Figure 12.2 (Tisserand 1985, Leclercq et al. 1994, Tisserand et al. 1997), shoes placed in the foot-flat position or at a fixed angle are tested against a stainless steel floor that moves sinusoidally. For LabINRS, the dynamic COF is measured at the instant when the speed reaches the maximum at 0.2 m/s. For PSRT (Redfern and Bidanda 1994), the Stevenson (1997) device, the STM603 slip tester (Wilson 1990), and the step simulator (M&T Slip Resistance Shoes, Final report 1997), as shown in Figures 12.3 through 12.6, respectively, the footwear is positioned at a fixed angle with the floor and is lowered to contact the floor. After a short dwell time, horizontal movement of either the footwear or the floor begins. For devices with a high normal force, the force is built up during the dwell time. The measured COF is averaged over a short interval shortly after the horizontal movement starts and the normal force reaches the threshold value. For the slip simulator, shown in Figure 12.7 (Grönqvist et al. 1989), the footwear is positioned at a fixed angle with the floor and moves horizontally. Then, the footwear is lowered to contact the floor still maintaining the horizontal movement. The measurements of the normal force and COF begin when the normal force reaches 100 N and lasts for 50 ms. The Stevenson et al. (1989) device, shown in Figure 12.8, has the shoe mounted on a pendulum. A hydraulic cylinder pushes the pendulum downward to contact the floor. The shoe is mounted at a fixed angle, so it has an angle with the horizontal at the instant of contact with the floor.

12.4.2 Portable Devices

Two drag-sled methods are classified as static portable devices. One uses a motor to apply the drag force and is called a *horizontal pull slipmeter* (HPS), shown in Figure 12.9 (ASTM F609-05 2013). The other uses a dynamometer pull meter to apply a horizontal force by hand and is based on ASTM C1028-07 (2007). Another static device is the portable articulated

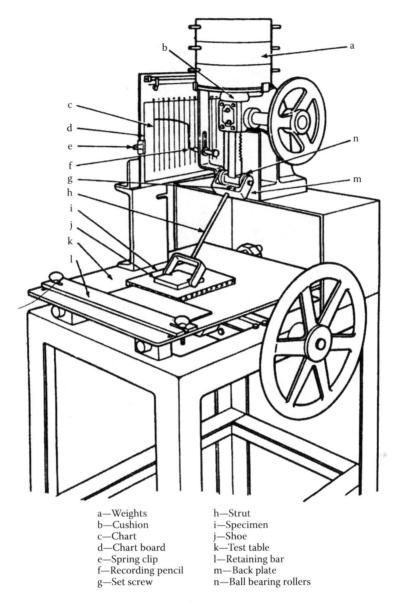

a—Weights	h—Strut
b—Cushion	i—Specimen
c—Chart	j—Shoe
d—Chart board	k—Test table
e—Spring clip	l—Retaining bar
f—Recording pencil	m—Back plate
g—Set screw	n—Ball bearing rollers

FIGURE 12.1
The James machine. (From ASTM D2047-11, *Annual Book of ASTM Standards, 15.04,* American Society for Testing and Materials, 2015.)

strut tribometer (PAST), known as the Brungraber Mark I, shown in Figure 12.10, which is an articulated strut slipmeter (ASTM F462-79 2007, ASTM F1678-96 2005). The HPS uses a motor to apply the drag force, but the ASTM C1028-96 uses a dynamometer pull meter to apply a horizontal force by hand. For the PAST, the COF is determined from the tangent of the angle between the strut and the vertical at which a drastic slip occurs at the interface between footwear sample and floor surface, similarly to the James machine.

The portable friction tester (PFT), the appareil de frottement à petite vitesse—low velocity skidmeter (AFPV), the Tortus, the BOT 3000E, and the Schuster are classified as steady-state dynamic devices. Their measurement characteristics are quite different. As shown

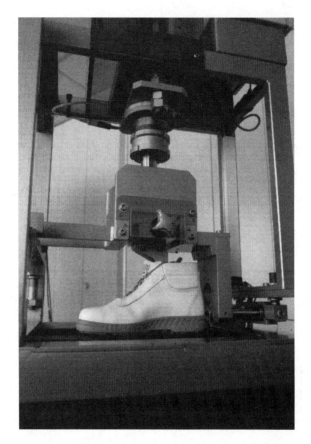

FIGURE 12.2
LabINRS. (From Chang, W.R. et al., *Ergonomics*, 44, 1233–1261, 2001.)

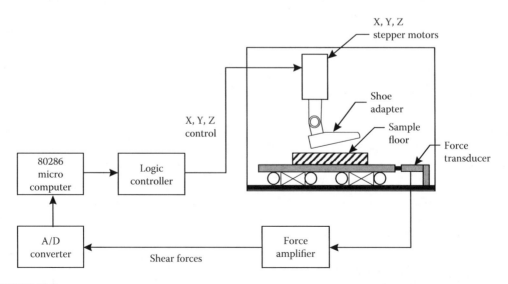

FIGURE 12.3
Programmable slip resistance tester (PSRT). (From Redfern, M.S. and Bidanda, B., *Ergonomics*, 37 (3), 511–524, 1994.)

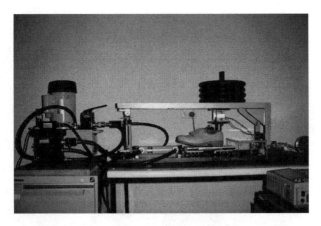

FIGURE 12.4
Stevenson 1997 device. (From Chang, W.R. et al., *Ergonomics*, 44, 1233–1261, 2001.)

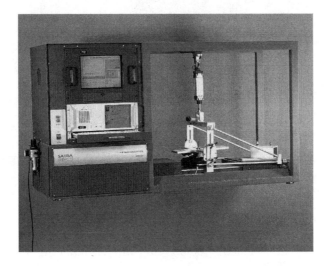

FIGURE 12.5
Slip resistance tester STM603. (From Chang, W.R. et al., *Ergonomics*, 44, 1233–1261, 2001.)

in Figure 12.11, the PFT is pushed at a constant speed by the operator on the floor surface (Strandberg 1985, Leclercq et al. 1993a,b, 1994, Tisserand et al. 1997). Dynamic COF is measured with a slip. The slip is controlled by the operator and occurs between a braked front wheel (test wheel) and the floor surface. For the AFPV, shown in Figure 12.12, the footwear sample is dragged on the floor surface by a guide system at a speed of 0.83 m/s, while normal force is applied through a carriage that slides on the guide rails (Majcherczyk 1978, Tisserand et al. 1997). The Tortus, shown in Figure 12.13, is a four-wheeled trolley driven across the floor surface. The footwear sample for COF measurement is attached to a shaft near the center of the trolley (Harris and Shaw 1988, Proctor and Coleman 1988, Scheil 1993, Tisserand et al. 1997, Grönqvist et al. 1999). The elastomer sample for COF measurement for the BOT 3000E, shown in Figure 12.14, is hemicylindrical (2.8 × 2.8 cm) (Powers et al. 2010, Kim 2012). The operating principle of this device is similar to that of the Tortus, except that there is an option to lower the shoe sample during the measurement to include impact loading for COF measurement. For the Schuster, shown in Figure 12.15, the operator

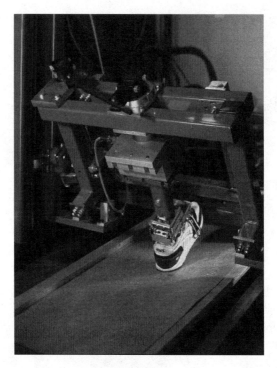

FIGURE 12.6
Step simulator. (From Chang, W.R. et al., *Ergonomics*, 44, 1233–1261, 2001.)

simply drags the device on floor surfaces to measure friction, and the drag speed depends on operator experience (Scheil 1993, Tisserand et al. 1997).

Both the Sigler and the British portable skid tester (BPST) are pendulum-swing devices that measure the energy loss of a pendulum swiping a path of a fixed length across a floor surface with a piece of spring-loaded heel material held at an angle with respect to the floor. The Sigler, shown in Figure 12.16, was developed in a successful attempt to eliminate the dwell time between the shoe and the walking surface (Chang 1999, Powers et al. 2010). It has been succeeded by other more recent devices and is rarely used. The BPST is an updated version of this type (Scheil 1993, Tisserand et al. 1997, Grönqvist et al. 1999). The leveling and height-adjusting functions of the BPST, shown in Figure 12.17, are independent, so that setup time is significantly reduced.

The variable incidence tribometer (VIT) and the portable inclineable articulated strut tribometer (PIAST), as well as its subsequent generations, measure friction during impact between footwear material and the floor. PIAST, also known as the Brungraber Mark II, shown in Figure 12.18a, is an inclined-strut slipmeter driven by gravity (ASTM F1677-05 2005, Li et al. 2009), while its newer version, the Mark III, shown in Figure 12.18b, is driven by spring force. As shown in Figure 12.19, VIT is driven by pneumatic pressure (ASTM F1679-04 2005, Chang 2002). In all of these devices in this category, the shoe sample impacts the floor surface at an inclined angle from the vertical direction. The COF is obtained from the angle at which a nonslip transitions to a slip. Although the standards for these articulated strut devices have been withdrawn, the test methods remain valid without regular updates.

A portable version of the slip simulator (Grönqvist et al. 1989) has been developed (Aschan et al. 2005) with the same operating principles as the laboratory version. However, the device is not as portable as other portable devices summarized in this section.

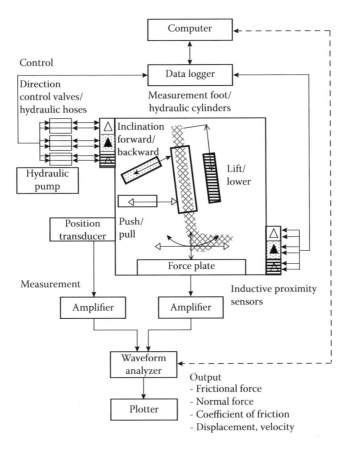

FIGURE 12.7
Slip simulator. (From Grönqvist, R. et al., *Ergonomics*, 32 (8), 979–995, 1989.)

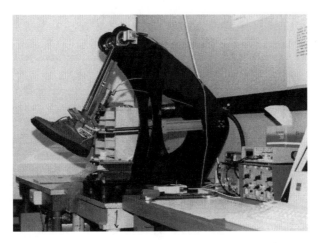

FIGURE 12.8
Stevenson et al. 1989 device. (From Chang, W.R. et al., *Ergonomics*, 44, 1233–1261, 2001.)

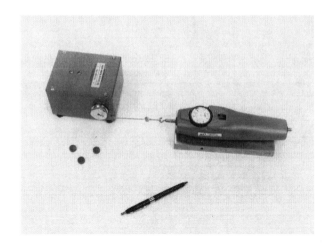

FIGURE 12.9
Horizontal pull slipmeter (HPS). (From Chang, W.R. et al., *Ergonomics*, 44, 1233–1261, 2001.)

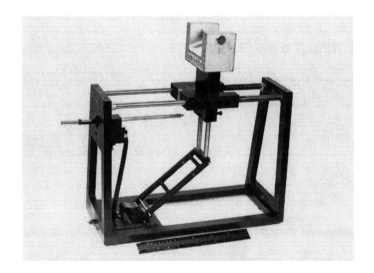

FIGURE 12.10
Portable articulated strut tribometer (PAST). (From Chang, W.R. et al., *Ergonomics*, 44, 1233–1261, 2001.)

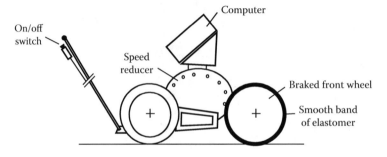

FIGURE 12.11
Portable friction tester (PFT). (From Leclercq, S. et al., *Safety Science*, 17, 41–55, 1993.)

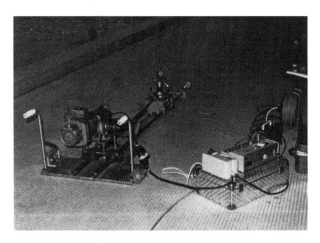

FIGURE 12.12
Appareil de frottement à petite vitesse—low velocity skidmeter (AFPV). (From Chang, W.R. et al., *Ergonomics*, 44, 1233–1261, 2001.)

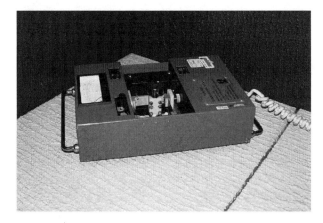

FIGURE 12.13
Tortus device. (From Chang, W.R. et al., *Ergonomics*, 44, 1233–1261, 2001.)

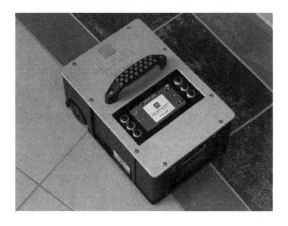

FIGURE 12.14
BOT 3000E.

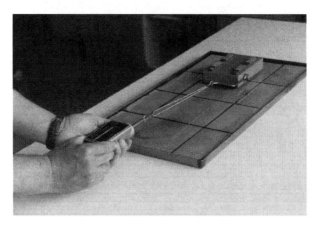

FIGURE 12.15
Schuster. (From Chang, W.R. et al., *Ergonomics*, 44, 1233–1261, 2001.)

12.5 Validity of Friction Measurements

It is generally agreed in the literature that static friction measurement, using a traditional drag-type device, is only suitable for dry and clean surfaces due to its lack of lubrication effect to properly reflect what happens at the shoe–floor interface. Dynamic and impact friction methods are needed to properly estimate the potential risk on contaminated surfaces (Chang et al. 2001b). Friction measured with most of the devices has been shown to have a significant correlation with other measurements. They include objective measurements based on biomechanics, the ratio of forces measured at the actual interface with a force plate, COF measured with other devices, and time-based friction use values, as well as subjective measurements, such as perception of slipperiness and paired comparison, as summarized by Chang et al. (2001a, 2006). Only the COF obtained with a slipmeter and the ratio of forces measured at the actual interface with a force plate can be directly compared by numbers. All other comparisons were performed by calculating correlation coefficients. More recently, Powers et al. (2010) compared the rankings obtained from slipmeters with those obtained from a human subject experiment based on four reference surfaces: polished black granite, porcelain, ceramic tile, and vinyl composition tile. In addition, the authors evaluated whether the slipmeters could distinguish whether there was a statistically significant difference between the COFs of the surfaces. Among 11 slipmeters evaluated, the BPST, the Sigler, and the PIAST (also known as Brungraber Mark II, and its updated version Mark III) correctly ranked and differentiated all four surfaces.

12.6 Discussion

Although most of the output from these mechanical devices has a significant correlation with the output from other measures, such as those based on biomechanics or psychophysics, or output from other mechanical devices, many problems remain. Tisserand (1985) pointed out

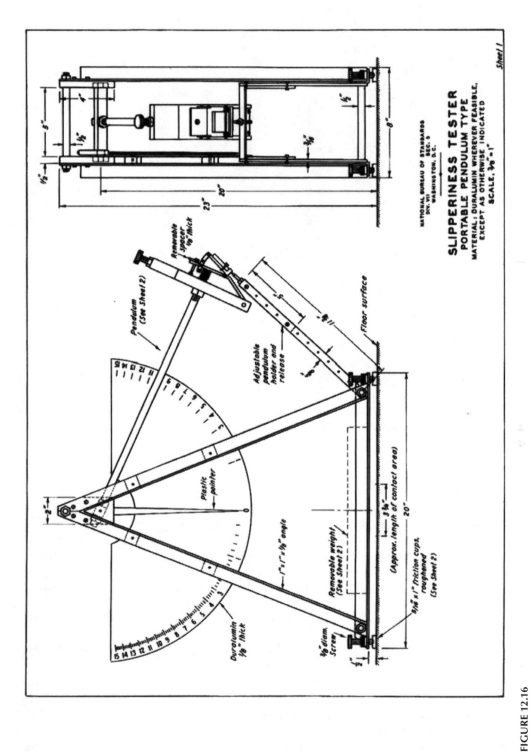

FIGURE 12.16
Sigler. (From Chang, W.R. et al., *Ergonomics*, 44, 1233–1261, 2001.)

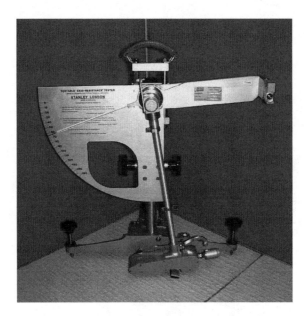

FIGURE 12.17
British portable skid tester (BPST). (From Chang, W.R. et al., *Ergonomics*, 44, 1233–1261, 2001.)

that LabINRS was by no means a biomechanical model for walking or slipping. It was simply a model reproducing the ranking made by human participants; that is, even devices lacking bio-fidelity could produce outputs that have the same ranking as human participants. Although most of these devices could produce outputs with the same ranking, their measured values could be different even if the same samples were used. As indicated in Section 12.2, in determining whether a slip will happen, the required COF, also known as friction demand, is typically compared with the available COF (Hanson et al. 1999, Chang 2004). The measurement conditions of these devices, summarized in Section 12.4 in this chapter, are still far from perfect as compared with the biomechanical data reported in the literature and are inconsistent across the various devices. For the laboratory-based whole-shoe devices, the issue is bio-fidelity. For the portable devices, the issues are bio-fidelity and tribo-fidelity. The question about tribo-fidelity is whether the tribological phenomena at the shoe–floor interface of slip events are properly reflected at the measurement interface with these devices. Till these issues about bio-fidelity and tribo-fidelity have been properly addressed, discrepancies will still exist in the outputs from these devices, and the results still cannot be compared with the required COF measured from biomechanical experiments.

For laboratory-based devices, one of the common issues is that the heel contact angle is fixed for almost all the devices. This limitation is usually based on the consideration of the improved repeatability for measurement results, as pointed out by Grönqvist et al. (1989). The second issue is that the forward sliding speed might be too high. Although a slip and fall incident usually results from a severe slip, a more critical instant could be around slip initiation at a low speed. The third issue is that the measurement of COF might be too late in the process, considering that the prime consideration is to capture slip initiation. The fourth issue is the dwell time right before the start of the movement. Based on biomechanical observations, the ankle rotates continuously from heel strike till the foot is flat. Right after heel strike, the heel contact angle, which is the angle between the floor and the shoe bottom, is reduced as the ankle continues to rotate, and the heel can move backward

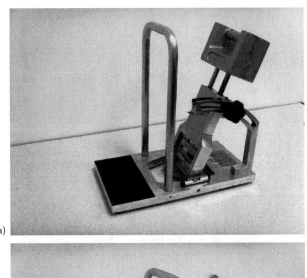

(a)

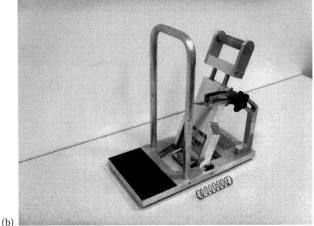

(b)

FIGURE 12.18
Portable inclineable articulated strut tribometer (PIAST) (a) II and (b) III. (From Li, K.W. et al., *Safety Science*, 47, 1434–1439, 2009.)

when walking on slippery surfaces (Perkin 1978). Then, the heel slides forward at the end of the backward movement, while the heel contact angle continues to reduce. This characteristic of backward movement could have a significant effect on the measured available friction, since the contaminant is redistributed during the backward movement, and the lubrication effect at the shoe–floor interface could be quite different with and without this backward movement and changing contact angle. In most of the laboratory-based devices, this movement has been either eliminated or simplified as a stationary position. The friction mechanisms involved are more complex than the wedge and squeeze-film effects that have been widely cited in the literature.

In addition to bio-fidelity, tribo-fidelity could be more important for field-based devices. Ideally, friction measurement devices should meet the requirements of both bio-fidelity and tribo-fidelity. Compared with field-based devices, it is easier for laboratory-based devices to meet these requirements due to their abilities to use the whole shoe and generate larger contact forces with complicated movements. Due to the requirement for portability, the contact force applied with the portable slipmeters would not be as high as that at the actual

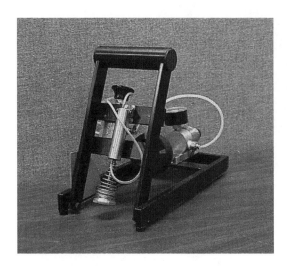

FIGURE 12.19
Variable incidence tribometer (VIT). (From Chang, W.R., *Safety Science*, 40 (7–8), 593–611, 2002.)

shoe–floor interface. To maintain the same contact pressure and lubrication conditions, the contact area needs to be reduced. Contact area and contact pressure at the footwear–floor interface during walking were investigated by Harper et al. (1961). Assuming that the shoe sole had a plain surface, the contact area at 0.1 s after heel strike was approximately 11 cm^2, and the corresponding contact pressure was approximately 410 kPa (Harper et al. 1961). The contact pressure from 0 to 0.1 s after a heel strike was extremely high. According to this result, Chang et al. (2001b) specified that the contact pressure should be within the range of 200–1000 kPa. The contact pressures of most of the slipmeters are well below this range. To reflect correct tribo-fidelity, other parameters should be adjusted, such as an increase in the contact area or impact speed. Accommodations made for portability could cause the measurement conditions to deviate significantly from those observed in biomechanical experiments, that is, to lose bio-fidelity, so we should focus on tribo-fidelity under these circumstances. Tribo-fidelity could be more useful than bio-fidelity to properly reflect what actually happens at the shoe–floor interface under lubricated conditions. Unfortunately, what actually happens at the shoe–floor interface during a slip event is still not well understood. Beschorner et al. (2014) attempted to measure fluid pressure at the shoe–floor interface during a slip event, and Singh and Beschorner (2014) attempted to measure it during friction measurements with the portable version of the slip simulator. They were able to measure only the hydrodynamic fluid pressure. However, the lubrication regions include boundary lubrication, hydrodynamic lubrication, and a mixture of both. Measuring hydrodynamic lubrication alone, without the contribution of boundary lubrication, cannot account for the whole picture at the shoe–floor interface.

12.7 Conclusions

The measurement characteristics and conditions of the currently available friction measurement devices are very different among themselves and different from slips observed in biomechanical experiments. They also produce very different results, but most of these devices can still produce meaningful results that have been accepted by users. As we improve the bio-fidelity and tribo-fidelity of these devices, we can also bring the characteristics and conditions of these devices closer to what actually happens at the shoe–floor interface at the critical instants and closer to each other.

Acknowledgments

The author would like to thank Taylor and Francis, Elsevier, and American Society of Testing and Materials (ASTM International) for permission to reproduce Figures 12.1 through 12.19, and Regan Scientific Instruments for providing the picture of BOT 3000E. Figure 12.1 was reprinted, with permission, from ASTM D2047-11 Standard Test Method for Static Coefficient of Friction of Polish-Coated Flooring Surfaces as Measured by the James Machine, copyright ASTM International, 100 Barr Harbor Drive, West Conshohocken, PA 19428. The complete standard may be obtained from ASTM at www. astm.org.

References

Aschan, C., Hirvonen, M., Mannelin, T. and Rajamäki, E. 2005, Development and validation of a novel portable slip simulator, *Applied Ergonomics*, 36 (5), 585–593.

ASTM C1028-07 2007, Standard method for determining the static coefficient of friction of ceramic tile and other like surfaces by the horizontal dynamometer pull-meter method, *Annual Book of ASTM Standards, 15.02* (West Conshohocken, PA: American Society for Testing and Materials).

ASTM D2047-11 2015, Standard test method for static coefficient of friction of polish-coated floor surfaces as measured by the James machine, *Annual Book of ASTM Standards, 15.04* (West Conshohocken, PA: American Society for Testing and Materials).

ASTM F462-79 2007, Consumer safety specification for slip-resistant bathing facilities, *Annual Book of ASTM Standards, 15.07* (West Conshohocken, PA: American Society for Testing and Materials).

ASTM F609-05 2013, Standard test method for using a Horizontal Pull Slipmeter (HPS), *Annual Book of ASTM Standards*, 15.07 (West Conshohocken, PA: American Society for Testing and Materials).

ASTM F1677-05 2005, Standard test method for using a Portable Inclineable Articulated Strut Slip Tester (PIAST), *Annual Book of ASTM Standards, 15.07* (West Conshohocken, PA: American Society for Testing and Materials).

ASTM F1678-96 2005, Standard test method for using a Portable Articulated Strut Slip Tester (PAST), *Annual Book of ASTM Standards, 15.07* (West Conshohocken, PA: American Society for Testing and Materials).

ASTM F1679-04 2005, Standard test method for using a Variable Incidence Tribometer (VIT), *Annual Book of ASTM Standards, 15.07* (West Conshohocken, PA: American Society for Testing and Materials).

Barquins, M. 1982, Influence of dwell time on the adherence of elastomers, *Journal of Adhesion*, 14, 63–82.

Beschorner, K. E., Albert, D. L., Chambers, A. J. and Redfern, M. S. 2014, Fluid pressures at the shoe-floor-contaminant interface during slips: Effects of tread and implications on slip severity, *Journal of Biomechanics*, 47, 458–463.

Cham, R. and Redfern, M. S. 2002, Heel contact dynamics during slip events on level and inclined surfaces, *Safety Science*, 40 (7–8), 559–576.

Chang, W. R. 1999, The effect of surface roughness on the measurements of slip resistance, *International Journal of Industrial Ergonomics*, 24 (3), 299–313.

Chang, W. R. 2002, The effects of slip criterion and time on friction measurements, *Safety Science*, 40 (7–8), 593–611.

Chang, W. R. 2004, A statistical model to estimate the probability of slip and fall incidents, *Safety Science*, 42 (9), 779–789.

Chang, W. R., Grönqvist, R., Leclercq, S., Brungraber, R., Mattke, U., Strandberg, L., Thorpe, S., Myung, R., Makkonen, L. and Courtney, T. K. 2001a, The role of friction in the measurement of slipperiness, part II: Survey of friction measurement devices, *Ergonomics*, 44, 1233–1261.

Chang, W. R., Grönqvist, R., Leclercq, S., Myung, R., Makkonen, L., Strandberg, L., Brungraber, R., Mattke, U. and Thorpe, S. 2001b, The role of friction in the measurement of slipperiness, part I: Friction mechanisms and definition of test conditions, *Ergonomics*, 44, 1217–1232.

Chang, W. R., Li, K. W., Huang, Y. H., Filiaggi, A. and Courtney, T. K. 2006, Objective and subjective measurements of slipperiness in fast-food restaurants in the USA and their comparison with the previous results obtained in Taiwan, *Safety Science*, 44 (10), 891–903.

Elrod, H. G. 1988, Granular flow as a tribological mechanism: A first look, in D. Dowson, C. M. Taylor, M. Godet, and D. Berthe (eds), *Interface Dynamics*. Amsterdam. (Elsevier), 75–88.

Grönqvist, R., Hirvonen, M. and Tohv, A. 1999, Evaluation of three portable floor slipperiness testers, *International Journal of Industrial Ergonomics*, 25, 85–95.

Grönqvist, R., Roine, J., Järvinen, E. and Korhonen, E. 1989, An apparatus and a method for determining the slip resistance of shoes and floors by simulation of human foot motions, *Ergonomics*, 32 (8), 979–995.

Hanson, J. P., Redfern, M. S., and Mazumdar, M. 1999, Predicting slips and falls considering required and available friction, *Ergonomics*, 42 (12), 1619–1633.

Harper, F. C., Warlow, W. J., and Clarke, B. L. 1961, The forces applied to the floor by the foot in walking, National Building Research Paper 32, DSIR, Building Research Station (London: Her Majesty's Stationary Office).

Harris, G. W. and Shaw, S. R. 1988, Slip resistance of floors: Users' opinions, Tortus instrument readings and roughness measurement, *Journal of Occupational Accidents*, 9, 287–298.

Heshmat, H., Godet, M. and Berthier, Y. 1995, On the role and mechanism of dry triboparticulate lubrication, *STLE Lubrication Engineering*, 51, 557–564.

James, S. V. 1944, What is a safe floor finish?, *Soap and Sanitary Chemicals*, 20, 111–115.

Kim, J. 2012, Comparison of three different slip meters under various contaminated conditions, *Safety and Health at Work*, 3 (1), 22–30.

Kummer, H. W. 1966, Unified theory of rubber and tire friction, Engineering Research Bulletin B-94 (Pennsylvania: The Pennsylvania State University).

Lanshammar, H. and Strandberg, L. 1983, Horizontal floor reaction forces and heel movements during the initial stance phase, in H. Matsui and K. Kobayashi (eds), *Biomechanics VIII* (University Park Press, Baltimore, MD), 1123–1128.

Leclercq, S., Tisserand, M. and Saulnier, H. 1993a, Quantification of the slip resistance of floor surfaces at industrial sites. Part I. Implementation of a portable device, *Safety Science*, 17, 29–39.

Leclercq, S., Tisserand, M. and Saulnier, H. 1993b, Quantification of the slip resistance of floor surfaces at industrial sites. Part II. Choice of optimal measurement conditions, *Safety Science*, 17, 41–55.

Leclercq, S., Tisserand, M. and Saulnier, H. 1994, Assessment of the slip-resistance of floors in the laboratory and in the field: Two complementary methods for two applications, *International Journal of Industrial Ergonomics*, 13, 297–305.

Li, K. W., Chang, W. R. and Chang, C. C. 2009, Evaluation of two models of a slipmeter, *Safety Science*, 47, 1434–1439.

M&T Slip Resistance Shoes 1997, Development of a test method for measuring the slip resistance of protective footwear, unpublished final report (October 20, 1997) for the Commission of the European Communities, Contract no. MAT1 CT 940059, 60 pp.

Majcherczyk, R. 1978. A different approach to measuring pedestrian friction: The CEBTP skidmeter, in C. Anderson and J. Senne (eds), *Walkway Surfaces: Measurement of Slip Resistance, ASTM STP 649* (Philadelphia, PA: American Society for Testing and Materials), 88–99.

Moore, D. F. 1975, *The Friction of Pneumatic Tyres* (Amsterdam: Elsevier Scientific).

Perkins, P. J. 1978, Measurement of slip between the shoe and ground during walking, in C. Anderson and J. Senne (eds), *Walkway Surfaces: Measurement of Slip Resistance, ASTM Special Technical Publication 649* (Philadelphia, PA: American Society for Testing and Materials), 71–87.

Powers, C. M., Blanchette, M. G., Brault, J. R., Flynn, J. and Siegmund, G. P. 2010, Validation of walkway tribometers: Establishing a reference standard, *Journal of Forensic Science*, 55 (2), 366–370.

Proctor, T. D. and Coleman, V. 1988, Slipping, tripping and falling accidents in Great Britain: Present and future, *Journal of Occupational Accidents*, 9, 269–285.

Redfern, M. S. and Bidanda, B. 1994, Slip resistance of the shoe-floor interface under biomechanically-relevant conditions, *Ergonomics*, 37 (3), 511–524.

Scheil, M. 1993, Analyse und Verlgleich von instationären Reibzahlmessgeräten. [Analysis and comparison of nonstationary friction coefficient measurement tools.] Fachbereich Sicherheitstechnik der Bergischen. [Department of Safety Technique]. Universität-Gesamthochschule. Wuppertal, Doctoral Dissertation in German with English summary.

Singh, G. and Beschorner, K. E. 2014, A method for measuring fluid pressures in the shoe-floor-fluid interface: Application to shoe tread evaluation, *IIE Transactions on Occupational Ergonomics and Human Factors*, 2 (2), 53–59.

Stevenson, M. 1997, Evaluation of the slip resistance of six types of women's safety shoe using a newly developed testing machine, *Journal of Occupational Health and Safety, Australia and New Zealand*, 13 (2), 175–182.

Stevenson, M. G., Hoang, K., Bunterngchit, Y. and Lloyd, D. 1989, Measurement of slip resistance of shoes on floor surfaces. Part 1: Methods, *Journal of Occupational Health and Safety, Australia and New Zealand*, 5 (2), 115–120.

Strandberg, L. 1985, The effect of conditions underfoot on falling and overexertion accidents, *Ergonomics*, 28, 131–147.

Strandberg, L. and Lanshammar, H. 1981, The dynamics of slipping accidents, *Journal of Occupational Accidents*, 3 (3): 153–162.

Tabor, D. 1974, Friction, adhesion and boundary lubrication of polymers, in L-H. Lee (ed.), *Advances in Polymer Friction and Wear, Polymer Science and Technology*, Volume 5A (Berlin: Plenum), 5–30.

Tisserand, M. 1985, Progress in the prevention of falls caused by slipping, *Ergonomics*, 28 (7), 1027–1042.

Tisserand, M., Saulnier, H. and Leclercq, S. 1997, Comparison of seven test methods for the slip resistance of floors: Contributions to developments of standards, in P. Seppälä, T. Luopajärvi, C-H. Nygård and M. Mattila (eds), *Proceedings of the 13th Triennial Congress of the IEA: From Experience to Innovation*, Volume 3 (Helsinki: Finnish Institute of Occupational Health), 406–408.

Wilson, M. P. 1990, Development of SATRA slip test and tread pattern design guidelines, in B. E. Gray (ed.), *Slips, Stumbles, and Falls: Pedestrian Footwear and Surfaces, ASTM STP 1103* (Philadelphia: American Society for Testing and Materials), 113–123.

13

Stairway Safety Research

Hisao Nagata

CONTENTS

ABSTRACT Falls involving level floors and stairways have become the leading cause of hospital-treated injuries in most advanced countries. Stairway safety research has been conducted to reduce the rate of casualties from falls involving stairways. Research to prevent stair-related falls is holistically presented in this chapter. Studies of casualties caused by falls from stairways, risk assessment of stairway use, classification of missteps, and suggested combinations of tread depth and riser height are included. The author also introduces the inherent potential risks of human walking that cause stair-related falls and fundamental concepts to understand principles of safety on stairways, focusing on tread depth and riser height. Recent literature has identified some etiological factors relating to stair-related falls. Accordingly, some safety codes for individual dwellings and other buildings have recently been revised. When adopting these codes for stairway design, designers and building owners need to understand the principles that decrease stair-related falls, especially tread depth and riser height.

KEY WORDS: *stairways, safety, falls, injuries, design, tread depth, riser height, risk.*

13.1 Introduction

Fatal and nonfatal falls involving level floors and stairways will increase as the population of people aged 65 and over increases. Subsequent long-term care and institutionalization cause increased medical and nursing care costs and loss of family income. At the same time, level falls and stair-related falls are becoming such an economic burden that their impacts cannot be ignored. The effects of falls from stairways have become better known since the hazard information provided by the US National Electronic Inquiry Surveillance System (NEISS) began in 1973. Stair-related injuries requiring hospital treatment are consistently ranked at or near the top of probability samplings by NEISS.

People often blame themselves for being careless when they trip or misstep on stairways, but those missteps may not necessarily be the fault of the stair user. Four decades ago, one of the leading articles for stairway safety research, entitled "The Dimension of Stairs," was published in *Scientific American* (Fitch et al., 1974). This article, summarized in a doctoral dissertation (Temler, 1974), has had an influential impact worldwide on safety researchers, building designers, builders, ergonomists, advocates, practitioners, and so on. Intensive research to decrease stair-related falls has applied an etiological approach to define the dimensions of stairways, as changes in dimensions relate to lower rates of missteps while ascending or descending stairways by human gait analysis of foot movements on an experimental flight of stairways.

These early studies pointed out some experimental findings regarding the geometry of stairways. They also attracted attention to stairway safety and initiated research to seek safer design of stairways (Archea et al., 1979). Since then, fundamental findings on safe stairways have been studied in detail, and a considerable amount of stairway safety research has been carried out from the aspects of various disciplines to decrease fatal and nonfatal injuries while ascending/descending stairways.

Stairway safety is one area used to modify individual surroundings to decrease potential risk in dwellings and other buildings. When stairways are designed in public facilities, hospitals, and nursing care homes, special attention should be paid to decreasing potential risk by considering every risk factor for children, the elderly, and impaired persons. Consideration must be given to individual causes of loss of balance, such as reduced physical, visual, and cognitive abilities associated with aging, intoxication, and the effects of medication. Stairways in hospitals, residential care centers, and nursing homes should be considered one of the most likely sites for falls to happen, even if the stairways are built to optimal dimensions and with the safest designs. Physically and mentally impaired users should be restricted from using stairways by setting up barriers at the entrance to stairways that could be accessed by hospital patients, the elderly, and toddlers. Another option, the installation of elevators and, in the case of emergencies, escape chutes to evacuate from higher floors to ground level for impaired people should be considered. Stairway safety research to decrease potential risk for the elderly mainly focuses on building risk awareness in the individual. At the same time, awareness campaigns to change risky stair behavior should be used. In this chapter, physiotherapeutic countermeasures, such as proper exercise for muscle strengthening and balance training and use of protectors for those at risk of hip fractures and head injuries, are not considered, but fundamental overview topics especially for stairway safety and their solutions are comprehensively presented.

13.2 Fatal and Nonfatal Falls on/from Stairways

13.2.1 Fatal Falls on/from Stairways

Many researchers have undertaken field, demographic, or epidemiological surveys of stair-related falls (Svanström, 1974; Wild et al., 1981; Hay and Barkow, 1985; Webber, 1985; Pauls, 1991; Jackson and Choen, 1995; Wyatt et al., 1999; Ragg et al., 2000; Preuß et al., 2004; Mitchell et al., 2013). The exact annual number of fatal falls from stairways in each country can be obtained from mortality statistics from the International Classification of Diseases recommended by the World Health Organization (WHO). In 2001, there were 1917 deaths due to falls on/from stairways and steps in the United States and 693 deaths in England and Wales, and in 2012, there were 679 deaths in Japan. One case of an actual fatal fall is shown in Figure 13.1.

The occurrence of fatal falls is higher in residential homes. People aged 65 and over suffer the greatest number of fatal falls and serious injuries. Most inadvertent fatal falls are related to physical, sensory, and cognitive deterioration associated with aging. Global fatalities due to falling have had a tendency to increase yearly in developed countries as the ratio of senior people in the population has increased.

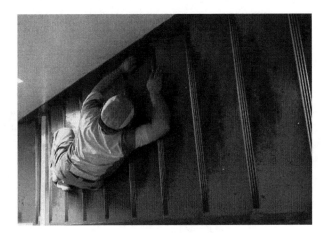

FIGURE 13.1
Reenacted photograph of a worker's fatal fall on a stairway. Death was caused by several rib bones penetrating his lung cavity.

TABLE 13.1

Percentage of Injury of Fatal Falls by Age Group and Gender

	Fall on the Same Level				Fall on/from Stairways or Steps			
	Male Age Group		Female Age Group		Male Age Group		Female Age Group	
Nature of Injury	0–64 (%)	65 and Over (%)	0–64 (%)	65 and Over (%)	0–64 (%)	65 and Over (%)	0–64 (%)	65 and Over (%)
Intracranial injury excluding those with skull fracture	55.2	27.3	62.4	12.1	51.7	47.9	57.3	42.3
Fracture of skull	27.3	10.8	16.2	2.1	35.0	25.1	24.6	14.1
Fracture of spine and trunk	3.0	6.4	3.4	5.4	4.7	8.5	6.4	6.7
Fracture of upper limb	0.2	2.3	0.9	4.7	0.0	0.0	0.0	3.9
Fracture of lower limb	1.8	36.2	6.8	66.2	0.2	6.2	0.9	19.2
Internal injury of chest, abdomen, and pelvis	4.1	3.2	2.6	1.0	1.1	1.6	4.6	2.9
Contusion and crushing with intact skin surface	3.4	9.3	3.4	7.3	1.3	3.3	2.7	6.4
Injury to nerves and spinal cord	3.0	3.1	4.3	0.5	5.3	6.8	3.6	3.5
Other nature of injury	2.0	1.4	0.0	0.7	0.7	0.6	0.0	1.0

According to the author's statistical survey of 1278 fatal falls on/from stairs/steps and 2815 fatal falls on the same level, the nature of injuries attributed to fatal falls by age group clearly differs, as shown in Table 13.1 (Nagata, 1991a). As many published papers have already shown, most fatal falls on the same level caused fracture of the lower limbs of people aged 65 and over because of bone fragility of the lower limbs. Most fatal falls on the same level involving people below 65 years old caused intracranial injuries and fractures of the skull, not fractures to lower limbs (male: 82.5%, female: 78.6%). Meanwhile, most fatal falls from stairways resulted in head injuries.

Preuβ et al. (2004) reported that skull injuries occurred in 105 of 116 fatal falls from stairways (90.5%), and the injuries were mostly located on the back of the skull and the forehead (92 individuals: 87.6%). Skull fractures were found in 75 cases (71.4%) of skull injuries, and the majority of these were basal skull fractures. The majority of skull injuries resulting from falls from stairways were above "the hat brim." In contrast, most head injuries from falls on the same level are below "the hat brim." Ragg et al. (2000) also reported that head injuries account for the majority of serious injuries caused by falls from stairways. Major anatomical serious injuries of both fatal and nonfatal falls are shown in Table 13.2.

The percentage of fatal falls by males in residential houses is relatively higher among groups from the age of 20 to 60 years old (Nagata, 1991a). Males are more likely than females to suffer fatal falls on/from stairways even in residential houses. The assumed reasoning behind this phenomenon is male risk-taking behaviors and habits such as alcohol

TABLE 13.2

Major Serious Injuries Caused by Falls from Stairways

Injured Region	No. Patients	Injury	No. Injuries
Head and neck	99	Subdural hematoma	64
		Extradural hematoma	18
		Skull vault fracture	25
		Base of skull fracture	29
		Other intracranial hematoma	20
Face	11	Facial fracture	11
Thorax	15	Fractured rib(s)	12
		Others	6
Extremities	15	Upper limb fracture/dislocation	11
		Lower limb fracture including pelvis	4
Others	16	—	18

Source: Based on data from Ragg, M., et al., *Emergency Medicine*, 12, 45–49, 2000.

consumption. Many researchers have proven that heavy drinking habits are included in the contributory factors leading to serious falls from stairways (Svanström, 1974; Waller, 1978; Jackson and Choen, 1995; Wyatt et al., 1999; Ragg et al., 2000; Preuß et al., 2004).

13.2.2 Nonfatal Falls on/from Stairways

Many surveys of stair-related falls in homes have been conducted by various researchers (Miller and Esmay, 1961; Carson et al., 1978; Webber et al., 1979; Wild et al., 1981; Kose, 1986; Jackson and Choen, 1995). Some articles have dealt with occupational falls from stairways (Allcott, 1979; US Department of Labor, 1984; Cohen and Templer, 1985; Templer et al., 1985; Nagata, 1991b), but the actual number of nonfatal casualties cannot be estimated accurately. One typical case of a nonfatal fall is shown in Figure 13.2.

The rates of nonfatal fall casualties resulting in hospitalizations for the elderly and for those under five are higher, according to hazard information provided by the NEISS data. But the rate of fatal falls on/from stairways is very low for children, presumably because of their smaller stature, leading to lower drop heights and "rolling over" just after falls to soften the impact to the body.

The author surveyed 1476 nonfatal stair-related falls based on occupational casualty reports (Nagata, 1991b). Most healthy adults received injuries to the legs/feet, followed by the trunk, then the head and arms/hands. Fewer than half of injuries to the trunk are suffered to the lower back. Nearly 60% of all victims of stair-falls were found to be descending stairways hastily, as shown by results of other researchers' field surveys (Miller and Esmay, 1961; Svanström, 1974). Particularly, females aged between 18 and 24 were injured while wearing high- or semi-high-heeled footwear. According to the analysis of injuries while walking on stairways (Svanström, 1974; US Department of Labor, Bureau of Labor Statistics, 1984; Cohen and Templer, 1985; Hay and Barkow, 1985; Templer, 1985; Nagata, 1991b; Jackson and Choen, 1995), users are more likely to receive injuries while descending stairways. The rates of falls while descending and ascending stairways are reported as 92% (Cohen and Templer, 1985) and 76% (Svanström, 1974), respectively. The author obtained similar rates of falls in descent: 85% (92% for females and 78% for males, respectively) (Nagata, 1991b).

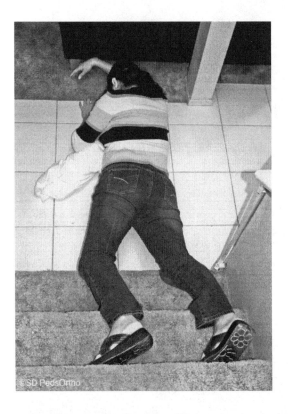

FIGURE 13.2
Reenacted photograph of a caregiver's nonfatal fall while descending with a baby in her arms. (From Pennock, A.T., et al., *J. Child. Orthop.*, 8, 77–81, 2014. Open Access. This article is distributed under the terms of the Creative Commons Attribution License, which permits any use, distribution, and reproduction in any medium, provided the original author(s) and the source are credited.)

13.3 Potential Risk while Ascending/Descending Stairways

13.3.1 Inherent Risks of Stairways

13.3.1.1 Fall Risk and Kinesthetic Risk in Descending Stairways

A human walks stairways upright, using bipedal locomotion, with the head always positioned at the highest point of the body. Consequently, human bipedal locomotion itself provides potential risks when falling, because the skull might be easily broken if it impacts hard surfaces, even from the height of a meter. Walking with bipedal locomotion can be easily disturbed by unstable footing, losing balance, or even applying a few kilograms of horizontal force against the body.

Falls while descending stairways cause more severe injuries than falls on a level surface because of the consecutive protruding edges of the treads, which cause serious injuries and higher drop height. Because of the gravitational energy in ascending stairways, people will mostly fall forward if they trip against a step edge or if the foot is awkwardly placed on a tread. Therefore, the gravitational energy of falls while ascending stairways will not be higher than that while descending. Severe injuries caused by impact to the head are more likely to occur on steeper stairways and straight, longer flights of stairways than on gentle stairways, U-shaped two-flight stairways, and spiral stairways. The latter stair configurations result in comparatively lower impacts to the body just after falls (Svanström, 1974; Nagata, 1991a). Major risk factors that cause stair-related falls should be focused on descending stairways.

Natural bipedal gaits on stairways maintain regular rhythm and gait locomotion; therefore, irregular tread and rise dimensions will disturb a user's steady gait rhythm. Stair users cannot visually recognize tiny irregularities in dimensional differences.

13.3.1.2 Foot Movements in Descent and Possible Causes of Loss of Balance

When the track of a small bulb attached to the heel tip of a shoe is recorded with a camera, the motion of the heel tip in descent is as shown in Figure 13.3 (Nagata, 1979, 1984). The following variables are observed to be relevant to stair-related falls:

1. G_1: The shortest clearance between the edge of the upper step and the tip of the heel
2. G_2: The shortest clearance between the edge of the lower step and the tip of the heel
3. A_f: The foot contact angle between the shoe sole and the tread surface
4. L_f: The ratio of the foot contact length to the shod foot length.

According to the author's experimental results (Nagata, 1979, 1984), the G_1 and G_2 clearance values are considered relevant causes of tripping. The G_1 values for male subjects increase from 48 to 106 mm, and from 22 to 64 mm for female subjects wearing high heels, as the incline of stairways increases from 26.6° to 46.3°, and the G_2 values for both male and female subjects, on average, remain almost constant at 28–38 mm, increasing to 53 mm with the use of high heels only on a very steep incline (46.3°). Female subjects wearing high heels were apt to descend stairways more cautiously to avoid catching their heels on the nosing. Lockwood and Braaksma (1990) also measured G_1 and G_2 values on experimental stairways. They ascertained that the G_2 value remained constant. The G_2 value increased with increasing tread length. Their results for G_1 are consistent with the author's data except for the results for steep inclined stairways with high heels. Cohen

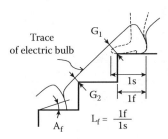

FIGURE 13.3
Track of the heel tip in descending stairways.

(2000) observed and videotaped six male users' behaviors to measure the clearance distance between the leading point of the heel of the trailing foot and the nose of successive steps on an actual gentle stairway (16 risers, tread depth: 27.9 cm, riser height: 17.8 cm, incline: 32.5°), on which falls allegedly occurred in descent at work. The clearance was 18.3 mm at the 50th percentile, with only 5.1 mm as a minimum clearance and 58.4 mm as a maximum clearance. Users who appear confident in descending moderate declining stairways seem to place their foot on the minimum clearance distance between heel placements on successive steps. This implies that a misstep may occur even on moderately declining stairways if a user is overconfident. According to the present codes, the tolerance level between the largest and smallest riser height is within 9.5 mm. Variation in depth of adjacent treads or in heights of adjacent risers shall be within 4.8 mm. Those tolerance levels seem to be reasonable to prevent tripping on the edge of a step just before placing the foot on the tread.

The L_f value is relevant to overstep. The foot is positioned inside the step when the L_f value is greater than 1.0. The tiptoe protrudes from the step when the L_f value is lower than 1.0. The L_f value remains almost constant for various walking speeds except with shorter tread depth. The foot angle, A_f, increases proportionally to the incline of stairways. A_f values are distinctly influenced by differences in the height of heels. The A_f value in descent differs between low and high heels, as shown in Figure 13.4. A high heel will come into contact with the tread more quickly than a low heel. The A_f value indicates the rotating degree of the foot joint and related shock absorption caused by the ankle bending. Footwear with high heels results in lower angles, with poor shock absorption, and can be more awkward on steep stairways.

Stair users are apt to lose balance and fall on/from stairways most easily due to the following six fundamental causes:

1. *Tripping*: The toe contacts the step nosing in ascent, or the heel contacts the step nosing in descent just before contact with the step.

2. *Overstepping*: The foot does not sufficiently contact an undersized tread in descending. During descent, overstepping the tread was a major factor associated with stair incidents.

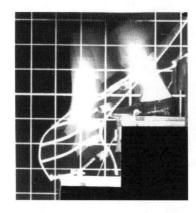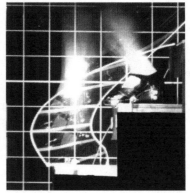

FIGURE 13.4
Photos taken with intermittent flash while descending stairways.

3. *Understepping*: The foot does not sufficiently land on the next tread when ascending stairways.

4. *Ghost step (air step)*: Users unaware of the location of the final step take an additional step that does not exist, caused by misrecognition of the gait mode at the last step of a stairway. Ghost steps are liable to occur just after adjusting a viewpoint from the foot to a forward view.

5. *Unstable footing*: This is caused by steps in the presence of debris, objects such as pebbles, sand, mud, algae, leaves, toys, and so on,

6. *Slipping*: Falls occur on lubricated tread surfaces, such as wet, oily, or icy stairways. True slipping is, in general, not a major factor that causes stair-related falls except in extreme cases, that is, icy or lubricated steps. Most stair-related fall victims first described their missteps as "slips"; even missteps by overstepping in descent or understepping in ascent. Slips are the easiest concept to comprehend, but least likely to occur (Carson et al., 1978; Templer, 1992; Jackson and Choen, 1995; Pauls, 2001). The ball of the foot touches down on the nosing at first in descending or the tread surface in ascending. Just after overstepping or understepping, foot rotation begins around the nosing, and subsequently, a foot slips off the step nosing. Then, stair users generally are apt to delude themselves about slipping as the major cause of missteps.

13.3.2 Interactive Triggering Factors that Cause Stair-Related Falls

Triggers causing loss of balance while walking on stairways are attributed to the interaction between a user's gait characteristics, stair design, environments, and maintenance. At least four categories for inducing stair-related falls can be listed as users' behavioral characteristic factors, stair design–induced factors, environment-related factors, and maintenance factors.

1. *Behaviorally induced risk factors by users*
   a. Descending/ascending in a hurry
   b. Descending/ascending with a hand-carried object, a baby, or a bulky object
   c. Descending/ascending with small objects, making it difficult to grab a handrail
   d. Descending/ascending while skipping steps
   e. Descending/ascending with high heels, slippery footwear, or loose footwear
   f. Descending/ascending with bifocal glasses, dark glasses, or poor eyesight
   g. Descending/ascending while fixating on a cell phone or watch or reading a newspaper or book
   h. Descending/ascending while chatting
   i. Descending/ascending wearing poorly fitting attire, making it hard to walk
   j. Descending/ascending wearing a long dress that covers the feet
   k. Descending/ascending under the influence of alcohol or medication
   l. Descending/ascending while staggering, attributed to a user's physiological impairments: dizziness, visual field loss
   m. Descending/ascending with deteriorated equilibrium and/or poor stato-kinetic reflexes

2. *Design-induced risk factors*

    a. Triggering factors that initiate missteps

        i. As tread depth becomes narrower than a foot length, missteps become more frequent. Shorter treads give insufficient foot support and cause postural instabilities.

        ii. Inconsistent dimensions of tread or rise cause missteps.

        iii. Slippery and rough treads cause missteps.

        iv. Inappropriate combinations of tread depth and riser height will cause an awkward walking mode and missteps.

        v. One or two isolated steps may be located in walkways, which provide no cues to their presence.

        vi. There may be no graspable, reachable handrail.

        vii. There may be a discontinuous handrail.

        viii. There may be confusing color patterns on the tread or poor visibility of nosings.

        ix. The nosing strip may project above the tread.

    b. Triggering factors that increase the severity of falls on/from stairways

        i. Long straight flights of stairways will possibly cause higher impact forces and gravitational energy to users just after falls by missteps.

        ii. If there is no reachable, graspable handrail on stairways, it is difficult to interrupt falls after losing balance.

3. *Environmentally induced factors*

    a. Lighting and color schemes that do not allow a user to distinguish steps or a clear step edge. False illusions created by shadows on the steps, glare, and sudden change of ambient illumination are liable to cause missteps because of insufficient visual perception.

4. *Maintenance-induced factors*

    a. Inadvertently dropped objects on the tread surface

    b. Obstacles or objects on the steps

    c. Broken or dirty handrail

    d. Eroded tread surface, loose nosing strip, worn or bulged carpet on the tread

    e. Broken step edge, abrasive surfaces, uneven surfaces and bumps

    f. Insufficient illumination, high-contrast shadows, reflected glare

    g. Distracting objects, such as a wall-clock or a publicity poster

13.3.3 Risk Assessment to Estimate Potential Risk to Cause Stair-Related Falls

13.3.3.1 *Estimation of Individual Risk*

Mainly in hospitals, residential care centers, and nursing homes, it is very important to assess an individual's potential risk for fall prevention. The potential risk score (I) for an individual person (j) could be obtained from past records of fall experience (M), postural instability (N), score for physical fragility of bones (F), and daily activities in mobility (D).

In this case, tailor-made countermeasures for an individual to prevent falls from stairways should be taken (Nagata and Kim, 2007). The following conceptual formula could be suggested for an individual user (j):

$$I_j = \left(M_j + N_j + F_j\right) \cdot D_j \tag{13.1}$$

where:

  I_j: Potential risk score for an individual user (j)
  M_j: Score estimated by frequency of previous incidents or falls by missteps for an individual user (j)
  N_j: Score for postural instability for an individual user (j)
  F_j: Score for physical fragility of bones and vulnerability of internal organs for an individual user (j)
  D_j: Probable daily frequency rate of use of stairways for an individual user (j)

If D_j is nearly zero, for example, a bedridden patient, the potential risk score for an individual person (I_j) is almost nil. An elderly person with poor physical fragility (F_j) is highly accident-prone even if they do not use stairways (D_j). If intoxicated users or the elderly are descending stairways, the scores for postural instability (N_j) become very high.

Specifically, in hospitals, nursing care homes, and residential care homes, average individual potential risk (I_j) will be comparatively higher than at other venues because of the advanced ages of users and their physical incapability and fragility. Risks for each individual should be considered as much as possible. Even if a better stair design is used, the potential risk still depends on an individual's physical capabilities and the characteristics of users on each specific stairway.

In the field of public health, fall prevention strategies should be comprehensive and multifaceted. Stairway safety is one way to modify the individual's surroundings to decrease potential risk. Nonetheless, when stairways are designed for public facilities, hospitals, and nursing care homes, overall attention should be paid to decreasing potential risk by considering every risk factor for children, the elderly, and impaired persons. Stairways in hospitals, residential care centers, and nursing homes should be considered some of the riskiest sites for falls to happen, even if the stairways are built at optimum dimensions and with the safest designs. The use of stairways should be limited for physically and mentally impaired users, such as those with dementia as well as hospital patients, the elderly, and toddlers, by setting up barriers at the entrances to stairways. Another option, installing elevators, should be considered for physically impaired people. In case of emergencies, escape chutes to evacuate from higher floors to the ground level should be considered. Stairway safety research to decrease potential risk for the elderly mainly focuses on individuals to build risk awareness. Physiotherapeutic countermeasures such as proper exercise for muscle strengthening, balance training, and the use of protectors for those at risk of hip fractures and head injuries are not considered in this chapter.

13.3.3.2 Estimation of Interactive Risk between a Stairway and an Individual

Potential risks and their interventions to decrease stair-related falls should be further considered. Stair-related falls should be investigated and classified by environmental factors such as stair geometry, handrail, illumination, nosing, surface material, color, and so on, along with the characteristics of the stair users, such as the physical, sensory, and cognitive deterioration associated with aging. In general, the risk of stair-related falls could be estimated by multiplication of the magnitude of a latent hazard and its probability. Accurate estimations of potential risks are often difficult. Uncommon catastrophes can be hard to estimate. Human activities are sometimes considered to be beyond estimation.

A common concept to assess potential risk factors is essential in setting up preventive measures to reduce potential risks. The risk of probable stair-related falls (E) on a certain stairway (k) depends on the probability of stair-related falls (P) on the stairway (k) multiplied by the magnitude of latent hazard (H) for the stairway (k). The following conceptual formula for fall-related risk for a certain stairway (k) can be derived as

$$E_k = P_k \cdot H_k \qquad\qquad (13.2)$$

where:

E_k: Risk of stair-related falls of a certain stairway (k)
P_k: Probability of stair-related falls at a certain stairway (k)
H_k: Magnitude of latent hazards of a certain stairway (k)

Fall prevention strategies should be individually comprehensive and multifaceted. The individual potential risk score (I_j) of a stair user can be basically assessed by possible impact forces from falls and possible slipping, tripping, or stumbling on a certain stairway (k). The possible interactive risk score for a certain stairway (E_k) can be derived from the score of physical fragility (F_j) and the score of postural instability (N_j) of an individual user (j). The following conceptual interactive formula is suggested:

$$E_{jk} = P_k\left(F_j\right) \cdot H_k\left(N_j\right) \qquad\qquad (13.3)$$

where:

E_{jk}:   Possible stair-related risk for an individual user (j) at a certain stairway (k)
$P_k(F_j)$:   Interactive function for probabilities of stair-related falls at a certain stairway (k) while a user (j) with the score for physical fragility (F_j) is descending
$H_k(N_j)$:   Interactive function for magnitude of latent hazards at a certain stairway (k) while a user (j) with the score for postural instability (N_j) is descending

Even if better environmental designs are standardized, the potential risk of a certain stairway still depends on physical factors and the number of users at each specific site. The latent hazard of a certain stairway should be estimated by probable drop height or falling impact forces or harmful or risky materials on stair surfaces and their interactions with users. The theoretical interactive risk score for a certain stairway (E_{jk}) should be derived from the integration of individual interactive users' risk scores at a certain stairway. Stair-related falls would not occur, even on very steep and risky stairways, if no one used them. On the contrary, stair-related falls will occur even on a safer stairway if numerous users, including children, the elderly, and impaired people, are using the stairway, such as at railway stations and public facilities. Stairway safety research should be applied to individual physical properties and high-traffic stairways to reduce rates of stair-related falls. Therefore, the risk of a certain stairway partially depends on the number of users and their physical risk scores. By introducing these formulas for intrinsic and extrinsic values, we could holistically focus the importance of points to discuss regarding stairway safety to reduce fall risk while descending stairways. A holistic approach to the design of stairways should be taken to prevent stair-related falls.

13.4 Consideration of Safer Tread Depth

13.4.1 Critical Tread Depth to Support Upright Posture in Descent

The tiptoe is likely to protrude from the tread in descending stairways, especially in cases where the tread depth is shorter than the shoe length, but the metatarsal heads of a foot should always be in contact with the tread surface, even on a shorter tread depth. Therefore, very short tread depth will impose crabwise gaits on stair users. As the proportion of the shoe that can be placed on the stair tread becomes greater, the protrusion of the tiptoe from the tread will be less likely to occur in descent (Wright and Roys, 2005). Safer tread depth should have sufficient length to accommodate the contact length of a shoe on tread enough to keep a user standing upright and balanced in descent. Templer (1974) suggested that the tread depth should be between 27.9 and 29.2 cm as a minimum to accommodate 99% of the population, considering maximum male foot length (30.0 cm) plus 3.0 cm of additional length for a street shoe. The projection of tiptoe of an average shoe length is 4.4 cm, and 0.6 cm for the clearance distance between the back end of a heel and a riser. He also remarked that for users with large feet, narrower treads less than 27.9 cm would produce more arrhythmic incidents in descent. Sufficient tread depth to support upright posture should satisfy the stable foot contact depth as a minimum dimension to reduce the probabilities of overstep. This implies that taller users or users wearing longer shoes will require longer minimum tread depth. The experimental results have shown that the mean ratio of the distance by which a shoe overhangs a nosing increases as tread depth decreases. Subjects managed to put a significantly greater part of their foot on a tread depth over 30.0 cm (Wright and Roys, 2005).

13.4.2 Safer Visible Tread Depth

13.4.2.1 Visual Cues to Adjust Walking Rhythm at Entrances to Stairways

Incomplete visual information is one of the major reasons attributed to human error that cause missteps due to a lapse of adjustment to gait mode in case of hurried ambulation, inappropriate dimensions, poor lighting, and so on. A disproportionately high percentage of missteps were observed at the top and the bottom of flights by video recording (Templer et al., 1978). It is crucial that stairways be designed so that users' sensory cues for correct perception of stairways are not blocked. Users walk naturally on a level floor while directing their attention a few meters ahead. However, while ascending or descending stairways, especially at entrances, users must carefully watch their feet to adjust their walking rhythm to put a foot correctly on the allotted tread depth. One step length on stairways must be adjusted to one tread depth and, to some extent, by riser height.

Stair users adjust their gait by visualizing the initial placement of their foot on the first step at the entrance of stairways. Some users are liable to fall because of lack of attention at the first or second step (Hay and Barlow, 1985). Visual deception or distractions disrupt the visual scans associated with safe ambulation on stairways, and are the leading causes of missteps (Carson et al., 1978; Templer et al., 1978; Pennock et al., 2014). This article discusses inaccurate visual or tactile information regarding stairways while users descend from an upper horizontal floor. Many missteps occur at entrances to stairways due to an abrupt change of a user's walking rhythm. The fewest missteps were observed while subjects were walking at a pace slow enough to spend sufficient time to pay attention to correct foot placement. This is the reason why many falls occur at the entrance to stairways when people are hurrying down them. Stairways with few steps are most risky, with slight changes in elevation, whereby users are not apt to take notice of visual cues to adjust their gait mode. Building designers should eliminate stairways with few steps as much as possible.

13.4.2.2 Required Visual Tread Depth to Adjust Steps at the Entrance of Stairways

The size of the necessary tread depth can be determined by adding the minimum dimension required for placing the shoe sole on the tread depth and the extra dimension of the inner part of the tread depth in a blind spot with consideration of the field of sight in descent. Factors causing visual errors due to hand-carried objects, design patterns, or the color scheme of the tread depth and the like have not been mentioned in this section.

When users are approaching the entrance of a stairway, they adjust their pitch of walking based on peripheral visual information. Users usually watch the entrance to a stairway and the first step of a stairway to ensure a safer footing. A specific illustration of a user's field of view is shown in Figure 13.5. When approaching the stairway, a user positioned at a distance (L_s) at view height (L_e) can begin to overview the lowest part of the stairway. At that time, the user unconsciously starts to adjust their walking rhythm to fit their length of stride to the tread depth. If the user's line of view is directed within the area A in Figure 13.5, the user might be able to view the entrance to the stairway, but would not be able to overview the whole stairway. The user begins to overview the whole of the stairway down to the bottom only when the viewer reaches the area B. The tip of the step comes into the sight of a user starting from the position in area B. Figure 13.6 shows how the first step is detected in this case. When a user stands in front of a stairway and looks down at the step, the nosing of the tread may be seen, but the inside of the shadowed part

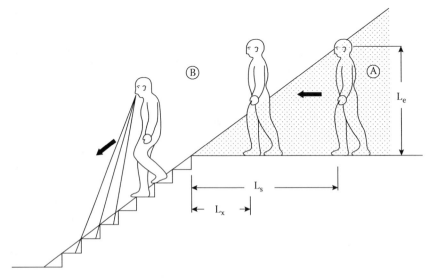

FIGURE 13.5
Field of view in descending stairways.

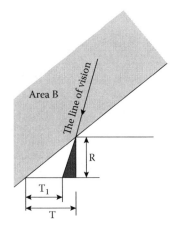

FIGURE 13.6
Blind spot and visual area of the first tread in descending stairways.

of the tread will be in a blind spot. The wider the visible part of the tip of the step, the more accurate foot placements will be. The visible depth of the first step (T_1) and the depth of the blind spot at the first step $(T-T_1)$ can be theoretically derived from Equation 13.4:

$$T - T_1 = R\left(L_x / L_e\right) \tag{13.4}$$

where:
   L_x is the horizontal distance from the standing point to the entrance of the stairway
   R is the riser height
   T is the tread depth

The necessary distance L_x for adjustment in front of a stairway can be derived from Equation 13.4:

$$T_1 = T - R\left(L_x / L_e\right) \tag{13.5}$$

The distance L_x is fixed by height of viewpoint of an individual (L_e), dimensions of tread depth (T), riser height (R), and visible tread depth for targeting mark (T_1). At the position of distance L_x from the stair entrance, users can detect part of the tread by T_1 as a visual cue. Then, the user can start to adjust his or her step length to match the tread depth as much as possible.

To avoid missteps caused by making a false foot step, it is necessary for a user to be able to view the width of a step available for his or her foot in advance. This poses the question of the appropriate distance from the top of stairways to see the tread available for safely placing feet. To sum up, it is possible to determine the size of the step necessary for safety by adding the minimum visible tread depth needed for safely placing feet and the inner step space that creates a blind spot. The size of the blind spot on the first step is $R(L_x/L_e)$. The necessary size of the step will be calculated by the following equation:

$$T_{req} = L_f S + R\left(L_x / L_e\right) \tag{13.6}$$

where:

T_{req}: necessary tread depth

L_f: ratio of shoe sole contact length on the tread depth divided by shoe length

S: Shoe length

L_x/L_e: Approach ratio of the horizontal distance from the standing point to the entrance of the stairway divided by the height of the user's viewpoint

In Equation 13.6, the necessary tread depth T_{req} in the case of $L_x/L_e = 0$ at the value $L_x = 0$ just at the entrance is the minimum necessary tread depth obtained from shoe length (S) and foot contact ratio (L_f), and the safety performance to place the foot on the tread will presumably increase proportionally as the L_x/L_e value becomes greater. If the tread depth is smaller than the T_{req} value at the approach ratio $L_x/L_e = 0$, the step may be not wide enough for placing the shoe safely, causing the user to descend in an awkward manner, which could cause missteps. Theoretical calculations of the range of tread depth specifications are feasible from the visual depth. The minimum required tread depth T_{req} could be derived numerically if the minimum ratio (L_f), the shoe length (S), and the safer approach ratio (L_x/L_e) can be hypothesized from the actual behavior of users, types and length of shoes, how stairways are used, and so on.

The author experimentally measured the ratio of L_f values of male adults as 0.76 and that of female adults as 0.91 for low-heeled footwear and 0.92 for high-heeled footwear for ordinary descending gaits (Nagata, 1979, 1984). Lockwood and Braaksma (1990) also measured the L_f for high heels, which was approximately 0.8–0.87, or 10%–12% higher than for low heels. Therefore, the L_f value of 0.9 can be permissible for the minimum foot contact area. Assuming that the minimum safe distance to adjust a stride before descending stairways is 20% of the height of the eye (approximately half the step length), the ratio of L_x/L_e will be approximately 0.2, and the L_f value will be 0.9. The recommended minimum tread depth can be derived from the following equation:

$$T_{req} = 0.9S + 0.2R \qquad (13.7)$$

The required safe tread depth is a combination of minimum shoe contact length (0.9S) and safety depth (0.2R) for covering a blind spot. Safe tread depth increases as riser height increases. The L_f values should be less for the young and greater for the elderly for stable footing. This principal equation can be applied to ascertain the differences in safe tread depth for children and adults.

13.4.3 Visual Obstruction Just before Foot Contact with the Tread

Steps visibly obscured by poor lighting, abrupt changes of lightness level, visual obstruction from holding a baby or carrying objects, attire such as a long dress, and so on can also cause missteps. A directly obstructed view toward the foot will often cause erroneous steps while descending stairways. Most people do not recognize the risks inherent in bipedal locomotion. With regard to the visual field just before placing a foot on the tread while passively descending stairways, the tiptoe of a shoe as a visual cue for placing a foot correctly on a tread becomes obscured. The extent of vision toward the tiptoe being obstructed by thigh movement on steep stairways is shown in Figures 13.7 and 13.8. This could lead to an erroneous step on a tread. Since thigh movement obstructs the visual field to a footstep, the influence of the dimensions of the tread and rise and the height of the user are examined.

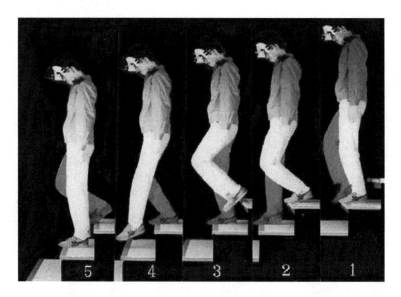

FIGURE 13.7
Movements of a thigh in descending stairways. (1) The left tiptoe of the shoe starts to be hidden by the left thigh movement; (2) the left tiptoe of the shoe is completely hidden by the left thigh movement; (3) the left knee is largely bending and the vision to the steps is obstructed by the left thigh movement; (4) the left tiptoe for placing the foot starts to be seen; (5) the left shoe is placed on the tread.

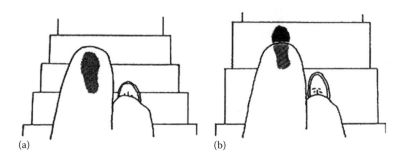

FIGURE 13.8
Vision of lower treads obstructed by the thigh extension. (a) Steep stairways; (b) gentle stairways.

In the author's research regarding view during descent (Nagata, 1993, 2006), several experiments were conducted using stairways with six steps of 90 cm width that can be mechanically set up with various combinations of tread depth and riser height. Two subjects were used in the experiment: a male subject A (170 cm tall and 25 years of age) and a male subject B (163 cm tall and 25 years of age). The subjects wore a small camera on their heads, as shown in Figure 13.9. The experiment included combinations of 24 different setups for six sizes of the tread depth (15–36 cm) and four sizes of the riser height (14–23 cm) at 3 cm intervals. The experiment was conducted with each subject descending the stairways five times for each of the different dimensional combinations. All the scenes including views to the tread were recorded by video recorder with a precise time stamp.

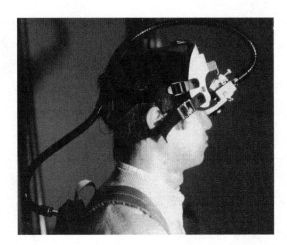

FIGURE 13.9
Fixing the camera on the subject's head.

The following values have been calculated from the videotape image-recording experiments:

- The ratio of the time from vision of the shoe tip being obstructed by the thigh till the shoe comes into sight again, divided by the stride time.
- The maximum ratio of the tread depth obstructed by the thigh. This value is the ratio (%) of the length of the step obstructed by the thigh divided by the size of the whole tread depth. If the ratio of the step obstructed by the thigh is 150%, it means that the whole tread depth just before placing a foot and 50% of the following tread depth is also obstructed. If the value is 300%, it means that three tread depths downward are totally obscured.

These values were calculated from the data read from the video images for each movement of the left and right leg. Time measurements were read from the video images based on the frame-by-frame advance at the rate of 1/30 of a second, and the lengths of projection were visually read from the scale marked in advance on the tread by using the images recorded on the videotape. All the 480 pieces of data were summarized in terms of the dimensions of the steps and the experiment subjects.

Vision obstruction ratios were summarized based on the data of a distribution map drawn as shown in Figure 13.10. The results are shown for the 163 cm tall subject in Figure 13.10a and for the 170 cm tall subject in Figure 13.10b. Judging from the contour map, there are characteristics probably arising from the difference in the statures of the experiment subjects. The obstruction ratios are higher by 15%–20% for the taller subject between the obstruction ratio ranges of 100% and 150% even in the same experimental dimension. This means that taller users are liable to suffer oversteps while descending stairways.

As shown in Figure 13.10, when the stairway slope is around 45°, the distribution curves of the obstruction ratios become similar to the slant line of incline of the stairway. On the contrary, if the stairway slope is around 30°, the contour lines of the obstruction ratio are variable as the tread depth increases, but rather stable as the riser height increases. The effects of reducing vision obstruction ratios are greater by widening the tread depth than

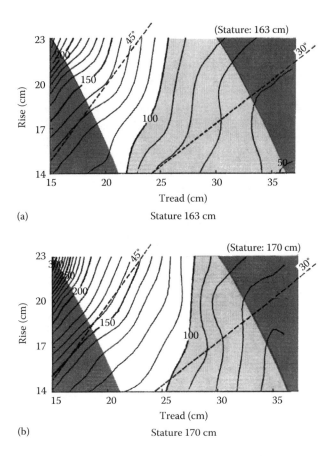

(a) Stature 163 cm

(b) Stature 170 cm

FIGURE 13.10
Contour map of the ratios obstructed by the thigh extension in descent. (a) Stature 163 cm; (b) stature 170 cm.

by changing the riser height. The differences in statures negatively affect visual range. The obstruction ratio by the thigh movements is greater for a taller person. In other words, on the same steep stairway, a taller person has a smaller range of sight toward the footstep obstructed, and the risk of falling down by false stepping increases.

13.5 Safer Combinations of Tread Depth and Riser Height

13.5.1 Stairway Safety from Building Design

Physiological loads such as oxygen consumption and heart rate have been used to obtain suitable tread and rise combinations for stairways (Lehmann and Engelmann, 1933; Ward et al., 1967; Ward and Beading, 1970; Templer and Corcoran, 1972; Ramanathan and Kamon, 1974). Steep stairways with higher risers and shorter treads demand no greater metabolic loads than less steep stairways with much lower risers and larger treads (Corlett et al., 1972). Moreover, physiological loads may hide differences in performance caused by small changes in stair geometry. Design priority should not be put on physiological loads in ascent, but on safety performance in descent.

Tread depth and riser height measurements of stairways have historically been based on empirical design rules of thumb. Fitch et al. (1974) raised questions about the 300-year-old empirical rule entrenched in many building and fire codes, which specified that the tread depth should be one step length when walking on a flat surface minus two times the riser height (one step length from 61 to 63.5 cm). According to this rule, as the riser becomes higher, tread depth should be narrower. This produces risky stairways not sufficient to maintain a safe footing length in descending. It is apparent that this empirical rule was considered only for ascending stairways to decrease physiological loads. Most stair-related falls occur while descending stairways. Bipedal locomotion in descent should be considered for safety performance. Templer (1974) stated: "The empirical formula is too restrictive for human adaptability and the range of options for combining tread depth and riser height at any level cannot be expressed satisfactorily by a linear equation."

Safety researchers for stairways have been challenged to create safer combinations of tread depth and riser heights and to reduce risk related to falls from stairways. Building researchers have intensively engaged in developing codes of practice for constructing stairways and in specifying allowable dimensions and design (Templer et al., 1978; Fitch et al., 1974; Pauls, 1991, 2001; Roys, 2001; Roys and Wright, 2005; Wright and Roys, 2005). Pauls (1991) has summarized three leading characteristics of safer stairways:

1. Visibility of steps: Steps that can be readily seen
2. Appropriate step geometry: Treads large enough to provide adequate footing
3. Provision of handrail: Reachable and graspable handrail

13.5.2 Less Risky Combinations of Tread Depth and Riser Height

13.5.2.1 Suggested Dimensions

In this section, less risky dimensions of tread and rise are discussed. Better-designed stairways contribute to decreasing stair-related falls. Building codes and standards have drastically influenced effects to improve the quality of actual environments. Based on past research, building codes, such as detailed dimensional requirements of stairways in the International Building Code (IBC) adopted throughout most of the United States, were established. The IBC-2012 specifies dimensions of tread depth and riser height, dimensional uniformity of tread depth and riser height, nosing projection size, nosing projection uniformity, incline of tread surface, handrails, and so on. According to the IBC-2012, riser height shall be 17.8 cm maximum and 10.2 cm minimum, and tread depth shall be 27.9 cm minimum, except for individual dwellings: 19.6 cm for maximum riser height and 25.4 cm for minimum tread depth where stair-related serious falls most frequently occur among senior inhabitants. The International Residential Code (IRC-2012) for one- and two-family dwellings also follows the same allowable dimensions for tread depth and riser heights as the IBC-2012 code. The US Life Safety Code (LSC) specifies less restrictive dimensions of tread depth and riser height for existing stairways and industrial access as the means of egress. By estimating possible stair-related risk and minimum tread depth for keeping stable posture as previously mentioned, this seems to be one example of compromise between safety research and practice. We should be more cautious in adopting these codes for stairway design in individual dwellings.

TABLE 13.3

Suggested Combinations of Tread Depth and Riser Height

Researcher and Code	Year	Method	Tread Depth (cm)	Riser Height (cm)
Lehman et al.	1933	Oxygen consumption	29	17
Fitch et al.	1974	Less observed missteps	27.9–35.6	10.2–17.8
Irvine et al.	1990	Acceptable dimensions	27.9–30.5[a]	18.3[b]
Templer et al.	1985	Least observed missteps	27.9	15.2
		Less observed missteps	25.4–27.9	15.2–17.8
Nagata	1995	Least perceived difficulties	29[d]	18.0[d]
			30[e]	15.5[e]
International Building Code	2012	For building	Above 27.9	10.2–17.8
		For residential house	Above 25.4	Below 19.6

[a] Tread depth below 25.4 cm and above 33.0 cm should not be allowed.
[b] Riser height below 15.2 cm and above 20.3 cm should not be allowed.
[c] For both younger and older males.
[d] For low-heeled footwear below 4.5 cm heel height.
[e] For high-heeled footwear with 9 cm heel height.

Lehman and Engelmann (1933) suggested optimum combinations of tread depth 29 cm and riser height 17 cm obtained from the energy demand of the human metabolism for different tread and rise dimensions. Fitch et al. (1974) suggested that a low rate of missteps should be between 27.9 and 35.6 cm for tread depth and between 10.2 and 17.8 cm for riser height, as shown in Table 13.3. Irvine et al. (1990) suggested that the optimum tread depth was between 27.9 and 30.5 cm and the optimum riser height was 18.3 cm. These dimensions are acceptable to males and females, young and old, and subjects of different physiques. They recommended that a riser height below 15.2 cm and above 20.3 cm, and tread depths more than 33 cm and less than 25.4 cm, should not be allowed. According to observations of actual users' behavior captured by video-recorders, which focused on the relationships between occurrence of incidents and dimensions (Templer et al., 1985), it was cited that the safest stairways should have maximum 27.9 cm tread depth and minimum 15.2 cm riser height. From their conclusions, a stairway designed within this range will result in a fairly low rate of missteps.

Safety researchers have not presented any indices for overall relations between tread depth and riser height. The author has investigated the perceived difficulty for elderly males, young males, and females for 42 tread/riser combinations while descending stairways to obtain a contour map of tread/riser dimensions using experimental stairways, as shown in Figure 13.11 (Nagata, 1995). Missteps will decrease as stair geometry becomes more precise. A series of perceptual tests with ten young female subjects (average age 19.7 years old) with four different types of footwear (slipper, low heel [heel height: 1 cm], mid heel [4.5 cm], and high heel [9.0 cm]) were conducted.

Both younger and elderly male subjects perceived least difficulty around 30 cm tread depth and 18 cm riser height. Combinations of tread and riser dimensions with less difficulty exist within a specific range.

For females, combinations of tread depth and riser height with least difficulty when descending stairways are around 29 cm tread depth and 18.0 cm riser height for lower-heeled footwear and around 30 cm tread depth and 15.5 cm riser height for high-heeled footwear. There are substantial differences in the sum of scaled values of perceived difficulties between high-heeled footwear and the other three heel heights for 42 experimental

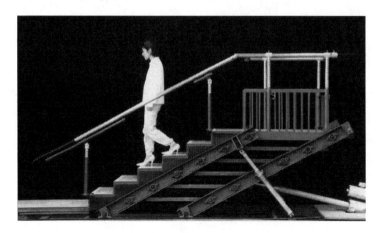

FIGURE 13.11
Experimental stairways.

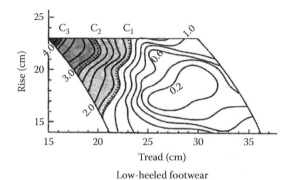

Low-heeled footwear

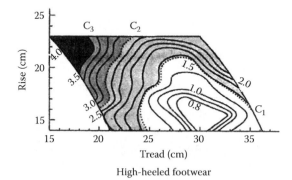

High-heeled footwear

FIGURE 13.12
Contour map of mean scaled values for younger female group with low-heeled footwear and high-heeled footwear. C_0: not at all difficult; C_1: slightly difficult; C_2: difficult; C_3: considerably difficult; C_4: very difficult.

combinations of tread depth and riser height. The perceived difficulty value gradually increases as the measurements deviate from these least difficult combinations, as shown in Figure 13.12 for high-heeled and low-heeled footwear. This implies that excessively shallower and wider tread depth or lower or higher riser height will cause awkward bipedal locomotion and loss of balance. These suggested dimensions are very consistent with other researchers' suggested combinations of tread depth and riser height, as shown in Table 13.3.

13.5.2.2 New Formula to Evaluate Combinations of Tread Depth and Riser Height

Female subjects with high-heeled footwear experienced considerable difficulty in every tread and riser combination. Many stair-related falls occur while females wearing high-heeled footwear are descending stairways, due to a risk of stumbling on the tread nosing. Walking with high heels is very unstable and prohibits bending the ankle as the foot touches the tread surface, resulting in lower shock absorption (Nagata, 1992). From a safety point of view, dimensions should be designed for risk-prone users wearing unstable footwear in descent, which causes more frequent stair-related falls. Hence, an index for designing safer stair dimensions should be used on the basis of perceptual tests with high-heeled footwear. To obtain an index for assessing perceived difficulty in descent, the relationship between scaled values (Y), dimensions of tread depth (T), and riser height (R) can be obtained by multiple regression analysis. The following equation has been derived:

$$Y = 0.0140 \cdot (T - 30)^2 + 0.0191 \cdot (R - 15.5)^2 + 1.05 \tag{13.8}$$

where Y are scaled values for each tread depth (T) and riser height (R). The multiple regression factor is 0.947, which is very significant: F-value = 168.1 $>F$ (2,39;0.001). Next, a simplified equation can be derived from Equation 13.8:

$$Y / 0.0140 = (T - 30)^2 + 1.364 \cdot (R - 15.5)^2 + 75 \tag{13.9}$$

$$(Y/0.0140) - 75 = (T - 30)^2 + 1.364 \cdot (R - 15.5)^2 \tag{13.10}$$

If the left-hand side of this equation is replaced into the index Z, and rounding the factor 1.364–1.5 because rounding errors are very negligible. The value of Z can be derived from

$$Z = (T - 30)^2 + 1.5 \cdot (R - 15.5)^2 \tag{13.11}$$

As the index increases, the tread and riser dimension combinations deviate from the center of the ovals, as shown in Figure 13.13. Tread depth differences produce greater

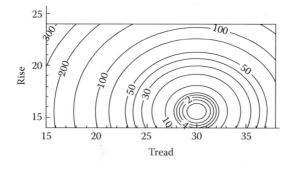

FIGURE 13.13
Contour map of the evaluation index of the Z value.

changes in the index values, especially in the region below around 25 cm tread depth and between around 14 and 24 cm riser height. This suggests that building designers should widen the tread depth to decrease the Z value as much as possible to improve safety on steeper stairways. The Z value should be below 10 to be least risky for public stairways by alleviating foot rotation in descent. This suggested index is more etiological than the traditional empirical rule, which specified that the tread depth should be one step length when walking on a flat surface minus two times the height of the riser.

13.6 Conclusion

Serious injuries that impact heads are more likely to occur on steeper stairways and straight longer flights of stairways than on gentle stairways, U-shaped two-flights, and spiral stairways when considering drop height and its gravitational energy. Head injuries account for the majority of fatal injuries caused by stair-related falls. The occurrence of fatal falls is higher in residential houses. People aged 65 and over suffer the greatest number of fatal falls. Particularly, heavy drinking habits are one of the contributory factors leading to serious falls from stairways. The field survey results of falls from stairways indicate that most stair-related falls occur when a user's walking speed is high.

Minimum tread depth sufficient to cover a shoe length will reduce the number of missteps on stairways. Tread and riser dimensions can be checked against the critical tread depth to support upright posture in descent, plus additional safety clearance to cancel the blind spot of the tread in descent to prevent visual deception. Taller stair users or people wearing longer shoes will require longer minimum tread depth. The size of the necessary tread depth can be determined by adding together the minimum dimension required for placing the shoe sole on the tread depth and the extra dimension of the inner part of the tread depth in a blind spot with consideration of the field of sight in descent. Tread depth is more important to stair safety than riser height. Therefore, it is recommended that the tread dimension should be increased, rather than the riser height being reduced, when improving stairways.

To achieve safer design of stairways, during risk assessment, designers should take into account users' actual movements, behavioral characteristics, footwear, and so on. The lowest perceived difficulties for combination of tread depth and riser height converge into single points (30 cm tread depth and 15.5 cm riser height for unstable footwear; 29 cm tread depth and 18.0 cm riser height for other, lower footwear). Perceived difficulties increase as measurements deviate from these combinations of tread depth and riser height.

Building designers must consider adequate dimensions and safety designs, reducing the potential risk of causing stair-related falls to the greatest extent possible. At the same time, we should recognize that each approach has certain limitations in reducing stair-related falls. For example, many stair-related falls occur on stairways with adequate combinations of tread depth and riser height because of behaviorally induced factors. The severity of injuries would be as low as possible if stair users were to grasp or touch handrails while descending stairways. The resolution may be an issue of user education more than one of stairway design or maintenance (Templer et al., 1985). An initiative to raise social awareness for preventing falls is imperative.

References

Allcott, G. A., *Safety information profile: Slips, trips and falls, working surfaces and industrial stairs*, PB84-154285, National Institute of Occupational Health and Safety, West Virginia, 1979.

Archea, J. C., Collin, B. L., Stahl, F. I., *Guideline for stair safety*, NBS: Building Science Series 120, National Bureau of Standards, Gaithersburg, US Department of Commerce, Washington, DC, 1979.

Carson, D. H., Archea, J. C., Margulis, S. T., Cason, F. E., *Safety on stairs*, NBS BSS 108/PB296732, National Bureau Standards, Washington, DC, 1978.

Cohen, H. H., A field study of stair descent: Videotapes of stair descent at an accident site attempt to reveal why and how people fall down stairs, *Ergonomics in Design: The Quarterly of Human Factors Applications*, 8(2), 11–16, 2000.

Cohen, H. H., Templer, J. A., An analysis of occupational stair accident patterns, *Journal of Safety Research*, 16, 171–181, 1985.

Corlett, E. N., Hutcheson, C., Delugan, M. A., Rogozenski, J., Ramps or stairs: The choice using physiological and biomechanic criteria, *Applied Ergonomics*, 3, 195–201, 1972.

Fitch, J. M., Templer, J., Corcoran, P., Dimension of stairs, *Scientific American*, 231(4), 82–90, 1974.

Hay, T. F., Barkow, B., A study of stair accidents, International Conference on Building Use and Safety Technology, 1985.

Irvine, C. H., Snook, S. H., Sparshatt, J. H., Stairway risers and treads: Acceptable preferred dimensions, *Applied Ergonomics*, 21(3), 215–225, 1990.

Jackson, P. L., Choen, H. H., An in-depth investigation of 40 stairway accidents and the stair safety literature, *Journal of Safety Research*, 26(3), 151–159, 1995.

Kose, S., Safety requirements of stairs during traverse with special emphasis on domestic stairs, *Report of the Building Research Institute*, 109, 1986.

Lehmann, G., Engelmann, B., Der zweekmäßigste Bau einer Treppe, *Arbeitphysiologie*, 6, 271–282, 1933.

Lockwood, I. M., Braaksma, J. P., Foot accommodation on various stair tread sizes, *Journal of Architectural and Planning Research*, 7(1), 1–12, 1990.

Miller, J. A., Esmay, M. L., Nature and causes of stairway falls, *Transactions of American Society of Agriculture*, 4(1), 112–114, 1961.

Mitchell, S. E., Aitken, S. A., Court-Brown, C. M., The epidemiology of fractures caused by falls down stairs, *ISRN Epidemiology*, Volume 2013, 6 pages, 2013.

Nagata, H., Experimental study of human motion on stairs, Research Institute of Industrial Safety, Research Note, No. 27–3, 1979 (in Japanese).

Nagata, H., Human factors contributing to slipping on stairs and development of slip resistance measurements on tread, *Proceedings of International Conference on Occupational Ergonomics*, Toronto, Canada, 1, 582–586, May 7–9, 1984.

Nagata, H., Analysis of fatal falls on the same level or on the stairs/steps, *Safety Science*, 14, 213–222, 1991a.

Nagata, H., Occupational accidents while walking on stairways, *Safety Science*, 14, 199–211, 1991b.

Nagata, H., Fundamental study on factors to cause falls on stairs: Evaluation of combination of tread and rise in regard to safety, *Journal of Architectural Planning and Environmental Engineering*, Trans. AIJ 439, 73–80, 1992 (in Japanese).

Nagata, H., Fatal and non-fatal falls: A review of earlier articles and their developments, *Safety Science*, 16, 379–390, 1993.

Nagata, H., Rational index for assessing perceived difficulty while descending stairs with various tread/rise combinations, *Safety Science*, 21, 37–49, 1995.

Nagata, H., Evaluation of safety dimensions of stairways based on human peripheral vision, *Proceedings of the 16th World Congress on Ergonomics*, Maastricht, the Netherlands, 6 pages, July 10–14, 2006.

Nagata, H., In-Ju Kim, Fall accidents in Japan and the classification of fall-risk factors, *International Conference on Slips, Trips, and Falls 2007: From Research to Practice*, Hopkinton, USA, 108–112, 2007.

Pauls, J. L., Safety standards, requirements and litigation in relation to building use and safety, especially safety from falls involving stairs, *Safety Science*, 14, 125–154, 1991.

Pauls, J. L., Life safety standards and guidelines focused on stairways, in *Universal Design Handbook*, 1st edn, ed. Preiser, W. F. E., Sostroff, E., New York, McGraw-Hill, 23.1–23.20, 2001.

Pennock, A. T., Gantsoudes, G. D., Forbes, J. L., Asaro, A. M., Mubarak, S. J., Stair falls: Caregiver's "missed step" as a source of childhood fractures, *Journal of Children's Orthopaedics*, 8, 77–81, 2014.

Preuβ, J., Padosch, S. A., Dettmeyer, R., Driever, F., Lignitz, E., Madea, B., Injuries in fatal cases of falls downstairs, *Forensic Science International*, 141, 121–126, 2004.

Ragg, M., Hwang, S., Steinhart, B., Analysis of serious injuries caused by stairway falls, *Emergency Medicine*, 12, 45–49, 2000.

Ramanathan, N. L., Kamon, E., The application of stair climbing to ergometry, *Ergnomics*, 17, 13–22, 1974.

Roys, M., Serious stair injuries can be prevented by improved stair design, *Applied Ergonomics*, 32, 135–139, 2001.

Roys, M., Wright, M., Minor variations in gait and their effect on stair safety, in Bust P.D. and McCabe P.T. (eds.), *Contemporary Ergonomics 2005*, Taylor and Francis, London. 427–431, 2005.

Svanström, L., Falls on stairs: An epidemiological accident study, *Scandinavian Journal of Social Medicine*, 2, 113–120, 1974.

Templer, J. A., Stair shape and human movement, Doctoral dissertation, New York, NY, Columbia University, 1974.

Templer, J. A., The unforgiving stair, *Proceedings of the International Conference on Building Use and Safety Technology*, Los Angeles, 122–126, March 12–14, 1985.

Templer, J. A., *The Staircase: Studies of Hazard, Falls and Safer Design*, MIT Press, Cambridge, MA, 1992.

Templer, J. A., Archea, J., Cohen, H. H., Study of factors associated with risk of work-related stairway falls, *Journal of Safety Research*, 16, 183–196, 1985.

Templer, J. A., Corcoran, P. J., Energy cost and stair design: Preliminary report, *Proceedings of Conference of Man/Transportation Interface*, Washington, DC. 67–86, May 31–June 2, 1972.

Templer, J. A., Mullet, G. M., Archea, J., Margulis, S. T., *An Analysis of the Behavior of Stair Users*, Washington, DC, US Department of Commerce, 1978.

US Department of Labor, Bureau of Labor Statistics, *Injuries resulting from falls on stairs*, Bulletin 2214, US Government Printing Office, Washington, DC, 1984.

Waller, J. A., Falls among the elderly: Human and environmental factors, *Accident Analysis & Prevention*, 10, 21–33, 1978.

Ward, J. S., Beadling, B., Optimum dimensions for domestic stairways, *Architects' Journal Information Library*, 25, 513–520, 1970.

Ward, J. S., Randall, P., Optimum dimensions for domestic stairways: A preliminary study, *Architects' Journal Information Library*, 5, 29–34, 1967.

Webber, G. M. B., Accidental falls on stairs or steps in England and Wales: A study of time trends of fatalities, *Journal of Occupational Accidents*, 7, 83–99, 1985.

Webber, G. M. B., Clark, A. J., Building related home accidents: A preliminary study, *Journal of Consumer Studies & Home Economics*, 3, 277–287, 1979.

Wild, D., Nayak, U. S. L., Isaac, B., Prognosis of falls in senior people at home, *Journal of Epidemiology & Community Health*, 35, 200–204, 1981.

Wright, M., Roys, M., Effect of changing stair dimensions on safety, *Contemporary Ergonomics*, Taylor and Francis, London. 469–474, 2005.

Wyatt, J. P., Beard, D., Busuttil, A., Fatal falls down stairs, *International Journal of the Injured*, 30(1), 31–34, 1999.

14

Improving Balance Control: Current State and Practices

Kari Dunning, Ashutosh Mani, and Amit Bhattacharya

CONTENTS

14.1 Introduction

Falls are multifactorial, due to both internal and external factors. Balance is an important intrinsic factor to prevent falls and injury. This chapter will review strategies that improve balance, specifically those that train the internal physiological systems, and provide recommendations for those who work at elevation or inclined surfaces.

14.2 Background and Significance of Fall Prevention

14.2.1 Need for Fall Prevention in the Workplace: A Mechanism-Based Strategy

Fall risks are most prevalent in aging workers and workers who work at elevated and inclined surfaces, such as roofers and sheet metal workers.[1-7] In the aging workers (who are assumed to be healthy), the natural compensatory mechanisms (i.e., visual, vestibular, and proprioceptive afferents) necessary for maintenance of safe upright balance are compromised due to the normal aging process.[8-12] In addition, work-related risks associated with working on elevated and inclined surfaces have been shown to compromise the functionalities of healthy workers' afferents (vision, vestibular, and proprioceptive), which in turn, detrimentally impacts their postural balance.[3-6,13-15] Therefore, there is a need to develop innovative balance control training strategies, which are specifically focused to enhance the functionalities of workers' afferents, that is, visual, vestibular, and proprioceptive systems.

Falls from roofs are a common cause of nonfatal injuries in the construction industry and are the leading cause of fall fatalities.[16-18] Falls are the second highest cause of nonfatal injuries in the construction industry.[16-18] In 2005, in comparison with other industries, on average, nonfatal fall-related injuries were twice as frequent among construction workers. The construction industry has the highest frequency of falls from elevation. Injury due to a single fall from elevation usually cost at least $500,000.[18] In the construction industry, roofers, sheet metal workers, and ironworkers are considered high-risk occupations, having the three highest rates of fall-related deaths and nonfatal injuries.[16] Because of high rates of fatality and nonfatal injuries in the construction industry, there is a critical need for a comprehensive fall prevention program, particularly in the high–fall risk occupations.

Therefore, to minimize the risk of falls in this industry, traditional fall-protection devices/strategies have to be supported with innovative and physiologically/biomechanically appropriate intrinsic training so that workers' postural balance is improved and conditioned to effectively respond to workplace-associated perturbations to their postural stability. This chapter will provide useful and innovative fall-prevention strategies adapted from evidence-based clinically effective balance-improvement programs.

14.2.2 Workplace Risk Factors for Falls and the Need for Improving Balance Capacity for Workers at High Fall Risk

As per Liberty Mutual Workplace Safety Index analysis,[19] in 2005, fall on the same level ranked as the second leading cause of disabling injury, costing $6.6 billion. In 2005, the impact of overall cost burden due to falls of all kinds (same level and to lower level) collectively shares the first place ranking with overexertion totaling about 25% of the total cost of all disabling injuries.

Biomechanically and physiologically speaking, falls and/or near-falls occur for many reasons: both *extrinsic* factors at the workplace (e.g., type of task being performed, environmental lighting, standing/walking on inclined surface properties, and shift work) and *intrinsic* factors (e.g., neuromuscular functional abilities and health status) of the workers' ability to maintain safe upright postural balance when exposed to these external factors. Previous studies from our laboratory and others have shown that postural stability is detrimentally affected by task performance on inclined/elevated surfaces (e.g., residential roofs), ladders, slippery surfaces, and dark environments.[7,14,20-25] The interplay among external fall risk factors and workers' intrinsic factors determines whether a fall can be prevented. Therefore, a comprehensive fall-prevention program must include fall-prevention devices via engineering control as well as innovative evidence-based currently available techniques (but not applied to construction workers yet) to enhance workers' intrinsic capacity to maintain safe upright postural balance under exposure to fall risk factors at their workplace. Although significant efforts have been applied to develop fall-arresting devices, there is a lack of application of existing evidence-based techniques for enhancing the intrinsic capacity of workers' postural balance.

One of the leading causes of workplace falls/near-falls is the *slip event* (usually >60% of cases).[26–32] Previous studies from our laboratory and others have shown that accurate a priori slip perception is associated with better postural balance maintenance during task performance on a slippery surface.[22,33–36] A recent study supports the notion that *anticipatory postural adjustments* (APA) (i.e., feed-forward postural control) are associated with activation of postural muscles in advance of perturbation to balance, thereby providing better postural control.[37] Since slip perception ability varies with inherent differences in the capacity of individuals' physiological afferents' (e.g., proprioception), it is reasonable to expect different types of compensatory responses to be used by different subjects while carrying out a task on a slippery surface. Also, with aging, the proprioception, visual, and vestibular systems become impaired, thereby causing age-associated changes in the compensatory responses used while negotiating a slippery surface at the workplace. Field-based studies in restaurant workers and laboratory-based studies from our group provide evidence that older workers have reduced perception of the slipperiness of a surface.[13,26,27,38–41] As shown in Figure 14.1, older workers demonstrate decreased ability to adequately gage the slipperiness of a work surface as the COF decreases.[13] In fact, as shown by the solid line in the graph, older workers show a plateau effect, whereby, despite a rapid decrease in the slipperiness, their perception of the slipperiness does not decrease accordingly. On the other hand, younger workers' perception of slipperiness decreased along with the decrease in actual COF, as shown by the dashed line in Figure 14.1. This suggests that with increasing age, workers may not be able to adequately assess the risk of loss of

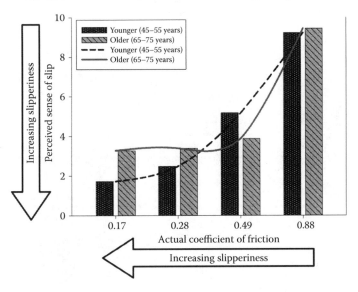

FIGURE 14.1
Workers' perception of slipperiness.

balance and falling when working on a slippery surface. Previous studies have shown that the proprioception system is amenable to improvement with appropriate conditioning/ training in patient populations, but it has not been applied in the working population of all ages.[42–60] Since there are numerous occupations (e.g., restaurant workers, grocery workers, construction workers, delivery workers, agricultural workers, and mining workers) for which the uncontrollable nature of the workplace environment does not always lend itself to proper and continuous management of slippery surfaces, it is reasonable to investigate the role of slip perception training in minimizing slips/falls.

The overall focus of this chapter is on investigating the types of training modes most appropriate for enhancing the functional balance of aging workers and those who work on elevated and inclined surfaces and on surfaces with slippery contamination.

14.3 Mechanisms of Balance Control

To maintain upright posture and avoid falls, the neuromotor control system in the human body receives inputs from three afferent systems to assess the risk of loss: visual, vestibular, and proprioception (Figure 14.2). Once the risk of balance loss has been assessed by the higher motor control centers and/or the spinal reflex control system, output (efferent) signals are sent to the musculoskeletal system to take corrective measures and avoid loss of balance. These corrective measures include anticipatory and reactive postural adjustments (ankle, knee, and hip strategies), taking a step in the anticipated direction of fall (thereby increasing base of support), and whole-body reactions that involve bilateral coordination of the legs, arms, and trunk.[61]

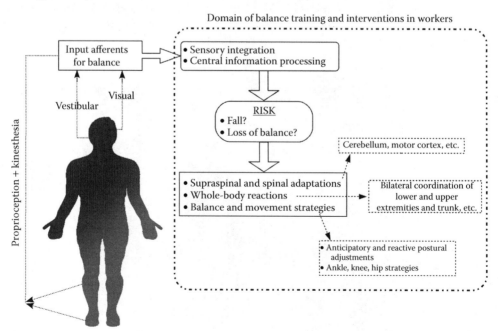

FIGURE 14.2
Neuromotor control system for the maintenance of postural balance.

Anticipatory controls involve internal feedback loops (internal to the person)—they allow a person to "anticipate" movement and react in a manner that avoids loss of balance. Reactive controls, on the other hand, are in response to external input—they allow a person to "react" to external conditions (e.g., perturbations, stepping in a hole) to allow a person to either maintain or recover balance.

Sensory integration of the visual, vestibular, and proprioception systems is critical; however, healthy and responsive motor output systems are also needed, including adequate strength, flexibility, coordination, and reaction speeds for movement strategies of ankles, knees, and hips. In addition, healthy nonmotor systems are important, including cognition (attention, learning), orientation, and perception.

Any impairment in these systems has the potential to impair balance: visual, vestibular, proprioception, strength, flexibility, coordination, reaction speed, perception, and cognition. Medical conditions that impair balance include hypo- or hypertension, heart disease, diabetes, and neurological diagnoses (e.g., Parkinson's disease, multiple sclerosis, stroke). Specific types of medications can impair balance, especially those that work via the central nervous system, including medications for sleep, depression, and anxiety; diuretics; hypnotics/sedatives; digoxin; and cardiovascular, anti-parkinsonian, and psychoactive drugs, including benzodiazepines. Over-the-counter medications can also impair balance, including those that have anticholinergic and sedating effects, specifically Benadryl and Tylenol PM.

Falls generally occur due to an interaction between three factors: the individual's predisposition to falling, the task being performed, and the environment (Figure 14.3). Intrinsic factors can increase an individual's propensity to fall, including diminished motor control, weakness, older age, cognitive impairment, and impaired perception. Extrinsic work factors that increase fall risk can be categorized into the environment and the task (Figure 14.3). Environmental conditions that challenge the balance system include performing a task on unstable, unlevel, or slippery surfaces and in poor lighting. Tasks that involve high fall risk include working to

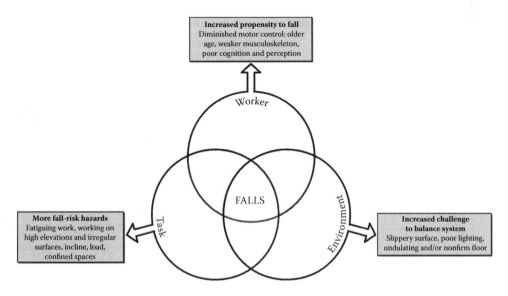

FIGURE 14.3
Fall risk categorized into worker, environment, and task.

fatigue and on elevations and inclines. These extrinsic factors can be minimized by using safe working practices such as keeping the work area clean, using fall-protection personal protective equipment (PPE) (harness, appropriate footwear, etc.), and fall-arrest equipment.

Most workers have healthier cognitive and musculoskeletal systems than populations with a higher propensity to falling, such as those with medical conditions such as Parkinson's disease and multiple sclerosis. Therefore, workers are typically better equipped to avoid loss of balance and falls, *provided* they assess and perceive the risk accurately. Minimizing the intrinsic fall risk factors in workers may require focus on training the afferent systems of balance to better assess fall risk.

The ability to perceive the risk of loss of balance and fall is critical for maintaining upright balance in static and dynamic conditions. Inability to accurately gage the risk of balance loss can lead to inadequate deployment of compensatory mechanisms for avoiding falls (Figure 14.4). Examples of such situations are (1) when an individual fails to accurately assess (especially, underestimates) the slipperiness, measured by the COF between the bottom of the shoes and the floor, and (2) underestimation of postural sway in the mediolateral and anterior–posterior direction. The technology and knowledge base are now available to quantify such mismatches between actual and perceived risk of environmental factors (e.g., slipperiness of standing/walking surface) and/or individuals' perception of threat to their postural balance. COF-μ can be objectively quantified for any two given surfaces using force platform technology (μ = horizontal force/vertical force; these forces are created by the subjects during task performance), and the subjective perception of slipperiness can be quantified using an established perception scale.[20,23,62] A measured (with a force plate) value of $\mu = 1$ is associated with the COF of a "dry" surface, while decreasing values approaching $\mu = 0$ are associated with a "very-very" slippery surface. On the other hand, a subjective perception scale for slipperiness[62] of a surface ranges between 10 ("dry") and 0 ("very-very" slippery). Essentially, using such a rating scale, an individual reports the perceived slipperiness (of friction) between his/her shoe sole and the walking/standing surface. Therefore, a higher value of COF-μ should be associated with a higher score on the perceived slipperiness scale. Similarly, force plates can also be used to objectively quantify the postural sway (sway length and sway area) of an individual as a measure of their postural balance, while perceived sense of postural sway and instability (PSPSI) can be used to capture their perception of postural sway/balance.[20] The PSPSI scale ranges between 0 (no perception of postural sway) and 8 (maximum perception of postural sway). On the other hand, an increase in postural sway (i.e., increase in sway length and/or sway area) measured with a force platform is associated with poorer balance. An increase in objectively measured postural sway (with a force platform) without a corresponding increase in PSPSI rating suggests a mismatch between actual and perceived states of postural balance. Since our response to a risky situation depends on our assessment (of nature and magnitude) of the risk, it is essential to include measures of potential mismatch between actual and perceived risk while evaluating the chances of balance loss and falls.

14.4 Strategies to Improve Intrinsic Balance

There is limited research regarding improving balance for workers. Therefore, we will begin by presenting evidence in other populations. Before we move on, however, it is important to differentiate between improving balance and preventing falls. Balance

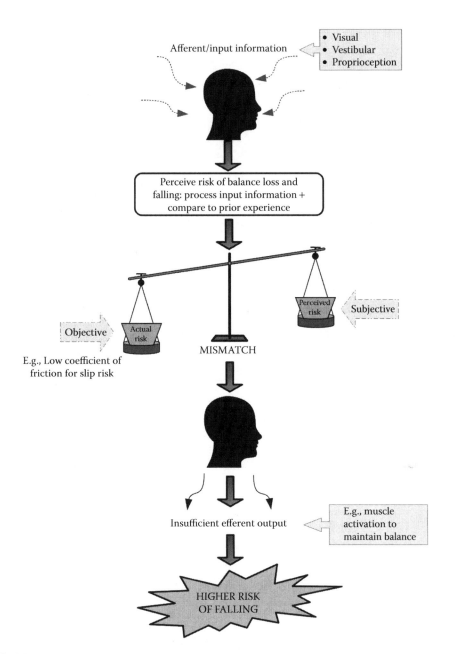

FIGURE 14.4
Sources of MISMATCH between actual and perceived risk of balance loss and fall: inaccurate afferents and inaccurate processing of input information. Healthy workers may be more capable of deploying appropriate postural muscle groups to avoid balance loss and falls, *provided* the risk is perceived accurately. Hence, workers should be trained on accurately perceiving risk of balance loss and falling. For an aging work force, afferent input systems deteriorate, which can increase the chances of a MISMATCH between actual and perceived risk. e same is true for workers with movement disorders, such as Parkinson's disease.

specifically refers to the ability to maintain upright posture, whether static, dynamic, anticipatory, or reactionary. Balance training improves balance but, by itself, does not prevent all falls. The prevention of falls involves many factors in addition to balance, for example, safe working conditions, environmental controls, fatigue, medications, and drugs/alcohol.

14.4.1 Neurophysiological Balance Training Targeting Vision, Vestibular and Proprioception Systems

Balance training that targets the vision, vestibular, and proprioception systems has been referred to as *sensorimotor training* and *neuromuscular training*. There is very little research regarding this neurophysiological balance training approach among workers. However, balance training improves postural stability in persons with neurological diagnoses, athletes, and elite athletes. Balance training also increases strength and jumping ability.

Neurophysiological balance training targeting the vision, vestibular, and proprioception systems is achieved through supraspinal and spinal adaptations, including the cerebellum, the basal ganglia, and the motor/sensory cortex.[63] An understanding of these systems provides the foundational information to develop balance training based on individual impairments and needs.[64] Balance training should be based on individual abilities and needs, should be conducted with at least moderate intensity, and should progress to be challenging as the physiological system adapts and the client's balance improves.

An important concept in maintaining balance and preventing a fall and injury is static versus dynamic abilities and anticipatory versus reactive balance controls. Static and dynamic abilities refer to the ability of a person to maintain balance while standing in one place with no movement (static) and during movement (dynamic), respectively. A strategic approach to balance training is essential and, based on motor learning principles, should be progressive to remain challenging to the client. As such, balance training typically starts easily (e.g., static) and progresses to more complicated tasks (e.g., dynamic), based on client abilities. If a client performs well with dynamic abilities, the training is progressed to more challenging tasks including environmental changes (e.g., decreased lighting, unlevel surfaces), dual tasking (e.g., walking while carrying items or climbing ladders), and cognitive challenges (e.g., walking/performing activities while performing a cognitive task).

14.4.2 Fall Prevention and Improving Intrinsic Balance in Older Adults

An area of fall-prevention research we can learn from is the older adult literature and the efforts to translate findings to practical use. In older adults, falls are a leading cause of injury, hospital admission, institutionalization, and death. Much research has focused on this problem for the past 30 years, providing established guidelines regarding how to screen for fall risk and prevent falls. Recent systematic reviews including up to 159 randomized controlled trials involving over 79,000 participants feature effective multifactorial fall-prevention programs. This plethora of evidence has resulted in the translation of research to practice, including several systematic reviews, clinical practice guidelines, and online resources for consumers and healthcare professionals.[65–69] Multifactorial fall prevention programs are the most successful, because the causes of falls are multifactorial. These programs include regular exercise; reviewing and minimizing medications—both prescribed and over the counter; individual tailored exercise and balance training programs; tai chi; yearly vision exams and treating vision impairment; managing postural hypotension and heart rate and rhythm abnormalities; vitamin D; managing foot and footwear problems; modifying the environment to reduce tripping hazards, providing grab bars, rails, and adequate lighting; special shoes for walking in snow and ice; and providing education and information.

Similarly to fall prevention, there is also a lot of evidence regarding treatments that improve intrinsic balance among older adults. A recent systematic review[70] including 94 randomized controlled trials and involving 9821 participants identified the following treatment strategies to improve balance in older adults: functional task training emphasizing balance, gait, and coordination; strengthening (resistance or power training); Tai Chi, qu gong, dance, yoga; and computerized balance training using visual feedback.[70] Programs involving multiple combinations of these approaches also improve balance, including dynamic balance training, agility and reaction training, strengthening, flexibility, aerobic exercise, jumping, muscle power training, and load-bearing functional activities.[70]

14.4.3 Healthy Adults and Athletes

Sports-specific training improves balance and balance reactions, decreases fatigue, reduces injury, and improves performance among healthy adults and athletes. A recent systematic review summarized 16 studies and concluded that balance training improves static and dynamic balance in healthy adults, athletes, and elite athletes on stable and unstable surfaces.[71] A training program duration of at least 10 minutes per session, 3 days/ week for 4 weeks is recommended. Various devices used include tilt boards, tilting platform, wobble boards, foam pads, unstable surfaces, mini trampoline, balance sandals, ankle disk, and instrumented balance systems that provide visual feedback. Examples of activities include dynamic body movements, including jumping with a focus on holding a stable position when landing; single-leg balance with contralateral limb and trunk motion; and single-leg balance with external perturbations. Balance exercises can be performed in isolation or in combination with other exercises such as plyometrics and resistance training. Programs that combined other exercises had longer durations (e.g., 60–90 minute sessions).

A recent systematic review of seven high-quality studies showed that programs including proprioceptive/neuromuscular balance training also reduced lower extremity (knee and ankle) injury among athletes.[72] Balance training alone resulted in a significant risk reduction of ankle sprain injuries and a nonsignificant risk reduction for injuries overall.[72]

Balance training under unstable surface conditions (compared with stable conditions) may be most effective by maximally challenging the neuromuscular and physiological systems.[73–75] This may be an important consideration when designing a balance training program for workers, considering the high probability of unstable conditions in the occupational environment. Unstable surface training can be achieved in many ways, including Swiss balls, wobble boards, and balance boards (e.g., BOSU). These studies also suggest that combining balance training under unstable conditions with resistance training (e.g., tubing, cables, free weights) may maximize efficiency and application to real-life situations. Based on these studies, it is recommended that sport- specific programs incorporate both stable and unstable surface training to maximize overload forces and "offer the highest degree of carry over into a real world setting."[73]

14.4.4 Other Approaches to Improve Intrinsic Balance in Nonworker Populations

14.4.4.1 Alternative Approaches

Tai chi improves balance and decreases falls in older adults and persons with Parkinson's disease.[76–78] Pilates also has limited evidence of improving dynamic balance in healthy people.[79]

14.4.4.2 Virtual Reality and Visual Feedback Systems

While the research is new, evidence suggests that virtual reality improves balance in older adults and persons with neurological diagnoses (e.g., stroke, Parkinson's disease, or vestibular dysfunction).[80–86] Specific to workers, computerized virtual reality systems have the potential to challenge sensory integration in different environments, including surface tilt and dynamic visual flow, training postural stability mechanisms, especially when visual dependence is present.[87]

Evidence also suggests that *visual feedback systems* improve balance among older adults[88–91] and persons with Parkinson's disease[92–93] and stroke.[94–96] Examples include the Neurocom Balance Master, the Kinesthetic Ability Trainer, Kinect, and the Nintendo Wii Fit.[97] A new device that provides an immersive system offering vestibular challenge is the Bertec Dynamic CDP (http://bertec.com/bertecbalance/resources/videos).

There are many benefits to virtual reality or computerized systems. Virtual reality can provide challenging real-life environments, integrate vestibular components, and maximize repetition, while being fun and motivating. Reduced treatment cost is also possible due to less supervision being required. Computerized systems can measure objective balance in different situations, including moving surfaces. There are also devices that specifically train motor and oculomotor reflexes (which may be essential for working at elevations and on inclined surfaces).

14.5 Strategies and Recommendations to Improve Intrinsic Balance Control in Workers

There has been limited research regarding treatments to improve balance for workers. A recent study investigated the effect of individualized exercise training on aerobic capacity and muscle strength among construction workers,[98] and there are two ongoing trials investigating exercise among workers with high–physical demand jobs[99] and sedentary jobs.[100] None of these studies assess balance as an outcome. Therefore, we will integrate current knowledge of other study populations with workload demand to suggest strategies that may improve balance in workers, with an emphasis on elevation and inclined surfaces.

For workers performing tasks at elevation and on inclines, visual spatial perception of vertical and horizontal orientation plays a significant role in the maintenance of upright balance. Working at heights compromises visual input, resulting in altered and unstable visual input. A combination of inclination and elevation results in a synergistic effect with greater instability.[13,14] Elevation and inclined surfaces commonly result in a "mismatch" between the perceived risk and the objective balance, increasing the risk of fall.[13,14] Balance training for workers exposed to elevations and inclined surfaces, therefore, should focus on strengthening the vestibular and proprioceptive systems. Further, training should integrate risk factors including confined and inclined work surfaces, varying loads, physical exertion, fatigue, task complexity, and unexpected changes in work surface.[101]

There are several studies showing that workers with more experience demonstrate better balance, suggesting that focused training may improve worker ability to maintain balance in challenging environments. Kincl and colleagues[24] tested visual spatial perception among 60 roofers using a computer-based program that generated random inclines in a darkened room in a black enclosure. Experienced workers were more accurate at determining the incline.[24] Similarly to Kincl, Mangharam[102] and colleagues found that increased fatigue and decreased experience were associated with reduced anticipatory and voluntary reactions to fall. Similar results were shown by Rietdyk and McGlothlin[103] when challenging workers' balance during dual tasking (carrying loads on elevated surfaces and different surfaces). In these dual-task studies, older, more experienced workers demonstrated better balance compared with those who were younger and less experienced—experience actually mitigated age-related differences in balance and ability.[103] More recent research[104] also found that less experienced workers had greater postural instability at heights on scaffolding. Interestingly, these less experienced workers also demonstrated greater cardiovascular stress (increased heart rate) at heights compared with experienced workers, and the presence of safety rails improved postural stability and decreased cardiovascular stress.[104]

14.6 Recommendations and Considerations to Increase Intrinsic Balance among Workers

Balance training improves balance and balance reactions, decreases fatigue, decreases injury, and improves performance among healthy adults and athletes.[71] Although research is limited, this suggests that balance training will also improve these outcomes in workers. We offer the following recommendations and considerations specific to workers, especially those who perform tasks at elevation or on inclined surfaces.

- A baseline screening evaluation may be helpful in developing a customized training program including vision, vestibular, proprioception, strength, and flexibility. A rehabilitation specialist (e.g., physical therapist, occupational therapist) can do this evaluation.
- Based on motor learning principles, balance training programs must be challenging and continually progressive based on the client's abilities. Ideas to increase challenge include training on unstable surfaces, dual tasking, and using instrumented balance systems. Also, consider adding job-specific demands, including resistance, confined spaces, awkward positions, and fatigue.
- Balance training programs should target neurophysiology: the integration of the vision, vestibular, and proprioception systems. To train specifically for elevated surfaces, the program may wish to emphasize vestibular and proprioception.
- Low back and neck pain is associated with impaired motor control and greater postural instability, especially when performing challenging or dual tasks.[105–112] Therefore, workers with musculoskeletal pain and injuries may benefit from balance training. Rehabilitation specialists (e.g., physical therapists, occupational

therapists) should test higher-level balance and provide focused balance training as needed for workers with musculoskeletal injuries.

- In general, postural stability decreases with age. Kincl also found that visual spatial perception decreased among older workers.[24] Older workers may benefit from training.

- Experienced workers demonstrate better balance in occupationally challenging settings. Therefore, new hires may benefit from focused balance training.

- Specific medications, drugs, and alcohol affect postural balance. Workers should be educated about the effects of certain medications, including over the counter (e.g., sleep aids, Benedryl).

- Programs such as Tai Chi in the workplace may provide an opportunity for cost-effective group training.

14.7 Future Areas of Growth

Considering the extremely limited research in this area, we recommend that future studies focus on worker-specific balance training programs. Sport-specific concepts, shown to be effective, can be modified into an occupation-specific training program. Studies should focus on high-risk worker populations such as those who work at elevation and on inclined surfaces. Considering the importance of visual perception while working at elevated and/ or inclined surfaces, a training program that especially targets the proprioception and vestibular systems and that integrates slip perception is recommended.

14.8 Conclusions

There has been little research regarding intrinsic balance training for workers. However, based on nonworker populations (e.g., sport-specific training), there is much promise for balance training to be effective in workers, including those who are exposed to elevation and inclined surfaces. Research is needed in this area.

References

1. Bureau of Labor Statistics. Fatal occupational injuries by industry and event or exposure. Bureau of Labor Statistics, US Department of Labor, 2008.
2. Bureau of Labor Statistics. Incidence rates of nonfatal occupational injuries and illnesses by industry and case types. Bureau of Labor Statistics, US Department of Labor, 2010.
3. Wade C, Davis J. Postural sway following prolonged exposure to an inclined surface. *Safety Sci.* 2009;47:652–8.
4. Wade C, Davis J, Weimar WH. Balance and exposure to an elevated sloped surface. *Gait Posture* 2014;39:599–605.

5. Simeonov PI, Hsiao H, Dotson BW et al. Height effects in real and virtual environments. *Hum. Factors* 2005;47:430–8.
6. Simeonov P, Hsiao H, Powers J et al. Postural stability effects of random vibration at the feet of construction workers in simulated elevation. *Appl. Ergon.* 2011;42:672–81.
7. Simeonov PI, Hsiao H, Dotson BW et al. Control and perception of balance at elevated and sloped surfaces. *Hum. Factors* 2003;45:136–47.
8. Vander AJ, Sherman JH, Luciano DS. *Human Physiology: The Mechanisms of Body Function.* McGraw-Hill, New York, 1970.
9. Woollacott MH, Inglin B, Manchester DL. Response preparation and posture control: Neuromuscular changes in the older adult. *Ann. N. Y. Acad. Sci.* 1988;515:42–53.
10. Woollacott MH, Manchester DL. Anticipatory postural adjustments in older adults: Are changes in response characteristics due to changes in strategy? *J. Gerontol.* 1993;48:M64–70.
11. Woollacott MH, Shumway-Cook A, Nashner LM. Aging and posture control: Changes in sensory organization and muscular coordination. *Int. J. Aging Hum. Dev.* 1986;23:97–114.
12. Woollacott MH, Von Hosten C, Rosblad B. Relation between muscle response onset and body segmental movements during postural perturbations in humans. *Exp. Brain Res.* 1988;72:593–604.
13. Bhattacharya A, Succop P, Modawal A et al. Impact of mismatch between actual and perceived risks on slip/fall while negotiating a ramp. In *Proceedings of International Conference on Slips, Trips and Falls: From Research to Practice.* Liberty Mutual Research Institute for Safety, Hopkinton, MA, August 23–24, 2007.
14. Bhattacharya A, Succop PA, Kincl LD et al. Postural stability during task performance on elevated and/or inclined surfaces. *Occup. Ergon.* 2003;3:83–97.
15. Wade C, Garner JC, Redfern MS et al. Walking on ballast impacts balance. *Ergonomics* 2014;57:66–73.
16. Center for Construction Research and Training. *The Construction Chart Book: The U.S. Construction Industry and Its Workers,* Fourth Edition. CPWR: The Center for Construction Research and Training, Silver Spring, MD, 2007.
17. National Academy of Sciences Report-Pre-Publication. *Traumatic Injury Program at NIOSH.* National Academies Press (US), Washington, DC. 2008. http://www.nap.edu; http://www.ncbi.nlm.nih.gov/books/NBK214739/.
18. National Institute for Occupational Safety and Health. *NIOSH Traumatic Injury Research and Prevention Program Evidence Package (NAS03-07).* Traumatic Injury Research and Prevention Program Evidence Package (NAS03-07), National Academies, Washington, DC. 2007.
19. Liberty Mutual Research Institute for Safety. Research to reality. *Liberty Mutual Research Institute for Safety,* Winter 2008;11:3–4.
20. Chiou SY, Bhattacharya A, Lai CF et al. Effects of environmental and job-task factors on workers' gait characteristics on slippery surfaces. *Occup. Ergon.* 2003;3:209–23.
21. Chiou SY, Bhattacharya A, Succop PA. Effect of workers' shoe wear on objective and subjective assessment of slipperiness. *Am. Ind. Hyg. Assoc. J.* 1996;57:825–31.
22. Chiou SY, Bhattacharya A, Succop PA. Evaluation of workers' perceived sense of slip and effect of prior knowledge of slipperiness during task performance on slippery surfaces. *Am. Ind. Hyg. Assoc. J.* 2000;61:492–500.
23. Chiou SY, Bhattacharya A, Succop PA et al. Effect of environmental and task risk factors on workers' perceived sense of postural sway and instability. *Occup. Ergon.* 1998;1:81–93.
24. Kincl LD, Bhattacharya A, Succop P et al. The effect of workload, work experience and inclined standing surface on visual spatial perception: Fall potential/prevention implications. *Occup. Ergon.* 2003;3:251–9.
25. Punaxallio A, Lusa S, Luukkonen R. Protective equipment affects balance abilities differently in younger and older firefighters. *Aviat. Space Environ. Med.* 2003;74:1151–6.
26. Courtney TK, Huang YH, Verma SK et al. Factors influencing restaurant worker perception of floor slipperiness. *J. Occup. Environ. Hyg.* 2006;3:592–8.

27. Courtney TK, Verma SK, Chang WR et al. Perception of slipperiness and prospective risk of slipping at work. *Occup. Environ. Med.* 2013;70:35–40.

28. Manning DP. Deaths and injuries caused by slipping, tripping and falling. *Ergonomics* 1983;26:3–9.

29. Manning DP. Slipping and the penalties inflicted generally by the law of gravitation. *J. Soc. Occup. Med.* 1988;38:123–7.

30. Manning DP, Ayers IM. Disability resulting from underfoot first events. *J. Occup. Accidents* 1987;37:37–9.

31. Manning DP, Mitchell RG, Blachfield LP. Body movements and events contributing to accidental and nonaccidental back injuries. *Spine* 1984;9:734–9.

32. Manning DP, Shannon HS. Slipping accidents causing low-back-pain in a gearbox factory. *Spine* 1981;6:70–2.

33. Cham R, Redfern MS. Lower extremity corrective reactions to slip events. *J. Biomech.* 2001;34:1439–45.

34. Cham R, Redfern MS. Changes in gait when anticipating slippery floors. *Gait Posture* 2002;15:159–71.

35. Chambers AJ, Margarum S, Redfern MS et al. Kinematics of foot during slips. *Occup. Ergon.* 2003;3:225–34.

36. Chambers AJ, Cham R. Slip-related muscle activation patterns in the stance leg during walking. *Gait Posture* 2007;25:565–72.

37. Mohapatra S, Aruin AS. Static and dynamic visual cues in feed-forward postural control. *Exp. Brain Res.* 2013;224:25–34.

38. Verma SK, Chang WR, Courtney TK et al. Workers' experience of slipping in U.S. limited-service restaurants. *J. Occup. Environ. Hyg.* 2010;7:491–500.

39. Verma SK, Chang WR, Courtney TK et al. A prospective study of floor surface, shoes, floor cleaning and slipping in US limited-service restaurant workers. *Occup. Environ. Med.* 2011;68:279–85.

40. Verma SK, Courtney TK, Corns HL et al. Factors associated with use of slip-resistant shoes in US limited-service restaurant workers. *Inj. Prev.* 2012;18:176–81.

41. Verma SK, Lombardi DA, Chang WR et al. Rushing, distraction, walking on contaminated floors and risk of slipping in limited-service restaurants: A case–crossover study. *Occup. Environ. Med.* 2011;68:575–81.

42. Morioka S, Fujita H, Hiyamizu M et al. Effects of plantar perception training on standing posture balance in the old old and the very old living in nursing facilities: A randomized controlled trial. *Clin. Rehabil.* 2011;25:1011–20.

43. Morioka S, Yagi F. Effects of perceptual learning exercises on standing balance using a hardness discrimination task in hemiplegic patients following stroke: A randomized controlled pilot trial. *Clin. Rehabil.* 2003;17:600–7.

44. Morioka S, Yagi F. Influence of perceptual learning on standing posture balance: Repeated training for hardness discrimination of foot sole. *Gait Posture* 2004;20:36–40.

45. Nakano H, Nozaki M, Ueta K et al. Effect of a plantar perceptual learning task on walking stability in the elderly: A randomized controlled trial. *Clin. Rehabil.* 2013;27:608–15.

46. Abrahamova D, Mancini M, Hlavacka F et al. The age-related changes of trunk responses to Achilles tendon vibration. *Neurosci. Lett.* 2009;467:220–4.

47. Akizuki H, Uno A, Arai K et al. Effects of immersion in virtual reality on postural control. *Neurosci. Lett.* 2005;379:23–6.

48. Andersson G, Persson K, Melin L et al. Actual and perceived postural sway during balance specific and non-specific proprioceptive stimulation. *Acta Otolaryngol.* 1998;118:461–5.

49. Capicikova N, Rocchi L, Hlavacka F et al. Human postural response to lower leg muscle vibration of different duration. *Physiol. Res.* 2006;55 Suppl 1:S129–S134.

50. Caudron S, Boy F, Forestier N et al. Influence of expectation on postural disturbance evoked by proprioceptive stimulation. *Exp. Brain Res.* 2008;184:53–9.

51. Dozza M, Chiari L, Horak FB. Audio-biofeedback improves balance in patients with bilateral vestibular loss. *Arch. Phys. Med. Rehabil.* 2005;86:1401–3.

52. Dozza M, Wall C, III, Peterka RJ et al. Effects of practicing tandem gait with and without vibro-tactile biofeedback in subjects with unilateral vestibular loss. *J. Vestib. Res.* 2007;17:195–204.

53. Haddad JM, Rietdyk S, Claxton LJ et al. Task-dependent postural control throughout the lifespan. *Exerc. Sport Sci. Rev.* 2013;41:123–32.

54. Haddad JM, van Emmerik RE, Whittlesey SN et al. Adaptations in interlimb and intralimb coordination to asymmetrical loading in human walking. *Gait Posture* 2006;23:429–34.

55. Hiyamizu M, Morioka S, Shomoto K et al. Effects of dual task balance training on dual task performance in elderly people: A randomized controlled trial. *Clin. Rehabil.* 2012;26:58–67.

56. Horak FB. Postural compensation for vestibular loss. *Ann. N. Y. Acad. Sci.* 2009;1164:76–81.

57. Horak FB. Postural compensation for vestibular loss and implications for rehabilitation. *Restor. Neurol. Neurosci.* 2010;28:57–68.

58. Horak FB, Jones-Rycewicz C, Black FO et al. Effects of vestibular rehabilitation on dizziness and imbalance. *Otolaryngol. Head Neck Surg.* 1992;106:175–80.

59. Rege S, Joshi A. The effects of remedial therapy on visual perception, depth perception and balance on a community dwelling older population. *Indian J. Occup. Ther.* 2005;XXXVI:57–62.

60. Shumway-Cook A, Horak FB. Rehabilitation strategies for patients with vestibular deficits. *Neurol. Clin.* 1990;8:441–57.

61. Marigold DS, Misiaszek JE. Whole-body responses: Neural control and implications for rehabilitation and fall prevention. *Neuroscientist* 2009;15:36–46.

62. Swensen EE, Purswell JL, Schlegel RE et al. Coefficient of friction and subjective assessment of slippery work surfaces. *Hum. Factors* 1992;34:67–77.

63. Taube W, Gruber M, Gollhofer A. Spinal and supraspinal adaptations associated with balance training and their functional relevance. *Acta Physiol. (Oxf.)* 2008;193:101–16.

64. Horak FB. Postural orientation and equilibrium: What do we need to know about neural control of balance to prevent falls? *Age Ageing* 2006;35 Suppl 2:ii7–ii11.

65. Gillespie LD, Robertson MC, Gillespie WJ et al. Interventions for preventing falls in older people living in the community. *Cochrane Database Syst. Rev.* 2012;9:CD007146.

66. Robertson MC, Gillespie LD. Fall prevention in community-dwelling older adults. *JAMA* 2013;309:1406–7.

67. Agency for Healthcare Research and Quality (AHRQ). *AGS/BGS Clinical Practice Guideline: Prevention of Falls in Older Persons.* National Guideline Clearinghouse (NGC), Rockville, MD, 2015. Agency for Healthcare Research and Quality (AHRQ). http://www.guideline.gov/content.aspx?id=37707.

68. CDC Fall prevention website. CDC STEADI (Stopping Elderly Accidents, Deaths & Injuries) Tool Kit for Health Care Providers including downloadable PDFs, video instructions and webinars, 2015. http://www.cdc.gov/HomeandRecreationalSafety/Falls/index.html.

69. NICE (National Institute for Health and Care Excellence). *Falls: Assessment and Prevention of Falls in Older People.* NICE Clinical Guideline. NICE National Institute for Health and Care Excellence, 2013. ISBN: 978-1-4731-0132-6; http://www.nice.org.uk/guidance/cg161.

70. Howe TE, Rochester L, Neil F et al. Exercise for improving balance in older people. *Cochrane Database Syst. Rev.* 2011;CD004963.

71. Distefano LJ, Clark MA, Padua DA. Evidence supporting balance training in healthy individuals: A systemic review. *J. Strength Cond. Res.* 2009;23:2718–31.

72. Hubscher M, Zech A, Pfeifer K et al. Neuromuscular training for sports injury prevention: A systematic review. *Med. Sci. Sports Exerc.* 2010;42:413–21.

73. Anderson K, Behm DG. The impact of instability resistance training on balance and stability. *Sports Med.* 2005;35:43–53.

74. Behm D, Colado JC. The effectiveness of resistance training using unstable surfaces and devices for rehabilitation. *Int J. Sports Phys. Ther.* 2012;7:226–41.

75. Behm DG, Colado Sanchez JC. Instability resistance training across the exercise continuum. *Sports Health* 2013;5:500–3.

76. Leung DP, Chan CK, Tsang HW et al. Tai chi as an intervention to improve balance and reduce falls in older adults: A systematic and meta-analytical review. *Altern. Ther. Health Med.* 2011;17:40–8.

77. Li F, Harmer P, Fitzgerald K et al. Tai chi and postural stability in patients with Parkinson's disease. *N. Engl. J. Med.* 2012;366:511–19.

78. Yang Y, Li XY, Gong L et al. Tai Chi for improvement of motor function, balance and gait in Parkinson's disease: A systematic review and meta-analysis. *PLoS One* 2014;9:e102942.

79. Cruz-Ferreira A, Fernandes J, Laranjo L et al. A systematic review of the effects of Pilates method of exercise in healthy people. *Arch. Phys. Med. Rehabil.* 2011;92:2071–81.

80. Adamovich SV, Fluet GG, Tunik E et al. Sensorimotor training in virtual reality: A review. *NeuroRehabilitation* 2009;25:29–44.

81. Cho GH, Hwangbo G, Shin HS. The effects of virtual reality-based balance training on balance of the elderly. *J. Phys. Ther. Sci.* 2014;26:615–17.

82. Duque G, Boersma D, Loza-Diaz G et al. Effects of balance training using a virtual-reality system in older fallers. *Clin. Interv. Aging.* 2013;8:257–63.

83. Hsieh WM, Chen CC, Wang SC et al. Virtual reality system based on Kinect for the elderly in fall prevention. *Technol. Health Care* 2014;22:27–36.

84. Pavlou M, Kanegaonkar RG, Swapp D et al. The effect of virtual reality on visual vertigo symptoms in patients with peripheral vestibular dysfunction: A pilot study. *J. Vestib. Res.* 2012;22:273–81.

85. Wright WG. Using virtual reality to augment perception, enhance sensorimotor adaptation, and change our minds. *Front. Syst. Neurosci.* 2014;8:56.

86. Yen CY, Lin KH, Hu MH et al. Effects of virtual reality-augmented balance training on sensory organization and attentional demand for postural control in people with Parkinson disease: A randomized controlled trial. *Phys. Ther.* 2011;91:862–74.

87. Slaboda JC, Keshner EA. Reorientation to vertical modulated by combined support surface tilt and virtual visual flow in healthy elders and adults with stroke. *J. Neurol.* 2012;259:2664–72.

88. Laufer Y, Dar G, Kodesh E. Does a Wii-based exercise program enhance balance control of independently functioning older adults? A systematic review. *Clin. Interv. Aging* 2014;9:1803–13.

89. Pluchino A, Lee SY, Asfour S et al. Pilot study comparing changes in postural control after training using a video game balance board program and 2 standard activity-based balance intervention programs. *Arch. Phys. Med. Rehabil.* 2012;93:1138–46.

90. Wolf SL, Barnhart HX, Ellison GL et al. The effect of Tai Chi Quan and computerized balance training on postural stability in older subjects. Atlanta FICSIT Group. Frailty and Injuries: Cooperative Studies on Intervention Techniques. *Phys. Ther.* 1997;77:371–81.

91. Zijlstra A, Mancini M, Chiari L et al. Biofeedback for training balance and mobility tasks in older populations: A systematic review. *J. Neuroeng. Rehabil.* 2010;7:58.

92. Mhatre PV, Vilares I, Stibb SM et al. Wii Fit balance board playing improves balance and gait in Parkinson disease. *PM. R.* 2013;5:769–77.

93. Zalecki T, Gorecka-Mazur A, Pietraszko W et al. Visual feedback training using Wii Fit improves balance in Parkinson's disease. *Folia Med. Cracov.* 2013;53:65–78.

94. Barcala L, Grecco LA, Colella F et al. Visual biofeedback balance training using Wii Fit after stroke: A randomized controlled trial. *J. Phys. Ther. Sci.* 2013;25:1027–32.

95. Bateni H. Changes in balance in older adults based on use of physical therapy vs the Wii Fit gaming system: A preliminary study. *Physiotherapy* 2012;98:211–16.

96. Van Peppen RP, Kortsmit M, Lindeman E et al. Effects of visual feedback therapy on postural control in bilateral standing after stroke: A systematic review. *J. Rehabil. Med.* 2006;38:3–9.

97. Goble DJ, Cone BL, Fling BW. Using the Wii Fit as a tool for balance assessment and neurore-habilitation: The first half decade of "Wii-search." *J. Neuroeng. Rehabil.* 2014;11:12.

98. Gram B, Holtermann A, Sogaard K et al. Effect of individualized worksite exercise training on aerobic capacity and muscle strength among construction workers: A randomized controlled intervention study. *Scand. J. Work Environ. Health* 2012;38:467–75.

99. Holtermann A, Jorgensen MB, Gram B et al. Worksite interventions for preventing physical deterioration among employees in job-groups with high physical work demands: Background, design and conceptual model of FINALE. *BMC Public Health* 2010;10:120.

100. Sjogaard G, Justesen JB, Murray M et al. A conceptual model for worksite intelligent physical exercise training—IPET—Intervention for decreasing life style health risk indicators among employees: A randomized controlled trial. *BMC Public Health* 2014;14:652.

101. Hsiao H, Simeonov P. Preventing falls from roofs: A critical review. *Ergonomics* 2001;44:537–61.

102. Mangharam J, Bhattacharya A, Succop P et al. The effects of lower limb muscular fatigue and work experience on patterns of falling in workers. In Straker LM, Pollack CM (Eds.), *Proceedings of Cyberg 2nd International Conf on Ergonomics*. The International Ergonomics Association Press, Curtin University of Technology, Perth, WA, 1999.

103. Rietdyk S, McGlothlin JD, Knezovich MJ. Work experience mitigated age-related differences in balance and mobility during surface accommodation. *Clin. Biomech. (Bristol, Avon)* 2005;20:1085–93.

104. Min SN, Kim JY, Parnianpour M. The effects of safety handrails and the heights of scaffolds on the subjective and objective evaluation of postural stability and cardiovascular stress in novice and expert construction workers. *Appl. Ergon.* 2012;43:574–81.

105. Jorgensen MB, Skotte JH, Holtermann A et al. Neck pain and postural balance among workers with high postural demands: A cross-sectional study. *BMC Musculoskelet. Disord.* 2011;12:176.

106. Mazaheri M, Salavati M, Negahban H et al. Postural sway in low back pain: Effects of dual tasks. *Gait Posture* 2010;31:116–21.

107. Michaelson P, Michaelson M, Jaric S et al. Vertical posture and head stability in patients with chronic neck pain. *J. Rehabil. Med.* 2003;35:229–35.

108. Salavati M, Mazaheri M, Negahban H et al. Effect of dual-tasking on postural control in subjects with nonspecific low back pain. *Spine (Phila Pa 1976)* 2009;34:1415–21.

109. Silva AG, Cruz AL. Standing balance in patients with whiplash-associated neck pain and idiopathic neck pain when compared with asymptomatic participants: A systematic review. *Physiother. Theory Pract.* 2013;29:1–18.

110. Sjolander P, Michaelson P, Jaric S et al. Sensorimotor disturbances in chronic neck pain: Range of motion, peak velocity, smoothness of movement, and repositioning acuity. *Man. Ther.* 2008;13:122–31.

111. Treleaven J. Sensorimotor disturbances in neck disorders affecting postural stability, head and eye movement control. *Man. Ther.* 2008;13:2–11.

112. Woodhouse A, Vasseljen O. Altered motor control patterns in whiplash and chronic neck pain. *BMC Musculoskelet. Disord.* 2008;9:90.

15

Ladder Safety: Research, Control, and Practice

Peter Simeonov

CONTENTS

ABSTRACT   This chapter summarizes the causes, mechanisms, and risk factors for ladder falls and the range of available and most promising control and prevention strategies, with an emphasis on portable ladders. The focus is on proximal factors associated with the most common user–ladder interactions, discussed from the perspective of mechanics, biomechanics, and human factors. The chapter reviews the current ladder safety standards, regulations, and practices and summarizes the latest ladder safety research. The chapter includes suggestions for ladder design improvements, research needs, and measures for preventing falls from ladders.

15.1 Ladder Fall Injury Problem

Ladders are the most common equipment for access to elevation and are generally considered simple to use. However, ladders are also associated with considerable risk of injury both when used in the workplace and at home. Ladder-related injuries are persistent and yet represent a preventable public-health problem with a significant economic impact on society. The Consumer Product Safety Commission (CPSC) estimated that in 2013, approximately 511,000 people in the United States were injured in ladder-related incidents and were treated in hospital emergency rooms, doctors' offices, clinics, and other medical settings, and the financial cost of these injuries was $24 billion, including work loss, medical, legal, liability, and pain and suffering expenses (CPSC, 2014).

Ladder fall injuries are a well-recognized problem in the U.S. workplace. In 2011, there were 113 fatal ladder fall injuries identified by the Census of Fatal Occupational Injuries; an estimated 15,460 nonfatal ladder fall injuries, involving at least one day away from work, were reported by employers to the Survey of Occupational Injuries and Illnesses; and approximately 34,000 (±6,800) ladder fall injuries were treated in emergency departments, according to the National Electronic Injury Surveillance System—Occupational supplement (NEISS-Work) (Socias et al., 2014).

Successful prevention of ladder fall injury requires a comprehensive analysis of the mechanisms, causes, and risk factors for ladder falls, combined with a good understanding of ladder-user behavior and ladder mechanical performance during ladder–user interactions. Ladder mechanical performance is defined to a great extent by ladder type and characteristics.

15.2 Ladder Types, Classes, and Characteristics

15.2.1 Common Ladder Types

Various job types, and the associated work environments and tasks at elevated locations, impose physical size restrictions and support conditions requirements and thus define the need for different ladder types. The underlying desire to create a more versatile ladder has further resulted in a number of ladder designs with variable geometry. The American Ladder Institute (ALI) lists the following most common standard ladder types: stepladder, single ladder, articulated ladder, combination ladder, extension ladder, extension trestle ladder, job-made ladders, fixed ladders, mobile ladder stands, and ladder stand platforms (ALI, 2014a). Other ladder types include multipurpose, telescopic, sectional, folding, and rope ladders; and specialized ladder types such as library, escape, attic, dock, and orchard ladders (Ladders.net, 2014; Wikipedia, 2014).

15.2.2 Major Ladder Classification

Based on their purpose, design, structure, support conditions, and portability, all ladder types can be classified into the following three major classes: fixed, mobile, and portable. Fixed ladders are permanently attached to a structure or a vehicle and are used exclusively for access. Most fixed ladders are sufficiently strong to be used with an integrated fall-protection system, which can stop a user from falling in case of lost balance during climbing. Mobile ladders are used mainly as work platforms and require even and smooth floors to be moved from one location to another. They are heavy and have a large base of support, and thus they are generally very stable and safer to use. Portable ladders include all other ladder types that can be lifted and carried from one location to another, and they can be used for a variety of tasks, including for access and as work platforms. Because portable ladders are often improperly set up and misused, much of this chapter addresses matters of portable ladder safety.

15.2.3 Portable Ladder Classes

Portable ladders can be classified according to their structural geometry and their support conditions. Two major classes are *self-supporting* and *non-self-supporting*. In addition, some portable ladders can be attached and supported only at the top (e.g., escape ladders) and could be regarded as *suspended* ladders. The self-supporting ladders are usually *A*-shaped, have four legs, and can stand erect on their own as an independent structure (Figure 15.1). They include all stepladders, trestle ladders, and articulated and combination ladders. Some stepladders used in orchard agriculture may have only three legs. The non-self-supporting or leaning ladders require a structure to lean on and use as the upper support, and they rely on friction under their feet at the base to maintain stability (Figure 15.2). Non-self-supporting ladders include all extension ladders, straight or single ladders, telescopic ladders, sectional ladders, and combination ladders in their straight configuration. Since self-supporting and non-self-supporting ladders have different structures and mechanical behaviors and are associated with different causes and mechanisms of falls, they are treated and addressed in the chapter as two separate groups when required. For convenience, the self-supporting ladders are referred to as "stepladders," and

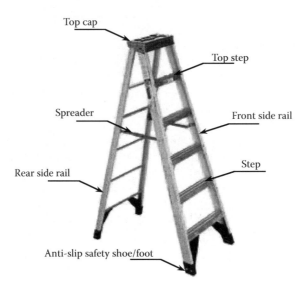

FIGURE 15.1
Stepladder: self-supporting ladder.

the non-self-supporting ladders are referred to as "leaning ladders" as this term is more inclusive and self-explanatory.

15.2.4 Portable Ladder Characteristics (Load Ratings, Sizes, Materials)

Portable ladders are designed in different categories according the working load they have to sustain. The working load is the maximum applied load, including the weight of the user, materials, and tools that the ladder is to support for the intended use. According to the working load, portable ladders are available in the following five categories:

Type	Duty Rating	Working Load
IAA	Special duty	170 kg (375 lbs.)
IA	Industrial—extra heavy	159 kg (350 lbs.)
I	Industrial—heavy	114 kg (250 lbs.)
II	Commercial—medium	102 kg (225 lbs.)
III	Household—light	91 kg (200 lbs.)

The ladder duty rating determines the attributes of its structural components (e.g., rails' and steps' cross-sectional dimensions), its overall weight, its structural properties, and ultimately its mechanical behavior. The duty rating determines also the available sizes for a ladder.

Type	Available Stepladder Sizes
IAA	0.92 m (3 ft.)–6.10 m (20 ft.)
IA	0.92 m (3 ft.)–6.10 m (20 ft.)
I	0.92 m (3 ft.)–6.10 m (20 ft.)
II	Up to 3.66 m (12 ft.)
III	Up to 1.83 m (6 ft.)

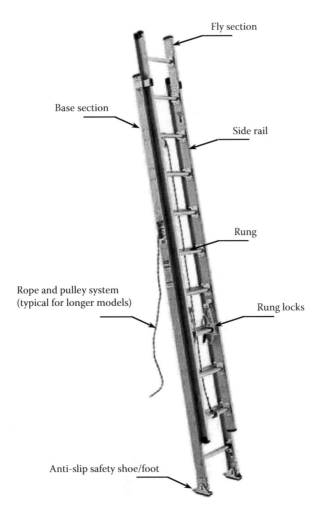

FIGURE 15.2
Extension ladder: non-self-supporting or leaning ladder.

Type	Available Extension Ladder Sizes
IA	Up to 18.30 m (60 ft.) (two-section) and 21.96 m (72 ft.) (three-section)
I	Up to 18.30 m (60 ft.) (two-section) and 21.96 m (72 ft.) (three-section)
II	Up to 14.64 m (48 ft.) (two-section) and 18.30 m (60 ft.) (three-section)
III	Up to 9.85 m (32 ft.) (two-section)

Ladders can be made of different structural materials, such as aluminum, fiberglass, or wood. A ladder's composition and type are key considerations in selecting the right ladder for the tasks to be performed. For example, nonmetal ladders may be used safely around electrical lines or chemicals. Lightweight aluminum ladders are easier to use in jobs requiring frequent ladder relocation, adjustments, and manual transport. Only ladders with an industrial duty rating of Type IA or Type I can be used on construction job sites. A straight ladder or extension ladder is best for reaching heights over 10 ft. Articulating ladders allow users to access elevated, difficult-to-reach areas.

A good knowledge of the available ladder types, their duty ratings, material properties, and geometrical characteristics, combined with a proper understanding of their function and most adequate areas of application, is required for proper ladder selection—improper ladder selection is often cited as a contributing factor in ladder fall injuries. Good safety practice requires that before using a ladder, the user should become familiar with the specific properties and safety rules available on the product data information labels and safety labels attached to the ladder.

15.3 Causes and Mechanisms of Ladder Falls

15.3.1 Theoretical Considerations

From the perspective of mechanics, biomechanics, and human factors, a fall can be defined as uncontrolled descent under the influence of gravity, and the causes of falls can be regarded as failures or disruptions in the control of dynamic postural stability during human interaction with the environment. Ladder-related falls can be broadly considered as resulting from failures or disruptions in the control of dynamic stability of the user-ladder system during its interaction with the environment. Some of the possible interactions include user with work surface, user with ladder, and ladder with support. During ladder use, the control of dynamic stability is most often compromised by internal forces generated by the user as self-induced perturbations. On some occasions, the disruption could also be caused by external forces (external perturbations), applied for example as an impact on the ladder or the user by a moving person, machine, or object. In most cases, ladder incident victims are not aware of the causes of their falls (Seluga et al. 2007). In order to develop a better understanding of the possible causes of ladder-related falls and to suggest effective preventive measures, a thorough analysis of ladder–user interactions is provided in this section.

15.3.2 Mechanical Behavior of Portable Ladders

Portable ladders are inherently unstable. The requirements for their portability set limits for their mass and geometry and thus define considerable limitations to their stability. Generally, the mass of the user is several times greater than that of the ladder, so the combined mass and the location of the center of mass (COM) of the ladder–user system will be greatly determined by the user mass and location on the ladder. Furthermore, during pushing or pulling tasks, the user can generate forces in any direction that can reach values equal to his weight. The limited ladder base of support (BOS) and the available friction at the ladder–support interface (between ladder feet and ground) is associated with severe limitations on the loading that a ladder can sustain while remaining stable. In general, for self-supporting ladders, the ladder will only remain stable if the projection of the user–ladder system's COM remains within the ladder stability limits (within the boundaries of its BOS), defined by the positions of the supporting feet. For non-self-supporting ladders, in addition to this requirement, the required coefficient of friction (RCOF) at the base must remain below the available coefficient of friction (ACOF). The unstable nature of the portable ladders requires vigilance and constant control, especially during their use, to maintain stability; this may be especially challenging while performing a task from the ladder, where the user's attention needs to be carefully managed in a dual control task—between the control of work task and the ladder–user system stability control task.

Most portable ladders are supported at four points—typical step ladders have four legs, and leaning ladders have two rails supported both at the base and at the top. Since only three support points are statically required to support an object on a surface, all portable ladders are inherently over-constrained (Seluga et al. 2007). Previous stepladder testing has shown that even when all four ladder feet are positioned properly on the ground, only three legs/feet experience a significant ground reaction force at any particular instant, and that these "foot triplets" carrying the load periodically and abruptly change as the user moves on the ladder (Clift et al. 2002). Theoretically, up to four triplets are possible with four support points, and the loading may shift between them, depending on the shifts in the dynamic loading applied to the ladder and the resulting location of the user–ladder system's COM (Figure 15.3). Structural rigidity affects the mechanical behavior of the ladder—more flexible configurations allow for more equal force distribution between the four support points and more gradual load transition between triplets. However, overly flexible ladder structures will be associated with excessive movement; therefore, the rigidity/flexibility of the ladder structure has to be optimized (Seluga et al. 2007). Three-point support and weight shifting between triplets is a condition that can create ladder and user instability and increase the risk of falls. While this issue has been well recognized for stepladders, it may be also a problem for straight and extension ladders, where a shift in the

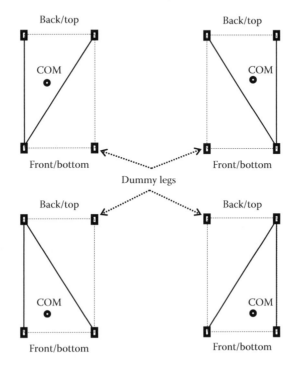

FIGURE 15.3
Four possible ladder base triplets as related to ladder-user center-of-mass (COM) location. "Front"–"Back" indicates a step ladder, and "Bottom"–"Top" indicates a leaning ladder.

reaction force between the two legs at the ladder base may lead to movement and increase the risk of slide-out events.

15.3.3 User–Ladder Indirect Interactions (Selection, Inspection, Positioning)

There are several phases that set the stage for the ladder–user interaction during ladder use: ladder selection, ladder inspection, and ladder setup. These three phases should be considered as indirect interactions, since the ladder is not loaded—the user has not climbed on the ladder and there is no risk of a fall. Furthermore, it is possible that the user is not directly involved in some or all of these phases—they may be performed, for example, by an employer or a coworker, or a neighbor in the case of home users. Such proxy indirect interaction indicates shared control, where the user relies on other parties for the proper performance of these stages. However, these interactions are crucial for the stability of the ladder and the user–ladder system. That is why it is advisable that the user always double check the proper performance of these steps to establish direct control. The following paragraphs provide information on the three phases.

15.3.3.1 Ladder Selection

The ladder selection process determines the ladder type, size, and rating and therefore the associated geometrical, structural, and mechanical characteristics of the ladder. The ladder has to accommodate the user's physical characteristics (weight) and also has to meet the requirements for the task(s) (weight of tool and materials, height and location of the job) in an optimal fashion. Therefore, proper ladder selection may substantially affect safety performance and the risk of falls. For example, the ladder type and geometric characteristics define its BOS and the associated stability limits; its rating, structure, and materials define its mechanical properties and load capacity; its effective height, as related to the task location, determines the need for reaching and thus affects the risk for tipping instability; and other characteristics, such as ladder feet and safety shoes, can also influence its sliding stability. However, very often the user does not have access to a wide selection of portable ladders or does not have the resources to purchase the appropriate ladder for the job and task at hand. In such cases, the user is frequently forced to make a compromise and use a suboptimal or inappropriate ladder, which can lead to excessive leaning and significantly increase the risk of a fall.

The ladder selection process may also include considerations related to the selection of different ladder accessories. Accessories attached to the ladder can also change its geometrical configuration and its mechanical behavior and as a result have profound effects on different aspects of its safety performance (Clift, 2004). More detailed discussion of different types of ladder accessories is available in Section 1.5.2.

15.3.3.2 Ladder Inspection, Care, and Maintenance

The ladder inspection phase and process is to ensure the ladder's structural integrity and proper operation before use. The ladder inspection should include the following steps: (1) inspect for damage or excessive wear the major structural components, such as rails, rungs, hinges, spreaders, and locks; (2) inspect for integrity and excessive wear the supporting components, such as rail top caps and safety shoes at the base; (3) inspect for proper operation all moving parts, such as hinges, spreaders, locks, pulleys, swivel safety feet and shoes; inspect for cleanliness the rails, rungs, and safety shoes; and (4) inspect the integrity and readability of all safety labels. Thorough inspection of the ladders should be done periodically and before each use. Ladder inspection is directly related to ladder care and maintenance, which include the immediate cleaning of spills and drips, periodic oiling of the moving parts, replacing damaged or worn components and labels, and ensuring proper storage away from damaging weather effects and corrosive agents. Inspection, care, and maintenance should be regarded as critical control activities in the ladder–user interaction, since failures to provide proper care and maintenance and to thoroughly inspect a ladder before use may lead to ladder structural failure, loss of ladder stability, or loss of user stability.

15.3.3.3 Ladder Setup

During the ladder setup stage, the ladder is not loaded and the user establishes the ladder support conditions, it structural/geometrical configuration, and its proper space orientation. This stage is critical for the ladder's structural integrity, proper operation, and overall stability. The ladder setup process involves several steps.

The first step in the process is selection and preparation of the support surface. The support surface must be level, firm, even, and slip-resistant to ensure secure contact between the ladder legs and the ground. Most often the ground conditions are not perfect—sometimes the ground is not level and frequently not sufficiently firm; in such cases, other objects (a board, a brick, or a stone), available on the site, are used as wedges and levelers, which may create unsafe conditions. Leaning ladders' safety shoes are constructed so they can swivel and accommodate uneven surfaces, and they have riveted rubber foot pads to improve the frictional resistance and spur plate ends to secure the ladder base on soft support surfaces. More recent ladder designs and ladder attachments feature extendable legs specifically designed to serve as levelers on laterally sloped and uneven surfaces.

For leaning ladders, this step involves also the selection (and preparation) of the upper support surface so that both rails are in contact with the supporting structure. Some of the requirements for the ladder top supporting structure include adequate structural stability to sustain the loading from the ladder, structural rigidity to minimize the ladder movement, and sufficient frictional resistance to reduce the risk of ladder tipping sideways. Numerous extension ladder top accessories have been developed to accommodate various upper support conditions or protect from damage structural elements, such as windows and wall openings, corners, poles and trees, wires, and gutters. Inadequate selection and preparation of ladder support conditions directly affect ladder stability and may set the stage for a ladder fall or structural collapse.

The second step in the ladder setup process is to establish the ladder structural/geometrical configuration. For a stepladder, this involves spreading the two articulated ladder sections and securely engaging the spreaders on each side. For an extension ladder, this involves extending the ladder to the desired length and securely engaging the locks on each side rail. Incorrect or incomplete performance of this step may lead to structural failure and ladder collapse. Furthermore, for extension ladders, the proper ladder length should be estimated based on the elevated level of the task location, the last available/allowable rung (three rungs from the top) for support, and the conditions at the top supporting structure. For elevated transitioning tasks, the ladder length should allow sufficient extension (minimum 1 m or 3 ft.) above the structure edge to ensure safe hand grasping and support in the transitioning process (Figure 15.4).

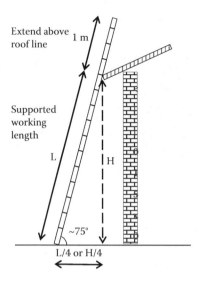

FIGURE 15.4
Setup of leaning ladders.

The last step in the ladder positioning process is its proper space orientation. The proper space orientation of a ladder requires considering the elevated location of the task and adjusting the ladder so that the user will normally be facing the location and will be able to complete the task without excessive reaching. For leaning ladders, this step involves also their proper angular positioning. The proper angular positioning of a leaning ladder is a critical step in establishing its stability, since it relies on friction at its base to maintain stability. The American National Standards Institute (ANSI) and Occupational Safety and Health Administration (OSHA) recommended angle for the positioning of extension ladders is approximately 75° from horizontal. This angle corresponds to a 4:1 ratio between the ladder supported-working length and its horizontal projection (Figure 15.4) (using the height instead the supported length in the ratio gives a similar result). Most ladder users are not familiar with this recommendation and generally tend to position ladders at suboptimal angle, which may increase the risk of ladder slide-out incidents. Furthermore, often the proper ladder angular positioning may not be achievable due to obstructions and inadequate support conditions.

From the description of the ladder positioning process, it becomes clear that a major issue is the need for greater flexibility in the ladder structural geometry to properly accommodate the different surface geometries and various support conditions available in the environment. Some of the barriers to addressing this need include the associated increases in ladder mass, structural and functional complexity, and overall cost. Therefore, the need for flexibility in ladder structural geometry is being addressed mainly by different ladder accessories. However, these ladder accessories are not always available, and multiple accessories are needed for different support conditions. Furthermore, some ladder accessories may create additional problems when not properly installed and used.

An alternative solution to addressing issues with suboptimal ladder setup conditions is to secure the ladder to a supporting surface/structure by tying it off using available structural elements or custom tools, such as clamps, hooks, and spikes in the ground.

15.3.4 User–Ladder Direct Interactions (Ladder Use) and Major Ladder-Related Fall Mechanisms

Portable ladders are designed to provide quick and easy access to elevated workplaces and to serve as temporary support for various short-term tasks at elevation.

From the perspective of mechanics and biomechanics, *ladder use* is defined as the phase of direct ladder–user interaction—when on the ladder, the user applies dynamic loading to the ladder, while the ladder transfers the loading to the supporting surface(s)/structure(s). Furthermore, for most tasks, the user also interacts with one of the supporting structures (e.g., while mounting or dismounting the ladder) or with an independent structure (to complete a task), thus potentially generating considerable destabilizing forces. According to the "control paradigm," failure or disruption in the control of these interactions may result in loss of stability (of the user or the system) and a fall. Different modes of failure and disruption in the control of dynamic stability during user–ladder interactions define the following three major types of ladder-related falls: loss of ladder (user–ladder system) stability, loss of user stability, and loss of ladder integrity or ladder structural failure.

Loss of user–ladder system stability occurs when the system's COM vertical projection leaves its stability limits (the boundaries of its BOS), defined by the ladder's four supporting legs. In addition, for leaning ladders, loss of stability may occur due to loss of traction as a slide-out event at the ladder base. For stepladders, most often the loss of stability occurs in the mode of tipping sideways and rarely by tipping forward or backward. In addition, twisting and racking movements can further destabilize the stepladder structure and lead to tipping or sliding at the base. For leaning ladders, loss of ladder stability can occur in four modes: ladder slides out at the base, top tips sideways, top tips backward, and ladder flips rotates alongside one of the rails (Clift, 2004). However, for leaning ladders, slide out is the most common stability failure mode, followed by top-tipping events.

To avoid a fall with the ladder, the user must maintain control over the stability of the whole system, in other words the user–ladder system, which uses the ground as support. To keep the whole user–ladder system in balance, the user must maintain control over the forces induced on the ladder at all time during different activities. However, the challenge for this control process is that the user does not receive feedback from the ladder about the proximity of the system's COM to its stability limits (the boundaries of the BOS), or when the friction requirements (RCOF) are approaching the available friction (ACOF) at the ladder base. That is why some ladder users will intuitively do a test when they first step on the ladder by shaking it side-to-side to get a better feel of the available stability limits of the system; in other words, to test how much force can be safely applied in different directions. However, such a testing approach is inadequate because it is usually done at a safer stage of the ladder climbing, when the user is on the first several steps, while the most dangerous loading conditions are when the user is at the top of the ladder (Hepburn, 1958).

Loss of user stability can occur during activities such as climbing up or down or while using the ladder as support and performing a task. The loss of stability may be triggered by self-induced (internal) perturbations, such as slipping on a rung, tripping, misstepping, and losing hold or losing balance while standing on a step or a rung and performing a task; or by external perturbations such as being knocked down by an object, an instrument, or a machine.

To avoid a fall from a ladder, the user must maintain balance both while climbing and when using the ladder as support for a task. Using a ladder structure as support is challenging for a number of reasons—narrow rung surfaces associated with reduced BOS and stability limits; visual exposure to elevation; fatigue which can induce instability;

and unstable ladder structure used as support, which can move, shake, and twist under dynamic loading conditions. In addition to all these challenging environmental factors, while on the ladder, the user may perform various tasks, such as climbing, reaching, pulling/pushing, and using different tools, which may involve generation of dynamic forces that may perturb and disrupt balance control. To ensure user stability in these challenging conditions, safety regulations and best-practice recommendations suggest that the user has to maintain three-point contact at all time while climbing and working from the ladder. However, these recommendations may not always be practical. Furthermore, balance can also be disrupted due to deficiencies in user hand-grip strength or in available friction at the hand–rung or hand–rail interface, as well as at the shoe-sole and ladder step/rung interface.

Ladder structural failure may occur as a result of excessive loading (exceeding the prescribed design load) or due to a damaged or defective structural element, component or system. Examples include the failure of a side rail, step or rung, hinges, spreaders, or extension locks. Some ladder structural failures have been attributed to excessive ladder twist flexibility and the associated tear and distress (Seluga et al., 2007). Proper ladder selection, adequate inspection and maintenance, optimal positioning, and appropriate loading during ladder use are key measures to prevent ladder structural failures.

15.4 Risk Factors for Falls from Ladders

Most incidents, including ladder falls, are nonrandom events with multiple causes. The major causes and risk factors for ladder falls have been summarized and described in the technical literature (Cohen and Lin, 1991; Axelsson and Carter, 1995; Hsiao et al., 2008; Grant and Hinze, 2013) and in the ladder safety standards (ANSI, A14.2 2007). The risk factors have been categorized according to an ergonomic systems model in an attempt to look at the person–equipment–environment interface (Cohen and Lin 1991); and according to the most common ladder fall mechanisms (Hsiao et al., 2008).

Analyses have demonstrated that factors closest to the incident event (associated with ladder use and working conditions) are stronger predictors than variables further away from the event, namely individual characteristics (Cohen and Lin, 1991). Tables 15.1 and 15.2 represent an attempt to summarize and organize the major causes and risk factors for ladder-related falls associated with the main ladder–user interactions and fall mechanisms enlisted and discussed in Section 15.3.

It is important to recognize that the sources of information used to determine the causes for ladder falls come from circumstantial reports of ladder fall incident investigations and interviews with ladder fall injury victims using structured questionnaires. There is a lot of subjectivity and bias in this information, since it is based on ladder users' perceptions and recollections (Axelsson and Carter, 1995). In addition, most users have limited understanding of the mechanical performance and the failure mechanisms of ladders. Nevertheless, in the absence of more accurate evidence, this epidemiological information continues to serve as the basis for developing preventive measures.

To help avoid the conditions and circumstances associated with ladder fall incidents, organizations at different levels have proposed and developed sets of guidelines and ladder safety rules. The rule-based control approach may not be the best strategy to eliminate ladder fall incidents, but it remains the main focus of ladder fall injury prevention efforts.

TABLE 15.1

Risk Factors for Falls from Stepladders (Self-Supporting Ladders)

	Selection	Inspection	Support	Setup		Orientation	Use
				Configuration			
Ladder stability—tipping (accounting for 17.9% of cases, in Lombardi et al., 2011)	Improper size, type, or style; ladder is not the proper equipment	Missing, worn, spreaders	Soft, uneven, unstable, slippery surface, irregular surface firmness, surface slope, one or more feet unsupported, unstable or insufficient supports	Unlocked spreaders		Ladder not close enough to work location, incorrect stepladder placement	Standing above highest standing level, reaching out too far laterally, climbing onto ladder from above, handling heavy loads or unstable objects, applying side load, walking the stepladder
Ladder stability—sliding (15.4% of cases, in Lombardi et al., 2011)	Ladder is not the proper equipment	Missing, worn or contaminated feet	Uneven surface, unstable surface, slippery surface—ice, snow, or wet	Using a folded stepladder as a leaning ladder		Not close enough to work location, position parallel to the task	Reaching out too far, stepping off ladder, applying side load
User stability—slip, trip, loss of balance, struck by object, lost handgrip (55.2% of cases, in Lombardi et al. 2011)	Ladder is not the proper equipment	Worn, slippery, contaminated steps	Soft, uneven, unstable surface	Unlocked spreaders		Position close to uninsulated electrical wires	Electrical shock, misstepping, slipping, misstepping the final step while descending, standing on the top step of ladder; age, health, shoes
Ladder structure failure (3.2% of cases, in Lombardi et al. 2011)	Improper selection, ladder does not fit the loading	Worn, damaged or defective elements	Soft, uneven, unstable surface	Unlocked spreaders		Incorrect placement	Ladder is subjected to overloading

TABLE 15.2

Risk Factors for Falls from Leaning Ladders (Non-Self-Supporting Ladders)

	Selection	Inspection	Support	Setup		Use
				Configuration	Orientation	
Ladder stability—sliding outward at the base (Accounting for 40.0% of cases, in Lombardi et al., 2011)	Ladder too long or extending too far, ladder is not the proper equipment; improper selection of feet or slip-resistant bearing surfaces	Worn, missing or slippery feet	Unstable or insufficient supports; base—unstable, loose surface; low friction slippery surface—ice, snow, or wet; top—overextension above top support	Ladder not footed, ladder not tied off or blocked; extension locks not engaged	Leaning angle too shallow	Standing above highest standing level, careless climbing onto or off ladder (from or to a roof), applying side load
Ladder stability—lateral sliding at the top (6.6% of cases, in Lombardi et al. 2011)	Too short or too long (size); ladder is not the proper equipment	Worn or missing top end caps/covers	Base support—uneven unstable surface, irregular surface firmness; top support—uneven, unstable surface, slippery, unstable surface, (pole/tree, corner of building), ice, snow, or wet surface, insufficient top support	Not tied off, not held at base; feet unsupported or unstable; extension locks not engaged	Leaning angle too shallow; inadequate or excessive extension above the top support; not close enough to work location	Reaching out too far laterally; stepping on or off ladder to roof; applying side load
User stability—slip, trip, loss of balance, struck by object (34.7% of cases, in Lombardi et al. 2011)	Ladder is not the proper equipment	Worn, slippery, contaminated (dirty, oily or icy) step surface	Uneven unstable surface, irregular surface firmness	Leaning angle not optimal	Leaning angle too steep (especially with flat rungs); position close to uninsulated electrical wires	Being struck by an object, or by electrical shock; excessive force, carrying objects, missteps while descending; age, health; shoes
Ladder structure failure (5.0% of cases, in Lombardi et al. 2011)	Improper selection, ladder does not fit the loading	Worn, damaged or defective structural elements	Soft, uneven, unstable surface	Extension locks not properly engaged	Suboptimal leaning angle;	Overloading

15.5 Current Measures to Control Falls from Ladders

15.5.1 Rule-Based Control

From the preceding analysis, it is clear that maintaining stability on ladders is not intuitive. To resolve the problem, a rule-based control strategy (also referred to as administrative controls) has been developed and implemented by organizations at different levels. Ladder safety standards, regulations and guidelines are rule-based control tools, which prescribe a set of rules for safe user–ladder interaction.

15.5.1.1 Ladder Safety Standards and Regulations

The OSHA, United States Department of Labor, develops, publishes and updates a standard (regulation) pertaining to ladders used in the construction industry. The portable ladder safety component resides in the OSHA Standards—29CFR Safety and Health Regulations for Construction subsection 1926.1053—Ladders (OSHA, 2014). The standard is based on information from the industry consensus standards and input from many stakeholders, including ladder user organizations. The provision for safe ladder use 1926.1053 (b) includes 22 rules addressing topics in the major user–ladder interaction categories.

The ANSI A14 Accredited Standard Committee develops, revises, and updates a number of industry consensus standards (*Ladders—Safety Requirements*), administered and published by the ALI. In addition to the technical requirement for manufacturing of ladders, the standards include a set of very detailed ladder-safety rules. The most essential safety rules are best summarized in the ANSI A14 Safety Labels developed for and attached to each ladder type. The current safety labels for stepladders include 25 safety rules and, for extension and straight ladders, 34 rules; furthermore, the rules are arranged in sections, which reflect the major user–ladder interactions: selection, inspection, setup, climbing and use, care, and storage.

In addition to the OSHA regulations and the ANSI standards, some ladder-safety practice guides have been developed by various organizations concerned with worker or public safety (Consumer Product Safety Commission [CPSC], 2011; Center to Protect Workers' Rights [CPWR], 2013; the Electronic Library of Construction Occupational Safety and Health [eLCOSH], 2014; the National Institute for Occupational Safety and Health [NIOSH], 2003; the National Safety Council [NSC], 2012; the American Academy of Orthopaedic Surgeons [AAOS], 2012). Most of these practice guides are based on the rules from the ladder-safety regulations and standards.

The following is a consolidated and simplified list of essential ladder-safety rules arranged by major user–ladder interactions.

Selection

1. Select ladder of proper size/length to reach working height.
2. Select ladder of proper duty rating to support the load of user plus materials and tools.
3. Select ladder of nonconductive material such as fiberglass or wood, if there is an electrical hazard.

Inspection

1. Inspect ladders before each use for broken, loose, missing, or inoperative parts.
2. Do not use damaged or worn ladders.
3. Keep ladders clean and free of slippery substances.

Proper Setup

1. Use ladders only on firm, level, and stable surfaces unless secured.
2. Do not use ladders on slippery surfaces without securing from movement.
3. For stepladders, set all four feet on the supporting surface.
4. For extension ladders, support both rails at top and base and tie off if possible.
5. Where tying off is not possible, use a second person to hold the ladder.
6. Do not let any ladder come in contact with electrical wires.
7. Keep clean the area around the top and bottom of ladders.
8. Secure ladder to prevent accidental displacement by work activities or traffic.
9. Do not set up and use ladder in high winds.
10. For stepladders, make sure the ladder is fully open and the spreaders secure.
11. For extension ladders, extend top section only from ground and make sure locks are secure.
12. Set extension ladder at 75° angle by using the ¼ length rule or the fireman's method.
13. Set extension ladder at least 1 m (3 ft.) above edge for roof access; tie top at support points.
14. Position ladder so that the user can face both ladder and task location.

Proper Climbing and Use

1. Always act carefully when climbing and using a ladder.
2. Never use ladders under the influence of alcohol, drugs, or medication or when in ill health.
3. Face the ladder and use both hands when climbing up or down.
4. Never climb a ladder from the side unless ladder is secured.
5. Grip and lean into ladder to maintain balance. Do not carry objects.
6. Keep the body's center of gravity between side rails. Do not overreach. Avoid pushing or pulling.
7. Keep ladder close to work location. Move ladder when needed.
8. Do not move, shift, or extend ladders while occupied.
9. Do not overload. Ladders are meant for one person only.
10. Use ladders only for the purpose they were designed.
11. Do not use ladder as brace, platform, or plank. Never use ladder on a scaffold.
12. For stepladders—do not climb, stand, or sit above second step from top of ladder.
13. For stepladders—do not use the rear section for climbing unless designed with steps.
14. For extension ladders—do not stand above third rung from top; never climb above top support.

Proper Transit and Storage

1. Properly secure and support ladder while in transit.
2. Store ladder where it is protected from foreign materials and corrosion damage.

15.5.1.2 Proper Use and Need for Education and Training

The proper use of portable ladders involves following closely all the requirements, recommendations, and guidelines listed in safety regulations and standards and practice guides. However, very often the ladder user is not familiar with some or most of the safety rules and recommendations. Furthermore, the average ladder user rarely reads the safety labels on the ladder. Occasionally, educated ladder users may find some of the safety rules impractical and thus ignore them. In most cases, users just follow their common sense to determine what is reasonable and may unknowingly use the ladder improperly.

For a rule-based control strategy to be effective, the users have to be educated and trained—the rule-based strategy is therefore a knowledge- and skills-based strategy. Numerous ladder-safety training courses and materials have been developed by different organizations, and some of them are available on the Internet. For example, ALI offers free access to its video-based training course (ALI, 2014b). More recently, training resources have become available as application for mobile devices—the NIOSH Ladder Safety app was released in 2013 and has been popular as a training tool among safety professionals and ladder users (NIOSH 2013).

15.5.1.3 Reasonably Foreseeable Misuse and Need for Further Design Improvements

Occasionally, educated users may be distracted and act under pressure to quickly complete a task without following the safety rules or take risks and knowingly compromise the conditions for safe use in order to complete a task. Frequently, knowingly or unknowingly, users buy ladders specifically to perform tasks that are considered unreasonable by the ladder industry. Some of these actions have been described as reasonably foreseeable misuse (Clift et al., 2002; Clift, 2004), and it has been argued that the ladder design should be improved to better accommodate users' expected behavior. Barriers such as requirements for simplicity, portability, low cost, and potentially increased manufacturer's liability prevent such improvements in ladder design. Therefore, some manufacturers have introduced ladder accessories to address these foreseeable misuses.

15.5.2 Design-Based Control (Human Factors and Ergonomics Considerations)

Integrating "safety-in-design" principles and solutions is the most efficient approach to reducing incidents and injuries associated with use of any product. Ladder-safety improvements can be achieved both through innovations in ladder structure design and in ladder accessories development.

The basic ladder design has remained relatively unchanged throughout history. The simple ladder geometry, defined by a set of side-rails connected with rungs or steps arranged at distances to allow comfortable climbing, effectively and efficiently fulfills its general function as a means of access to elevation. In the second half of the last century, with advancements in engineering materials and manufacturing technology, ladder structures have seen some significant improvements, resulting in lighter, stronger, and more durable ladder products.

While it is recognized that some improvement in ladder design may enhance its safety performance, further modifications in ladder design, beyond its basic function, have faced barriers. Some common sense ladder-design improvement needs include (1) increased stability through modified geometry, for example with wider base of support, adaptable legs/rails to accommodate various support conditions both at the bottom and at the top, and mechanisms for securing the ladder support points; (2) wider steps, providing secure standing support; and (3) handrails for improved stability during climbing and while standing and performing a task from the ladder.

Some of the barriers to incorporating the above-mentioned safety modifications into current ladder design include (1) increased ladder weight due to the additional structural components, which will compromise its portability and increase production costs; (2) increased base of support dimensions, which will limit the selection of appropriate support conditions; (3) increased structural complexity, which will increase production costs and increase the risk of system failure and thus the manufacturers' product liability; and (4) some safety improvements that may also increase user risk-taking behaviors.

Thus the existing need for ladder design modifications continues to be addressed by numerous ladder accessories. Thousands of patents and patent applications for ladder accessories have been published, and hundreds of products have been developed. Very few, however, have found a place in everyday practice. Some of these accessories have been manufactured without sufficient pretesting and standardization. To address this issue, the ANSI A14 committee recently developed and released the A14.8 standard for ladder accessories (ANSI, A14.8, 2013), which covers the most common accessory types and will gradually incorporate new classes of accessory products as they become available and established on the market.

This section provides some examples of ladder design modifications and accessories that address different ladder-safety issues.

15.5.2.1 Ladder Design Modifications and Improvements

The following are some examples of safety design improvements described in the research literature and implemented in products.

To reduce the risk of ladder slide-out incidents, some improvements have been made to portable ladder feet. Experiments by Pesonen and Hakkinen (1988) have shown that rubber-treated feet provide a better margin of safety than plastic or no treatment at all. Most extension ladders now have rubber-treated feet (Chang et al., 2005). In addition, most extension ladders have swiveling safety feet, incorporating a metal spike that can anchor the ladder base to prevent sliding on soft surfaces.

To improve the ease of climbing and reduce the risk of tripping, ladder geometry has been optimized to match the average ladder–user body dimensions and physical abilities. Investigators have speculated that a mismatch between ladder users' stature and ladder dimensions could contribute to incidents; very short or very tall persons could be more at risk than others (Dewar, 1977; Chaffin and Stobbe, 1979; Hammer and Schmalz, 1992). To address this issue, Chaffin and Stobbe (1979) evaluated the distance between ladder rungs and endorsed the ANSI recommendation of 30.5 cm (12 in).

To improve users' climbing comfort and reduce the risk of slipping, the simple round ladder rungs have been appropriately modified. The rungs of most extension ladders now are D-shaped with the flat upper surface at an angle of 75° to the rails. This design feature serves also as a guide for the user to a safe practice (Haakinen et al., 1988), since the rung becomes horizontal only when the ladder is positioned at the proper angle of 75°.

The following are some additional safety design modifications proposed recently in the research literature.

For stepladders, Seluga et al. (2007) suggested the following measures to control the risk of user losing balance: improve rigidity of stepladders to reduce twist flexibility and the risk of racking by making the front and rear side rails from tubular sections; redesign spreader bars to decrease twisting by using solid-plate or cross-shaped spreaders; and use a stiffer top cap for better stability and to resist twisting loads. To control the risk of falls from the top of stepladders, Clift and Navarro (2002) suggested that designs should not offer features permitting unsafe modes of use, such as top platforms on which one could step, and Shepherd et al. (2006) proposed removing the top step or ensuring that it cannot be stood upon and installing handholds and hand rails.

For extension ladders, Shepherd et al. (2006) proposed controlling the risk of electrocution by incorporating insulated segments; controlling the risk of slide out at the base by providing feedback for the ladder incline (e.g., by a bubble level or a hanging arrow) and methods to secure the ladder (e.g., by lashes, straps, or hooks that are fixed to the ladder); controlling the risk of user slipping by providing slip-resistant surfaces on rungs and providing barriers to prevent users from working off the side of the ladder; controlling the risk of falls during transition onto/off ladders by delineating the top 1 m of the ladder to help with proper above-edge extension during positioning and improving lateral stability by implementing splayed base.

In addition to the ladder design suggestions in the research literature, thousands of ideas directed toward improving different safety aspects of portable ladders have been described in the patent literature. One interesting example is the "smart ladder," designed with a tip-warning system that uses sensors to provide a feedback signal and warn the user of impending stability failure (Chandra, 2005). The majority of ideas relate to development of different ladder attachments and accessories rather than ladder-structure design modifications.

15.5.2.2 Ladder Accessories and Tools

A ladder accessory, as defined by the ANSI A14.8 standard, is "a device which may be factory installed by a ladder manufacturer or field installed, and which may expand its function, utility and safety, but without which the portable ladder still functions in its intended manner." The current standard recognizes three broad classes of accessories: top end (e.g., cable hooks, roof hooks, v-rungs, house pads, side rail end covers, pole chains/straps, stabilizers/stand-offs, walk-throughs) (Figure 15.5); bottom end (e.g., feet, spurs, levelers) (Figure 15.6); and miscellaneous (e.g., stabilizer straps, step brackets).

According to a study commissioned by the U.K. Department of Trade and Industry, in 1999 the U.K. market offered more than 80 accessories (safety devices) for extension (leaning) ladders (DTI, 1999). The study evaluation stage grouped the accessories into four major classes based on function and purpose and found that the "ladder stand-offs" offered some improvement in sideways slip resistance; most of the "levelers" reduced the risk of ladder base slide out; most of the "safety feet" offered some improvement in base-slip resistance; and most of the "stabilizers" offered some improvement in lateral stability at the top but not much in base-slip resistance.

A recent review on extension ladder safety (Hsiao et al., 2008) discussed some of the ladder safety accessories available on the U.S. market as they relate to the most common causes of falls and the associated risk factors. For example, accessories for reducing the risk of ladder slide out included inclination indicators, ladder base friction-enhancing devices,

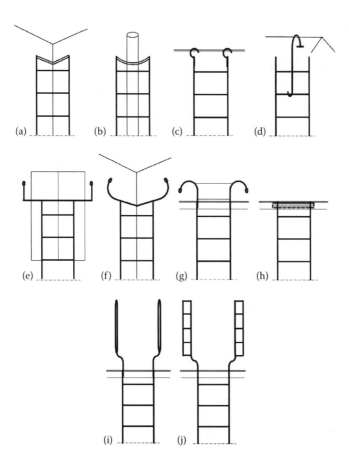

FIGURE 15.5
Schematic diagrams of ladder top-end accessories: (a) V-rung; (b) tree/pole chain; (c) cable hooks; (d) roof/ridge hook; (e) stand-off stabilizer; (f) corner stand-off stabilizer; (g) stand-off gutter-protector stabilizer; (h) gutter-protector stabilizer; (i) walk-through with vertical hand-rails; (j) walk-through with horizontal hand-holds.

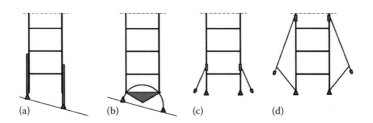

FIGURE 15.6
Schematic diagrams of ladder bottom-end accessories. (a) Adjustable-leg leveler; (b) circular leveler; (c) antislide stabilizer; (d) tripod stabilizer.

ropes and straps to secure the ladder base, and folding legs that engage in case of a slide. Accessories for reducing the risk of tipping sideways included hooks, straps, extender arms, and gutter stabilizers. While some accessories remain highly specialized (e.g., inclination indicators), many relate to more than one of the ladder-stability failure mechanisms (e.g., hooks, straps, gutter stabilizers).

Despite the multiple devices available on the market, few ladder accessories are being used in the field (Clift, 2004). Diversity of construction tasks and the time and effort required in carrying, assembling, and storing multiple accessories might hinder the wide use of these accessories. Furthermore, very few of these devices have been thoroughly evaluated. Systematic study of the effectiveness of ladder accessories and their possible integration with the ladder unit would be beneficial to ladder users (Hsiao et al., 2008).

The following evaluation criteria for leaning-ladder safety accessories have been suggested (Clift, 2004): a device would be considered to "enhance" safety if it increases the stability value in at least one of the four potential failure modes (slide out, side tip, back tip, or flip—see Section 1.3.4), while not causing the stability in the remaining modes to drop below the critical threshold. Furthermore, structural integrity under loading should be the primary safety concern for the device-augmented ladders, since many of the devices available on the market have been designed based on intuition rather than mechanics or engineering.

Engineering analysis demonstrates that most stability devices function by changing the ladder geometry and/or the available friction at the support points and, respectively, the direction and magnitude of the reaction force vector (Clift, 2004). In some instances, however, the changes in structural geometry may convert the leaning ladder–device system into a freestanding structure (a tripod) or a structure with multiple possible support points and stability states (defined by the possible triplets), which complicates the methodology for device effectiveness evaluation.

As long as the need for more adaptable and stable portable ladders is unmet, the development of ladder accessories will remain an important area in ladder safety. Thorough and adequate safety evaluation of the device-enhanced portable ladders may be complicated and may require significant efforts and resources. There is a need to further develop the classification, evaluation methodology, and standardization for ladder-safety devices and accessories. Developing and adopting robust criteria for inclusion of ladder accessories in the ladder-safety standards is an important step in this process.

15.5.3 Hazard Elimination and Substitution

The best strategy for preventing ladder fall incidents and injuries is to eliminate the need for work at elevation. Constructability analyses can be applied to identify tasks that can be finished on the ground. Furthermore, implementing safety-in-design principles may reduce the need for work at elevation, both in the short term during the construction process and in the long term during maintenance (Toole and Gambatese, 2008). If work at elevation cannot be eliminated, the next-best safety approach is to substitute the use of portable ladders with safer equipment for work at elevation, such as aerial lifts, rolling scaffolds, or mast-climbing scaffolds. While the substitution approach becomes more and more popular among large construction companies, it may be still infeasible for smaller construction and maintenance companies and homeowners.

15.5.4 Fall Protection Measures

The current OSHA regulations do not require fall protection for ladder use; however, using some fall-protection measures for work on ladders may be feasible under certain circumstances, such as availability of adequate and easily accessible anchor points. Securing the ladder and using a fall-protection system would be advisable especially when performing strenuous activities from the ladder such as pulling and pushing.

Fall-protection measures are directed and designed to reduce the dangerous consequences of a fall after it has initiated, in other words, to reduce the risk of impact injury by controlled transfer of the kinetic energy of the falling body to a supporting structure. The most common fall-protection measure is a fall-arrest system, which involves the use of a full body harness attached with a lanyard to an anchor point on a supporting structure. The fall protection harnesses and lanyards are commercial products, designed to transfer safely the dynamic forces generated during deceleration of the human body. The critical element in a fall-arrest system remains the anchor point—it has to be designed and engineered or selected and approved by a certified professional for the specific work environment. In many circumstances, adequate anchor points are not available, especially in light construction, where the partially completed structures are not capable of supporting the fall arrest loads. Accessing safely any available anchor points may also be a challenge, which further limits the use of fall-arrest systems.

When adequate and easily accessible anchor points are available, using a retractable lanyard may be beneficial while climbing and working on ladders, since it allows movement while reducing the free-fall distance and thus the fall-arrest load that needs to be transferred. It should be noted that portable ladders are not designed to serve as an anchor point for fall-arrest systems even when secured at the top and the base.

Available alternative fall-protection systems include inflatable mats or foam mats that can be positioned on the ground around the ladder base. However, these are associated with severe limitations and have not been widely adopted. Innovative fall-protection solutions, such as wearable and automatically deployable airbag jackets, which may be particularly appropriate for use on ladders, are not fully commercialized yet.

15.6 Recent Ladder Safety Research

15.6.1 Improving Extension Ladder Setup

A leading cause for extension-ladder fall incidents is a slide-out event usually related to suboptimal ladder inclination. An improved ladder positioning method or procedure could reduce the risk of ladder stability failure and the related fall injury. Recent studies conducted at the NIOSH laboratories compared the accuracy and efficiency of different anthropometric and instrumental methods to achieve optimal ladder angular positioning.

15.6.1.1 Anthropometric Methods Evaluation

The objective of the first study (Simeonov et al., 2012) was to evaluate the effectiveness of two anthropometric positioning methods: the ANSI A14 standard label (Figure 15.7) method ("stand-and-reach to hold the rung") and the "fireman" method ("stand-and-reach to hold the rail") (Figure 15.8). The results indicated that both anthropometric methods were similarly effective in improving extension ladder positioning; however, they required 50% more time than did the no-instruction condition and had a 9.5% probability of setting the ladder at a less-than-70° angle. Shorter ladders were consistently positioned at shallower angles. The study concluded that, when accurately and correctly performed, anthropometric methods may lead to safer ladder positioning than does no instruction. Workers tended to underperform as compared with their theoretical anthropometric estimates. Specific training or use of an assistive device may be needed to improve ladder users' performance.

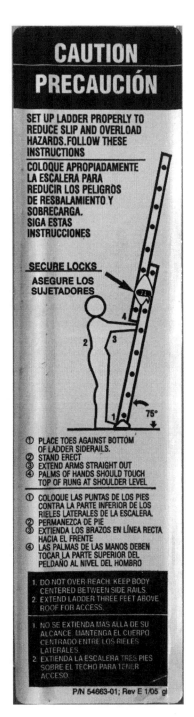

FIGURE 15.7
ANSI A14 Standard anthropometric sticker.

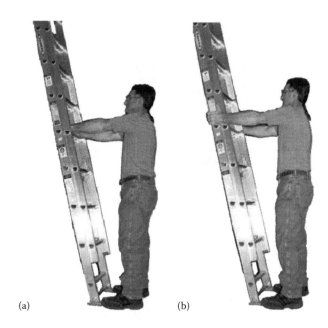

(a)   (b)

FIGURE 15.8
Two anthropometric methods for setting up leaning ladders: (a) ANSI A14 standard method; (b) fireman's method.

15.6.1.2 Instrumental Methods Evaluation

The second study (Simeonov et al., 2013) comparatively evaluated the effectiveness of a multimodal angle indicator, which provides direct feedback with visual and sound signals, with other existing methods for extension-ladder angular positioning, including the standard anthropometric method and a bubble-level indicator. The results indicated that the bubble-level method was very accurate but required more than double the time of the no-instruction method. The multimodal indicator improved the ladder angle setting as compared to the no-instruction and anthropometry methods and required the least time for ladder positioning among all tested methods. The main advantage of the new multimodal method is that it provides continuous feedback on the angle and hence does not require repositioning of the ladder. Such an indicator can be a valuable tool for training ladder users to correctly apply the current ANSI A14 standard anthropometric method in ladder angular positioning. The multimodal indicator concept has been extended to become a hand-held tool in the form of a smartphone application (see Section 15.6.2).

15.6.2 Innovative Mobile Technology Tools: The NIOSH Ladder Safety App

NIOSH recently released its first smartphone application, which is aimed at improving extension-ladder safety (Figure 15.9). The Ladder Safety phone app features an angle-of-inclination indicator that uses visual, sound, and vibration signals, making it easier for workers and other users to set an extension ladder at the proper angle of 75°. The app also includes a "Selection" tool which provides an interactive and easy-to-use procedure to select the minimum required ladder duty rating corresponding to the user characteristics and task. Furthermore, the app features an "Inspection" tool, which provides a comprehensive, graphic-based, interactive, and easy-to-use checklist for ladder mechanical

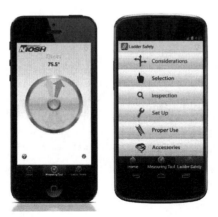

FIGURE 15.9
The NIOSH Ladder Safety smartphone app.

inspection. The app's "Proper Use" tool presents a set of standard-recommended rules in a clear graphic format, which is both informative and easy to understand.

Using smartphone technology, the Ladder Safety app delivers free and easy-to-use ladder safety tools and information, reference materials, and training resources into the hands of individual ladder users wherever and when they are needed. NIOSH developed the app using, patented technology, innovative research, existing information from safety regulations and consensus standards, and input from industry. The application is available in English and Spanish as a free download for Apple iPhone/iPad and Google Android devices. Recently, the application has been updated to include stepladder safety. Additional information on the app is available at the NIOSH webpage on Prevention of Fall Injury: http://www.cdc.gov/niosh/topics/falls/mobileapp.html.

15.6.3 Enhancing User Stability on Extension Ladders: Hand-Grip Issues and Three-Point Control

The ability to break a fall due to a slip or loss of balance on the ladder by grasping and holding onto the ladder may be a critical control mechanism to reduce the risk of ladder fall incidents. It has been previously reported that most people prefer holding the ladder side rail while ascending or descending on a portable ladder (Irvine and Vejvoda, 1977). Most likely, this preference is due to the convenience of being able to slide the hand on the ladder side rail for continuous lateral control. Since vertical support and climbing is exclusively done with the legs, the hands are used mostly for sideways balance (Barnet and Poczynok, 2000). However, the importance of a correct holding strategy becomes evident in case of a lost footing, when a good grasp on a handhold becomes critical to break a fall (Barnet and Poczynok, 2000).

The most important feature for control when exposed to a fall hazard is being able to hold onto a properly positioned and designed handhold during a loss of balance so that one's grab hand prevents the fall without slipping off (Ellis, 2012). Holding side rails or vertically placed holds provides a hand grip based on friction, while holding a rung or horizontal bar is referred to as horizontal power grip (Barnet and Poczynok, 2000). A recent biomechanics study found that holding a horizontal round object or grab bar (similar to a rung) with a horizontal power grip provided a greater safety margin for preventing a fall as compared to holding onto a vertical side rail or object when the fall starts (Young et al. 2012).

Based on these findings, Ellis (2012) recommended using a "three-point control" climbing strategy instead of the well-known "three-point contact" ladder-climbing safety rule. For portable leaning ladders, the three-point control strategy recommends that the user climbs by holding the rungs and should always use one hand and grasp a rung for stability. In an earlier discussion of this issue, Haakinen et al. (1988) pointed out that in practice, the dirt on the rungs results in the user trying to avoid touching them, and they suggested improving the design of the side rails to make the grip as steady and comfortable as possible.

15.6.4 Enhancing Step-Ladder Safety

Two of the major causes for falls from stepladders, addressed by recent research, are loss of balance on the part of the user and stepladder lateral tipping, usually related to excessive reaching. The following subsections discuss appropriate training and behavior modification strategies as well as compliance assessment tools.

15.6.4.1 Balance Control on Step Ladders

In a review of the literature related to human balance control on stepladders, Tichon et al. (2011) identified conditions that may degrade balance. Among the risk factors for losing balance on stepladders, they pointed out the reduced base of support on the narrow steps, the increased risk of compliant surfaces on excessively flexible ladders, and the absence of stepping strategies (due to a restricted support surface) or handhold restraining control strategies for the recovery of lost balance. To improve balance, they suggested that ladder users should avoid looking or reaching above their heads while working, wear thinner hard-soled shoes, and lean forward into the ladder to rest their shins against the step immediately above the step being stood on.

15.6.4.2 Lateral Reaching and the Belt-Buckle Rule

Guidelines for work on ladders recommend that the center of gravity of the user's body should remain within the rails of the ladder (the "belly button" or the "belt buckle" rule). Research has indicated that novice ladder users might be expected to take fewer risks than more experienced ladder users and to increase their risk taking as experience increases. In an experimental study on lateral reaching from step ladders, DiDomenico et al. (2013) demonstrated that novice workers can acclimate very quickly to a challenging reaching task, especially when motivated to complete a task, resulting in dangerous overreaching, such as when the belly button (belt-buckle) is surpassing the rail. Ladder-specific safety training is recommended to continuously reinforce the emphasis that safety is more important than task completion speed.

15.6.4.3 Quantifying Best Practices in the Field

To assess the extent to which users comply with the best-practice guidelines for portable ladder use in construction industry, Dennerlein et al. (2009) developed and tested an audit tool using a hand-held computer. The auditing tool consisted of a series of checklists organized in four groups: ladder condition, ladder setup, moving on a ladder, and completing a task from a ladder. The results indicated that the tool is reliable and offers a practical method to quantify the best practices associated with ladder use.

15.7 Conclusions

Portable ladders remain the most common and widespread equipment for access to elevation, despite the increasing availability of alternative equipment for work at height, such as aerial lifts, rolling scaffolds, and mast-climbing scaffolds. They are the tool of choice in small construction and maintenance projects and for home use. Portable ladders are lightweight, affordable, and relatively simple devices; however, their use is associated with considerable risk of fall injury and thus a substantial burden on society.

Manufacturers have attempted to improve portable ladder design; however, most of the ladder-safety improvements are being introduced as accessories. Despite the perceived simplicity, the mechanical behavior of portable ladders is complex and difficult to model and assess, especially in the field. The current rule-based control strategies are not sufficiently effective. To reduce the burden of ladder fall injuries, there is a need for (1) further improvements in ladder design by integrating effective safety concepts and devices, combined with (2) continuous improvements in ladder-safety rules, and supported by (3) thorough ladder user training, and (4) rigorous field compliance assessment.

To prevent ladder falls, employers should consider the following steps: (1) Plan the work to reduce or eliminate the need for using ladders by applying safety-in-design and constructability principles to finish as much of the work as possible on the ground; (2) provide alternative, safer equipment for extended work at elevation, such as aerial lifts, supported scaffolds, or mast-climbing work platforms; (3) provide properly selected and thoroughly inspected ladders that are well-matched to employee weight, task, and location; (4) when applicable, provide proper accessories to supplement safe ladder use; and (5) provide adequate ladder-safety information and training for employees.

15.8 Disclaimers

The findings and conclusions in this report are those of the author and do not necessarily represents the views of NIOSH. Mention of any company or product does not constitute endorsement by NIOSH. In addition, citations to websites external to NIOSH do not constitute NIOSH endorsement of the sponsoring organizations or their programs or products. Furthermore, NIOSH is not responsible for the content of these websites. All web addresses referenced in this document were accessible as of the publication date.

References

AAOS (American Academy of Orthopaedic Surgeons). *Ladder Safety Guide*. Rosemont, IL: American Academy of Orthopaedic Surgeons, 2012. http://orthoinfo.aaos.org/topic.cfm?topic=a00235

ALI (American Ladder Institute). *Ladder Safety Training*. Chicago, IL: American Ladder Institute, 2014b. http://www.laddersafetytraining.org/

ANSI (American National Standards Institute) A14.2. *American National Standard for Ladders: Portable Metal—Safety Requirements*. Chicago, IL: American Ladder Institute, 2007.

ANSI (American National Standards Institute) A14.8. *American National Standard for Ladders—Safety Requirements for Ladder Accessories*. Chicago, IL: American Ladder Institute, 2013.

Axelsson, P.-O., and Carter, N., Measures to prevent portable ladder accidents in the construction industry. *Ergonomics*, 38 no. 2, (1995): 250–259.

Barnet, R. L., and Poczynok, P. J., Ladder rung vs. side-rail hand grip strategies. *Safety Brief*, 16 no. 4, (2000): 1–15.

Chaffin, D. B., and Stobbe, T. J., *Ergonomic Considerations Related to Selected Fall Prevention Aspects of Scaffolds and Ladders as Presented in OSHA Standard 29 CFR 1910 Subpart, D*. US Department of Labor. Ann Arbor, MI: University of Michigan, 1979.

Chandra, S. Smart ladder. US Patent no. 6966403, 2005.

Chang, W.-R., Chang, C.-C., and Matz, S., Available friction of ladder shoes and slip potential for climbing on a straight ladder. *Ergonomics*, 48 no. 9, (2005): 1169–1182.

Clift, L. Evaluating the Performance and Effectiveness of Ladder Stability Devices. Contract Research Report 205. Loughborough University, UK. London, UK: Health and Safety Executive, 2004.

Clift, L., and Navarro, T. Ergonomics Evaluation into the Safety of Stepladders: User Profile and Dynamic Testing. Phase 2. Contract Research Report 423. Loughborough University, UK. London, UK: Health and Safety Executive, 2002.

Clift, L., Navarro. T. B., and Thomas, D.A.B., How reasonable is reasonable use? The search for safer stepladders. *Injury Control and Safety Promotion*, 9 no. 3, (2002): 175–184.

Cohen, H.H., and Lin, L., A retrospective case-control study of ladder fall accidents. *Journal of Safety Research*, 22, no. 1, (1991): 21–30.

CPSC (US Consumer Product Safety Commission). Ladder safety 101. US Consumer Product Safety Commission, 2011, http://www.cpsc.gov/onsafety/2011/12/ladder-safety-101/.

CPSC (US Consumer Product Safety Commission). Unpublished data from the National Injury Information Clearinghouse (CPSC) using the CPSC's Injury Cost Model, 2014.

CPWR (Center to Protect Workers' Rights). *Hazard Alert—Ladders*. The Center for Construction Research and Training, 2013. Silver Spring, MD. http://www.cpwr.com/sites/default/files/publications/Ladders%202013.pdf

Dennerlein, J. T., Ronk, C. J., and Perry, M. J., Portable ladder assessment tool development and validation-quantifying best practices in the field. *Safety Science*, 47 no. 5, (2009): 636–639.

Dewar, M. E. Body movements in climbing a ladder. *Ergonomics*, 20 no. 1, (1977): 67–86.

DiDomenico, A. T., Lesch, M. F., Blair, M. F., and Huang, Y.-H., Reaching on ladders: Do motivation & acclimation affect risk taking? *Professional Safety*, 58 no. 2, (2013): 50–53.

DTI (Department of Trade and Industry). *Assessment of Leaning Ladder Safety Devices*. London: Department of Trade and Industry, 1999.

eLCOSH (Electronic Library of Construction Occupational Safety and Health). *Ladder Safety*. 2014; http://www.elcosh.org/document/1976/d000170/Ladder%2BSafety.html?show_text=1

Ellis, N. J., Three-point control—Analysis and recommendations for climbing ladders, stairs and step bolts. *Professional Safety*, 57 no. 11, (2012): 30–36.

Grant, A., and Hinze, J. Underlying causal factors associated with construction worker fatalities involving stepladders. *Australasian Journal of Construction Economics and Building*, 13 no. 1, (2013): 13–22.

Hakkinen, K.K., Pesonen, J., and Rajamaki, E., Experiments on safety in the use of portable ladders. *Journal of Occupational Accidents*, 10, (1988): 1–19.

Hammer, W., and Schmalz, U., Human behaviour when climbing ladders with varying inclinations. *Safety Science*, 15 no. 1, (1992): 21–38.

Hepburn, H. A., Portable ladders: Part 1—The quarter length rule. *British Journal of Industrial Safety*, 4 no. 46, (1958): 155–158.

Hsiao, H., Simeonov, P., Pizatella, T., Stout, N., McDougall, V., and Weeks, J., Extension-ladder safety: Solutions and knowledge gaps. *International Journal of Industrial Ergonomics*, 38, (2008): 959–965.

Irvine, C. H., and Vejvoda, M., An investigation of the angle of inclination for setting non-self-supporting ladders. *Professional Safety*, 22 no. 7, (1977): 34–39.

Ladders.net. Types of ladders. http://www.ladders.net/type, 2014.

Lombardi, D. A., Smith, G. S., Courtney, T. K., Brennan, M. J., Young Kim, J., and Perry, M. J., Work-related falls from ladders—A follow-back study of US emergency department cases. *Scandinavian Journal of Work, Environment and Health,* 37 no. 6, (2011): 525–532.

NIOSH (National Institute for Occupational Safety and Health). *NIOSH Ladder Safety Mobile Application.* Division of Safety Research, Morgantown, WV: U.S. Department of Health and Human Services, Centers for Disease Control and Prevention, National Institute for Safety and Health, 2013. http://www.cdc.gov/niosh/topics/falls/mobileapp.html.

NIOSH (National Institute for Occupational Safety and Health). Portable ladders for construction: Self-inspection checklist. DHHS (NIOSH) Publication Number 2004-101. 2003. http://www.cdc.gov/niosh/docs/2004-101/chklists/r1n73l~1.htm

NSC (National Safety Council). A safe climb: 20 steps for portable ladder use. *Safety and Health Magazine,* March 1, 2012. http://www.safetyandhealthmagazine.com/articles/a-safe-climb-2

OSHA (Occupational Safety and Health Administration). Regulations (Standards-29 CFR), Ladders.: 1926.1053, 2014. https://www.osha.gov/pls/oshaweb/owadisp.show_document?p_table=standards&p_id=10839

Pesonen, J. P., and Hakkinen, K. K., Evaluation of safety margin against slipping in a straight aluminum ladder. *Hazard Prevention,* 8, (1988): 6–13.

Seluga, K. J., Ojalvo, I. U., and Obert, R. M., Analysis and testing of a hidden stepladder hazard—Excessive twist flexibility. *International Journal of Injury Control and Safety Promotion,* 14 no. 4, (2007): 215–224.

Shepherd, G. W., Kahler, R. J., and Cross, J. Ergonomic design interventions—A case study involving portable ladders. *Ergonomics,* 49 no. 3, (2006): 221–234.

Simeonov, P., Hsiao, H., Kim, I.-J., Powers, J., and Kau, T.-Y., Factors affecting extension ladder angular positioning. *Human Factors,* 54 no. 3, (2012): 334–345.

Simeonov, P., Hsiao, H., Powers, J., Kim, I.-J., Kau, T.-Y., and Weaver, D. Research to improve extension ladder angular positioning. *Applied Ergonomics,* 44 no. 3, (2013): 496–502.

Socias, C., Chaumont Menéndez, C., Collins, J., and Simeonov, P., Occupational ladder fall injuries—United States, 2011. *MMWR,* 63 no. 16, (2014): 341–346.

Tichon, D.,. Baker, L. L., and Ojalvo, I. U., The role of human balance in stepladder accidents. *Proceedings of the Human Factors and Ergonomics Society Annual Meeting,* 55 no. 1, (2011): 1701–1705.

Toole, M. T., and Gambatese, J. The trajectories of prevention through design in construction. *Journal of Safety Research,* 39, (2008): 225–230.

Wikipedia. Ladder. http://en.wikipedia.org/wiki/Ladder, 2014.

Young, J. G., Wooley, C. B., Ahton Miller, J. A., and Armstrong, T. J., The effect of handle orientation, size and wearing gloves on hand/handhold breakaway strength. *Human Factors,* 54 no.3, (2012): 316–333.

16

Aerial Lift Safety Research and Practice

Christopher S. Pan

CONTENTS

ABSTRACT The increasing industrial use of aerial lifts has resulted in a corresponding increased risk of incidents with attendant injury and death. This chapter identifies factors contributing to those incidents, including hazardous surface conditions, aerial lift and worker motions, and the lack of use of safety systems. The chapter also describes current safety research on aerial lifts and other similar equipment.

16.1 Research on Aerial Lifts

The increasing industrial use of aerial lifts has resulted in a corresponding increased risk of incidents with attendant injury and death; there were over 300 deaths associated with the industrial use of aerial lifts between 1992 and 2003 [1]. To better understand the cause of aerial-lift incidents, the National Institute for Occupational Safety and Health (NIOSH), the National Safety Council (NSC), and the Center for Construction Research and Training (CPWR) joined together to review aerial platform fall, collapse, and tip-over data from three sources of information concerning incidents involving aerial lifts: the BLS

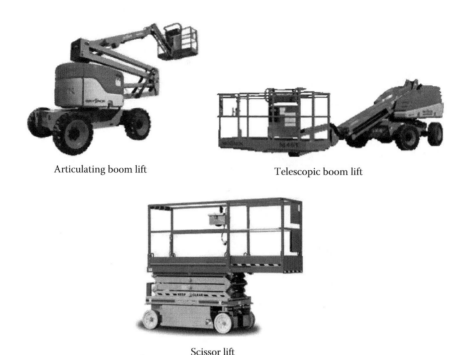

Articulating boom lift   Telescopic boom lift

Scissor lift

FIGURE 16.1
Types of aerial lifts. (Reprinted with permission of SkyJack Inc.)

Census of Fatal Occupational Injuries (CFOI) (1992–2003), Occupational Safety and Health Administration (OSHA) incident investigation records (1990–2003), and NIOSH Fatality Assessment and Control Evaluation (FACE) reports (1985–2002) [1]. Results presented in this chapter represent data taken from these three databases, unless a specific source is indicated.

Analysis of data from these sources identifies factors contributing to those incidents, including hazardous surface conditions, aerial lift and worker motions, and the lack of use of safety systems. The following sections explore the results of NIOSH research focused on the use of scissor lifts, a type of aerial lift that supports a work platform on top of an extendable, linked, and folding support assembly. Aerial lifts generally include scissor lifts and boom lifts (Figure 16.1). Although NIOSH's research presently focuses on scissor lifts, the following sections will also describe incidents arising from the use of the other major type of aerial lift—the boom lift—which supports a work platform at the end of an extendable boom.

16.1.1 Scissor Lifts

16.1.1.1 Background

Scissor lifts are self-propelled, mobile work platforms that can be raised or lowered to various heights [1–3] but lack the ability to rotate. Scissor lifts are popular because their small footprint permits their use in tight areas [4], and they are generally considered to be more productive than other forms of elevating device, which can require extensive assembly and disassembly time, lack mobility, and are commonly perceived as imposing constraints of reach, forceful loading, and postural instability upon users. Further, scissor lifts are generally perceived to effect reduction in physical demands on workers when compared to other traditional elevated devices, such as ladders [2], although the extent of physical demands on various body parts has not been extensively researched or comparatively established. However, despite the apparent reduction in exposure to some types of hazardous conditions, scissor lifts also present unique and substantial risks, particularly of falls to lower levels. Some of the hazards are inherent to the design and configuration of the lift itself; scissor lifts designed to fit through doorways can have narrow wheelbases, which decreases their stability. Rollout platform extensions on scissor-lift platforms also decrease stability, since they can reach beyond the wheelbase and thus affect the scissor lift's center of gravity. Further, horizontal worker motions and external kinetic forces can further destabilize the lift. For example, when a horizontal force of 623 newtons is applied while the lift is elevated over 5.49 meters, excess loading of the lift and subsequent tipover can occur [3]. These fall/collapse/tip-over hazards occur frequently and are easily overlooked by workers.

16.1.1.2 Factors Contributing to Scissor-Lift Injuries and Deaths

Descriptive results of a pertinent NIOSH study [1] shows that from 1992 to 2003, falls from scissor lifts caused 78 fatalities (CFOI data). Most of these deaths occurred in the construction industry (58 deaths, representing 74% of the total), at a construction site (41%), in an industrial zone (31%), or on a street or highway (30%). Consistent with the location of the incidents, the majority of scissor-lift falls recorded by OSHA and FACE investigations occurred while "constructing and repairing" (54%) or "painting and cleaning" (19%).

Tip-over and collapse of the scissor lift (known as *tip-overs*) caused over half of the falls (56% of the total, based on CFOI data), and falls from the scissor-lift platform caused the remaining incidents. The NIOSH/NSC/CPWR collaborative study collected information from the three source databases and identified several common factors associated with falls from scissor lifts. First, the study found that hazardous conditions largely contributed to falls from scissor lifts. For instance, the CFOI database shows that uneven or sloped ground or driving on or off a flatbed truck was cited as a factor in six tip-overs (14% of 44 scissor-lift tip-overs). That database also shows that driving into potholes, or over sidewalks or similar uneven edges, contributed to seven tip-overs (16%). In contrast, review of the information reported in the OSHA logs and FACE database show that 55% of fall reports cited surface conditions, and in the 16 fall incidents (55%) that cited surface conditions as contributing factors, seven cases involved potholes, and nine cases involved uneven or unstable ground [1].

The above-mentioned NIOSH/NSC/CPWR study also identified scissor-lift and worker movements as contributing to falls from scissor lifts. The OSHA/FACE databases cited scissor-lift motion in 42% of fall incidents. Also, scissor lifts had moved forward or backward in 18 of 78 (23%) of scissor-lift fatalities recorded in the CFOI database and in 18 (33%) of the 54 scissor-lift falls recorded in the OSHA/FACE databases. In addition, raising or lowering of the lift was cited in four (7%) of the total OSHA/FACE cases. Moreover, the study found that 25 (46%) of the OSHA/FACE fall reports cited worker movement as a contributory factor to the fall.

Surprisingly, the OSHA/FACE databases show that 83% of scissor-lift fall victims fell 3–8.8 m, yet only a small minority of the injury or fatality cases from the OSHA/FACE databases show that the workers were using safety protection, such as belts and harnesses.

In fact, only four of the 13 (31%) of the scissor-lift fall reports that mention fall protection show the use of such fall protection.

Indeed, the study found that mechanical failure was cited in only two scissor-lift cases (4%), suggesting that a majority of scissor-lift falls and resulting injuries and deaths may be considered to be related to operational variables and misuse scenarios and are preventable with appropriate training and safe-operation standardization procedures. When joined with careful analysis of the design variables of scissor lifts, and the inherent limitations of use under different conditions as a function of the design itself, virtually all of the injuries can be said to be preventable. Therefore, what is needed to effect the safe use of scissor lifts can be succinctly summarized as follows: A better understanding of scissor-lift design constraints under hazardous-exposure conditions; scissor-lift movements under normal and extreme conditions; worker movements, especially phase-amplifying movements that are cumulative and that contribute to tip-over and fall incidents; and the efficacy of safety systems designed to protect workers from such falls.

The current relevant regulations do not fully address these risk factors. Specifically, scissor lifts are "mobile scaffolds" as defined by 29 C.F.R. § 1926.451(g)(1)(vii) (OSHA) and thus require the use of guardrails or personal fall protection systems as a primary safety control system [1]. But these regulations were designed for the purpose of regulating scaffolding and not aerial lifts per se. In fact, the preamble to 29 C.F.R. § 1926.451 expressly states that the mobile scaffold section "does not apply to aerial lifts." Expert opinion suggests that this requirement may not fully address hazards presented by scissor lifts, which are generally operated at different heights and conditions and for different work tasks than such normal suspension scaffolds. Accordingly, NIOSH has investigated these risk factors and presents the findings from the relevant studies below.

16.1.1.3 Scissor-Lift Behavior in Hazardous Conditions

To conduct research into scissor-lift behavior under hazardous conditions without putting human subjects at risk, NIOSH researchers have developed computer simulations to model scissor-lift behavior under various potentially hazardous conditions. The NIOSH studies show that, although scissor lifts at static conditions are stable under certain circumstances, a static scissor lift may tip over when subjected to sufficient horizontal forces even if that scissor lift complies with all ANSI A92.6 safety limits [3]. The studies also show that decreasing the stiffness and increasing the tilt speed and tilt angle of a scissor lift generally reduces scissor-lift stability on sloped ground and during curb and pothole impacts. The studies further suggest that using a scissor lift on soft surfaces could cause tip-overs and that wind forces exceeding 20 m/s can potentially tip over a scissor lift.

16.1.1.3.1 Computer Simulations of Static Scissor-Lift Behavior in Hazardous Conditions

Nearly two-thirds of all scissor-lift tip-overs occur when the scissor lift is stationary, even when the scissor lifts at issue are designed and manufactured to withstand horizontal forces prescribed by ANSI safety standards [4]. To understand why such tip-overs occur, NIOSH studied how much horizontal force was required to tip over a scissor lift by developing a computer model of a stationary scissor lift, validating that model with experimental data, and then using this model to calculate the horizontal forces that would cause tip-over events. The results show that, although scissor lifts at rest are stable under certain circumstances, a static scissor lift may tip over when subjected to sufficient horizontal force even if that scissor lift complies with all ANSI A92.6 safety limits [4]. The results also show that the use of outriggers may substantially strengthen a scissor lift's ability to withstand horizontal forces.

More extensive and detailed information on the procedure followed by NIOSH is given below. The first action that NIOSH researchers undertook to determine the forces acting on a scissor lift was to develop a computer model using information from manufacturer specifications. Researchers then conducted center-of-gravity and horizontal-stability tests under the ANSI A92.6 (2006) standard to validate the results predicted by the preliminary model. In order to determine the empirical center of gravity, researchers placed four force plates (Bertec Corporation, Columbus, OH) under the wheels of the scissor lift and tilted the lift using hand force–activated pump jacks and jack stands. Researchers recorded the platform height using a cable-extension transducer (Model PT5A-250-N34-UP-500-C25, Celesco Transducer Products, Inc., Chatsworth, CA). The researchers used a horizontal actuator (Series 247, MTS Systems Corporation, Eden Prairie, MN) to apply horizontal loads through a cable-and-sheaf arrangement. The researchers hung the sheaf from a 4,535.9 kg-capacity overhead crane and took load readings with a load cell (Model 661.20e-02, MTS Systems Corporation, Eden Prairie, MN) integrated with the hydraulic actuator. The modeling predictions agreed well with the experimental data with an error margin of less than 1% for the whole range of the lift height variations in three orthogonal directions [4].

Second, the researchers used the validated and refined computer model to calculate the amount of horizontal force that a scissor lift could withstand at different heights. The results show that a scissor lift (model 3219, SkyJack Inc., Guelph, ON, Canada) can be safely extended to a height between 3.49 and 5.49 m if applied forces are between 623 and 889 N [4].

16.1.1.3.2 Further Computer Simulations of Dynamic Scissor-Lift Behavior in Hazardous Slope, Tilt, Curb Impact, and Pothole Conditions

NIOSH researchers also developed a dynamic computer model of the scissor lift to identify factors in hazardous conditions that contribute to tip-over events. The model shows that on sloped ground, increasing the height and flexibility of the lift structure also increases the scissor lift's tip-over potential [5]. Accordingly, the lift should not be elevated on soft or uneven surfaces. Also, scissor lifts should be designed to be as stiff as possible to avoid tip-overs during curb impact and pothole depression impacts and to potentially use lower pothole guards (to reduce the dynamic impact) so as to avoid tip-overs during the latter events. The computer model also shows that both ground slope and the tilt speed of the lift affect the stability of the lift, and thus both the tilt angle and tilt speed of the lift could be measured and used to help prevent tip-overs. Further, the computer model confirms that low-frequency disturbances (such as repetitive-motion tasks) may cause scissor-lift tip-overs, and thus workers should avoid making periodic horizontal motions that could amplify the rocking motion and result in a tip-over. Therefore, the study suggests that certain periodic movements and horizontal forces/moments applied by workers may excite (increase) the resonate frequencies of the lift and may subsequently contribute to tip-over incidents. The results also suggest that increasing the flexibility of the lift structure while it is on sloped surfaces increases its tip-over potential, and the lift should thus not be elevated on soft, uneven, or other sloped surfaces.

The researchers equipped a scissor lift weighing 1170 kg with a deck extension carrying a rated load of 113 kg. They also installed five in-house packaged triaxial accelerometers on the main frame of the base; the second, third, and fourth scissor frames; and the main frame of the platform. The accelerometers' signals were sent to an in-house packaged data-acquisition system, which sampled the accelerometer data at 128 Hz [5].

The researchers simulated a curb impact by driving the scissor lift, both forward and backward, into a curb at 30° and 90° at the maximum heights allowed by the lift at two different speeds—5.80 m high while at 0.29 m/s and 2.08 m high while at 0.89 m/s. The researchers also simulated a pothole impact by driving one of the scissor lift's front wheels into a standardized pothole (0.60 m square and 0.10 m depth). The collected data from both the curb and pothole impact tests suggest that when the platform is fully elevated (2.08 m), the major cause of movement in the platform is pitching and rolling, arising from resonant low-frequency vibrations, particularly from 0.3 to 2.08 Hz, and can cause significant deformations of the scissor-lift substructures. By contrast, the data also show that such low-frequency vibrations do not occur at the lower heights of the scissor lifts and that high-frequency vibrations quickly dissipate and therefore are not likely to cause tip-overs.

The researchers then created an ADAMS/View computer model based on the collected data; other measurements taken of the scissor lifts' wheels; and dimensions, connection points, mass properties, and centers of mass (CM) calculated through the scissor lifts' schematics. The researchers successfully validated the CM values generated by the model, which were consistent with CM values measured during a tilt-table experiment of the scissor lift at four different heights. The researchers further validated the computer model's predicted acceleration values upon curb and pothole impacts, which also closely agreed with experimental acceleration measurements. The researchers used the computer model to determine the tip-over threshold under four hazardous conditions. In so doing, the researchers treated the tip-over threshold as a function of the scissor lift's vertical stiffness because vertical stiffness controls the rolling and pitching motions of the scissor structure and platform. Thus, the researchers used the effect of the scissor structure's stiffness as an independent variable for most of the simulations.

In this study, the researchers first applied the model to determine the effect of scissor-lift stiffness on tip-over threshold when the scissor lift was on sloped ground. The results showed that, if the lift platform was elevated, the tip-over threshold primarily depended on the height of the platform but that a scissor lift's stiffness also affected its stability. Although increasing stiffness generally increases the tilt tip-over angle, once the stiffness value approaches the limit identified from physical experiments [5] to a stiffness value that is roughly double to that limit, the tilt tip-over angle remains constant and undifferentiated, equivalently recording the same level of stability. Further, the model shows that a marginal change (<15%) from normal stiffness results in only a slight change (<1.0%) in tilt tip-over angle but that reducing the scissor lift's normal stiffness by more than 60% significantly reduces the tilt tip-over threshold (>5.0%). Consequently, using the lift on soft soil and other deformable surfaces such as bridged wood boards or metal sheets—which are effectively sloped surfaces—could be hazardous, particularly if workers create periodic motions close to the resonance frequency of the scissor lift that amplify the rocking motion and can result in a tip-over.

Second, the researchers used the model to simulate the effect of a scissor lift's tilting and rocking speed on tip-over threshold. The results showed that if the tilt speed is low, the tip-over threshold is close to the quasi-static tip-over threshold. However, the tip-over threshold is substantially reduced when the tilt speed is greater than 2.5 degrees/second, because dynamic energy can increase the tip-over potential. Accordingly, both the tilt angle and tilt speed—not just the tilt angle—should be monitored to avoid tip-overs.

Third, the researchers used the model to determine the effect of stiffness on the tip-over threshold during curb impact. Although the stiffness of the scissor lift did not substantially affect the tip-over threshold of the impact speed, the results show that to reduce the tip-over potential, it is better to keep the scissor-lift structures as stiff as possible.

Finally, the researchers used the model to determine the effect of stiffness on the tip-over threshold of pothole guardrail height. The results show that reducing the stiffness of the scissor lift, in turn, requires lowering the pothole guardrail height to control the tilt angle within the stable limit, because reducing the stiffness makes the lift's center of gravity move further toward the tilt direction. Consequently, the results suggest that pothole guardrails should be designed to be as low as possible [5].

16.1.1.4 Drop Tests Evaluating Personal Fall Arrest System Efficacy, Personal Fall Arrest Systems' Impact on Workers, Fall Impact on the Stability of Scissor Lifts, and Methodologies for Evaluating the Biomechanical Risk Factors

Personal fall arrest systems, which prevent workers from falling by catching them on a lanyard attached to the scissor lift, are not required by regulation because guardrails on the platforms meet the OSHA requirements for fall injury prevention for scissor lifts. (See 29 C.F.R. § 1926.451(g)(4)). Additional requirements for using personal fall arrest systems currently are still under consideration by industry and standard committees (ANSI A92.6). Indeed, the impact of these fall arrest systems on the stability of a scissor lift is unknown. Further, the effectiveness of personal fall arrest systems for scissor lifts and their impact on the head, neck, and torso of a worker when activated is also largely unknown. The following studies show that personal fall arrest systems under the test conditions below are not likely to cause scissor lifts to tip over and that forces exerted on the human body fall within the acceptable limits defined by applicable industry standards. Given that workers did not use personal fall arrest systems in most falls from scissor lifts that resulted in fatalities, these results suggest that perhaps aerial lift standards should consider amending the use of personal fall protection equipment to include personal fall arrest systems.

16.1.1.4.1 Drop Test Results (Dead Weight Drop)

Presently available fall arrest systems prevent worker falls from scissor lifts by anchoring a harness worn by the worker to the scissor lift with an energy-absorbing lanyard. To determine whether the use of a fall arrest system imposes forces on a scissor lift exceeding 1800 lb (the maximum force allowed by ANSI Z359.1-2007) or can otherwise cause a scissor lift to tip over, another NIOSH study [6] measured the structural and dynamic stability of aerial lift work platforms by dropping different weights anchored to different anchorage points on a scissor lift from different heights and observing whether the scissor lift tip-over occurred or the structure subsequently experienced component and complete failure. The results showed that the specific scissor lift used in this study (model 3219, SkyJack Inc., Guelph, ON, Canada) can withstand many different levels of fall arrest forces when fully elevated and deployed on an incline and that the use of a personal fall system will not likely cause the scissor lift used in this study to tip over [6]. The results also showed that such fall arrest systems are not likely to cause the scissor lift to tip over even if anchored to locations unapproved by the scissor lift manufacturer, such as the mid- and top rails of a scissor lift [6].

For this study, the researchers first identified combinations of weights and free-fall heights that would generate specific fall arrest forces—2224 N; 4,448 N; 6,672 N; 8000 N; and 10,675 N—by tying weights to a rigid beam with Nystrom ropes, dropping those weights, and collecting fall arrest data. The researchers used a load cell (1361.8 kg, S-type, Interface Inc., Scottsdale, AZ) to record the maximum arrest force, a string potentiometer (635 cm, Model PT5D, Celesco Transducer Products, Inc., Chatsworth, CA) to record positions of the drop-test fixture, and an electromagnet (317.5 kg, Model SE-35352, Magnetic Products, Inc., Highland, MI) to activate the drop-test fixture. The researchers collected generated data with a laptop computer equipped with a data acquisition card (Model DAQCard-6036E, National Instruments Corporation, Austin, TX) running the LabVIEW data acquisition application (National Instruments Corporation, Austin, TX).

Using these same weights and heights and similar equipment, researchers repeated the experiment but dropped the weights anchored to the mid right point of a scissor lift (model SJIII3219, SkyJack Inc., Guelph, ON, Canada). Since the scissor lift neither tipped over nor suffered any structural failure, the researchers then applied the height and weight combinations generating the maximum 10,675-N arrest force for the five other anchor points—(1) mid left, (2) back right, (3) back left, (4) front right, and (5) front left. Once again, the scissor lift neither tipped over nor suffered any significant structural failure or deformation during any of these tests.

The researchers therefore repeated the experiment using the maximum 10,675-N arrest force but dropped weights anchored to the midpoints of the rails, which are the weakest points and thus the "worst-case anchorage points"—(1) right mid rail of the main platform, (2) left mid rail of the main platform, (3) right top rail of the main platform, (4) left top rail of the main platform, (5) right mid rail of the extension platform, (6) left mid rail of the extension platform, (7) right top rail of the extension platform, and (8) left top rail of the extension platform. Although all the anchor points on the respective rails deformed, the scissor lift did not tip over during any of these tests.

Next, the researchers repeated this experiment to evaluate the stability of the scissor lift where workers improperly stood on either the mid-rail or top rail of the scissor lift and fell from those heights. The researchers dropped a 128-kg weight from a height of 3.53 m while it was anchored to the (1) right mid rail of the main platform and (2) right top rail of the main platform, and dropped that same weight from a height of 3.10 m while it was anchored to the (3) right mid rail of the extension platform and (4) right top rail of the extension platform. Again, although all the anchor points on the respective rails deformed, the scissor lift did not tip over during any of these tests.

Finally, the researchers also tested whether the scissor lift would remain stable under three conditions when in its least stable orientation, at a tilt of 1.5° about the long axis of the lift. First, the researchers evaluated whether the tilted scissor lift met the Canadian Standards Association (CSA) B354.4-02 industry standard [7], which requires a scissor lift to remain stable when arresting the force from a 136-kg weight, falling 1.2 m while anchored to the least stable position (the front right point). Second, the researchers tested the tilted scissor lift's stability by applying 10,675-N arrest force to anchor points on its front right, mid span of the mid rail, and mid span of the top rail. Third, the researchers tested whether the tilted scissor lift would remain stable if a person weighing 128 kg and of 95th percentile nipple height (1.364 m) improperly stood on the mid rail of the lift and fell 3.53 m while anchored by an energy-absorbing lanyard to the mid span of the mid rail or 3.10 m from the mid span of the top rail of the tilted scissor lift. During these three tests, the tilted scissor lift neither tipped over nor experienced any significant structural failure or deformation [6].

16.1.1.4.2 *Drop Test Results from Alternative Anchor Points (Manikin Drop)*

Personal fall arrest systems work by attaching the worker with a lanyard to an anchor point on the scissor lift platform. Some scissor-lift work platforms contain lanyard anchor points on the floor of the platform, but using these floor anchor points may limit the worker's mobility since the worker may not be able to travel the length of the work platform without disconnecting the lanyard from either the floor anchor point or the worker's harness. Prior research suggests that the mid rail and top rail of a scissor lift work platform support forces associated with a person falling from within the platform and the lift is stable during such a fall and will not tip over [6]. The results here show that under certain (but not all) the test conditions here described, the use of unapproved scissor-lift anchor points may not result in a tip-over event.

In this study, NIOSH researchers investigated the performance of four personal arrest fall systems when those systems were attached to anchor points on the top rail of the work platform of a scissor lift. Specifically, the researchers used personal arrest fall systems from DBI/Sala (ISAFE™ Model 1102000 harness and 1240006 lanyard), Elk River (Construction Plus™ Model 48113 harness and lanyard), MSA (Workman™ Model 10072479 harness and Model 10072474 lanyard), SafeWaze (Safelight™ Model 10910 harness and Model 209512 lanyard), and Skyjack (model SJIII3219). The researchers attached each harness onto an Advanced Dynamic Anthromorphic Manikin (ADAM, Veridian, Dayton, OH), which was 1.88 m and weighed about 100 kg, and attached the respective harness and energy-absorbing lanyard to the top rail of the short axis of the scissor-lift work platform. The researchers dropped the manikin three times from two heights: 1.83 m (the standard drop height specified in ANSI/ASSE Z359.1-2007) and 3.35 m (to simulate a common misuse scenario in which operators stand on the mid rail of the scissor lift).

Preliminary analysis of the collected data showed that, during the standard 1.83-m drop height simulation, all four personal fall arrest systems kept the maximum arrest force (MAF) exerted on the manikin below 8700 N with 99% confidence and, therefore, met the ANSI and OSHA standards limiting MAFs to that amount. (See ANSI Z359.1-2007; OSHA § 1926.502(d)(16)(ii).) However, during the 3.35-m misuse simulation, only two of the four personal fall arrest systems met those ANSI and OSHA standards with 99% confidence [6].

Subject to further testing and validation, these preliminary results suggest that manufacturers may consider providing alternative anchor locations to permit better worker mobility through the work platform but that workers should be cautious when climbing the mid rail, since a fall from over 1.83 m could result in a MAF exceeding the ANSI and OSHA standards.

It should be noted that suspension trauma can occur while the worker is in a suspended position. Even though the MAF may not result in immediate health consequences, workers should not remain suspended for a sufficient period of time to engage trauma suspension; therefore, it may be necessary to work in pairs. Further information on this health hazard can be found in Turner et al. [8].

During the deceleration distance of a fall, the fall arrest system absorbs the kinetic impact energy, thereby reducing the impact force on the human body. The kinetic energy dissipated during the fall impact is an important parameter that characterizes the dynamic performance of the fall arrest system. The impact kinetic energy was either not considered or not correctly estimated in the literature. In the current study, a systematic approach was used to evaluate the energy dissipated in the energy-absorbing lanyard (EAL) and in the human body during the fall impact. The kinematics of the human body and the EAL during the impact were derived by using the data of the time histories of the arrest force, which was measured experimentally. The proposed method was used to analyze the experimental data of a 6-ft drop test and an 11-ft drop test. The preliminary results indicate that the distribution of the kinetic energy in the EAL and the falling body depends on the intensity of the impact: the portion of the kinetic

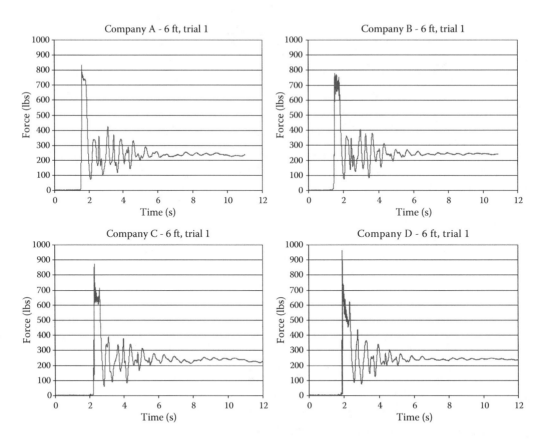

FIGURE 16.2
Arrest forces for four different lanyards/harnesses for 6-ft drops.

energy dissipated in the EAL for higher-impact force is more than that for lower-impact force. The following preliminary findings (Figures 16.2 through 16.7) are summarized as follows [9]:

1. Lanyard deployment forces among four manufacturers are all similar (~800 lbs) (Figures 16.2 and 16.3).

2. Maximum arrest forces vary but are all under 1800 lbs (6-ft and 11-ft drops) (Figures 16.2 and 16.3).

3. Deployment forces do not correlate to the drop distances (6-ft and 11-ft drops) (Figures 16.2 and 16.3).

4. Repeated test trials for the same harnesses/lanyards produce similar results (Figures 16.4 and 16.5).

5. Arrest forces calculated using the kinematic data agree well with those measured directly via a force sensor (Figure 16.6), and the accelerations calculated using the force data agree well with those measured directly (Figure 16.7). These analyses indicated that the kinematics of the falling surrogate can be determined using measured arrest force, and vice versa: the arrest force in the EAL can also be determined using the accelerations measured at the surrogate. Detailed calculations

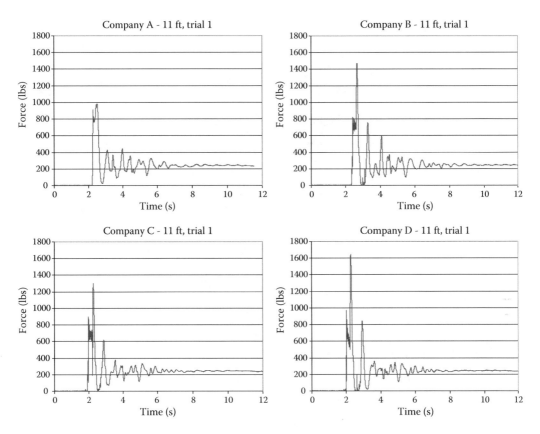

FIGURE 16.3
Arrest forces for four different lanyards/harnesses for 11-ft drops.

and equations (acceleration, velocity, and displacement) used for this component are listed in Wu's summarized manuscript [10].

16.1.1.4.3 Measuring Personal Fall Arrest System Performance By Dissipated Kinetic Energy

A personal fall arrest system reduces the impact force on the human body by absorbing kinetic energy resulting from a fall. Because the amount of absorbed kinetic energy is highly relevant to how well that safety system performs, NIOSH developed a systematic approach to evaluate the energy dissipated in the energy-absorbing lanyard and in the human body during a fall impact by deriving the kinematics of the human body and the EAL during impact from experimental arrest force data. The results confirm that arrest-force data can be used to predict the dynamics of a falling body. The results also show that increasing fall heights from 1.83 m to 3.35 m greatly increases the impact force on the human body even if a personal safety system is used [11].

The researchers first tested whether arrest-force data could be used to predict the dynamics of a falling body. In so doing, researchers equipped an Advanced Dynamic Anthromorphic Manikin (ADAM™, Veridian, Dayton, OH), which was 108 kg in weight and 1.88 m in height, with a harness and an EAL (Workman™ Model 10072479 harness and Model 10072474 lanyard, MSA the Safety Company, Cranberry Township, Pennsylvania). Using the harness and EAL, the researchers attached the manikin to a scissor lift (Model SJIII3219, SkyJack, Guelph, ON, Canada) at the scissor lift's maximum height of 5.79 m.

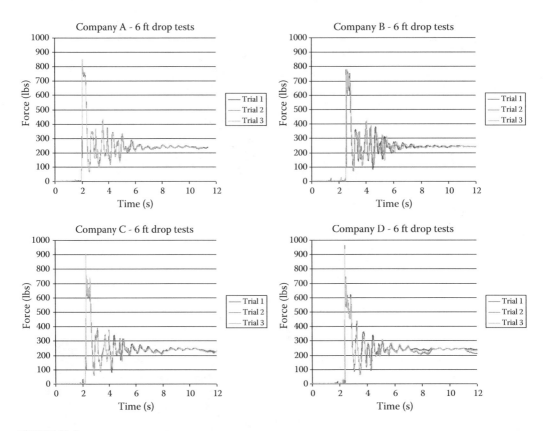

FIGURE 16.4
Arrest forces associated with three repeated trials for four different lanyards/harnesses for 6-ft drops.

The researchers then collected acceleration data from the manikin's three built-in uni-axial accelerometers (EAX series, Entran Devices Inc., Hampton, VA) located in the head, the middle of the spine, and the torso and arrest force data from a load cell (13.4 kN, S-type, Interface Inc., Scottsdale, AZ) connected inline to the lanyard. The researchers then dropped the manikin from heights of 1.83 m and 3.35 m, the latter being the drop distance that an operator standing on the mid rail of the scissor lift would fall.

The researchers found that the arrest force data collected from the load cell closely matched arrest forces calculated by using the acceleration data collected from the manikin's sensors. The researchers also used the arrest force data collected from the load cell to calculate the acceleration, speed, and displacement of the falling manikin. Those calculated values also closely agreed with the data collected directly from the manikin's sensors. Consequently, these results show that arrest force data can be used to predict the dynamics of a falling body.

Second, the data collected from the manikin and the load cell showed that increasing the drop height from 1.83 m to 3.35 m also increased the total impact energy by 42%, decreased the kinetic energy dissipated in the EAL from 92% to 84%, and increased the kinetic energy dissipated into the manikin by 193%. Consequently, increasing the drop height from 1.83 m to 3.35 m caused the amount of potential drop energy consumed in the manikin–harness–EAL system during a fall to decrease from 97% to 81%, causing the manikin to absorb much more energy. These results were confirmed by another drop test

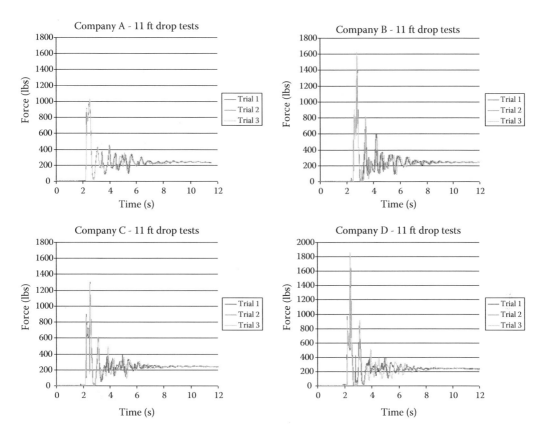

FIGURE 16.5
Arrest forces associated with three repeated trials for four different lanyards/harnesses for 11-ft drops.

using a rigid weight instead of the manikin. In other words, increasing fall heights greatly increases the impact force on the human body even if a personal safety system is used [11].

16.1.1.4.4 Drop Test Results Regarding Stability of Lift, Performance of Fall Arrest Systems, and Impact to the Head and Neck of a Scissor-Lift Operator (Manikin Drop)

This study evaluated lift the stability and performance of fall arrest harnesses and lanyards using manikin drop tests and a computer model. This study also predicted the dynamic loading to the head and neck of a scissor lift operator caused by fall arrest forces by using a dynamic simulation model including the scissor lift and the manikin. The results suggest that the particular personal fall arrest systems tested under the experimental conditions described below exert forces on the human body within acceptable limits defined by applicable industry standards [11].

To test the four personal arrest systems, researchers equipped the respective personal fall arrest system harnesses on an Advanced Dynamic Anthromorphic Manikin (ADAM™, Veridian, Dayton, OH), which had a height of 1.88 m and weight of 108 kg. The researchers attached each of the respective four energy-absorbing lanyards to the manikin's harness and anchored each EAL to the scissor-lift guardrail (top rail) of a model SJIII3219 scissor lift (Skyjack Inc., Guelph, ON, Canada). Each EAL was also connected to an interface load cell (Model SSM-S, Series 1000, Interface Inc., Scottsdale, AZ), which measured arrest forces. The researchers dropped the manikin three times from two heights: 1.83 m (the

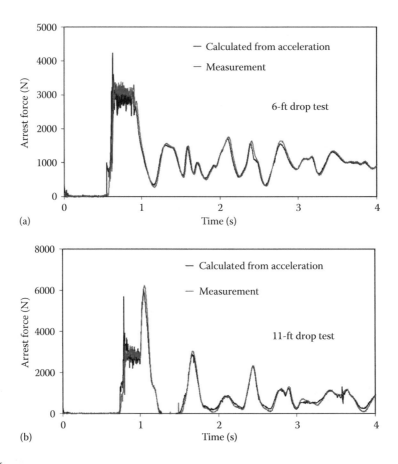

FIGURE 16.6
Calculated arrest forces and load cell measurement for 6-ft drop (a) and 11-ft drop (b).

standard drop height specified in ANSI/ASSE Z359.1-2007) and 3.35 m (to simulate a common misuse scenario in which operators stand on the mid rail of the scissor lift).

The researchers developed a scissor-lift simulation model using multibody dynamics software (ADAMS™, Version 2010, MSC Software Corporation, Santa Ana, California), which was refined and verified using experimental data obtained from dynamics tests. The simulated operator information was incorporated into a completed and validated scissor-lift model using the LifeMOD Biomechanics Human Modeler (Version 2010, LifeModeler, Inc., San Clemente, California), a plug-in to the ADAMS software. The researchers evaluated the stability of the simulated scissor lift in the fall arrest by applying the collected drop data from one of the widely used personal fall arrest systems to the simulation and predicting how much the rear wheel of the lift was vertically displaced and horizontally tilted about the short axis. From the collected data for one such widely used personal fall arrest system, the researchers also modeled the impact of the force on the joint and segments of a human body by applying the measured arrest force based on a computer model of the human torso divided into 15 body segments: head, neck, torso, left and right forearm and upper arms, left and right hands, left and right upper and lower legs, and left and right feet.

The results from the drop tests showed that the maximum arrest force exerted by the four personal arrest systems was less than 8000 N for both the 1.83 m and 3.35 m drops

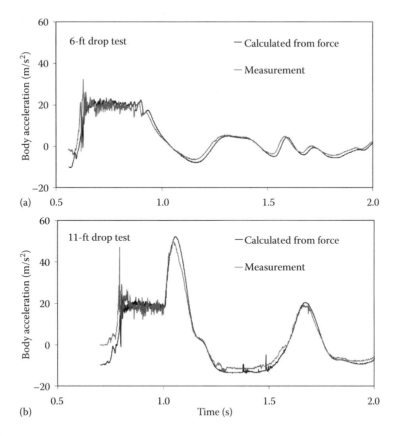

FIGURE 16.7
Calculated body accelerations and accelerometer measurements from ADAM for 6-ft drop (a) and 11-ft drop (b).

and therefore complied with the ANSI Z359.1 standard (2007), which requires all maximum arrest forces to be less than 8000 N for 1.83 m drops. Further, the data generated by the scissor-lift simulation model showed that the scissor lift was stable during the arrest of a fall under the test conditions of a scissor lift on a flat surface with one occupant in a static working position. Consistent with other NIOSH studies [4], the data also showed that reducing the stiffness of the scissor-lift structure decreases the stability of the scissor lift and may substantially increase the scissor lift's tip-over potential.

The data generated by the simulation of the arrest forces on a joint-and-segment model showed that, during the 3.35-m drop tests, the neck will be subject to a maximal compressive force of 360 N, a maximal shear force of 260 N, and a maximal joint flexion moment of 68 N-m, some of which are greater than forces imposed on the neck during vehicle-impact tests. The simulation of a 3.4-m drop also generates a neck injury criterion factor comparable to the figure observed in vehicle-impact tests and ambulance crash-test results [10,11]. Although some of these results are well below the injury threshold, the sudden arrest forces upon the neck and head could still potentially result in serious spinal cord injuries. Future studies that concentrate on soft tissue–injury outcomes might very well indicate dimensions of fall protection that could fruitfully be developed by focused research on this mechanism of injury and injury prevention. Research following the model of the Intervertebral Neck Injury Criterion [IV-NIC] might be considered [12,13]. Specifically, the contribution of improper adjustment of fall protection to injury mechanisms is undetermined, and research to quantify the role of this equipment adjustment factor is relevant and appropriate.

16.1.1.5 Future Scissor-Lift Studies

The draft ANSI standard A10.29 [14] provides that workers may enter and exit an aerial platform at heights greater than 1.8 m when the aerial platform surface is adjacent to the elevated surface. The draft standard further specifies that if the platform is adjacent to the elevated surface, no vertical gap will be larger than 20.3 cm or no horizontal gap will be larger than 35.6 cm between the aerial lift platform and the adjacent surface. But, to date, there has been no published scientific justification regarding the values of these gaps and how the distances between the lift platform and the adjacent surface may affect workers' postural stability and fall propensity.

NIOSH is presently testing whether interaction forces between workers and landing surfaces are different under various entrance or exit conditions and whether such differences affect workers' postural stability on an elevated lift [15]. To do this, NIOSH is investigating the postural instability and impact forces when a worker enters and exits elevated scissor lifts. First, this ongoing study examined the effects of vertical and horizontal gaps between the lift platform and the adjacent surface on workers' postural stability on two types of scissor lift entrance and exist systems. Second, this study examined the effect of an inclined landing surface on workers' postural stability.

The researchers used a 5.8-m electric scissor lift and its platform (Model SJIIIE 3219, Skyjack, Inc., Guelph, ON, Canada), which has a deck extension, a gate for entrance and exit, peripheral guardrails, and toe boards on all sides. This platform was about 162.6 cm wide and 73.7 cm long and had a deck that extended the platform's overall length to about 254 cm. The guardrails, which are composed of a top rail and a mid rail, were 99.1 cm in height, and the toe boards were about 15.2 cm high. The platform held a three-dimensional force plate (Kistler™, Amherst, New York) to measure the participants' baseline postural stability before exiting the scissor lift. The researchers also constructed a test platform with sides protected by guardrails, such that one end was adjacent to the scissor lift while the other open end was connected to a mezzanine. The test platform housed a three-dimensional force plate (Kistler™, Amherst, New York) to collect force data and was supported by a lift table (Bishamon Lift-2 K®, Bishamon Industries Corporation, ON, Canada) that could adjust the height of the test platform from 0 to 76.2 cm.

Since most aerial lift incidents occur when scissor lifts are elevated between 3 and 8.8 m, the researchers elevated the scissor lift to 3 m at all times. Force data was collected while 22 construction workers exited the scissor lift and entered the test platform, and alternatively, reversed the procedure so that they exited the test platform and stepped onto the scissor lift. Testing involved measurement of force exerted onto a force platform following the actions of researchers in removing a barrier, which depended upon the lift type (one with a gate, the other with a bar and a chain).

Measured force as an indicator of center of pressure and of postural instability was also a function of the test platform's vertical and horizontal landing distance. The vertical distance was chosen to represent five test conditions—the test platform was set at identical height as the scissor-lift platform (0 cm vertical displacement) and then adjusted to different vertical positions (10.2 cm lower, 20.3 cm lower, 30.5 cm lower, and 30.5 cm higher). Horizontal distance between the aerial lift test platform and the test structure (i.e., the construction building) was also a test variable, with the horizontal distance between the aerial lift and the test building set at 17.8 and 35.6 cm. All of these test conditions were chosen to represent various scenarios at a construction site. The researchers further collected data after adjusting the lift type (as before), the test platform's vertical landing distance (with the test platform at the same height, 20.3 cm lower or 20.3 cm higher than the scissor-lift platform), and the test platform's slope (0° and 26°). The researchers also traced the participants' shoe prints prior to the experiments and standardized them so that their heels were touching and feet were at a 30° angle.

Preliminary analysis of the collected impact force data suggests that positioning the scissor lift higher than the landing surface increases the vertical forces on the feet and the impact force to the ankles and knees. The preliminary results also suggest that workers experience more postural instability when they exit or enter from a sloped surface and that entering the scissor lift generally imposes more postural demands on the workers than exiting the scissor lift. The preliminary results also indicate that entrance or exit of scissor lifts with a bar/chain opening created greater postural instability in participants. The final results from this study will be used to suggest safer work practices to prevent injuries from scissor-lift falls [15].

16.1.2 Boom Lifts

16.1.2.1 Background and Injury Surveillance

Boom lifts are self-propelled, mobile work platforms, which, unlike scissor lifts, have platforms extending beyond the wheelbase of the supporting structure, which may be further extended with telescoping or articulating booms [1]. From 1992 to 2003, boom lifts accounted for nearly 60%–75% of fatalities arising from aerial lifts. The CFOI database shows that the plurality of these deaths occurred in the construction industry (45%), on a road (30%), or at an industrial location (15%) while "constructing and repairing" (42%) and "logging, trimming, and pruning" (26%).

16.1.2.2 Injury Surveillance

Tip-overs and collapse of the boom lifts (collectively, *boom tip-overs*) cause nearly half of the falls (46%). Falls from the basket, bucket, or platform of the boom lift caused about 27% of the remaining falls, and ejection from the boom lift caused about 28% of the remaining falls from 1992 to 2003. The NIOSH study [1] collected information from three different databases and identified several common factors associated with falls from boom lifts. First, the study found that mechanical failures, including failures of the lift structure, largely contributed to falls from boom lifts (33% of CFOI boom-lift events and 47% of OSHA/FACE investigations). The study also shows that collisions with vehicles and falling trees caused 14% of boom tip-overs and 13% of boom-lift ejections. Further, the study shows that failure to use a harness or belt and lanyard to tie off while performing tasks was reported in 18% of boom-lift fatalities. The OSHA/FACE databases also showed that surface conditions were cited in 35% of boom-lift cases, including the floor of a building, platform, ramp, sidewalk, or street (45%) or the ground or soil level (42%).

The fall height in 35% of boom-lift incidents recorded in CFOI and 42% recorded in OSHA/FACE ranged from 3 to 8.8 m. The OSHA/FACE database cited forward or backward boom-lift motion in 16% of fall incidents and elevating or lowering of the boom lift in 25% of all boom-lift falls. Moreover, the study found that 20 (22%) of OSHA/FACE fall reports cited worker motion (e.g., working postures) as a contributory factor to the fall.

Significantly, despite OSHA regulations mandating the use of fall protection in boom lifts (see § 1926.453[b][2][v]), the study shows that in 45% of boom-lift fatalities recorded in the OSHA/FACE reports, no such fall protection was used. Indeed, although fall protection was specifically mentioned in 55 (66%) of OSHA/FACE incident reports, fall protection was not in use during 82% of these incidents.

Boom-lift fatalities account for nearly 60%–75% of all aerial lift fatalities and warrant further investigation. Accordingly, these factors are potential avenues for future research.

16.2 Ongoing Aerial Lift Research and Practice Summary

A hazard recognition simulator has been developed by NIOSH using Unity simulation software (version 4.5.3, Unity Technologies, CA). This web-based simulation will allow users to perform simulated work procedures with a SkyJack 3219 scissor lift and SJ46 AJ boom lift (SkyJack, Inc., Guelph, ON, Canada). Task-based hazards will be generated using an actual model of an aerial lift as seen from the point of view of an operator or, alternatively, from a third-person point of view. Users will be able to load a web page from a remote location and use the simulator to remotely control the simulated aerial lift; frequently encountered hazards will be introduced into the simulation. Users will drive the lift to complete tasks such as (1) basic maneuvers driving the lift, (2) basic maneuvers including complications such as avoiding crushing and trapping areas, and (3) avoiding tip-over hazards (e.g., potholes). This simulator approach has potential applications to other models and types of aerial lifts. User manuals and practice tools for the computer simulation model are planned so as to generate a model user package for safety officers.

Acknowledgments

We would like to acknowledge the contributions of SkyJack Inc., which provided the NIOSH researchers with the use of a new scissor lift and other critical technical and design data. We would like to extend our appreciation for the contributions of the following companies: DBI/SALA, Elk River, Inc., MSA, and SafeWaze, who generously provided new harnesses/lanyards for use by the NIOSH aerial-lift researchers. We acknowledge the International Safety Equipment Association in providing constructive comments at various stages of this aerial-lift study. The authors also want to express their gratitude to Randall Wingfield and Gravitec Inc., who generously provided constructive comments on the drop-test component of the NIOSH aerial-lift study.

Disclaimer

The findings and conclusions presented herein are those of the authors and do not necessarily represent the views of NIOSH. Mention of any company names or products does not constitute the endorsement by NIOSH.

References

1. Pan, C.S., Hoskin, A., Lin, M., Castillo, D., McCann, M., Fern, K., and Keane, P. (2007) Aerial lift fall injuries: A surveillance and evaluation approach for targeting prevention activities, *Journal of Safety Research* 38: 617–625.

2. Pan, C.S., Chiou, S., Hsiao, H., and Keane, P. (2012) Ergonomic hazards and controls for elevating devices in construction, in Bhattacharya, A., and J. D., McGlothlin (Eds.), *Occupational Ergonomics: Theory and Applications*, Chapter 25, pp. 653–693.

3. American National Standards Institute. (2006). *Self-Propelled Elevating Aerial Work Platforms* (ANSI/ASSE A92.6). New York, NY: Author.

4. Ronaghi, M., Wu, J.Z., Pan, C.S., Harris, J., Welcome, D., Chiou, S., Boehler, B., and Dong, R. (2009) Modeling of the static stability of scissor lift and operators, *Professional Safety*, 43–48.

5. Dong, R., Pan, C.S., Welcome, D.E., Warren, C., Brumfield, A., Wu, J.Z., Xu, S. X., Lutz, T., and Boehler, B. (2012) An investigation on the dynamic characteristics of a scissor lift, *Open Journal of Safety Science and Technology* 2: 8–15.

6. Harris, J.R., Powers, J.R., Pan, C.S. (2010) Fall arrest characteristics of a scissor lift, *Journal of Safety Research* 41 (2010): 213–220.

7. Canadian Standards Association B354.4-02. (2002). Self-propelled, boom-supported, elevating work platforms. http://ohs.csa.ca/standards/construction/Elevated_Platforms/B354-4-02.asp

8. Turner, N., Wassell, J., Whisler, R., and Zwiener, J. (2008) Suspension tolerance in a full-body safety harness and a prototype harness accessory, *Journal of Occupational and Environmental Hygiene*, 5: 227–231.

9. Pan, C.S. (2009) Health impacts during the arrested falls, International Society of Safety Equipment Fall Meeting, Arlington, VA, 9–11 November 2009.

10. Wu, J., Powers, J., Harris, J., and Pan, C.S. (2011) Estimation of the kinetic energy dissipation in fall-arrest system and human body during fall impact, *Ergonomics* 54(4): 367–379.

11. Pan, C.S., Powers, J., Hartsell, J.J., Harris, J., Wimer, B., Dong, R., and Wu, J.Z. (2012) Assessment of fall arrest systems for scissor lift operators: Computer modeling and manikin drop testing, *Human Factors*, 54(3): 358–372.

12. Panjabi, M.M., Ito, S., Ivancic, P.C., and Rubin, W. (2005) Evaluation of the intervertebral neck injury criterion using simulated rear impacts. *Journal of Biomechanics*, 38, 1694–1701.

13. Panjabi, M., Wang, J., and Delson, N. (1999) Neck injury criterion based on intervertebral motions and its evaluation using an instrumented neck dummy. In *Proceedings of the IRCOBI Conference* (pp. 179–190). Zurich, Switzerland: International Research Council on Biomechanics of Injury.

14. American National Standards Institute. *Safe Practices for the Use of Aerial Platforms in Construction* (ANSI/ASSE A10.29). New York, NY: Author.

17

Falls from Commercial Vehicles: Safety Research, Control, and Practice

K. Han Kim and Matthew P. Reed

CONTENTS

ABSTRACT   Falls are one of the leading causes of injuries to truck drivers, accounting for 20–25% of the work-related injuries in the trucking industry, with an average compensation cost of $36,000 per claim. The common incident types are truck drivers slipping or falling during ingress or egress of a truck cab or trailer. This chapter discusses the multifaceted risk factors and prevention approaches for fall injuries with a focus on truck-step and handhold designs. Common designs in commercial trucks are critiqued in relation to design standards and guidelines. Recent systematic studies have provided new details on truck driver behavior and the effects of vehicle design and driver factors. Although design factors are important, worker training for safe ingress–egress tactics remains as a crucial part of prevention efforts.

17.1 Fall Incidents in Commercial Trucking Industry

17.1.1 Prevalence of Fall Injuries

Driving a heavy truck is one of the most dangerous occupations in the United States. Among truck drivers, 328.4 cases of nonfatal injury and illness were reported per 10,000 full-time workers during the year 2013, a rate more than three times greater than that for all private sector workers (Bureau of Labor Statistics, 2014). General freight truck drivers, for example, show a work-related injury rate of 5.4 (95% confidence interval 5.22–5.56) per 100 FTEs (full-time equivalent). This rate is significantly higher than the average rate of 3.9 (3.85–3.97) for vehicle drivers in all other industries (Smith and Williams, 2014).

On average, falls from height or on the same level account for approximately 20–25% of all work-related injuries to truck drivers (Helmkamp and Lundstrom, 2000; Rauser et al., 2008). Motor vehicle–related incidents, such as crashes, have the highest cost per claim ($45,500), but these incidents account for only 7% of all occupational injuries for truck drivers, while falls from elevation and on the same level occur more than twice as often (17%). The average cost is somewhat smaller at $36,700 and $30,300, respectively (Rauser et al., 2008).

Among different types of vehicles and workers in the trucking industry, the largest proportion of fall incidents occurs among truck drivers. Specifically, 87% of ingress–egress incidents are associated with car haulers, tractors, trailers, and cab-over-engine trucks (Lin and Cohen 1997), while 9% are associated with forklifts and other vehicles. Across workers in different job classes, truck drivers have the largest number of fall incidents (90.8%) followed by repair/maintenance crews and material handlers (6.3%) (Galavan 2012). Consequently, this chapter will focus on truck-driver ingress and egress.

17.1.2 Characteristics of Fall Injuries

Falls from trucks more frequently occur while drivers are exiting from the truck cab or trailer (egress) than while entering (ingress). Lin and Cohen (1997) reported that egress injuries occur about three times more often than ingress injuries. Falls occur as a result of one or more triggering events, including slipping on a truck step or having footwear catch on the steps (Shibuya et al. 2008). Rain, snow, or other contaminants, including motor oil or debris, can also contribute to slipping events (Lin and Cohen 1997). Trucking workers attribute slip and fall injuries to "not using proper equipment or procedures (32%)," "climbing in/out and falling off load/truck (25%)" and "weather and slippery walking surface (15%)" (Spielholz et al., 2008).

Falls can result in a wide range of injuries, including strains and sprains, contusions, abrasions, and fractures of the back, knees, wrists, ankles, and shoulders (Lin and Cohen, 1997). The Ontario Workplace Safety and Insurance Board database in 1997 indicated that the most common types of injuries with falls from a truck include sprain/strains (43%), contusions (24%), and fractures (20%), followed by abrasions, ligament injuries, concussions, lacerations, and dislocations (Jones and Switzer-McIntyre, 2003). The upper extremities are more frequently injured (34%) than other body regions (lower extremities 29% or spine 24%; Jones and Switzer-McIntyre, 2003). Driver efforts to protect the head and torso upon slipping or falling, possibly by reaching out the arms and hands to absorb impact energy, may increase the likelihood of upper-extremity injuries (Robinovitch, 1999).

17.2 Risk Factors for Fall Injuries

17.2.1 Ground Reaction Force

As with falls from other types of elevation, the likelihood and severity of injuries are associated with the magnitude of impact a person's body and lower extremities receive from contact with the ground (Robinovitch, 1999). Ground reaction force (GRF), which measures the magnitude of impact, primarily varies with the height of elevation a person exits from and the individual's body weight (McNitt-Gray, 1991; Robinovitch, 1999). Falling or jumping from a truck cab results in a large GRF. Fathallah and Cotnam (2000) measured GRF ranging from 2 to 12 times body weight for 10 men employing various vehicle exit strategies, with the highest force observed when the participants jumped from the truck cab or trailer. Although the relationship between GRF and injury likelihood has not been established, a higher GRF is associated with higher tissue loading (Funk et al., 2002; Grimston et al., 1991). The risks can be amplified by exposure frequency (Lipps et al., 2013), implying increased risks for short-haul, waste-collection or city truck drivers who frequently exit the vehicle.

17.2.2 Ingress–Egress System Configurations

The ingress/egress system is composed of steps and handholds, along with the door openings. Handholds for drivers include the steering wheel. Inappropriately designed handholds and steps may increase the risk of falls.

17.2.2.1 Step Configurations

Steps differ widely in their geometry, construction, and mounting, and some types of steps perform better than others for slip and contamination resistance. For example, perforated aluminum (Figure 17.1a) is a common step material. Holes punched from the underside of the step promote drainage and leave a raised rim that increases slip resistance. Grating steps (Figure 17.1b) are often constructed with steel and provide the best drainage and resistance to accumulated contaminants. Figure 17.1c shows a chrome steel box step with an overlay of nonslip stair treatment (grit). This step design would be sensitive to the buildup of contaminants, such as mud, snow, and fuel, and provides little slip resistance on the edge. Similarly, diamond-plate or other nonperforated step surfaces may not provide sufficient slip resistance both for cab entry/exit and for accessing the hookup area behind the cab.

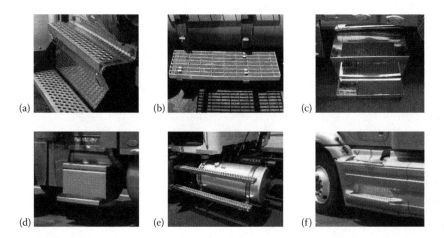

FIGURE 17.1
Truck steps in different construction and mounting types: (a) perforated step surface, (b) grating steps, (c) chrome steel box, (d) box type, (e) steps mounted on the fuel tank, (f) steps integrated into plastic fascia.

Step mounting also varies significantly among trucks. Box steps (Figure 17.1d) tend to have inferior surfaces lacking in perforations, gratings, or other contaminant-shedding characteristics. The edges of the steps are often smooth rather than sharp, potentially increasing the risk of slipping. A large number of trucks have steps mounted on the fuel tank (Figure 17.1e). Tank-mounted steps are usually made of perforated materials that provide better resistance to contamination than box steps. However, with their proximity to the fuel filter opening, these steps may be more likely than others to be contaminated with diesel fuel. Many modern trucks have steps that are integrated into the plastic fairing or fascia that extends rearward from the fender (Figure 17.1f). The fascia is both cosmetic and functional, improving the aerodynamics of the vehicle. Integrated steps are usually constructed of perforated metal, with a variety of edge treatments. The plastic surfaces fore and aft the steps have lower slip resistance than the steps, potentially creating a risk of slipping if a driver places a foot on the plastic rather than the step surface.

17.2.2.2 Handhold Configurations

Most trucks have at least one handhold placed behind or at the rear of the door opening. Most handholds are external (Figure 17.2a), mounted to the cab body, and extend vertically. Some external handholds are mounted on the shielding surrounding the exhaust stack. However, an increasing number of trucks are equipped with internal handholds (Figure 17.2b). Internal handholds can be at the rear of the door opening, replacing the external handhold; or at the front of the door opening, where they supplement the steering wheel and handholds on the door. Internal handholds have several advantages; in particular, they remain free of water and ice and may improve aerodynamics over external handholds. However, internal handholds are less accessible than exterior handholds during outward-facing egress. Most trucks have one or more handholds on the door (Figure 17.2c). A handhold directly below the window is common and is used both for ingress and to close the door once inside. These handholds are more difficult to use in outward-facing egress than lower handles. Additionally, manufacturers realize that the map pocket on the door may be used as a handhold (Figure 17.2d), even if it is not specifically designed for that purpose.

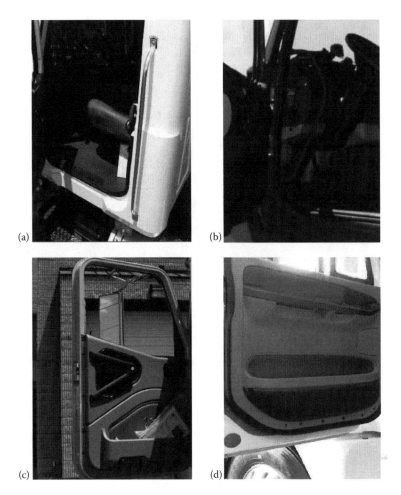

FIGURE 17.2
Handholds in different mounting positions: (a) external, (b) internal, (c) door-mounted, (d) map pocket that can be used as handhold.

17.2.3 Ingress–Egress Tactics

17.2.3.1 Inward- versus Outward-Facing Egress

While GRF primarily increases with the height of the cab and trailer, significant variations result from the tactics drivers use for ingress or egress. GRF can be reduced by as much as 80% with adequate use of steps and handholds compared to jumping straight from heights (Fathallah and Cotnam, 2000). Studies and field practice manuals generally recommend using a "three points of contact" technique, which utilizes handholds, steps, or ladders at all times during exit movements (Montante, 2008; van Dyne, 2002). *Three points of contact* means that two hands and one foot, or two feet and one hand, should be in contact with the truck at all times (Federal Motor Carrier Safety Administration, 2005). Further, even when truck drivers use steps and handholds, an egress tactic with the truck driver's body facing outward (Figure 17.3a) results in a 28% higher mean peak GRF compared to inward egress (Figure 17.3b) (Reed et al. 2011). Similar results were found for egress from a fire truck: when egressing from the crew cab (76 cm elevation from the ground) or rear

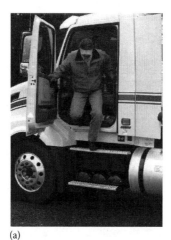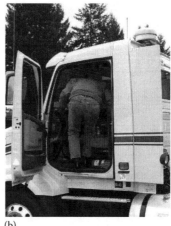

(a)   (b)

FIGURE 17.3
Egress tactics with the body facing outward (a) versus inward (b). (Washington State Department of Labor and Industries, 2011.)

running board (51 cm elevation), facing outward resulted in GRFs of more than three times body weight, while facing inward induced 1.6–1.8 times body weight. Outward-facing egress also increases lower back stresses: increased torque (96.6 Nm vs. 68.3 Nm) and compression forces (2,297 N vs. 1544 N) were estimated for the L5/S1 joint for the outward-facing egress (Patenaude et al. 2001).

17.2.3.2 Ingress–Egress Motion Kinematics and Dynamics

Even when a driver uses an inward-facing tactic while continuously maintaining three points of contact, the specific patterns of ingress–egress motions show significant variations depending on the specific configurations of handholds and steps. In a laboratory study, truck drivers entered and exited a reconfigurable truck cab mockup (Figure 17.4; (Reed et al. 2010b). The drivers' motions were recorded using a motion capture system. The contact location of the driver's hand and the force exerted on the handhold were measured for two different handhold-mounting positions (internal versus external) and eight different variations of step configurations (lateral positions).

Peak force on the handhold during ingress was 233 N (SD 67 N) on average, which corresponds to 25% (SD 7%) of body weight. Although hand forces were not significantly related to body weight, stature, or body mass index (BMI: ratio of body mass to squared stature), the mean external handhold force was significantly larger ($p < .05$) than internal handhold force for certain step configurations (step condition 1, 2, 7, and 8 in Figure 17.5a). Further, external handhold forces were larger than internal handhold forces when the lower step was displaced out farthest from the handhold (Figure 17.5b). These results indicate that the step configuration, particularly the lateral offset between the lower step and handhold, significantly affects hand force.

The patterns of handhold use are associated with foot movements. Using a mockup of a cab-over-engine truck, Chateauroux et al. (2011) measured egress motions for 22 different combinations of floor, step, and doorframe heights, door opening angle, and fore/aft positions of the step. The foot motions were classified into a "left foot first" (64% of trials) versus "right foot first" (33% of trials) strategy, depending on which foot first contacts the

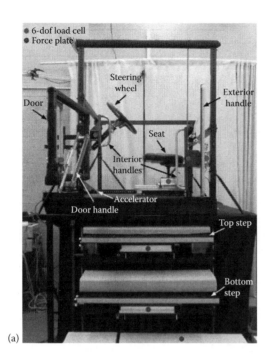
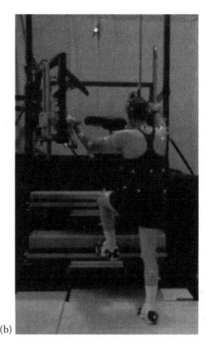

FIGURE 17.4
(a) Truck cab mockup with reconfigurable steps and handholds. (b) Driver performing ingress/egress while motions were recorded using a motion-capture system.

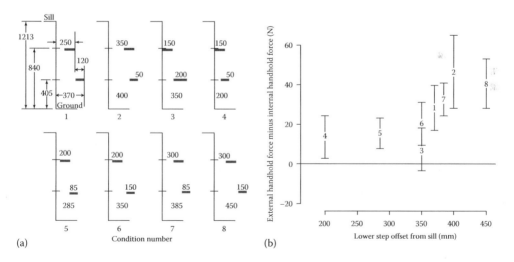

FIGURE 17.5
(a) Step configurations (mm units) from front view. (b) Handhold forces for different step configurations (external–internal handhold).

step just below the sill. Overall, drivers consistently chose one strategy, but in certain configurations, such as a cab without seats for increased clearance, the right-foot first strategy appeared more often than left-foot first.

Reed et al. (2010a) modeled foot trajectories of truck drivers' ingress motion using a Bezier parameterization. The effects of step configuration (lateral positions of the first and second step) and driver characteristics (stature and BMI) on foot movements were examined. Step configurations did not have a significant influence on the shape of the foot trajectory after accounting for the starting and ending locations. However, taller drivers tended to move their feet on a flatter trajectory, and drivers with a higher BMI show a steeper initial trajectory.

17.2.4 Anthropometric Characteristics of Truck Drivers

The National Institute for Occupational Safety and Health (NIOSH) systematically surveyed the body dimensions of the truck driver population in the United States (Guan et al., 2012). From the 1779 male and 171 female truck drivers sampled from 15 states, 33 anthropometric measurements were taken. The results demonstrated that the average body weight was 102.6 (SD 23.93) kg for male and 91.0 (SD 21.14) kg for female truck drivers. Compared to the general U.S. population statistics (McDowell et al. 2008), truck drivers are heavier by 13.5 kg for men and 15.4 kg for women ($p < .05$). However, the average stature for truck drivers was larger by only 1.2 cm for men ($p < .05$) and 0.3 cm shorter for women ($p > .05$). The corresponding BMI was 33.2 kg/m^2 for male and 34.4 kg/m^2 for female truck drivers, which exceeds the threshold level of obesity defined as 30 kg/m^2 by the World Health Organization (World Health Organization, 1995). Further, even when compared to the truck drivers measured 25–30 years ago (Sanders 1977; Sanders 1983), the mean body weight of male truck drivers is 12.0 kg larger and the mean male waist circumference is 6.2 cm larger.

The higher body weight and BMI for truck drivers may be due to their prolonged sedentary work patterns and the quality of nutrition available on the road (Whitfield et al. 2007). Increased body weight and BMI, and the associated lower levels of physical fitness, may contribute to the incidence and severity of fall injuries (Martin et al. 2009).

However, drivers with a higher BMI may compensate by choosing safer egress techniques. When the drivers were free to choose their egress tactics in laboratory truck cab mockup, those with a larger BMI ($\geq$30 kg/m^2) tended to use an inward-facing ("safer") tactic more often (73% of trials) than drivers having a smaller BMI (50% trials) (Reed et al. 2011).

17.2.5 Environmental Factors

Friction from the handholds, steps, and ground surfaces is an important factor in determining the likelihood of slip and fall incidents. Water, ice, debris, or lubricant contamination reduce friction from the contact surface (Gao and Abeysekera 2004). Among the slip and trip events that ultimately resulted in falls, 38.3% are associated with wet, icy, or snow-covered surfaces or oil spillage (Shibuya et al. 2010). In a survey of commercial truck drivers who had fall incidents during the previous 12 months, 68.8% identified ice, snow, mud, or rain as influencing factors (Shorti et al. 2014).

Slips occur when the friction available between the footwear and the ground surface (available coefficient of friction [ACOF]) is not sufficient for the task being performed. The required coefficient of friction (RCOF) is defined as the ratio of the horizontal to vertical components of GRF (Redfern et al., 1998; Chang et al., 2008; Hanson et al., 1999) . RCOF is generally reported for successfully completed trials without slippage, under the assumption that a person trying to perform the task in the same way would slip if the ACOF were less than the RCOF. When a driver jumps straight from a cab, the RCOF tends to be significantly larger (0.26–0.29) than if the driver exits slowly (0.13–0.22; Fathallah et al., 2000). The ACOF on dry tile is between 0.59 for footwear with a styrene-butadiene rubber sole and 0.89 with a nitrile-butadiene rubber sole (Perkins 1978). However, the ACOF can be as low as 0.180 on hard ice, 0.137 on lubricated steel, and 0.056 on melting ice (Gao et al. 2003). Drivers in fast or straight jumping egress are consequently at increased risks of slips and falls, particularly in inclement weather or in the case of contaminated surface conditions. Because drivers do not intend to fall, the risk results from an inconsistency between drivers' expectations of surface conditions and those that are actually present.

17.3 Practice and Control: Strategies to Reduce Fall Injuries

Although considerably more research is needed to improve our understanding of risk factors and mitigation strategies, the current state of knowledge is sufficient to offer recommendations to reduce fall injuries. The interventions suggested below are focused on avoiding situations believed to increase risk, although quantitative metrics are not available for many important variables. The recommendations are multifaceted and include system-wide approaches to address the range of factors affecting the risk of injury.

17.3.1 Improve Ingress–Egress System Design

17.3.1.1 Steps

17.3.1.1.1 Step Construction

Steps should be constructed to provide good slip resistance and to shed contaminants well. One glaring weakness in our current understanding is that we lack a suitable definition and measurement procedure for both slip resistance and shedding contaminants. Measurement procedures have been developed for footwear used for gait on relatively smooth surfaces (Chambers et al., 2014; Liu et al., 2013; Manning and Jones, 2001; Ziaei et al., 2013; Chang and Matz, 2001), but the nature of the interaction between footwear and steps used for ingress/egress is quite different. In particular, the standard definition for ACOF generally does not apply, because the maximum resistance to motion parallel to the step surface is generally not a linear function of the vertical force due to geometric interactions between the step features and those of the footwear. In what follows, we apply our knowledge gained from laboratory and field study of ingress/egress, but we recognize that we do not have data and methods that would allow us to rate slip resistance and contaminant shedding in a manner known to be associated with the risk of slip and fall.

Based on our understanding of system needs, grating-type steps provide both the highest slip resistance and best shed contaminants. If perforated metal steps are used, they should have large, well-located drain holes to minimize the buildup of water, snow, and ice.

The design of some truck steps appears to be influenced by the design of stair nosing. On stairs, trips due to sharp edges on the stair nose are a concern and thus round edges have been considered as alternative. Some drivers have expressed a similar concern: a sharp edge likely increases the risk of tripping for outward-facing egress. The driver's trailing foot may snag on the step, and a sharp step edge can also increase the severity of injury if a body part strikes the edge during a fall.

However, caution must be exercised in applying stair-design concepts to truck steps, because truck steps are used differently. For example, drivers facing inward on egress (the commonly recommended tactic) show substantially different foot motions compared to people walking forward down stairs. Even drivers who egress facing outward usually face sideways to the steps (either toward the rear of the truck or toward the open door) and move their feet differently from people walking down stairs. Hence, the risks and kinematic effects of tripping are different than on stairs.

Slips, including those of small magnitudes, occur commonly on ingress and egress motions and can act as triggering events for falls. As steps with smooth edges generally provide little slip resistance when the shoe sole is engaged only with the edge, an effort should be made to reduce the risk of slips rather than compromising slip resistance for reduced trip risk. Overall, our preferred design is a step having a relatively small (sharp) radius on the outer, upper edge rather than a rounded edge.

17.3.1.1.2 *Step Layout*

Step placement, as part of the ingress/egress system, may affect the tactics drivers choose. Conceptually, a ladder-like vertical arrangement of steps would be expected to induce a larger percentage of drivers to use an inward-facing egress tactic. Yet, such a step arrangement would not generally be considered safer because the consequences of a slip on either ingress or egress would be greater, and the overall difficulty of both ingress and egress would be much greater than with a more typical arrangement. Conversely, a stair-like arrangement with vertical step offsets similar to the horizontal offsets would probably not be desirable because it would be expected to increase the likelihood of drivers exiting facing outward and neglecting to use both hands for support. Overall, the ideal arrangement of the steps should encourage safer, inward-facing egress but also provide reasonable support for outward-facing egress.

17.3.1.1.2 *Step Visibility*

Drivers can have difficulty seeing the steps and the ground when they exit, particularly if they use the preferred inward-facing egress method. Consequently, visibility should be reasonably maintained over the steps. Contrasting colors on the edges of the steps can improve visibility, particularly for grating-type steps. Drivers should be trained to check the condition of the steps before exiting, and adequate lighting should be provided to detect accumulated snow, ice, or other contaminants at night. Lights should also be aimed at the ground adjacent to the steps so that drivers can inspect the area before exiting.

17.3.1.2 Handholds

Vehicle designers must assume that, in spite of training recommendations, many drivers will exit facing away from the truck. For drivers who use a rearward- and outward-facing tactic, the external handhold (Figure 17.2a) is the critical hand support. The handhold should extend upward approximately to the shoulder height of the seated driver. This may be difficult to achieve with an internal handhold (Figure 17.2b), which is one reason to prefer an external handhold. Further, internal handholds may not provide sufficient support for outward/rearward-facing egress compared to external handholds. External handholds must be mounted as close to the door opening as is practical, so that drivers do not have to move out of the cab before being able to grasp the handhold.

The friction provided by the handhold surface should be as high as possible. Many handholds are made from chromed metal rather than knurled metal or other surfaces with high friction. A high-friction surface will reduce the risk of a hand slip for both bare and gloved hands and maximize the benefits of the hand grasp in the event of a foot slip.

Door-mounted handholds (Figure 17.2c) vary much more than aft handholds. On some trucks, a map pocket may be used as a handhold (Figure 17.2d). At minimum, handholds are needed near the bottom of the door and near the top of the door trim, below the window. The handholds should extend fore–aft sufficiently that the driver can place both hands on each of them if necessary (similar to ladder rungs). These handhold locations could be integrated into a single Z-shaped handhold or otherwise built into the trim, but both the high and low handholds are needed.

17.3.1.3 Standards and Design Guidelines

Trucks in use vary widely in step and handhold configurations. Thus design standards and guidelines should provide specifications and regulations with which a baseline of safety requirements can be met for ingress and egress systems. In general, guidelines should specify requirements on materials, geometric configurations, accessibility, and construction quality. The following is a brief summary of existing standards and guidelines for ingress/egress system design. Table 17.1 summarizes the recommendations from the standards most widely used in the United States.

17.3.1.3.1 FMCSA Part 399, Subpart L

The Federal Motor Carrier Safety Administration (FMCSA) has promulgated 49 CFR (DOT), Part 399, Subpart L for cab-over-engine (COE) highway tractors (Federal Motor Carrier Safety Administration, 2005). The standard prescribes step, handhold, and deck requirements for commercial motor vehicles, with the intent of enhancing the safety of motor carrier employees. Although few COE trucks are currently produced or used in the United States, many heavy-truck manufacturers reference the FMCSA standard for all of their heavy-truck configurations. Section 399.205 defines handholds, fingertip grasps, and full grasps. Section 399.207 defines "three points of contact," step design to accommodate two feet, and slip resistance of steps. Section 399.207 also defines handhold dimensions, locations, and static loading requirements. Section 399.211 defines ingress/egress systems maintenance requirements.

17.3.1.3.2 TMC RP-404B

The Technology and Maintenance Council of the American Trucking Association has created the recommended practice RP-404B to enhance the safety of motor carrier employees by providing guidance regarding the use of access systems on heavy trucks and truck tractors and by developing design criteria to meet the performance objectives of the driver

TABLE 17.1

Summary of Geometry Recommendations from Representative Standards

| | Step Length | | Step Width | | Step Spacing | | | | Handle Height |
| | | | | | Step-Ground/ Step-Step | | Step to Sill | | — |
	min	rec	min	rec	max	rec	max	rec	—
FMCSA 399, Subpart L	—	254	—	127	—	609	—	609	—
TMC RP-404B	—	305	127	152	—	609	—	609	—
SAE J-185	320	400	130	200	700	400	400	300	900–1600
MILSTD 1472	300	460–530	150	200	380	300	—	380	—

(Rhoades and Miller, 1989; Technology and Maintenance Council, 1989). RP-404B defines "three points of contact," step and handhold design criteria, climbing methods, and future improvements.

17.3.1.3.3 SAE J185

The Society of Automotive Engineers (SAE) first published SAE J185 in 1970, and the latest revision was published in 2015 (SAE, 2015). The first landmark version in 1970 defined ingress and egress assist equipment for climbing irregular vertical surfaces to the operator's cab, such as those found on construction and industrial vehicles. Although J185 is not explicitly applicable to on-highway vehicles, many vehicle manufacturers reference its recommendations. SAE J185 also defines steps, handholds, "three points of contact," step height, step slip resistance, and handhold spacing. The latest revision (2015) recommends the coordination of steps and handholds to minimize foot slippage and to promote an "actively self-evident" climbing strategy without the need for special training. SAE J185 conforms in all significant details to ISO 2867-1980 (International Organization for Standardization, 1980).

17.3.1.3.4 MILSTD-1472

U.S. military standard 1472G includes dimensional specifications for steps and handholds on vehicles and other systems (U.S. Department of Defense, 2012). Because the military standard is publicly available, these recommendations are also widely referenced in U.S. truck design.

17.3.2 System Assessment

The steps and handholds, together with the steering wheel, seat, cab openings, and other features of the truck, function to form an ingress/egress system. No single component of the system functions independently, and consequently the performance of the system must be assessed as a whole. This section presents ideas for system-level assessment.

17.3.2.1 Virtual Assessments

Virtual assessment tools using digital human-figure models have become increasingly valuable for the design of ingress and egress system design. With advanced digital human-modeling tools, engineers can evaluate the motion kinematics and dynamics of ingress and egress motions (Figure 17.6) and also identify potential hazards and risk factors from proposed system designs. Further, such evaluation processes can be performed iteratively over a number of design variations and anthropometric characteristics of the driver population.

Although further work still needs to be done in this area, figure models can currently be used to assess handhold reach for each of the likely ingress and egress tactics in military (Reed, 2009; Baker et al., 2013) and civilian truck designs (Reed and Huang, 2008; Ait El Menceur et al., 2015; Monnier et al., 2009; Wang et al., 2013). The primary objective is to verify clearance for vision and reach to handholds for both hands at all times for all common tactics.

17.3.2.2 Driver Assessments

Testing with physical mockups with experienced drivers can provide useful input to system design. However, drivers may behave more conservatively when then know they are

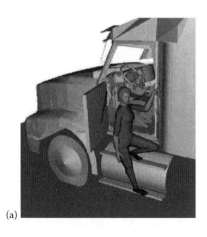 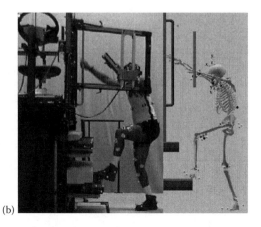

(a)   (b)

FIGURE 17.6
Simulation assessments of ingress–egress risk factors using digital human modeling software Siemens Jack (a) and AnyBody (b).

being observed. For example, they may be less likely to demonstrate outward-facing tactics than in the actual job context. Second, drivers' preferences for system layout may be contrary to the overall design objectives. For example, drivers may prefer layouts that are more "stair-like" (larger horizontal offsets), whereas a larger top-step-to-sill "landing" area is more desirable to promote the inward-facing egress tactic.

Given the large variability of truck drivers' body dimensions and demographic characteristics (Guan et al., 2012), a wide range of the driver population should be included for assessments. Drivers should also be encouraged to demonstrate various alternative tactics they may use on the job. Observations and testing should include a variety of environmental conditions, such as different lighting levels and inclement weather conditions.

17.3.3 Driver and Worker Training

In the following sections, we will discuss training for drivers and workers. Training is one of the most effective ways of intervention to reduce fall injuries. This section will address the specific messages training should include. Online training materials are available from a wide range of sources:

- www.cdc.gov/niosh/topics/falls
- www.KeepTruckingSafe.org/SlipsTripsFalls.html
- www.hse.gov.uk/FallsFromVehicles
- www.SafetyDriven.ca
- www.NapoFilm.net
- www.SafeWork.SA.gov.au

17.3.3.1 Three Points of Contact (3PC)

Studies and field practice manuals generally recommend using three points of contact (3PC) at all times during ingress and egress (Montante, 2008; van Dyne, 2002; Safe Work Australia, 2015). In addition to cab ingress and egress, 3PC is commonly recommended for other work tasks involving climbing or level transitions, such as climbing up/down the trailer or cargo for maintenance or load securement.

In surveys, drivers universally report having been trained to use three points of contact. Nonetheless, video and observational studies demonstrate that 3PC ingress or egress events are rare in the field (Reed 2008). Discussions with drivers indicate that they believe they are using 3PC even when they are not. Typically, they move both a hand and a foot at the same time; movements with two hands or two feet away from the truck simultaneously are rarer.

A driver using 3PC is more likely to catch a slip before a fall occurs. However, the most important benefit of 3PC is that it forces a driver to enter or exit slowly, reducing the momentum to be managed in the event of a slip or balance loss.

17.3.3.2 Use Two Hands (U2H)

The 3PC rule is often difficult to follow, even for those who show conservative egress patterns. We have observed a large number of drivers who enter or exit the vehicle with objects in one or both hands, which effectively preclude the use of those hands for support. Drivers demonstrate by their behavior that they find 3PC to be too slow.

While 3PC should be still stressed as general guideline, future safety messages can be directed toward a complementary and practical focus. Based on our research, we suggest an additional training guideline based on our field studies, namely "Use Two Hands" (U2H). Drivers will automatically use both feet when exiting but often use only one hand. U2H provides specific guidance that is easier for drivers to comply with than 3PC. Effectively, U2H tells drivers not to carry objects in their hands during ingress and egress, so the system must provide support for drivers who need to get log books, food, trash, and other objects into and out of the cab. This requires the provision of clean, dry locations in the cab that are accessible to the driver both when outside of the vehicle and while in the driver seat. Placing objects on the floor may not be practical in some occupational settings. Manufacturers should try to innovate in this area to reduce the risk drivers incur when they carry objects into and out of the cab.

17.3.3.3 Inward-Facing Egress

Drivers are more often able to use two handholds when facing inward, and they may be better able to use their hands to protect themselves if a foot slips. Further, inward-facing egress produces smaller GRF, which is associated with lower internal tissue forces (Reed et al., 2011). Thus, driver training should continue to emphasize inward-facing egress.

However, when descending facing inward, not being able to see the steps may create a perception of less control. Further, outward-facing egress helps drivers to look for certain hazards such as oncoming traffic, and this is particularly the case with drivers of emergency response vehicles (Giguère and Marchand, 2005) and military vehicles (Reed, 2009). Drivers should be trained to look carefully for hazards before exiting. Many injuries appear to be caused by slips due to unexpected ground surface conditions, such as ice, wet grass, or gravel.

17.3.4 Footwear

Driver footwear is critical for ingress/egress safety. Drivers should be instructed on the appropriate types of footwear. Some types of footwear, including cowboy boots or flip-flops, do not provide a sufficient interface with steps. The following recommendations are made for selections of footwear:

- Footwear should be fully enclosed (no open-toed sandals, for example) and well coupled to the foot (laces or Velcro, not slip-on).

- The sole should incorporate significant tread that can engage with the slip-resistant surface features on the steps. Shoe soles should be also inspected for wear as with other types of personal protective equipment (Williams 2013).

- A pronounced heel pocket should be avoided if possible to reduce the risk of tripping in outward-facing egress.

17.3.5 Maintenance and Retrofit

Poorly maintained steps having bent (Figure 17.7a), worn (Figure 17.7b), or corroded surfaces (Figure 17.7c) reduce the effectiveness of the slip-resistant features. Two types of maintenance should be emphasized: long-term attention to the overall functioning of the steps, particularly overt damage or wear; and immediate removal of any contaminants such as debris, ice, snow, mud, or oil. Using contaminant-resistant step designs will reduce the work required to maintain the steps. Similarly, truck lots, ramps, and loading docks should be maintained to remove pallet debris, oil contamination, snow, ice, and potholes on the surface.

Retrofitting can be also considered to provide additional handholds or steps that are not provided by original equipment manufacturer. For example, a flatbed operator may carry a detachable ladder on the truck and install the ladder for loading/unloading or cleaning the trailer, reducing the chances of the driver jumping from the trailer (Figure 17.8).

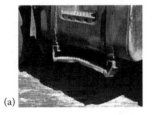
(a)
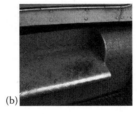
(b)
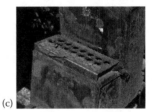
(c)

FIGURE 17.7
Steps showing bent (a), worn (b), or corroded surfaces (c). (Courtesy of Washington State Department of Labor and Industries.)

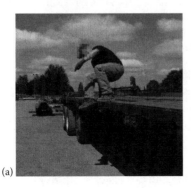
(a)
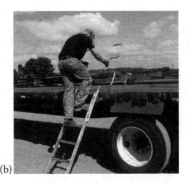
(b)

FIGURE 17.8
(a) A worker jumping straight from a flatbed trailer due to the lack of a proper egress point. (b) Egress using a detachable ladder. (Courtesy of Washington State Department of Labor and Industries.)

Retrofitting can also provide help to drivers having a small or large stature, heavy body weight, or certain injuries or disabilities.

17.4 Conclusion

Fall incidents in the trucking industry are a multifaceted problem. Among many other issues, ingress–egress system design, driver factors including anthropometry and physical fitness, behavior patterns, and environmental conditions are believed to influence the risk of falls and associated injuries. Other important issues not listed in this chapter, such as work organization, safety culture, laws and regulations, and drivers' physical fitness, will also affect behavior and injury risk. Given the complex nature of the problem, strategies to reduce the incidence of fall injuries should be explored in a system-wide and integrative approach spanning improved hardware design and maintenance as well as driver training.

Although considerable progress has been made in understanding ingress–egress behaviors and risks, some basic facts regarding injuries associated with ingress–egress systems are still unknown. For example, the risk of injury in egress is higher than in ingress, but we do not know when during the egress sequence the injury-producing event typically differs from an ordinary egress. We also have limited information about how ingress–egress system configurations affect risk. As discussed previously, step and handhold configurations, along with driver factors, affect the forces on the driver's body. But we do not know whether those increased forces correspond to a meaningful increase in either acute or chronic injury. Future research is expected to provide more insights into the listed problems and solutions.

References

Ait El Menceur, M O, P Pudlo, P Gorce, and F-X Lepoutre. 2015. A numerical tool to simulate the kinematics of the ingress movement in variably-dimensioned vehicles for elderly and/or persons with prosthesis. *International Journal of Industrial Ergonomics* 47 (May): 9–29.

Baker, E, S Budzik, and M P Reed. 2013. *Modeling Post-Accident Vehicle Egress*. Proceedings of the Ground Vehicle Systems Engineering and Technology Symposium. Troy, MI.

Bureau of Labor Statistics. 2014. *Nonfatal Occupational Injuries and Illnesses Requiring Days Away From Work, 2013*. U.S. Department of Labor, Washington DC.

Chambers, A J, A H Elizabeth, and R Cham. 2014. Shoe–floor frictional requirements during gait after experiencing an unexpected slip. *IIE Transactions on Occupational Ergonomics and Human Factors* 2 (1): 15–26.

Chang, W R., C C Chang, S Matz, and M F Lesch. 2008. A methodology to quantify the stochastic distribution of friction coefficient required for level walking. *Applied ergonomics* 39 (6): 766–771.

Chang, W R, and S Matz. 2001. The slip resistance of common footwear materials measured with two slipmeters. *Applied Ergonomics* 32 (6): 549–558.

Chateauroux, E, M Monnier, X Wang, and C Roybin. 2011. Strategy analysis of truck cabin egress motion. First International Symposium on Digital Human Modeling. Lyon, France.

Fathallah, F A, and J P Cotnam. 2000. Maximum forces sustained during various methods of exiting commercial tractors, trailers and trucks. *Applied Ergonomics* 31 (1): 25–33.

Fathallah, F A, R Grönqvist, and J P Cotnam. 2000. Estimated slip potential on icy surfaces during various methods of exiting commercial tractors, trailers, and trucks. *Safety Science* 36: 69–81.

Federal Motor Carrier Safety Administration. 2005. *Truck and Truck-Tractor Access Requirements.* Vol. 49 CFR §399.207.

Funk, J R, J R Crandall, L J Tourret, C B MacMahon, C R Bass, J T Patrie, N Khaewpong, and R H Eppinger. 2002. The axial injury tolerance of the human foot/ankle complex and the effect of Achilles tension. *Journal of Biomechanical Engineering* 124 (6): 750–757.

Galavan, E. 2012. Report on falls from non-moving vehicles. Trucking Safety Council of BC, Canada.

Gao, C, and J Abeysekera. 2004. A systems perspective of slip and fall accidents on icy and snowy surfaces. *Ergonomics* 47 (5): 573–598.

Gao, C, J Abeysekera, M Hirvonen, and C Aschan. 2003. The effect of footwear sole abrasion on the coefficient of friction on melting and hard ice. *International Journal of Industrial Ergonomics* 31 (5): 323–330.

Giguère, D, and D Marchand. 2005. Perceived safety and biomechanical stress to the lower limbs when stepping down from fire fighting vehicles. *Applied Ergonomics* 36 (1): 107–119.

Grimston, S K, J R Engsberg, R Kloiber, and D A Hanley. 1991. Bone mass, external loads, and stress fracture in female runners. *Applied Biomechanics* 7: 293–302.

Guan, J, H Hsiao, B Bradtmiller, T Kau, M P Reed, S K Jahns, J Loczi, L Hardee, and D Paul. 2012. U.S. truck driver anthropometric study and multivariate anthropometric models for cab designs. *Human Factors* 54 (5): 849–871.

Hanson, J P, M S Redfern, and M Mazumdar. 1999. Predicting slips and falls considering required and available friction. *Ergonomics* 42 (12): 1619–1633.

Helmkamp, J C, and W J Lundstrom. 2000. Work-related deaths in West Virginia from July 1996 through June 1999: Surveillance, investigation, and prevention. *Journal of Occupational and Environmental Medicine/American College of Occupational and Environmental Medicine* 42 (2): 156–162.

International Organization for Standardization. 1980. ISO 2867:1980: Earth-Moving Machinery— Access Systems. International Organization for Standardization, Geneva.

Jones, D, and S Switzer-McIntyre. 2003. Falls from trucks: A descriptive study based on a workers compensation database. *Work: A Journal of Prevention, Assessment and Rehabilitation* 20 (3): 179–184.

Lin, L-J, and H Cohen. 1997. Accidents in the trucking industry. *International Journal of Industrial Ergonomics* 20 (4): 287–300.

Lipps, D B, E M Wojtys, and J A Ashton-Miller. 2013. Anterior cruciate ligament fatigue failures in knees subjected to repeated simulated pivot landings. *American Journal of Sports Medicine* 41 (5): 1058–1066.

Liu, L-W, Y H Lee, C J Lin, K W Li, and C Y Chen. 2013. Shoe sole tread designs and outcomes of slipping and falling on slippery floor surfaces. *PloS One* 8 (7): e68989.

Manning, D P, and C Jones. 2001. The effect of roughness, floor polish, water, oil and ice on underfoot friction: Current safety footwear solings are less slip resistant than microcellular polyurethane. *Applied Ergonomics* 32 (2): 185–196.

Martin, B C, T S Church, R Bonnell, R Ben-Joseph, and T Borgstadt. 2009. The impact of overweight and obesity on the direct medical costs of truck drivers. *Journal of Occupational and Environmental Medicine/American College of Occupational and Environmental Medicine* 51 (2): 180–184.

McDowell, M A, C D Fryar, C L Ogden, and K M Flegal. 2008. Anthropometric reference data for children and adults: United States, 2003–2006. *National Health Statistics Reports*, no. 10 (October): 1–48.

McNitt-Gray, J L. 1991. Kinematics and impulse characteristics of drop landings from three heights. *Journal of Applied Biomechanics* 7 (2): 201–224.

Monnier, G, E Chateauroux, X Wang, and C Roybin. 2009. Inverse dynamic reconstruction of truck cabin ingress/egress motions. *SAE International Journal of Passenger Cars: Mechanical Systems* 2 (1): 1593–1599.

Montante, W M. 2008. Don't jump the potential effects of jumping from heights. *Professional Safety* 53: 32–35.

Patenaude, S, D Marchand, S Samperi, and M Bélanger. 2001. The effect of the descent technique and truck cabin layout on the landing impact forces. *Applied Ergonomics* 32 (6): 573–582.

Perkins, P J. 1978. Measurement of slip between the shoe and ground during walking. In *Walkway Surfaces: Measurement of Slip Resistance*, edited by Carl Anderson and John Senne, 71–87. Baltimore: ASTM International.

Rauser, E, M Foley, D Bonauto, S Edwards, P Spielholz, and B Silverstein. 2008. Preventing injuries in the trucking industry: Focus report 1997–2005. Technical Report 90-17-2008. Washington State Department of Labor and Industries.

Redfern, M S, J P Hanson, and M Mazumdar. 1998. Comparing required and available friction during walking to prevent falls. In *Advances in Occupational Ergonomics and Safety 2*, edited by Shrawan Kumar, 92–95. Amsterdam: IOS Press.

Reed, M P. 2008. *Truck Ingress/Egress Research at UMTRI*. Hopkinton, MA: LIberty Mutual Research Institute for Safety.

Reed, M P. 2009. *Simulating Crew Ingress and Egress for Ground Vehicles*. Proceedings of the Ground Vehicle Systems Engineering and Technology Symposium. Troy, MI.

Reed, M P, M E Sheila, and S G Hoffman. 2010a. Modeling foot trajectories for heavy truck ingress simulation. In *Advances in Applied Digital Human Modeling*, 19–27. Advances in Human Factors and Ergonomics Series. CRC Press.

Reed, M P, S G Hoffman, and S M Ebert-Hamilton. 2010b. Hand positions and forces during truck ingress. *Proceedings of the 2010 Human Factors and Ergonomics Society Annual Meeting*, San Francisco, CA.

Reed, M P, S G Hoffman, and S M Ebert-Hamilton. 2011. *The Influence of Heavy Truck Egress Tactics on Ground Reaction Force*. 2012-103. Morgantown, WV: National Institute for Occupational Safety and Health.

Reed, M P, and S Huang. 2008. Modeling vehicle ingress and egress using the human motion simulation framework. SAE Technical Paper 2008-01-1896. Warrendale, PA: SAE International.

Rhoades, T P, and J M Miller. 1989. Revisions of TMC recommended practice RP-404 "Truck and truck tractor access systems." SAE Technical Paper 892523. Warrendale, PA: SAE International.

Robinovitch, S N 1999. Fall-related occupational injuries. In *The Occupational Ergonomics Handbook*, edited by Waldemar Karwowski and William Steven Marras, 1139–1150. Boca Raton: CRC Press.

Safe Work Australia. 2015. *Managing the Risk of Falls at Workplaces Code of Practice*. Canberra ACT.

Sanders, M S. 1977. *A Nationwide Study of Truck and Bus Drivers*. Washington, DC: Department of Transportation, Federal Highway Administration, Bureau of Motor Carrier Safety.

Sanders, M S. 1983. *U.S. Truck Driver Anthropometric and Truck Work Space Data Study*. CRG/TR-83/002. Westlake Village, CA: Canyon Research Group.

Shibuya, H, B Cleal, and P Kines. 2010. Hazard scenarios of truck drivers' occupational accidents on and around trucks during loading and unloading. *Accident Analysis and Prevention* 42 (1): 19–29.

Shibuya, H, B Cleal, and K L Mikkelsen. 2008. Work injuries among drivers in the goods-transport branch in Denmark. *American Journal of Industrial Medicine* 51 (5): 364–371.

Shorti, R M, A S Merryweather, M S Thiese, J Kapellusch, A Garg, and K T Hegmann. 2014. Fall risk factors for commercial truck drivers. *Journal of Ergonomics* S3 (009). (9):1–9.

Smith, C K., and J Williams. 2014. Work related injuries in Washington state's trucking industry, by industry sector and occupation. *Accident; Analysis and Prevention* 65: 63–71.

Society of Automotive Engineers. 2015. J185: Access Systems for Off-Road Machines. Pennsylvanian, MI: Society of Automotive Engineers.

Spielholz, P, J Cullen, C Smith, N Howard, B Silverstein, and D Bonauto. 2008. Assessment of perceived injury risks and priorities among truck drivers and trucking companies in Washington state. *Journal of Safety Research* 39 (6): 569–576.

Technology and Maintenance Council. 1989. TMC Recommended Practice RP-404B: Truck and truck tractor access systems. Arlington, VA: The Maintenance Council.

U.S. Department of Defense. 2012. MIL-STD-1472G Department of Defense Design Criteria Standard Human Engineering. VA: United States Department of Defense.

Van Dyne, P. 2002. *Identifying and Controlling Worker Injuries in the For-Hire and Private Trucking Industries.* ASSE Professional Development Conference and Exposition, Nashville, TN.

Wang, N, K Kozak, J Wan, G Gomez-Levi, and G Strumolo. 2013. Enhancing vehicle ingress/egress ergonomics with digital human models. In *Proceedings of the FISITA 2012 World Automotive Congress,* edited by SAE-China and FISITA, 713–21. Lecture Notes in Electrical Engineering 195. Springer Berlin Heidelberg.

Washington State Dept of Labor and Industries, 2011. Don't fall for it. Publication No. 90-02a-2007. Olympia, WA.

Whitfield Jacobson, P J., A D Prawitz, and J M Lukaszuk. 2007. Long-haul truck drivers want healthful meal options at truck-stop restaurants. *Journal of the American Dietetic Association* 107 (12): 2125–2129.

Williams, J. 2013. Inspect your boots. 90-118-2013. Olympia, WA.: Washington State Department of Labor and Industries.

World Health Organization. 1995. Physical status: The use and interpretation of anthropometry. Report of a WHO Expert Committee. World Health Organization Technical Report Series 854: 1–452.

Ziaei, M, S H Nabavi, H R Mokhtarinia, and S F Tabatabai Ghomshe. 2013. The effect of shoe sole tread groove depth on the gait parameters during walking on dry and slippery surface. *The International Journal of Occupational and Environmental Medicine* 4 (1): 27–35.

Section IV

Practical Applications of Prevention and Protection Tools and Methods

18

Fall Rescue: Training and Practice

Loui McCurley

CONTENTS

ABSTRACT This chapter explores the concepts surrounding the rescue of persons after a fall from height in the workplace. Emphasis is placed on workplaces where employees are actively engaged in work at height using any manner of fall protection. It is the duty of the employer to prepare for such incidents and the duty of the employee to follow the employer's plan for both avoiding and reacting to falls from height. Solutions and resources are presented for consideration toward rescue planning, including established guidelines from existing standards and published materials. Recommendations for means and methods for personal escape, coworker-assisted rescue, and professional rescue are made using known incidents having successful outcomes.

KEY WORDS: *rescue, coworker-assisted rescue, personal escape, professional rescue, suspension intolerance.*

18.1 Introduction

While technologies and methods are advancing for work at elevation, the fact remains that any time an employee is working at height it is possible for a fall to occur. Decades of standards development, regulatory consequence, and legal ramifications have not stemmed the prevalence of such incidents. Year after year, falls continue to rank among the leading causes of mortality in the workplace (National Safety Council, 2014), along with accidents that involve employees being struck by or caught in between objects, and electrocuted.

18.1.1 Keys to Improved Safety

In traditional approaches to fall protection, regulatory language and standards have emphasized the definition and specification of fall-protection equipment and systems. The assumption, it seems, is that if equipment and systems are forced into compliance, accidents will not happen. As is evidenced by the continued prevalence of falls in the workplace, this approach has not had the desired outcome.

In a study published by Huang and Hinze (2003), 2955 Occupational Safety and Health Administration (OSHA)–investigated fall accidents from the construction industry were examined for cause. Huang and Hinze reported that across the span of their study, approximately 30% of falls were attributable to inadequate, inappropriate, or complete lack of personal protective equipment (PPE). Cross referencing their work with data from the U.S. Bureau of Labor Statistics (BLS), we find that during this time there were approximately 300 fatal falls per year, with 71% of those falls being falls from height. It is notable that this data spans a critical time period in 1996, when OSHA published significant revision to PPE regulations—yet neither the Huang/Heinz study nor the U.S. BLS statistics (U.S. Bureau of Labor Statistics, 2016) reflect any significant improvement in number of fatal falls from height, nor the reasoning behind the falls. In other words, the concept of improving mortality rates by forcing equipment and systems into compliance is not sufficient for fall fatality control.

Huang and Hinze (2003) went on to further examine these statistics in greater detail and also reported that the leading reasons for not using fall-protection equipment was that employers frequently cited fall protection as being "infeasible." This is to say that employers claimed that either the systems provided by existing standards and regulations were not adequate for the need, or the employer/employee did not have the knowledge and skills necessary to adapt the available resources to his or her needs.

In the prevailing approaches to fall protection to date, requirements for employee knowledge and skills training are largely left to the employer's discretion, with the idea that fall-protection training should be customized to the specific situation. The natural consequence of this approach is that there is little consistency and no standard verification of baseline knowledge in fall-protection training—and the result has been that accidents continue to happen.

Changing this pattern requires attention to improving worker's knowledge and skills specific to fall protection, as well as their preparation through the availability of proper equipment along with hands-on training. Fall rescue is in a similar situation and requires special training and practice.

18.1.2 When a Worker Falls

The following is an abstract about an incident in which an employee died from a fall from an elevated platform. "On January 24, 2012, Employee # 1 was working from an elevated area wearing a full face respirator and personal fall arrest harness with retractable lifeline. No one witness Employee # 1 fell. He was found suspended in his harness over the edge. Employee # 1 was rescued from the elevated work area by his coworkers. Employee # 1 was transported to Duality Hospital, where he later died. No other details were provided in the original abstract."

18.1.2.1 Risk Factors

Not every fall into fall arrest constitutes a crisis. The severity of the situation will depend largely on circumstances, including the reason the worker might have fallen, the force and nature of the fall, the manner in which the fall is stopped, possible impact with an obstruction or lower level, how the worker is suspended after the fall, and the ability of the worker to extract himself, or be extracted from, the resulting predicament.

If a worker has fallen as a result of a workplace accident, such as electrocution or trauma, or if they are suffering from a medical condition, potential rescuers should rule out the possibility of their being affected by the same or a resulting problem before responding. Sometimes it is unclear whether a fall might have precipitated, or been precipitated by, a medical condition. Either way, it is prudent to summon medical assistance as soon as possible after a fall has occurred.

Traditional fall-arrest methods might allow as much as 6 ft or greater free fall, but an arguably more important factor than free-fall distance is the impact force with which the fall was arrested. Also consider the nature of the fall and the orientation of the worker's body at the moment the fall was arrested. Even with modern fall-arrest equipment that limits impact force to 900 lbf, a worker may be injured if he strikes an object or swings into an obstruction during the fall. In addition, a whiplash effect might occur if the body is in a less-than-upright orientation when the fall-arrest system is deployed. The natural center of gravity being just behind the xiphoid process, it should be noted that a sternal attachment can reduce the rotational forces on the body during fall arrest and thereby minimize the whiplash effect (Lassia, 1991; Seddon, 2002).

Many commonly used fall-protection systems are designed to leave the worker hanging from a dorsal attachment after a fall. While it can be argued that being attached dorsally initially keeps equipment out of the way of the worker, this can make for a very difficult position from which to recover. It takes a well-trained, properly equipped worker, and one with a high level of physical fitness, to self-escape from dorsal harness suspension.

18.1.2.2 Suspension Intolerance

Any worker suspended after a fall is at further potential risk from a condition known as suspension intolerance. Also referred to as suspension trauma, this condition is precipitated by motionless suspension in a harness, such as might occur when a worker becomes unconscious or is immobilized from the effects of a fall. Research indicates that such a circumstance can result in unconsciousness, followed by death, in less than 30 min (Turner et al., 2008).

In a safety bulletin published in 2004 and subsequently updated in 2011, the U.S. Occupational Safety and Health Administration (OSHA) notes that risks associated with suspension in fall-arrest systems can be reduced by avoiding prolonged suspension, particularly motionless suspension, in a harness (Seddon, 2002). Employers should ensure that employees who work in fall protection are able to be rescued promptly after a fall so as to avoid prolonged suspension. Workers should also be trained to recognize signs and symptoms of orthostatic intolerance and to provide treatment as quickly as possible.

18.2 Planning for Rescue from Fall-Protection Systems

Any time a worker is exposed to a potential fall, the employer should consider what actions should be taken in the event of a fall and train employees accordingly. This is true regardless of what manner of fall protection is being used, whether passive or active.

Some employers believe they can rely on local emergency services agencies for rescue. However, this approach does not adequately address the natural proclivity toward spontaneous rescue attempts, nor does it necessarily adequately protect the fallen worker.

The ability of local emergency services to respond expeditiously to a workplace incident may be hampered by such things as delay in arrival, familiarity with site hazards, and being ill equipped to deal with a specific type of incident. Advance coordination with local municipal agencies will help to identify what capabilities they do (or do not) have, the minimum and maximum arrival window, and what role the employer should most appropriately expect them to have.

In some jurisdictions, regulatory requirements demand rescue provision (U.S. Department of Labor, 2016a), but a preplan achieves more than compliance. By helping to make the response to a fall disciplined and methodical, additional casualties can be prevented. Spontaneous rescue attempts by coworkers account for an alarming number of fatal injuries. Human nature will, more often than not, prompt a coworker to come to the aid of a fall victim, even if he is not specifically trained to do so. A written preplan can help to ensure that employees are consistently trained and equipped to react to an incident if it happens.

18.2.1 Example

Perhaps the most important point that an employer can emphasize in a preplan is that would-be rescuers must first protect themselves. This tendency is most noted in confined space incidents, where research indicates that up to 60% of all fatalities are would-be rescuers. One cannot help another if he becomes injured himself, so workers must be trained to establish safe working conditions for themselves before trying to help someone else. This might include consideration of environmental conditions, fall exposure, or other hazards.

The amount of time it takes for help to reach a fallen worker can contribute significantly to the survivability of a fall. National Fire Protection Association (NFPA) standards cite 6 min as the desired maximum response time for a municipal fire department to respond to any address within its jurisdiction (NFPA, 2016). However, a study performed by the *LA Times* newspaper (Linthicum et al., 2012) revealed that, even in a city with a large, well-staffed municipal department, fewer than 15% of responses actually met the standard. Of further concern is the fact that this response time is measured, at most, from the time that the responding unit is dispatched to the time it arrives at the address curb. It does not take into consideration the amount of time that may pass before someone is made aware that a fall has occurred, a coworker dials an emergency response number, and dispatch collects sufficient information to identify an appropriate resource. Nor does it take into consideration the time that will pass even after responders arrive at the address as they access the incident site, perform a hazard assessment, develop a plan of attack, and muster appropriate resources. Table 18.1 provides an estimate of elapsed time in a situation wherein all parts of the response are able to respond quickly and efficiently.

Even in the best of cases, it is unlikely that professional responders can be reasonably expected to reach a suspended worker in less than about an hour. This arguably does not achieve what should be the goal of the employer, which is to provide for prompt rescue of employees in the event of a fall. In fact, OSHA regulation mandates this (U.S. Department of Labor, 2016b) and further interpretations clarify that the word *prompt* requires that rescue be performed quickly—in time to prevent serious injury to the worker.

TABLE 18.1

Estimate of Elapsed Time of a Fall-Rescue Response

Best Case Target Expectations	Time to Accomplish	Total Elapsed Time (min)
Incident occurs	—	0
9-1-1 system activated	5	5
Dispatch collects info, initiates response	2	7
Vehicle begins moving	2	9
First vehicle arrives at curb	6	15
Scene is cleared, situation analyzed	3	18
Proper resources are mustered	5	23
Someone climbs to subject	10	33
Subject is packaged and evacuated	20	53

An essential part of any fall-protection and rescue preplan is a thorough and realistic determination of what capabilities local municipal agencies may or may not be able to provide, and how quickly they can assure a rescue.

In most cases, the prudent employer will elect to develop a preplan that involves capability at every level, starting with the ability of every worker to extricate himself from a suspended condition, progressing to at least some capability for coworker-assisted rescue, and eventually involving municipal resources at some level.

18.2.2 Rescue Plan

Adequate rescue training for an organization supporting workers in fall protection can be readily achieved with a simple combination of simple, prerigged rescue solutions, adequately trained personnel, and advance coordination with local municipal resources. Guidance is given in ANSI Z359.2 (American Society of Safety Engineers, 2007), which provides an excellent reference for inclusion of rescue preparation in a managed fall-protection program.

According to *Falls from Height: A Guide to Rescue Planning* (McCurley, 2013), the three levels of response to a fall incident are

1. Self-evacuation
2. Coworker-assisted rescue
3. Professional/municipal response

As soon as an incident occurs, all three levels should be activated. This allows each phase to be moving into position and preparing to act in the event that the preceding effort is unsuccessful. As soon as a fall occurs, the fallen worker should attempt to recover himself; this should prompt trained coworkers to begin to prepare their response, which should in turn prompt the notification of local emergency services.

The first responder to a fallen worker is that worker himself. With a limited amount of training and practice, and perhaps a couple of small bits of equipment, a worker should be capable of at least attaining a position of comfort within just a minute or two after a fall. In many cases, a properly trained worker will also be able to descend or ascend to safety. The goal should be for the worker to remove himself to safety within about 10 min.

In the event that self-evacuation is unsuccessful, workmates who are trained in coworker-assisted rescue should be prepared to assist. Unless specifically trained to do so, these responders should not enter the hazard but should use equipment and techniques that are prerigged specifically for that purpose, and they should do so from outside the hazard zone. The goal should be for coworkers to effect rescue within about 20 min.

If coworker-assisted rescue is unsuccessful within this amount of time, it is reasonable to expect that municipal responders should be beginning to arrive on scene and develop a plan. Equipment, techniques, and methods used for professional rescue differ from those for coworker-assisted rescue, so planning and training together in advance are imperative for smooth transition.

18.2.3 Training

According to a study performed at the University of Aberdeen (Fahmi, 2014), employees are likely to forget more than half their safety training in less than 1 year, regardless of experience or education level. Significant depreciation of safety knowledge begins to occur as little as two months after training and continues steadily if not reinforced. In Fahmi's estimation, consistent, repetitive behavior is key to the success of workplace safety programs.

Just as consistent, repetitive behavior is key to safety, consistent, repetitive training is key to consistent, repetitive behavior. An employer who establishes a well-crafted fall-protection program and then ensures that all employees consistently do things the same, safe way will experience fewer accidents as well as the increased productivity and efficiency that result from a safe, secure workforce. In order to succeed, workers must be working under a common set of guidelines and with a common baseline knowledge.

Fall-protection training should be organized so that it mimics as closely as possible actual work environment and practices. Employees should be given an opportunity to practice and apply learned knowledge and skills, and an evaluation should be performed to measure comprehension. Training can be said to have been effective only if workers understand the information well enough to use it on the job. This training and information should extend to what to do if a worker falls, and this is required even for employees who may not have a direct role in the response. Training should be such that their natural reaction to an emergency is to take the proper action as defined in the employer's emergency response plan.

18.3 Conclusion

Wherever employees are engaged in work at height, it is imperative that appropriate fall protection be provided. Further, wherever fall-protection equipment is being used, it is incumbent on the employer to plan and prepare for appropriate response in the event that a fall does occur.

It is the duty of the employer to prepare for such incidents and the duty of the employee to follow the employer's plan for both avoiding and reacting to falls from height. Various regulations, standards, and text resources are available to assist the employer in developing such a plan and should be utilized. Plans should include a means for personal escape of the fallen worker, coworker-assisted rescue by fellow workers, and professional rescue in the event that the other methods are not successful. Adequate training should be provided as well as practice on at least a quarterly basis.

References

American Society of Safety Engineers (2007). ANSI/ASSE Z359.2 Minimum Requirements for a Comprehensive Managed Fall Protection Program, Park Ridge, IL: American Society of Safety Engineers.

Fahmi, M. (2014). *The Importance of Regular Safety Training in Accident Prevention*, Scotland: University of Aberdeen (http://www.consist.com.my/v4/index.php?option = com_ content&view=article&id=89:the-importance-of-regular-safety-training-in-accident-prevention&catid=1:latest-news; accessed 13 March 2014)

Huang, X., and Hinze, J. (2003). Analysis of construction worker fall accidents. *Journal of Construction Engineering and Management*, 129:262–271.

Lassia, R. (1991). Voir la notice liée Essais de baudriers. Baudrier cuissard, baudrier complet attache dorsale et attache ventrale: Étude comparative des accelerations lors de la chute d'un mannequin.

Linthicum, K., Welsh, B., and Lopez, R. J. (2012). How fast is LAFD where you live? *Los Angeles Times*, 15 November 2012. http://www.latimes.com/local/lafddata/la-me-lafd-response-disparities-20121115-story.html.

McCurley, L. (2013). *Falls from Height: A Guide to Rescue Planning*, Hoboken, New Jersey: John Wiley & Sons.

National Safety Council (2014). *Injury Facts® 2014 Edition: A Complete Reference for Injury and Death Statistics*, Itasca, IL: National Safety Council.

NFPA (2016). NFPA 1710: Standard for the organization and deployment of fire suppression operations, emergency medical operations, and special operations to the public by career fire departments, National Fire Protection Association.

Seddon, Paul (2002). *Harness Suspension: Review and Evaluation of Existing Information*, Health and Safety Executive, UK.

Turner, N., Wassell, J., Zwiener, J., Weaver, D., and Whisler R. (2008). Suspension tolerance in a full body safety harness and a prototype harness accessory, *Journal of Occupational and Environmental Hygiene*, 5:227–231.

U.S. Bureau of Labor Statistics (2016). *Census of Fatal Occupational Injuries Summary, 1992–2013*, http://www.bls.gov/iif/oshcfoi1.htm.

U.S. Department of Labor (2016a). Personal Fall Arrest System, 29 CFR 1910.66 App C Sect I (e) (8) Subpart: F: Personal Fall Arrest Systems and 1926.502(d)(20) and Subpart: M—Fall Protection, https://www.osha.gov/pls/oshaweb/owadisp.show_document?p_table=STANDARDS&p_id=9730

U.S. Department of Labor (2016b). Fall protection systems criteria and practices: Construction Trade (29 CFR 1926.502 (d) (20)) General Industry (29CFR 1910.66 App C Sect I (e) (8)). https://www.osha.gov/pls/oshaweb/owadisp.show_document?p_table=STANDARDS&p_id=10758 Retrieved on 12 February 2016.

19

Slip and Fall Controls for Pedestrian and Community Safety*

Steven Di Pilla

CONTENTS

---

* Portions adapted from Di Pilla, S. (2009). *Slip, Trip, and Fall Prevention: A Practical Handbook*, 2nd ed. Hoboken, NJ: CRC Press.

ABSTRACT There are a wide range of influences on the potential of a given area to slips, trips, and falls involving the suitable design, inspection, maintenance, and management of walkway surfaces and their components. There are well established criteria for most dimensional design aspects, including sidewalks, curbing, curb cutouts, stairs, handrails, ramps, and parking-area elements including tire stops, speed bumps, and drainage. Likewise, there are tried and true best practices for controls such as lighting, signage, floor mats, and snow/ice removal. This chapter provides a concise discussion of each of these controls and their role in the cause and prevention of slips, trips, and falls.

KEY WORDS: *walkway surface, mobile device, walkway design, pedestrian behavior, floor, sidewalk, curb, ramp, handrail, stairs, steps, curb cutouts, parking, tire stops, speed bumps, changes in level, entryways, floor mats, lighting, signage, snow removal.*

19.1 Introduction

The National Safety Council (NSC) estimates that 25,000 slip and fall accidents occur daily in the United States and are estimated to cause almost 1 in 5 public sector injuries (NSC, 2007). However, falls are notoriously underreported because accidents are normally classified by injury type rather than injury cause in many statistics.

19.1.1 Expectation

When walkway surface conditions encountered are different from what is expected, the potential for an accident increases. For example, if we are aware of ice or water ahead, we can either attempt to avoid it or adjust our gait to compensate for the differing surface. We can slow down, take smaller steps, and walk flatter. Subtle adjustments like these are likely to allow us to safely cross a hazardous area. Thus, the most effective option for preventing falls is to either eliminate unexpected conditions that constitute slip and fall hazards or (which is less desirable) to assure that pedestrians receive clear notice of such conditions so they are adequately prepared to deal with them.

19.1.2 Trends

Few falls are due purely to carelessness. Rather, there are opportunities in the design and maintenance of walkways and their surroundings to reduce or eliminate the potential for many same-level falls. Among others, two trends are boosting the risk of the public to slips, trips, and falls: the susceptibility of the growing aging population and the expanding use of mobile devices.

19.1.2.1 Aging Population

The U.S. population is aging rapidly. Those 55 years and older, now at about 31%, are the fastest-growing segment of the population. By the year 2030, the number of people over 65 is expected to double (U.S. Bureau of the Census, 1996). The incidence of falls increases with age due in part to increasing fragility and decreasing visual acuity. Of older persons who fall, 20%–30% percent suffer serious injury. More than 60% of people who die from falls are aged 75 and over. Those who survive experience a greater functional decline in activities of daily living (ADLs) and physical and social activities and are at a higher risk of institutionalization than those at 65–74 years of age (Desai et al., 2001). Falls that do not result in serious injury may still have serious consequences for an older person. Fearing another fall can lead to reduced mobility and increased dependence through loss of confidence (Kalula et al., 2007).

19.1.2.2 Mobile Devices

In the United States, penetration of wireless devices is over 102% (number of active units divided by total population). Monthly wireless usage is almost 140 billion megabytes, and monthly text messages exceed 171 billion. This proliferation of mobile devices has significant implications due to the widespread distraction of pedestrians. A *Journal of Safety Research* study found that "eyes-busy" related accidents doubled over the prior year. Focused on their mobile devices, pedestrians fail to observe their surroundings (CTIA, 2009).

19.1.3 Walkway Design

There is substantial agreement on design dimensions for walkway surfaces and associated components. Most recognized are the model building codes and the life safety code. Effective safety begins with good design. When designing facilities and developing management programs, it is helpful to consider designing for the worst-case scenario. Pedestrians may be in any physical or mental condition. Once on site, management assumes at least some responsibility for the safety of the surroundings. Consider that someone under the influence of alcohol, drugs, prescription or over-the-counter medication, or illegal substances may be present. Consider that one or more people are distracted by pressing matters. Since these risk factors contribute to an increased risk of injury, it is prudent to take these variables into account when designing and implementing program components.

19.1.4 Inspect, Maintain, and Manage

A well-designed facility can still be subject to frequent fall accidents if it lacks sound management controls to maintain the facility as free from hazards as reasonably possible. The extent of management controls that are considered adequate depends on a variety of factors, including facility size, volume of foot traffic, and familiarity of building occupants with the facility.

Programs considered adequate for a small manufacturing facility would differ greatly from those suitable for a large hotel. The manufacturing facility likely has low foot traffic, mostly from employees familiar with the facility, while the hotel likely has very high foot traffic, mostly from visitors unfamiliar with their surroundings.

19.1.5 Distractions

It is important to recognize the impact that embedded distractions can have on pedestrians. Avoid extensive signage and eye-catching images and designs in areas where pedestrians need to be aware of where they are walking. Unfortunately, this advice may be at odds with other objectives, such as in retail establishments where great effort is expended to capture the attention of customers in order to sell products. In such cases, the immediate area surrounding placement of displays should be reasonably free of slip and trip hazards. Other areas of significant concern include stairs, escalators, at floor-surface transitions, changes in level (such as short flights of three steps or less), entryways where contaminants and moisture can accumulate, and congested areas.

19.1.6 Anticipating and Influencing Pedestrian Behavior

Areas of high foot traffic are especially vulnerable to falls because there is more congestion and exposure. These areas should be observed and traffic flows should be determined at various times of the day. Analyze losses according to time and day, relation to activities, and similar criteria to determine any correlations to fall incidents.

Consider putting controls in place to guide crowds safely through walkway areas. Use fencing for outside conditions and similar pedestrian guidance inside. Understand that barriers and visual cues, such as lighting and signage, may not be adequate to achieve the desired behavior. It is human nature to take the shortest and easiest path to a destination.

After identifying highest exposure periods, spend some time watching pedestrian movement and note evidence of heavy foot traffic such as worn pathways cutting across open areas where the sidewalk changes direction and wear on hard floor surfaces and carpeting.

It is generally most effective to adopt the path created by human behavior. For example, consider paving worn paths to make them safer. In the design and construction phase, arrange sidewalks and other pedestrian routes to use the most efficient route to reduce the potential for shortcuts into unintended and potentially hazardous areas. Optimally, determine where and how people tend to walk and then design routes based on that behavior. Once known, alternatives can be developed and again tested through observation (Figure 19.1).

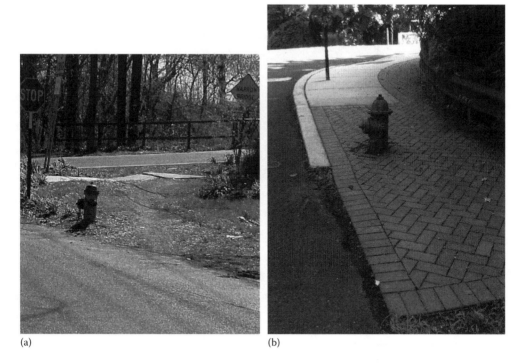

(a)   (b)

FIGURE 19.1
(a) Indications of pedestrian shortcut through unpaved area; (b) adoption of the path via paving.

19.2 Exterior Walkways

19.2.1 Level Surface Geometry

A seemingly insignificant but abrupt change in the walkway surface can readily result in a trip. A trip hazard is a change in elevation in a walkway that is not a proper ramp or stairway, with a vertical face ¼ in. (6.4 mm) or greater; or a change in elevation of more than ¼ in. (6.4 mm) with an inclined face steeper than two horizontal on one vertical (NFPA, 2012). Stride studies have shown that subjects in low-heeled shoes clear the ground by a mere ¼ in. (6.4 mm), and less by those in higher-heeled shoes (*Slip, Trip, and Fall Prevention: A Practical Handbook*, 2009).

19.2.2 Conventional Sidewalks

Conventional concrete sidewalks present a host of maintenance issues, most prominently the heaving and breakage of panels due to tree roots, weather, and temperature extremes. Patching is at best a temporary solution.

Identify surfaces with cracks, potholes, or other conditions that could contribute to a fall. Settlement of asphalt and concrete surfaces can often create these conditions, as can concrete spalling. Walkway surfaces should be free of debris and other slippery material (e.g., gravel, mud, sand, food spills) (Figure 19.2).

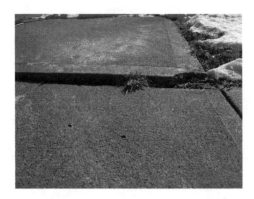

FIGURE 19.2
Unmarked sidewalk tripping hazard (unevenness exceeding ¼ in.). (Courtesy of Chris Janson.)

19.2.3 Rubber and Plastic Sidewalks

Rubber and plastic sidewalks can be an effective way to reduce the frequency and severity of trips, and they can mitigate injuries resulting from falls. Produced as modular panels, which in some cases are interlocking, the material is typically recycled plastic or recycled tire rubber with a polyurethane binder. These installations are durable, absorb shock, and are more resilient than concrete, and they appear otherwise indistinguishable from concrete panels. The life of reversible panels averages at least 14 years. Unlike concrete, rubber and plastic sidewalks resist cracking, indentation, chipping, breakage, or other damage in freezing temperatures, making them low-maintenance options.

Rubber and plastic sidewalks can be removed and replaced for tree root maintenance. Because these materials are lighter and more resilient than concrete, tree roots receive sufficient water and oxygen through paver seams. Note: Although slip resistance is reportedly high, the test method used was ASTM C1028, which is not a recognized method for wet or nonceramic surfaces (Table 19.1 and Figure 19.3).

TABLE 19.1

Comparison of Concrete, Rubber, and Plastic Sidewalks

	Concrete	Recycled Rubber	Recycled Plastic
Life cycle near tree roots; in freeze–thaw climates	2–5 Years	15+ Years	20+ Years
*Installed cost	$12–16/sf	$16/sf	<$13/sf
Labor	4 person crew	2 person crew	2 person crew
Install time	Minimum 2 days	500 sf/day	1200 sf/day
Size	Poured to form	2′×2.5′×1.875′	2′×2.5′×1.875′
Appearance change	Cracking, staining, cracks	Darkens over time	None
Mass changes	Lifting, breaking	Possible settling	Expected expansion/contraction

Source: Adapted from TERRECON.com.

* Installed costs include break out, demo, arborist services, consulting, contingency, management, and wait time (concrete).

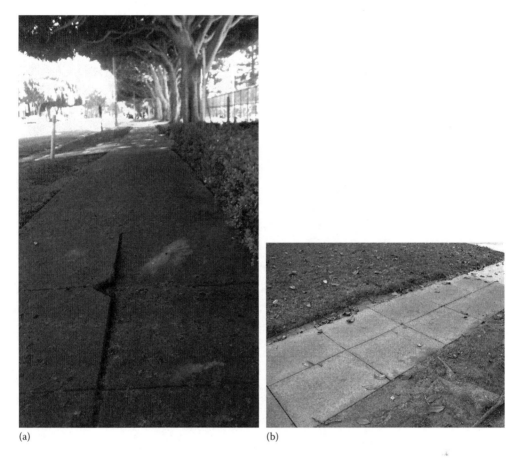

(a)   (b)

FIGURE 19.3
Side-by-side comparison of the original concrete sidewalk (a) and a recycled plastic replacement (b). (Courtesy of TERRECON, Inc. www.terrecon.com.)

19.2.4 Curbing

The standard height for curbs in the United States is 6 in. (15.24 cm) (English, 1996). Differing curb heights can result in an unexpected condition for pedestrians, increasing fall potential.

Curbing can be constructed in several ways. Less preferred is an extruded piece of concrete independent of the sidewalk. This method is susceptible to settling and can result in uneven surfaces between the curb and the sidewalk. Extruded curbing, sometimes identified by a concrete gutter extending into the roadway, and monolithic pour or doweling of adjoining slabs are preferred. These methods result in a unified curb and sidewalk, minimizing the potential for gaps and unevenness as well as heaving due to settlement or weather. Curved or rolled curb forms do not provide a distinct edge (offering unclear visual cues) and present a higher risk of footing instability.

There is no nationally recognized standard for curb marking. In terms of best practice, curbing leading to sidewalks and entrances should be painted a contrasting color to ensure this change is not unexpected by casual pedestrians (ASTM F1637, 2013). Unless painted yellow to denote "no parking" areas, good choices are white or red (Figure 19.4a,b).

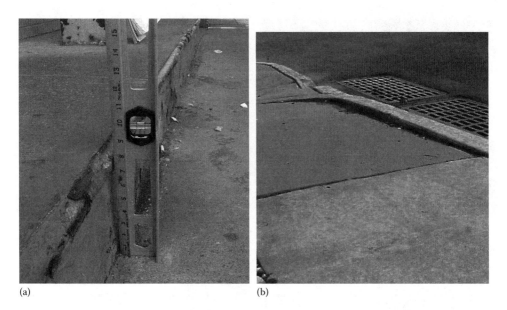

(a)   (b)

FIGURE 19.4
(a) Aside from the deteriorated condition of this curb, the height is excessive at 9 in. (Courtesy of K. Vidal.) (b) In addition to the cracking and unevenness, a major concern of this sidewalk is the extreme settlement. The curbing (a separate piece) remains as it was constructed, which presents a significant trip hazard. The presence of drainage grades in the path increases the risk of falls.

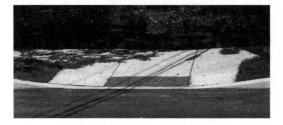

FIGURE 19.5
Properly sloped and marked curb cutout with good contrast with the asphalt street.

19.2.5 Curb Cutouts

Curb cutouts are intended to make exterior walkways accessible to persons with disabilities. However, if improperly designed, cutouts can become fall hazards to other pedestrians as well. Whenever possible, building approaches should be graded to preclude the need for cutouts by making the sidewalk and parking lot vertically seamless.

The American National Standards Institute (ANSI) A117.1 standard, "Accessible and Usable Buildings and Facilities," specifies that cutouts should not exceed a slope of 1:12 and that curb edging may not extend above the cutout slope. Instead, ramps should have flared sides (a maximum slope of 1:10). If edging is present, a landscaped area or other barrier should be provided to prevent crossing over the raised curb area (ANSI A117.1, 2009).

Painted cutouts should be coated with a slip-resistant paint, which usually entails adding grit to the mix to increase surface roughness. Although there are no marking requirements, expectation suggests there should be a visual prompt of a change in the walkway surface (Figure 19.5).

19.3 Water Accumulation

Facilities should be designed and maintained to minimize the accumulation of water in walkway areas and around buildings. Aside from the slip hazard posed by the water alone, cold weather often transforms liquid accumulations to ice, increasing the hazard. Among conditions that can contribute to water accumulation are:

- Land grading toward the building allowing water to travel toward and collect around the building
- Depressions, holes, and other concave areas due to settling or repaving
- Inadequate gutter or storm drain capacity, blocked drains, or clogged piping
- Drainage of gutters onto pedestrian paths

19.4 Parking Areas

19.4.1 Factors

Parking areas have design needs beyond those related to level surfaces mentioned previously. Notably, they are a challenge to maintain primarily because they are subject to concentrated heavy foot and vehicle traffic. Sealing parking lots reduces susceptibility to damage, reducing potential for falls. Weather, vehicle accidents, and snow plows can cause damage. Left unrepaired, these conditions become more severe, increasing injury potential for pedestrians. Assuring exterior lighting is maintained can also help reduce the risk of falls.

19.4.2 Drainage Grates

Optimally, parking-lot drainage grates should be situated away from natural and expected pedestrian paths. Grates often have excessively wide openings, as wide as 3 in. (76 mm). Some gratings are convex, making them even more hazardous to traverse. ASTM F-1637 and ADA Accessibility Guidelines for Buildings and Facilities specify openings be no wider than 1/2 in. (13 mm) in the predominant direction of travel (ASTM F1637, 2009, ADA, 1990). Grates are normally recessed to allow water from other areas to drain. Some are excessively graded, and settlement further increases the slope or creates depressions that cause pooling. Visually, grates tend to blend into parking lots. For pedestrian safety, consider marking grates a contrasting color to increase pedestrian awareness (Figure 19.6).

19.4.3 Tire Stops

Parking lots can be designed without tire stops. Tire stops are often damaged by vehicles and are a common tripping hazard. Where present, consider several precautions (ASTM F1637, 2013):

- Do not exceed a height of 6 1/2 in. (16.5 cm) with at least 3 ft (91 cm) between wheel stops.
- Tire stops should not protrude beyond tire width.

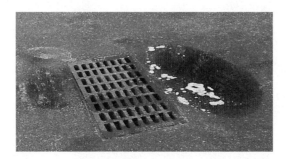

FIGURE 19.6
Note the large openings and uneven surface of this typical drainage grade design.

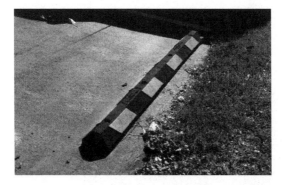

FIGURE 19.7
This tire stop is well-marked, strongly contrasting with its surroundings, and it is in good repair. Constructed of recycled rubber, it is also more durable and resilient than concrete. (Courtesy of K. Vidal.)

- Mark tire stops with a contrasting color to avoid blending with the parking lot.
- Avoid railroad tie construction as it deteriorates quickly.
- Reinforcing bar should not be above or extend beyond the tire stop (Figure 19.7).

19.4.4 Speed Bumps

Speed "bumps" found in parking lots differ from speed "humps" encountered on public roadways, which are wider and more gradual than speed bumps. According to ASTM F-1637 Practice for Safe Walking Surfaces, the use of speed bumps should be avoided, as the design and arrangement of the lot should make it impractical to drive at high speeds (ASTM F1637, 2013). Usually made of asphalt, speed bumps can be damaged by snowplows and other vehicles, and severe weather can accelerate their deterioration.

Because speed bumps pose a tripping hazard, they should be located out of natural and expected pedestrian paths, especially entrance and exit areas. Where speed bumps are present, they should be painted a contrasting color (ANSI Z-535.1 Safety Color Coding provides specifications). It is also advisable to provide signage indicating the presence of speed bumps. The Manual on Uniform Traffic Control Devices for Streets and Highways (MUTCD) provides marking and signage details but not design or dimensional criteria (FHA, 2001) (Figure 19.8).

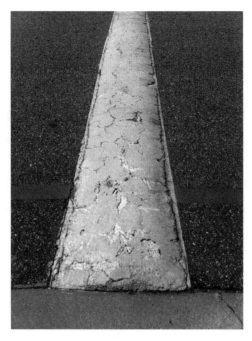

FIGURE 19.8
This speed bump is well marked, although it is in deteriorating condition.

19.5 Changes in Level

In general, building codes offer no requirements for short flights (e.g., three risers or fewer), but there is some agreement on designs to avoid an unexpected change in level from a doorway. The International Building Code specifies that the landing on both sides of a doorway should be as long as the doorway is wide, and at least 44 in. (112 cm) in the direction of travel (ICC, 2009). According to ADA Accessibility Guidelines for Buildings and Facilities (ADAAG, 4.5.2): "Changes in level up to 1/4 in. (6 mm) may be vertical and without edge treatment. Changes in level between 1/4 in. and 1/2 in. (6 mm and 13 mm) shall be beveled with a slope no greater than 1:2. Changes in level greater than 1/2 in. (13 mm) shall be accomplished by means of a ramp that complies with 4.7 or 4.8."

Where practical, convert short flights to a suitable ramp. If not, consider using contrasting colors, supplemental lighting, and signage to provide visual cues to make pedestrians aware of the change.

19.6 Stairways

19.6.1 Stair Design

Stairs should be uniform in tread width and riser height. The human body can detect subtle changes in elevation and distance. Thus, a change in riser height as small as 3/16 in.

(5 mm) can disrupt walking rhythm (Maynard and Brogmus, 2007). Stair design guidelines include (NFPA, 2012):

- The rise angle of stairways should be 30–35° of slope.
- Stair riser height should be 7 in. (18 cm) (new) or 8 in. (20 cm) (existing), with no deviation between adjacent risers exceeding 3/16 in. (5 mm) (the International Building Code permits 3/8 in. [9.5 mm]).
- Stair riser height should deviate no more than 3/8 in. (9.5 mm) over the entire flight.
- Stair tread depth should be 9 in. (23 cm) or 10 in. (25 cm) (existing), or 11 in. (28 cm) (new), with no deviation exceeding 3/16 in. (5 mm).
- Stair width should be at least 44 in. (112 cm) clear width, 36 in. (91 cm) if serving fewer than 50 occupants.
- Nosing should protrude no more than 1 1/2 in. (38 mm) and should be beveled. Having the entire tread of uniform slip resistance is optimal. When slip-resistant strips are used, they should extend to the edge of the nosing.

19.6.2 Stair Visibility

As people descend a stairway, the view of risers is impaired, which can make it difficult to accurately judge the vertical distance the foot must travel to the next step. Treads should be made more visible using contrasting nosings and adequate lighting. Illumination of at least 20 fc (200 lx) should be available in the stairway and the approaching floor, assuring that tread edges are properly illuminated, shadows do not impede the view, and glare does not disrupt visibility (Maynard and Brogmus, 2007).

19.7 Handrails

19.7.1 Geometry

Handrails provide visual cues, help pedestrians keep their balance, and provide support when using stairs. Properly designed and installed handrails can reduce the risk of falls and limit the severity if one falls. Per NFPA International 101 7.2.2.4, handrails should be accessible within 30 in. (76 cm) (for new buildings) and 44 in. (112 cm) (for existing buildings) of all portions of stair width (NFPA, 2012). This is to ensure that, even if standing as far away as possible from a handrail, a person should be able to grasp it. If a handrail is on only one side of the stairs, it is preferable to place it on the right side descending the stairs. Handrails should be between 34 in. (86 cm) and 38 in. (97 cm) in height, maximizing the ability of users to grab and exert the necessary force to stop a fall (NFPA 101, 2012) (Figure 19.9).

19.7.2 Graspability

Handrails are often seen primarily as aesthetic elements rather than essential safety features. Thus, handrails are often too wide or otherwise poorly designed to grasp.

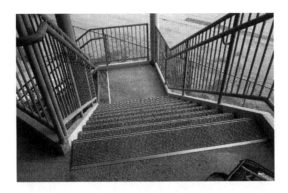

FIGURE 19.9
Example of a well designed and constructed set of stairs, including handrails. (Courtesy of Chris Janson.)

Handrails should allow continuous holding without being impeded by supports or other obstacles.

The optimal shape and size of the handrail is circular with a 32–50 mm (1.26–2.0 in) diameter or oval with a thickness 18–37 mm (0.71–1.46 in) horizontally 32–50 mm (1.26–2.0 in) vertically (NFPA, 2012). New handrails should be given a clearance of at least 2 1/4 in. (57 mm) to the wall. Handrails should extend at least 12 in. (30 cm) beyond the bottom of the stairway when descending so the user can maintain a hold on it until reaching the floor. They should also extend at least 12 in. (30 cm) beyond the top of the stairway to provide a visual cue to the presence of stairs and permit users to grasp the rail before beginning their descent (NFPA, 2012) (Figure 19.10).

19.8 Ramps

Because they are intended to provide access to facilities for persons with disabilities, there are rigid design requirements for ramps. Optimally, facilities should be designed with the fewest possible changes in level. By situating handicap parking spaces on opposite sides of an entrance from the primary pedestrian path, mobility-impaired individuals can often be accommodated while minimizing the exposure to other pedestrians.

Ramp slopes are calculated by rise (vertical distance) over run (horizontal distance). The slope should be no greater than one (vertical) × eight (horizontal), or 7.1°. Ramps for individuals with disabilities should have a slope no greater than 1 × 12 (4.8°), with slopes between 1:16 (3.6°) and 1:20 (2.9°) being optimal (NFPA, 2012).

In general, ramp width should be at least 36 in. (91 cm) with no projections extending into that space. NFPA 101 requires new ramps to be at least 44 in. (112 cm) clear width but allows some existing ramps to be as narrow as 30 in. (91 cm). Clear width and other ramp dimensions can also vary depending on occupancy (NFPA, 2012) (Table 19.2).

Unless there is an intermediate landing, the slope must be continuous and uniform. In addition, handrails are to be provided for ramps with a rise greater than 6 in. (15 cm).

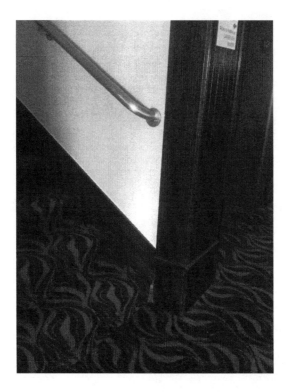

FIGURE 19.10
This handrail does not extended far enough to allow pedestrians to maintain a hold on it until reaching the floor.

TABLE 19.2

Ramp Slope Conversions

Slope Ratio	Degrees	Notes
1:8	7.1	Maximum pedestrian ramp slope
1:12	4.8	Maximum handicap, new construction
1:20	2.9	Walkway

19.9 Entryways

19.9.1 Importance

Building entryways are critical in controlling slips and falls for many reasons. There is a high concentration of foot traffic. There is often variation in the slip resistance of surfaces due to transitions between the outside, foyers, and lobby/interior areas. Congestion is greater. A high degree of surface wear occurs, making walkway surfaces smoother and less tractive. Finally, a greater concentration of water, dirt, and other contaminants from footwear develops in this often confined area.

To reduce the potential for falls in entry/exit areas, consider the impact of transitions between different types of floor surfaces, particularly transitions to extremes (e.g., from excessively low to very high traction or vice versa), which may present unexpected conditions.

19.9.2 Floor Mats

Ideally, a grate system with a catch basin should be used to remove moisture from footwear. If this is not possible, mats should be used. Proper mat selection and maintenance is crucial. If floor mats are not engineered for wear or properly cleaned, their ability to control contaminants is impaired. Over a 20-day period, 1000 people will deposit 24 lb (11 kg) of dirt. As much as 80% of dust, dirt, and other contaminants in buildings are tracked in from the outside (*Commercial Building Entrance Care*, 2007). One square yard of commercial carpet can accumulate 1 lb (453 g) of dirt a week and up to 2 lb a week in wet weather, and vacuuming removes only 10% of dirt from floor mats. Within the first six ft (1.8 m), 42% of a floor's finish will be removed after only 1500 people have entered (Tricozzi, 2009).

Properly cleaned floor mats can catch approximately 70% of the dust tracked into a facility. Floor mats protect high-traffic areas and carpets from wear and tear. Because they absorb water, mud, and internally generated soil, floor mats also minimize conditions that can contribute to slips and falls.

19.9.3 Floor Mat Design

Floor mats designed to remove dust, dirt, and moisture from footwear are distinct from other floor coverings such as carpet and rugs. Floor mat edges should be beveled for a smooth transition from floor to mat. Mats should be replaced when damaged and before they become excessively worn.

The Carpet and Rug Institute's (CRI) *Commercial Carpet Maintenance Manual* defines an entrance (or soil wipe-off) area as the 90 ft^2 (27 m^2) or 6 ft. (1.8 m) × 15 ft. (4.6 m) at building exterior entrances, where most tracked-in soil is deposited (CRI, 2014). Unfortunately, use of undersized mats is common. Entry mats should be understood as a system involving three distinct elements and totaling a length of at least 15 ft (*Commercial Building Entrance Care*, 2007). This approach allows most contaminants to be removed by abrasive mats, with absorptive mats removing much of the remaining moisture.

19.9.3.1 Scraper Mats

Scraper mats are designed for outdoor use but are also used in entryways. Their abrasive surface rakes the footwear bottom to remove gross contaminants. Because they are non-absorbing, moisture runs off and the debris settles to the bottom of the mat. The first 5 ft. (1.5 m) of scraping can remove as much as 40% of dirt from footwear.

19.9.3.2 Wiper/Scraper Mats

Wiper/scraper mats are designed to moderately dry and wipe the footwear bottom, scraping away remaining debris. The irregular pattern of the mat surface forces dirt particles into crevices, serving as an ongoing cleaning process. The 5 ft. (1.5 m) of a scraping/wiping mat can remove up to an additional 30% of dirt from footwear.

19.9.3.3 Wiper Mats

Wiper mats dry the footwear bottom. Because the heavy dirt and debris has been removed, wiper mats can make good contact with the footwear bottom (Figure 19.11).

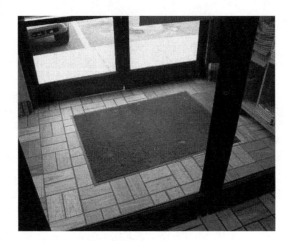

FIGURE 19.11
A typically undersized carpet mat in a foyer, providing no more than 3 ft of coverage.

19.9.4 In-Service Mats

Mats designed with cleats on the underside are intended to retard movement when used over carpet. When used on hard surfaces, cleats can compress, break, and create ripples. Avoid stacking mats in use. This tends to happen when a mat has become saturated instead of removing and replacing it. This increases the potential for tripping due to the higher and/or uneven edge and potential for rippling. Mats are more likely to slide when dust and dirt is permitted to accumulate under the mat. Smooth-backed mats are most susceptible.

19.10 Environmental and Operational Controls

19.10.1 Lighting

Poor lighting significantly increases the risk of falls. By age 40, visual acuity is reduced by 10% and is down 26% by age 60. Between the ages of 70 and 79, only 25% of people retain normal 20/20 vision; only 14% of those over age 80 have normal vision (Desai, et al., 2001). This loss is more pronounced under low-light conditions. The ability to perceive color and depth also decreases with age, negatively impacting the ability to identify nonstandard stairs and ramps. Avoiding glare becomes more important for older individuals because the aging eye is less able to detect contrasts and does not adjust as rapidly to changes in levels of lighting. Recognized standards for lighting are published by the Illuminating Engineering Society of North America (IESNA, 2011). Guidelines do not contemplate age but do recognize that requirements for older individuals are markedly different.

19.10.1.1 Lighting Levels and Transitions

Following are general IESNA guidelines on lighting levels, considered the "absolute minimum for safety alone." Substantially higher levels of lighting are needed for many reasons, such as work activities and security.

Interior lighting guidelines are relative to the level of activity:

- Two fc (22 lx) for areas where there is a low level of activity
- Five fc (54 lx) for areas where there is a high level of activity

In general, exterior areas of high pedestrian usage should be at least 0.9 fc (10 lx), and 0.2 fc (2 lx) should be provided in areas of less use. Enclosed garages should be provided with at least 5 fc (54 lx).

Transitioning between well-lit and low-light requires time for the eye to adjust, even for individuals with normal vision. Transitions between bright and dark areas should be as gradual as possible. Visual cues and barriers designed to slow pedestrian traffic flow can provide more time to adjust to new light levels.

19.10.2 Signage

Signage should be provided where appropriate. Criteria include changes in the type of floor surface, levels, trip hazards, and other conditions that pedestrians may not expect. Consideration should also be given to areas where pedestrians need special warnings. Subjects might include prohibiting the use of strollers and the wearing of high heels, reminders to use handrails, warning of icy conditions, and drawing attention to a step up or down.

Effective signage must be legible, understandable, visible, and in compliance with legal standards. Where there are populations that include non-English-speaking and illiterate individuals, pictorial or multilingual signage may be most effective.

Care should be taken to make signage prominent. Facility designers are often inclined to subtly integrate signage into an environment to maintain good aesthetics. Unfortunately, this defeats the purpose of signage, which is to draw attention.

19.10.3 Snow Removal

Planning and preparation for snow removal can be complicated by harsh conditions during and after each storm. Variables in moisture content, temperature, wind, depth of snow, and rate of snowfall influence the speed and effectiveness of removal efforts. For example, when there is ice buildup under the snow, it may be prudent to leave the snow on the ice until warmer weather arrives. If snow is wind-driven, removal is a judgment call.

Because pedestrians expect a broom-clean and dry pavement 24/7, the goal should be to achieve this condition as closely as possible. If parking areas and walkways cannot be cleared properly prior to the start of the day, the opening of the facility should be delayed to allow the removal to be completed.

19.10.3.1 Priorities for Removal

Recommended snow-removal priorities are as follows:

- First, assure fire lanes are available to emergency equipment and fire hydrants are free of snow and accessible.
- Next, clear main entrances, ADA ramps and curb cutouts, weather-exposed stairs, and primary sidewalks and parking before the facility opens.
- Finally, clear secondary parking lots, entrances, and other low-usage areas by noon.

Removal should begin when there is more than 1 in. of snow accumulation or sleet and iced-over conditions. Once snow stops falling and major walks and roadways are clear, concentrate on clearing snow in remaining areas and deicing as needed.

Maintain a hot list of problem areas to assure they are addressed. Close to provide warnings for areas that cannot be sufficiently cleared.

19.10.3.2 Anti-Icing, Deicing, and Sand

In many cases, ice-melt chemicals have displaced traditional salt and sand. Although some are effective and appropriate, others can create unexpected slipping hazards. Anhydrous chemicals are hydrophilic. Under certain conditions, as ice melts, these chemicals combine with water to create a slippery surface. Factors determining the effective life of an application include pavement temperature, application rate, precipitation, beginning concentration, and chemical type, so one application rate will not fit all storm events.

19.10.3.3 Before the Storm

Consider anti-icing as part of a prevention strategy for dealing with anticipated snow/ice accumulations. Applying chemical freezing-point-depressant materials prior to accumulation can retard the bonding of snow and ice to the pavement.

19.10.3.4 During the Storm

Deicing is a reactive measure applied to an accumulation of snow, ice, or frost already bonded to the pavement. Removing ice already bonded to the pavement can be difficult, and removing it mechanically can damage equipment and roads. Use winter sand and other abrasives when temperatures are too cold for deicing chemicals to be effective. However, sand only provides temporary traction, and only when it is on top. Consider abrasives in slow-moving traffic areas such as intersections and curves. Note that salt loses its effectiveness in extremely low temperatures.

19.10.3.5 After the Storm

After the event, evaluate what was done, its effectiveness, and what improvements can be made.

References

Americans with Disabilities Act (ADA) of 1990, Pub. L. No. 101-336, 104 Stat. 328 (1990), http://www.usdoj.gov/crt/ada/adahom1.htm.

ANSI A117.1 (2009), *Standard on Accessible and Useable Buildings and Facilities*, New York; American National Standards Institute (ANSI).

ASTM F1637 (2009), *Practice for Safe Walking Surfaces*, ASTM International.

ASTM F1637 (2013), *Practice for Safe Walking Surfaces*, ASTM International. West Conshohocken, PA.

Commercial Building Entrance Care (2007), Crown Mats and Matting and Mat Tech, http://www.mat-tech.ca/eng/products/entrance/index.html.

CRI (2014), *Commercial Carpet Maintenance Manual*, Dalton, GA: Carpet and Rug Institute (CRI), http://www.carpet-maint.com.

Desai, M., Pratt, L., Lentzner, H., and Robinson, K. (2001), *Trends in Vision and Hearing among Older Americans*, Centers for Disease Control, http://www.cdc.gov/nchs/data/ahcd/agingtrends/02vision.pdf. Washington, DC.

English, B. (1996), *Pedestrian Slip Resistance*, Alva, FL: William English.

IESNA (2011), *The IESNA Lighting Handbook Reference and Application*, New York: Illuminating Engineering Society of North America (IESNA).

NSC (2007), *Injury Facts*, Itasca, IL: National Safety Council (NSC).

ICC (2009), *International Building Code* (2009), International Code Council (ICC), http://publicecodes.cyberregs.com/icod/ibc/2009/icod_ibc_2009_10_sec001.htm. Washington, DC.

Kalula, S. Z., (2007), A WHO Global Report on Falls among Older Persons: Prevention of falls in older persons: Africa case study, World Health Organization, www.who.int/ageing/projects/AFRO.pdf.

FHA (2001), *Manual on Uniform Traffic Control Devices for Streets and Highways (MUTCD)*, U.S. Federal Highway Administration (FHA), http://mutcd.fhwa.dot.gov.

Maynard, W., and Brogmus, G. (2007), Reducing slips, trips and falls in stairways, *Occupational Hazards* 69(10), 81–86.

NFPA (2012), *NFPA 101, Life Safety Code*, Quincy, MA: NFPA International.

U.S. Bureau of the Census (1996), *Projections of the Population by Age and Sex: 1995 to 2050*, U.S. Bureau of the Census. Washington, DC.

Tricozzi, C. (2009), Getting mats down pat: Matting as part of a floor maintenance program, *ISSA Today*.

CTIA (2009), Wireless quick facts, CTIA-The Wireless Association, http://www.ctia.org/your-wireless-life/how-wireless-works/wireless-quick-facts.

20

Research Approaches to the Prevention and Protection of Patient Falls

Janice Morse, Andrew Merry, and Don Bloswick

CONTENTS

Since the 1970s, patient falls and, in particular, patient injuries from falls have been a concern to acute-care hospitals, rehabilitation centers, and long-term care institutions. It is estimated that annually "somewhere between 700,000 and 1,000,000 people in the United States fall in hospitals" (Ganz et al., 2013, p. 1). Approximately 5.1%* experienced a major injury; 137,255–196,078 patients per year received a major injury, such as a fracture or major head injury.

In the last five decades, the practice and research approaches to the problem of preventing patients from falling have changed dramatically. Falls were first considered a normal consequence of aging, a random event, or an unavoidable accident. But today, patient falls are considered both predictable and preventable. Despite various approaches to fall intervention and advances in technology, patient fall rates have not decreased significantly. Fall injuries have become the anathema of the health-care industry.

Here, in Sections 20.1 through 20.5, we describe and summarize the problem of patient falls. We examine the changes in fall interventions that have occurred over time and discuss the present approaches to fall intervention. In Sections 20.6 and 20.7, we discuss advances in biomedical and ergonomic approaches to fall intervention research and how they affect patient care. In particular, we present current biomechanical and ergonomic research to facilitate understanding patient ingress, egress, and in-bed movements as they contribute to fall potential, research approaches, and patient safety. We present slip/fall issues related to the design of bathrooms in Section 20.8 and a summary of the chapter in Section 20.9.

20.1 The Problem of Patient Falls

20.1.1 What Is a Patient Fall?

One of the difficulties in reporting and monitoring patient falls is that the commonly accepted definition of a *fall* is clinically inadequate: "the patient comes to rest unintentionally on the floor" (Morris and Isaacs, 1980). This definition causes confusion: Does it include a "saved" (intercepted) fall in which the patient is "caught" by a caregiver and lowered to the floor, and the risk of injury is reduced? Does it include falls when the patient does not "come to rest" on

---

* Rate reported by Schwendiman et al. (2008).

the floor, for instance, falls into a chair or other object? If the patient slides down a wall to the floor, is a slide a fall? Does "falling" include falls from the commode or wheelchair or chair or if a patient rolls out of bed, or must the person be in a standing position?

To complicate matters further, fall records often contain extraneous instances: falls by staff members and visitors and when a patient (or even an infant) is *dropped* by caregivers. A *drop* is not a fall.

The severity of a fall injury is dependent on (1) the distance of the free fall (i.e., impact velocity), (2) the trajectory of the fall (i.e., the part of the body landing on the floor), and (3) the deceleration distance (cushioning of the fall). If an institution has a "no fall" policy, there is an underlying belief that falling itself is dangerous and must not occur at any cost. The institution supports fall *prevention strategies*—strategies to prevent falls, the ultimate of which is the use of restraints or an enclosed bed. Patients are reminded constantly not to fall, so "fear of falling" (Butcher, 2013; Zijlstra et al., 2007) may impede rehabilitation.

On the other hand, institutions that are tolerant of falls (often rehabilitation units or nursing homes that prioritize mobility and independence) take precautions to prevent injury—fall protection strategies. They emphasize passive prevention strategies and are particular about the position of handrails, for instance, and use hip protectors, vigilance, walking aids, and assistance. These institutions focus on the injury rate rather than the fall rate as indicators of success. Of course the nature of the patient population also "drives" the type of interventions (preventive or protective), because facilities with cognitively impaired patient populations must primarily use fall preventive interventions.

This focus on prevention versus protection begs an important question: Should institutions be primarily concerned about fall rate or injury rate? Fall rates reported by institutions are erratic and imprecise, subject to reporting error and misreporting. Compounding the problem of an unclear definition of fall, nurses are reluctant to report *all* falls. When a patient for whom they are responsible falls, it is often considered the result of "poor care" and their personal responsibility, regardless of the cause of the fall. The reporting process is perceived as punitive, and this may be compounded if the incident is followed by legal action, which is carried out against the institution but may also implicate individual staff members.

Falls within health-care institutions are usually reported as the number of falls per 1000 patient bed days (Morse and Morse, 1988). Fall rates vary according to the patient population, the age of the institution (with increased rates in older hospitals), restraint use, the availability of fall prevention strategies, and the quality of nursing care. In fact, fall rates are used as an indicator of the quality of care as a nurse-sensitive patient outcome (Cho et al., 2003). Patient factors, such as patient acuity and mental status and treatments, also affect the fall rate. National databases have been established so that institutions can monitor their rates and compare their institution's rates nationally with institutions of a similar size and patient population (Gajewski et al., 2007). Conversely, injury rates provide a much more accurate indication of "what is going on." Nevertheless, an injury is a much less common occurrence, and because of its link to "quality of care" and legal action, injury reports are released reluctantly by the institution. However, the bottom line is that, whether institutions are prevention or protection oriented, the goal of fall intervention programs is to prevent patient injury.

20.1.2 Types of Patient Falls

There are three types of falls as classified by the cause of the falls*: anticipated physiological falls, unanticipated physiological falls, and accidental falls.

---

* We are excluding *developmental falls*, that is, toddlers falling in the process of learning to walk.

20.1.2.1 Anticipated Physiological Falls

Anticipated physiological falls are falls that occur in patients who have some type of impaired gait or cognitive impairment and/or a history of falling. These falls can be predicted by fall-risk triage scales, and they comprise 78%–82% of hospital falls (Morse, 2009). Anticipated physiological falls do not occur randomly but occur in fall-prone patient populations. The highest rates are among nursing-home residents, especially the frail elderly, with rates of approximately 3–13 falls per 1000 patient bed days (Oliver et al., 2007). Rehabilitation hospitals have falls rates ranging from 4 to 9/1000 patient bed days (Nyberg and Gustafson, 1997; Vassallo et al., 2004) and include some very high-risk groups, such as stroke patients (Macintosh et al., 2005). In acute-care hospitals, oncology patients are at high risk because of extreme weakness and fatigue, and medical centers have rates 3.6/1000 patient bed days (Donaldson et al., 2005).

20.1.2.2 Unanticipated Physiological Falls

Unanticipated physiological falls comprise 8% of all falls and occur in patients who otherwise have a normal fall score but experience an "event" (Morse, 2009). These patients may faint or have a drug reaction, a hypovolemic episode, a knee that "gives way," or a seizure. The first fall cannot be predicted and therefore cannot be prevented, but the patient should be protected from injury, lest the condition, and a second fall, occur.

20.1.2.3 Accidental Falls

Accidental falls occur in patients with normal gait and who have a normal fall score. The fall may be due to slipping or tripping (Morse et al., 1987; Morse, 2009), and prevention strategies are primarily enacted through ensuring a safe environment.

Does this mean that those who score at risk of falling do not fall accidentally? Those who score at risk of falling and have a shuffle, for instance, are more inclined to trip on a raised part of the floor; those with an impaired balance are more likely to slip, and those who are cognitively impaired are more likely to exit the bed without permission. They are an "accident about to happen." We expect these patients to fall and therefore put interventions in place to avoid conditions of an accidental fall. Importantly, we do not code these falls as accidents but as *unanticipated physiological falls*.

20.1.3 Consequences of Patient Falls

Injuries from falls are reported as minor, moderate, severe, or resulting in death (see List 20.1). Because these falls are from standing height or from the bed, the elderly, frail patient is more likely to be injured in a fall.

LIST 20.1

Classification of Injuries

Minor injuries (28% of falls) are bruises or abrasions, and there is usually no long-term consequence.

Moderate injuries (3%) consist of contusions, infiltrated IVs.

Serious injuries (0.01%–5.1%) are fractures, head injuries, burst wounds, or death. Death may result from a fractured skull or subdural hemorrhage or occur as a result of complications of a fractured hip and secondary to pneumonia, approximately 6 weeks after the fall (Donaldson et al., 2005).

As noted earlier, patient injury is generally the result of the trajectory of the fall, the height of the fall, the impact, the part of the body being impacted, and the deceleration distance. From standing height, patients may slip and fall backward, fracturing the occiput and/or causing a subdural hemorrhage; slip sideways and fracture a hip, or manage to "break" the fall with their hand and suffer a fractured wrist or arm; or impact their shoulder or chest, fracturing ribs, by falling against an obstacle. Falling forward, they may also fracture an arm or wrist or injure their face and fracture their nose. Abrasions are common, and frequently patients may dislodge and infiltrate an IV, dislodge drainage tubes or catheters, or rupture a surgical wound. Patients may hit their head on the furniture or other obstacles as they fall. They may fall by rolling out of bed, or by climbing over the side rails or the end of the bed and then falling onto the floor. Because a patient may incur several injuries in one incident, the most severe injury per fall is recorded.

20.1.3.1 Repeated Falls

Hospitals often consider a patient fall an independent event, yet repeated falls (patients who fall more than once) may quickly inflate the fall statistics. Of concern, 55% of patients who fall a second time were doing the same activity as in the first fall (Morse et al., 1985). Tracking patients who fall by activity and time of fall may assist in the identification of interventions and the prevention of falls.

20.1.4 Cost of Fall Injuries to the Health-Care System

Nationwide, the cost of moderate and serious injuries from falls has become so high that in 2008, Medicare stopped reimbursing hospitals for hospital-acquired conditions developed during the patient's stay, including injuries from hospital falls (Inouye et al., 2009). These nonreimbursable costs were estimated at between $4,000 (Inouyne et al., 2009) to $13,316 (Ganz et al., 2013) per fall. The injury costs of hospital falls are not covered by insurance; hospitals are responsible for the cost of care. Underlying this rationale is the value that patient falls are preventable and occur because of poor care practices.

Besides the financial cost, there is the cost to an individual of a fall injury, disability, and loss of independence. Even if a fall does not result in injury, psychological consequences, for example, the fear of falling (Zijlstra et al., 2007), often inhibits rehabilitation.

20.2 Historical Approaches to Fall Prevention

Over the past five decades, there have been shifts in patient acuity and length of stay, so that patients in the 2000s are much sicker than those in hospitals 20 years earlier. Along with this increasing acuity, the length of hospital stays has been reduced, so that patients are discharged earlier; the average length of stay (LOS) in acute-care institutions is now only 3.5 days. Recognizing the health risks of bed rest, patients are also mobilized more quickly and are often out of bed on the same day as surgery. Changes in rehabilitation include a reduced reliance on staff assistance and an increased emphasis on independence.

There have also been changes in the institution itself, with hospital design from the Nightingale wards (where all beds were in one large room, and patients could be easily surveyed by staff), to four-bed and two-bed wards, to a single room. This change resulted in increased patient privacy but made staff monitoring of the patients more difficult. Side rails, originally high and full length, became shorter, and they have been removed altogether from nursing-home beds. Hospitals introduced "sitters," that is, minimally trained staff, to observe patients. The removal of restraints resulted in the development of bed alarms, chair alarms, and alarms to alert staff if a patient climbed out of bed or door alarms if the patient wandered from the unit. Video surveillance is now being added to these technological advances for monitoring patients.

20.2.1 Changes in Fall Rates over Time

In the 1970s, hospitals began to track the number of falls and fall injuries, but the primary intervention made to prevent patient falls was the use of restraints; little else was available. Astonishingly, despite extraordinary efforts and fall prevention strategies that have become highly technical and have expanded over the decades, fall rates have remained relatively stable (or even increased) over the decades (see Table 20.1). This may be due to dramatic increases in patient acuity, with patients now being much sicker (and therefore weaker and more fall prone) than in previous decades. As mentioned, attitudes toward rehabilitation have changed, with the patients out of bed sooner (and therefore more fall prone); changes in fall reporting within the institution have also become more sensitive, and therefore fall rates are more accurate.

Patient fall rates and injury rates are used as a benchmark of the quality of care. The California Nursing Outcome Coalition (CalNOC) reported patient falls as a nurse-related quality indicator from 48,485 falls over 24 consecutive quarters (to March 2004); 74% occurred in medical–surgical units. (Gajewski et al., 2007).

Patient fall-injury rates often vary in different studies. In the CalNOC report, Gajewski et al. (2007) note that 32% sustained an injury (28% mild, 3.0% moderate, 1.0% major injury or death), and Schwendiman et al. (2006) report that 33.6% sustained an injury, 29.7% a minor injury, and 3.9% a major injury.

20.2.1.1 Hospital Beds and Falls

Adult hospital beds were originally built in one size, with a deck height of 36 in. Bed heights were designed primarily to accommodate medical examinations and nursing treatments, at a height so that nurses could lift patients without causing back strain or injury. However, this deck height was such that a step stool was sometimes required for patients to climb in and out of bed—thus resulting in a secondary hazard if patients subsequently slipped off the step stool. Further, a hazard existed should a patient roll out of bed from that height.

In 1948, Hill Rom developed the first variable height (*the Hi-lo*) adjustable bed.* Initially, the bed was hand-cranked (thereby increasing workload for nurses and in itself leading to back injuries); this system was subsequently replaced by a foot pedal. In 1952, the first variable-height electric motor bed was introduced, enabling the bed to be adjustable from a deck height of 17 in to 36 in. The low position was intended for patient ingress and egress, and the bed was adjusted to the high position for patient care and in-bed lifting. This low bed-deck height of 17 in remained the standard low height for all patients, regardless of patients' height or physical ability.

---

* From brochure: "The Hill-Rom Difference" (No author, ND).

TABLE 20.1

Fall Rates by Institution Type for Decades 1980 to Present

Years	Acute Care		Rehabilitation		Nursing Home	
	#/1000 pt bed days	Author (Year)	#/1000 pt bed days	Author (Year)	#/1000 pt bed days	Author (Year)
1980–1989	2.3	Morse et al., 1989a	46/143	Mion et al., 1989	4.27	Berry et al., 1981
	3.35	Morgan et al., 1985			5.7	Myers et al., 1989
	2.18	Raz and Baretich, 1987				
	3.8	Llewellyn et al., 1988				
1990–1999	4.1,4.7	Kilpack et al., 1991	178/1000 pts per year	Vlahov et al., 1990		
	3.8	Cohen and Guin, 1991				
2000–present	2.3–7.0	Lake and Cheung, 2006	12.46	Forrest et al., 2013	3.73	Lake and Cheung, 2006
	3.6	Menéndez et al., 2013			17.9	Healey et al., 2004
	6.12	Hitcho et al., 2004			11.7[d]	Schwendiman et al., 2006
	9.6	Barnett, 2002				
	10	von Rentein-Kruse et al., 2007				
	9.1[a]	Schwendiman et al., 2006				
	11.3[b]	Dykes et al., 2010				
	2.9[c]					
	3.15–4.18					

[a] Entire sample.
[b] Internal medicine.
[c] Surgery.
[d] Geriatrics.

By 2000s, the concern regarding patients who "fell" out of bed while sleeping or reaching for objects resulted in a demand for low-low beds with a 6–10 in. deck height, which, while reducing injury resulting from "rolling" out of bed, results in an unstable sit-to-stand process and increased likelihood of falling on egress. In addition, beds at this height were biomechanically more stressful for attending staff.

20.2.1.2 Side Rails

Side rails were installed on hospital beds to prevent the patient from rolling out of bed. Initially, these attachments were used only when necessary to "confine" a restless or confused patient in bed, but later they were adopted as a standard part of beds in the United States, folding down for ingress and egress. However, these side rails failed as a method of *confining* a patient in the bed and did not serve as a restraint: patients climbed over the rail or over the end of the bed and fell. As rails increased the distance of the fall, they therefore increased the severity of injury. Another risk occurred when patients attempted to climb *through* the rails, suffocating or even being found hanging with their head trapped between the rails (Todd et al., 1997).

To prevent these accidents, the design of side rails changed over the decades. Originally, side rails were high and full length. In 1949, the first short side rails were developed but were installed on the beds as two partial-length rails. [2] Thus, even when rails were "split" length, when both sets of rails were raised, they could be used as full-length rails. Shorter side rails (¾ length) were safer, offering the patients a safe route to egress. When ¾-length split rails were used with the top rails up and the foot rails down, the top rails served to provide support for the patient's in-bed mobility and support (especially when the top of the bed was raised to a sitting position) as well as access to bed controls. Even so, side rails have now been removed altogether from beds in nursing homes. Most problematically, the absence of side rails interferes with and shortens the bed-alarm response time and removes the advantage of providing a hand support for the sit-to-stand process during egress.

The Food and Drug Administration (FDA) issued a warning regarding the safety of side rails (Burlington, 1995) and recommended regular inspection of all rails, bed frames, and mattresses. While federal regulations did not specify specific dimensions, recommendations included that

> Additional safety measures should be considered for patients identified as high risk for entrapment. Such patients include those with altered mental status (organic or medication related) or general restlessness. Increased risk also occurs when the patient's size and/or weight are inappropriate for the bed's dimensions. (Burlington, FDA, 1995)

Old-style rails were not withdrawn from circulation. Although caregivers may use full bed-length side rails as a restraint, the FDA noted that

> Bed side rails should not be used as a substitute for patient protective restraints. Patients who need a protective restraint, such as a vest or wrist/leg device, must be monitored frequently while wearing it. (Burlington, FDA, 1995).

Deaths from old-style side rails continued, with 550 deaths occurring between 1995 and 2011, mainly among those aged 60 or older and often with cognitive impairment. Although the style of rail was not recorded, incidents continued because of mismatch between the components of the rails, bed, and mattress in the case of "portable" rails; or in instances when there was a mismatch between these features and outmoded design. The systematic review conducted by these authors concluded that there was no evidence that bed rails affected falls from the bed or increased fall-related injuries (Healey et al., 2008). The design of side rails continues to be updated, and they are primarily used in acute-care and rehabilitation hospital beds.

20.2.1.3 Physical Restraints

In an attempt to prevent patients from falling out of bed or from climbing out of bed, until the late 1980s, patients were *tied* with restraints in the bed, in wheelchairs, or chairs. Patients considered at risk of falling were also restrained on toilet chairs or placed in chairs with tabletops fixed across their laps. The use of such restraints failed to meet the goal of keeping the patients safe. While patients were less likely to fall from beds or chairs, the restraints had other negative effects: they often made the elderly enraged at being "tied down." Fighting against the restraints and struggling to be free of the restraints even resulted in deaths from strangulation (Brush and Capezuti, 2001; Todd et al., 1997). In addition, those who were restrained lost muscle mass and experienced increasing weakness with forced bedrest; they also developed pressure ulcers and sometimes pneumonia.

In the 1990s, political action led by the Quakers in Philadelphia lobbied for the removal of restraints. In addition, researchers documented patient responses to being restrained (Morse and McHutchion, 1991) and staff attitudes to restraints (Bourbonniere et al., 2003). Researchers also developed programs demonstrating that safe care could be provided without restraints. Kayser-Jones (1990) documented the safe care of the elderly in Scotland, where restraints were not used. Gradually, political pressure resulted in legislative recommendations against the use of restraints and side rails in nursing homes (Capezuti et al., 2007), without a physician's order, and frequent surveillance.

20.2.1.4 Pharmaceutical Restraints

As physical restraints were used less frequently, there was an increase in the use of medication to keep patients, quiet, sedated, and in bed. One side effect of these drugs was the fact that they increased the patient's fall risk by impairing gait and balance and causing postural hypotension and therefore increasing fall risk. In-bed patients were less likely to move so that the iatrogenic risks of bed rest were increased. Thus, chemical restraints as a fall intervention were discouraged, and the definition of a *restraint* was expanded to include chemical restraints (Mott et al., 2005).

20.2.1.5 Bed Alarms

As restraints were removed, concern about patient management and the prevention of falls became a primary concern. One technical intervention was the development of bed alarms to alert the nurse when a patient moved to the side of the bed to egress. The first of these alarms was a workaround developed by nursing staff—simply pinning a patient's call bell to his or her gown. Then as the patient moved forward to climb out of bed, the call bell pulled from the wall connection, sounding the emergency alarm.

Bed alarms have evolved through various styles and modes of operations since the early 1980s (see List 20.2).

LIST 20.2

Development of Bed Alarms (1980–present)

1982: Air pressure alarm: a sensor under the end of the mattress and an air pressure switch

1985: *Ambularm*: A mercury switch worn on the patient's thigh, which sounded as the patient stood up (http://www.familymedsupply.com/Catalog/Online-Catalog-Product/1346/Ambularm1000)

1985: Prototype of the *Bedcheck* alarm, a pressure-sensitive strip across the top of a mattress or seat or the chair

1985: Bed alarms built into the bed (NA, Hill Rom)

2004: Video alarm systems (Cucchira et al., 2007; Sixsmith and Johnson, 2004)

These alarms all shared a common problem: while alarms proved reliable in laboratory testing, they were not feasible in practice; that is, when a bed alarm sounded to indicate that a patient was getting out of bed, nurses had only 9 s or less to reach the bedside in order to support (i.e., "catch") the patient. Obviously, nurses were often not available or close enough to reach the patient before the fall occurred, especially if the patient had impaired gait or balance. Later, alarms could usually be programmed to give the patient instructions ("Hold on—I am coming!") in an effort to reach the patient in time.

20.3 Present Fall Intervention Programs

Since 2000, fall intervention programs consist of three arms: (1) fall triage to identify the patient at risk of a physiological anticipated fall, (2) fall prevention strategies, and (3) fall protection strategies.

20.3.1 Triage of the Fall-Prone Patient

The Joint Commission's 9th National Patient Safety Goal was "Reducing the risk of harm resulting from falls to inpatients and nursing home residents":

> Falls account for a significant portion of injuries in hospitalized patients, in long term care residents, and home care recipients. …the organization should evaluate the [patient's] risk for falls and take action to reduce the risk of falling, as well as the risk of injury should a fall occur. (Joint Commission, 2009)

The Joint Commission required institutions to "evaluate the [patient's] risk for falls" (p. 22) using short instruments designed to triage the fall-prone patient and to "take action to reduce the risk of falling, as well as the risk of injury" (p. 22). The major scales used in the United States are the Morse Fall Scale (MFS, of 6–10 items) (Morse et al., 1989b; Morse, 2007); Hendrich II, of eight items (Hendrich et al., 2003); and, in Britain, the STRATIFY scale, of five items (Oliver et. al., 1997), developed for use in nursing homes. The MFS and the Hendrich II were developed both by the identification and weighting of the items from a comparison of patient falls and a control group. The weights (i.e., scores) for the STRATIFY scale were subjectively selected until 2004, when added weighted scores were added (Papaioannou et al., 2004). Other scales in use have been developed statistically but have the item *weights* subjectively assigned, for instance, the Downton Index, Hendrix I,

Fall Prediction Index (Nyberg and Gustafson, 1997), and Scott & White Risk Screener (Yauk et al., 2005). In many cases, scales have been constructed qualitatively by identifying items from the literature, by freely adapting or combining other scales, or by using the nurses' "intuition" (Oliver, 2006, 2008; Uden et al., 1999). Item scores are also subjectively assigned (Kelly and Dowling, 2004). Although some of these may have been published in clinical journals, no reliability or validity statistics are available.

While triage scales are intended to identify the fall-prone patient and predict a fall, the main limitation is that the scales themselves do not prevent the fall—the fall interventions do. Problematically, these two major areas of fall prediction and fall intervention have not been systematically linked. That is, while we can now predict with reasonable accuracy the patients or residents who are likely to experience a physiological anticipated fall, the recommendations for fall intervention strategies remain subjective, haphazard, and undifferentiated and, at best, linked to categories of fall risk (high, medium, or low fall risk) rather than being associated with or linked to particular patterns of fall risk scores, (i.e., *patient fall profiles*) and items scored on the triage scales. Clearly, until intervention strategies are applied appropriately and consistently to particular patterns of patient profiles, fall intervention programs will remain unnecessarily expensive, fall strategies will be applied unnecessarily or will not be applied at all, and programs that are less than optimally effective will place patients at risk of injury from falls.

Fall prevention strategies are those intended to *prevent the patient from falling*. Unfortunately, there is confusion about the risk of a *fall* per se: Some institutions score infants and small children for anticipated physiological falls, yet their own records would show that these children are prone to injury from *accidental falls* (not anticipated physiological falls). They usually fall while climbing on playroom equipment, from cribs, or, as mentioned previously, when dropped by caregivers. Many nursing homes and rehabilitation units also recognize that overprotection may result in *fear of falling* (Zijlstra et al., 2007) and argue that the patient has a "right to fall," and must fall, if they are to rehabilitate. For these reasons, fall protection strategies are a primary concept in nursing homes and rehabilitation hospitals, and fall prevention strategies are of primary significance in acute-care institutions.

20.3.2 Fall Prevention

Fall prevention strategies are twofold: (1) environmental scans to remove the risk of an accidental falls, and (2) prevention strategies, or interventions, to *prevent* the patient from falling.

20.3.2.1 Environmental Scan

The environmental scan is an annual walk-through of an institution to inspect the institution hazards that may result in an accidental fall. The nurse specialist responsible for falls, the chief nursing officer, the chief engineer, and the head of housekeeping carry out the inspection. As this team moves into each unit, the head nurse for that area joins them. During the inspection, there is

- A random inspection of beds, wheelchairs, waking aids, and other equipment
- Inspection of patient rooms for the "flight path" between the bed and the bathroom, absence of clutter, and availability of walking aids and rails

- A visual inspection of bathrooms, positions of rails, flooring, security of shower curtains, ledges on the floor to contain water but that may also trip patients, and so forth
- Inspection of hallways for use of nonglare floor sealer, handrails, and clutter

20.3.2.2 Fall Prevention Strategies

Fall prevention strategies may be classified into those that enhance patient vigilance and those that are intended to prevent a fall. For example, some patient vigilance strategies *monitor the patient* by facilitating nurse surveillance of the patient and work by alerting the nurse when the patient is restless and egress is inevitable. Sometimes, hospitals employ *sitters*—people with minimal training who are employed to watch the patient and to call the nurse if the patient tries to get out of bed. Evaluating the need for and the activities of sitters, Tzeng et al. (2008), found that sitters were an alternative to the use of restraints but that fall rates were higher when sitters were used. Hiring sitters is expensive; many large urban medical centers spend more than $1,000,000 per year. At other times, hospitals may request that a relative sit with their loved one, also to monitor against falls. Many hospitals are now instituting *comfort rounds*, one- or two-hourly checks on all patients to see if they have bathroom or other needs (Tzeng et al., 2008).

Bed alarms are the most common methods of increasing patient surveillance. They now are available in various styles:

- An alarm built into the bed, which alarms when the patient's weight moves off the edge of the bed
- A separate pressure-sensitive strip placed under the patient's sheet, which alarms when the patient's buttocks move off the strip
- A clip attached to the patient's shirt, which alarms when the magnet detaches from the alarm as the patient moves out of bed
- An infrared beam detector, which alarms when the patient moves to the perimeter of the bed

Bed alarms may sound in the emergency call bed system or at the bedside. They may even have recorded announcements providing the verbal instructions "Get back to bed," or "Hold on and stand still." While these alarms pass the manufacturers' tests for reliability, they are subject to human error: staff forget to turn them on, staff do not hear the alarm, or staff cannot get to the patient in time to prevent a fall—it generally takes only 9 s for the patient to get out of bed.

Capezuti et al. (2009) conducted a study testing two types of bed alarms in a nursing home: a pressure-sensitive strip and a pressure-sensitive strip combined with an infrared beam. They concluded that the combined alarm reduced false alarms but that neither alarm was "a substitute for staff availability." This conclusion was endorsed by Hubbartt et al. (2011), who reported that the "University Health System Consortium (UHC) Patient Safety Net" aggregated falls data for 2008 examined more than 20,000 submitted fall reports that occurred in 2008 in 39 organizations. Data showed that bed-exit alarms were one of the fall prevention strategies in place at the time of the fall in the case of more than 3000 fallers, and that the UHC did not find any evidence supporting the use of monitoring devices (bed/chair or exit alarms) in preventing falls. However, the UHC also noted that "alarms on" were associated with a "slightly lower percentage of harmful events (11.4%–12%)

among those who fell" (Aggregated data, Web seminar report, University Health System Consortium, 2009, in Hubbartt et al., 2011, p. 199).

Side rails are intended to prevent the patient from rolling out of the bed and to provide support and a handhold as patients exit the bed. At first glance, this appears to be logical fall prevention strategy. However, as noted earlier, historically the side rail was a hazard, leading to strangulation. A British study by Healey et al. (2008) noted that problems with bed rails were due to outmoded designs and "incorrect assembly" and that "bed rails do not appear to increase the risk of falls or injury from falls" (p. 368).

Despite this resistance, side rails continue to be manufactured on beds and used primarily in acute-care and rehabilitation hospitals. A study showing how the rails may be used during ingress, egress, and turning will be discussed at the end of this chapter.

Video surveillance for general observation of the patient is relatively new—especially in patient rooms. Software has only recently been developed that will protect the patient's privacy by altering the image. Video technology allows the visual inspection of the bed with an alarm sounding if the patient breaks the perimeter of the bed, and enables the visual inspection of the bed from the nursing stations.

Walking aids include canes, crutches, and walkers that support the patient during ambulation. If used correctly, they reduce the patient's risk of falling. However, if the patient forgets to use the cane or walker or uses it incorrectly, the patient may fall. Thus these walking aids are not suited to patients with impaired cognition. Hand rails on the walls of bathrooms, patient rooms, and corridors may also be considered walking aids that support ambulation and prevent falls. Because they are always in place and do not require technology, they may be considered a *passive intervention*.

20.3.3 Fall Protective Strategies

Fall protection strategies are intended to *prevent injury* should a fall occur. From this perspective, the patient is permitted to ambulate, and the side effects of immobility are prevented. Alternatively, if the patient does make an illegal exit from the bed and fall, injury is minimized.

20.3.3.1 Hip Protectors

Hip protectors are items of underwear with pads that fit over each hip. They were originally plastic shields, but later, for reasons of in-bed comfort, they were made from dense foam. The pads fit over the hip and are inserted into underwear, so that if the patient falls sideways, the hip is protected and the impact on the hip is minimized. Early reports of hip protectors suggested they were effective, and they were adopted into nursing homes. However, more recently, their efficacy has been questioned.

A Cochrane review of nine randomized studies and six cluster randomized studies revealed that the "original protective effect was not confirmed in individually randomized studies… but marginal significance effect of hip protectors on reducing the incidence of hip fracture amongst participants in nursing homes and in residential care" (Parker et al., 2005, p. 8 was obtained).

20.3.3.2 Helmets

Helmets come in two forms: a hard helmet (rather like a bicycle helmet) and a "soft" helmet that may be used in bed, while sleeping. Helmets are primarily used by epileptics to protect the head during a seizure, and those who need helmets may refuse to wear them.

20.3.3.3 Floor Mats

Floor mats are padded mats placed beside the bed, so that if a patient rolls out of bed, the impact will be lessened and the opportunity to fracture a hip reduced. Independent tests in a laboratory (Bowers et al., 2008) using mannequins and simulated falls from six heights, both head and feet first, onto a tiled floor and onto a floor mat showed that both a low bed height and a floor mat decreased the risk of injury when falling from a bed.

However, in a study published by Doig and Morse (2010), it was noted that the beveled edge of the mat produced a hazard when patients walked across the mat, particularly when entering the bed. The patients experienced instability when their heels were placed on the beveled edge of the mat. This caused patients to stumble and presented a fall risk. It was recommended that the mat not be used.

20.3.3.4 Rails

There has been considerable amount of research conducted into the optimal height and circumference of rails. While dimensional and installation guidelines are provided in reference material, it is important that hand supports be designed and installed to facilitate use by those with reduced grip strength. This is required to prevent instability and increase the likelihood of fall arrest in the case of a fall initiation. It has also been found that the preferred positions of hand supports for toilet use by the elderly depends on individual preferences (Dekker et al., 2007). Railings are usually found in bathrooms and hallways. Oddly, they are not routinely installed in bedrooms, where they may be most needed. It is proposed that the use of grab bars on every patient-room wall would facilitate movement from the bedside to the bathroom (Tzeng and Yin, 2010).

20.4 Therapies to Reduce Risk of Falling

Fall risk assessment is an examination of the patient, by a physical therapist or a physician, to determine if the patient has a medical diagnosis that may be contributing to the fall-prone behavior or if the patient would benefit from exercise therapy (Tinetti et al., 1986). It differs from fall triage, as it seeks to uncover the *cause* of the fall-prone behavior and prescribes physical therapy or medications to correct deficits.

20.4.1 Vitamin D

There has been no evidence of the efficacy of vitamin D supplementation for the geriatric populations overall, although a subgroup with vitamin D sufficiency did show a significant reduction in the rate of falls (Gillespie et al., 2009; Kalyani et al., 2010). In one case, Cameron et al. (2010, p. 16) showed a significant positive effect of vitamin D supplementation on the rate of falls (0.57 [95% CI 0.37–0.89]) and the risk of falling (0.65 [95% CI 0.46–0.91]).

20.4.2 Muscle Strengthening

Because of the short length of stay in hospitals, strengthening exercises are not usually a part of therapy. However, physical therapy has shown that muscle strengthening has beneficial effects, improving gait and balance in the fall-prone elderly. A randomized control trial of the Otago home-based program showed a reduction in physiological fall risk and an improvement of functional mobility and executive functioning in older adults over a period of 6 months (Lui-Ambrose et al., 2008). In this study, 43% of the fall group and 67% of the control group fell, showing that a home-based exercise program significantly reduced fall risk.

Tai chi is another strategy used to improve balance and cardiorespiratory function and to reduce falls in the elderly. However, a systematic review (Verhagen et al., 2004) consisting of seven studies and 505 participants determined that evidence was "limited" in reducing falls and blood pressure in the elderly.

20.5 Summary

While these three approaches (fall prevention, fall protection, risk reduction therapies) form a logically complimentary fall intervention program in health-care institutions, there are tensions between these three facets of fall interventions. Researchers have tried to assess the efficacy of each intervention separately, but in reality, patient falls are caused by multiple factors. At the center is human error on the part of both the patient and the caregivers. Patients are expected to call for help before they get out of bed, yet this expectation is unrealistic. Patients are in a hurry to get to the bathroom; they do not want to be assisted with this intimate task and do not feel that such assistance is necessary. Nurses are busy with a large caseload and cannot immediately respond to calls for help or call bells or even be responsible for vigilantly and constantly observing patients. Institutions cannot afford one-on-one sitters for all restless patients. Correcting fall proneness using physical therapy or medication such as vitamin D or by correcting drug interactions to prevent hypotension or confusion are not usually immediate fixes.

Considering the *Swiss Cheese* model of causation (Reason, 2000), falls occur when series of factors "line up" (like the holes in Swiss cheese) and sequentially allow a series of events to lead to an accident. For instance, the patient climbs out of bed; the bed alarm fails or is not turned on, or the nurses cannot reach the bed in time. The patient is incontinent and slips on the urine; he then falls backward and his head hits the floor, fracturing his skull.

Astonishingly little attention has been given in the hospital environment to making the bed safe should a patient egress, placing rails and handholds in the patient's room, and attending to hazards in the bathroom. Ergonomic research and biomechanical solutions to making in-bed mobility easier, bed exit safer, and the route between the bed and the bathroom less hazardless appear to be the next step in fall intervention programs. This approach is addressed in the next section.

20.6 Review of Research Related to Biomechanical Parameters

Biomechanics, or the application of the basic principles of physics and mechanics to the biological system, is not new. A review of the notebooks of Leonardo da Vinci indicates that as early as the fifteenth century, scientists recognized the importance of understanding the physics and mechanics of living organisms. Biomechanical principles have been used in the analysis of how humans interact with their working and living environment. In this section, we discuss areas of research that would make the hospital environment safer and biomechanical research performed relating to human safety in the health-care setting. This discussion starts with a brief review of how biomechanics has been used in the analysis of patient handling. The section then focuses more specifically on the elderly and deals with the biomechanical analysis of mobility and gait, slips/falls and the potential for injury, and fall recovery/injury prevention in the hospital. We conclude with an example of such research—an interim report of a major research effort funded by the Agency for Healthcare Research and Quality (AHRQ) to determine the effect of bed design on slip/fall potential in a diverse group of older disabled adults.

20.6.1 Biomechanical Analysis of Patient Handling

Biomechanical principles have been used extensively in the analysis of the injury potential in persons handling or assisting patients in the health-care environment. In a comprehensive analysis, Marras et al. (1999) used a risk analysis and a biomechanical spinal loading model to evaluate the risk of low-back disorders in participants performing patient transfer and repositioning tasks carried out by one and two people. They found that, even with a light and cooperative patient, these tasks were "extremely hazardous" with a "substantial risk" for low-back injury, even when performed by two people. In a biomechanical analysis of patient transfer from bed to wheelchair and wheelchair to bed, Garg et al. (2007) found that pulling techniques required significantly lower hand forces and significantly lower low-back compressive forces than lifting techniques. They found that low-back shear forces and trunk moments were lower, and the percentages of females able to perform the tasks were higher, for pulling than lifting techniques.

In a biomechanical analysis of patient transfer from shower chair to wheelchair and wheelchair to shower chair, Garg et al. (2007) found that techniques based on pulling the patient resulted in lower trunk-flexion moments, erector spinae muscle forces, compressive forces, and shear forces than techniques utilizing lifting. Biomechanical analysis has also been used to evaluate the effectiveness of mechanical patient handling systems. In an evaluation of lift-assist systems, Keir and MacDonell (2007) found that erector spinae, latissimus dorsi, and trapezius muscle activity was lower during the use of the ceiling lift than during the use of the floor lift. Silvia et al. (2002) performed a biomechanical analysis of a manual patient transfer using a sling suspension lift (similar to a "Hoyer" lift) and a novel system involving a translation of the bed sheet to a gurney that converts to a moveable chair. They found that both mechanical systems resulted in lower back-compressive forces than manual patient transfer.

20.6.2 Biomechanical Analysis of Elderly Mobility and Gait

Biomechanical analysis techniques can be used to describe and quantify mobility issues in the elderly. In a detailed analysis, Schultz (1992) reviewed the potential for biomechanical analysis to quantify changes in gait, fall potential, and difficulty in bed and chair transfers as a function of increasing age. He notes that "physical disabilities ultimately express themselves as changes in the biomechanics of physical-task performance" and emphasizes that the needs for biomechanical research into mobility impairment in the elderly "clearly constitute new and major challenges for biomechanics research." Older participants slipped longer and faster and fell more often than younger subjects, and changes in gait as a function of age (particularly higher heel-contact velocity and slower movement of the center of mass of the upper body) may increase slip potential (Lockhart et al., 2003). It is interesting to note, however, that in an analysis of the biomechanical walking patterns of fit, when compared to a database of young adults, elderly adult subjects demonstrated shorter step length, increased double stance-support stance period, decreased push-off power, and more flat-footed landing, all of which are indicators of a more stable and safe gait pattern (Winter et al., 1990). Clearly, this is a fertile area for additional research.

20.6.3 Biomechanical Analysis of the Potential for Injury in Slips/Falls of the Elderly

In a biomechanical analysis of the injury severity potential resulting from falls from the bed onto a mat and hard floor using mannequins, Bowers et al. (2008) found that the likelihood of a serious head injury resulting from a feet-first fall from a bed height of 38.4 in. (97.5 cm) onto a tiled floor was 25% and approximately 1% when falling onto a mat. In a review of fall-impact biomechanics, the peak impact forces of a fall from standing height averaged 1260 lb (5600 N), which is well above the 900 lb mean force required to fracture the femur in an elderly person (Robinovitch et al., 2000). These authors also suggest that compliant surfaces can reduce the potential for wrist injuries during a fall from standing height or lower.

20.6.4 Biomechanical Analysis of Fall Recovery/Injury Prevention for the Elderly

Biomechanical research and analysis can be used not only to quantify slip-and-fall potential but also to minimize the adverse effects of these events. In a review of biomechanical issues related to age-related upper-body injuries in older adults, DeGoede et al. (2003) note that there is evidence that fall-related impact forces can be reduced by appropriate volitional strategies. They also suggest that further experimental and theoretical research is needed to determine the best fall-arrest strategies for older adults. In a discussion of the prevention of fall-related fractures through biomechanics, Robinovitch et al. (2000) suggest that "safe landing responses" may be an effective way to reduce injuries resulting from falls. Grabiner et al. (2008) discussed the translation of experimental biomechanical results to the clinic setting. They found that through task-specific training, elderly adults can be taught to limit trunk motion, and this learned motor skill has been shown to decrease the likelihood of a trip/fall risk. They conclude that traditional exercise-based fall prevention training can reduce fall-related injury in older adults.

Liu and Lockhart (2009) performed a biomechanical analysis of successful recovery from slips and found that there were age-related differences in joint moments during the recovery action. DeGoede and Ashton-Miller (2003) performed biomechanical simulations of forward fall arrest and found that the age-related decline in arm-muscle strength substantially reduces the ability to use the arms to arrest a fall and increases the potential for torso or head impact. They also note that elderly women with below-average bone strength are at risk of a colles fracture (fracture of the distal radius in the forearm) if they attempt to arrest a fall with an extended arm. In a biomechanical analysis of fall arrest, Kim and Ashton-Miller (2003) indicate that any fall prevention strategy that increases the time available for arm movement prior to impact would help reduce fall injuries, particularly for older males. In an analysis of the effects of ageing on slip/fall biomechanics, Lockhart et al. (2005) propose that the ability to recover from a slip is lower in the elderly due to reduced lower-extremity strength and sensory degradation. Interestingly, in a biomechanical analysis of lower-extremity joint moments, Wojcik et al. (2001) did not find conclusive evidence that age-related decline in lower-extremity strength was associated with a decreased capacity of adults to recover their balance after a forward fall. In a somewhat different approach, Gatts and Woollacott (2006) analyzed the biomechanics of recovery after a slip and found that, for gait-impaired seniors, Tai Chi training resulted in an increase in the ability to control stepping strategy and center-of-mass anterior–posterior motion, two key balance-control mechanisms.

There is a need to place what is known in the context of the hospital room and the patient's problem of safely moving off the bed, standing, and moving across the room to the bathroom.

20.7 Application of Biomechanical Research to the Hospital Bed, the Hospital Room, and the Bathroom

At the beginning of this chapter, we noted that each year in the United States, almost 200,000 hospital patients are seriously injured. In the previous sections, we noted that a great deal was known about the biomechanical movements of the elderly and disabled and fall proneness. But when hospitalized, the environment is planned for the movements of staff, that is, the space required for patient transfer and for caregiving. Little research has been done into the way patients may safely ambulate away from the bed; relatively little is known about the biomechanics and mobility support needs of safely "getting to the bathroom."

20.7.1 Bed Height and Safe Egress

As noted previously, bed height has changed over the past five decades, but beds are still constructed according to standards of "one size fits all." That is, despite the ability to adjust the height, the low height is usually approximately a 16 in. deck height for all patients (Morse et al., 2015). Yet research related to the safe bed height for ingress or egress according to individual disability, and anthropometric measurements had not been conducted, and results from an ongoing study are not yet available. Interim results are presented in Box 20.1.

Our interim results show that the lowest height of the bed must be adjustable, so that caregiver may "set" the low height for the patient who is entering and for exiting. Once these two standard measures are known and may be adjusted for each individual and the bed height "set" accordingly, falls from the bed while exiting will be reduced. Patients will be less likely to slip and will maintain better balance when exiting the bed or slip from the deck while entering (Chrisman et al., 2015). As most falls in the hospital involve the bed, injuries will be dramatically reduced.

20.7.2 Balance/Support on Standing

When patients exit the bed, there is nothing to provide balance support except the bed rail. These rails have 2–3 in. of "play" and, despite their strength, they *feel* to be a poor support to the patient. The gap across the floor from the bed to the bathroom door has been measured up the 16 ft without a handhold—much too far for a patient with an impaired gait to navigate.

BOX 20.1   EXAMPLE: BIOMECHANICAL AND ERGONOMIC ANALYSIS OF THE EFFECT OF BED HEIGHT

Interim Report of AHRQ #1R01HS018953-01, Linkages Between the Safety of the Hospitals Bed, patient falls and immobility (Morse et al., 2015)

BACKGROUND

The work noted above was the impetus for a comprehensive study into biomechanical parameters and other issues related to slip/fall risk for the elderly during movement to bed, bed entry, repositioning in bed, bed exit, and movement away from the bed in a simulated health-care setting. The major goal of this research effort is to determine the effect of bed height on biomechanical parameters and slip/fall potential during the above activities for fall-prone and control elderly subjects. Bed heights were set as low, medium, and high and were represented by 95%, 110%, and 125% of the lower leg length with lower leg length defined as by a measurement that is taken to the tibial plateau with the knee at 90° and the foot flat on the floor.

SUBJECTS

The present analysis is based on a subject population of 53 older adults ranging in age from 50 to 95 (mean = 59.3, SD = 10.6), with a Morse Fall Scale (MFS) (Morse, 2009) range from 15 to 100 (mean = 59.3, SD = 20.7). Height and weight ranged from 153.7 to 194.3 cm and 60.3–153.7 kg respectively, and the BMI ranged from 18.2 to 46.9 (mean = 29.4, SD = 5.7). Within the total subject population, 36 were categorized as "fall-prone" or "at risk" of falling (MFS >45 and/or significant gait and mobility impairment) and 17 were controls. Exclusion criteria were (1) unilateral strength deficit > 50%, (2) lower limb amputations, or (3) height >200 cm or other medical conditions (morbid obesity, osteoporosis) that prevented the use of the fall arrest system. Descriptive information for the fall-prone subjects: average age of 69 (SD = 12), average height of 172.2 cm (SD = 10.7), average weight of 88.4 kg (SD = 21.9), and average MFS = 67 (SD = 13.6). Descriptive information for the control subjects: average age of 65 (SD = 10.6), average height of 174.0 cm (SD = 7.9), average weight of 83.0 kg (SD = 16.3), and average MFS = 32 (SD = 8.4).

METHODS

The study was conducted in a biomechanics laboratory created specifically for this project at the George E. Wahlen Salt Lake City Veterans Administration Hospital. Two force plates were installed flush with the floor next to the bed and one force measurement system was mounted to record forces applied to the hand rails. Three-dimensional body motion data was captured from 70 retroreflective markers on key anatomical landmarks and limb segments. The combination of force plate and motion data allowed the calculation of shear forces at the foot–floor interface, joint torques, and parameters related to balance. To prevent falls, all subjects wore a safety harness attached to a climbing rope with a locking carabiner and were belayed from a steel frame. A registered nurse monitored each subject's stability prior to and during each trial and stopped the trial if a subject demonstrated excessive fatigue or indications of balance loss or instability.

(Continued)

BOX 20.1 (CONTINUED)   EXAMPLE: BIOMECHANICAL AND ERGONOMIC ANALYSIS OF THE EFFECT OF BED HEIGHT

RESULTS

Results to date indicate that for bed entry, the high bed presented the greatest slip potential and the low bed presented the least as it relates to the frictional forces at the foot–floor interface. For bed exit, the low bed presented the greatest slip potential using this same measure. The time to first step after bed exit, which may be a measure of stability, was the longest for the low bed and shortest for the high bed. The low-height bed required greater joint moments in the lower extremities. Participants with lower leg strength used movement patterns that increased the slip potential at the foot and increased leg strength moment requirements, both of which are potential indicators of increased slip or fall potential.

In summary, it is proposed that bed height should be adjusted for different patients to reduce slip/fall potential. Low beds required greater effort to rise and reduced slip potential on ingress. High beds made it difficult to sit securely on ingress but reduced slip potential and required effort on egress.

It is unrealistic to expect a patient—in particular a patient with cognitive impairment—to remember to stay in bed when instructed. It is therefore our responsibility to provide a means for safe exit from the bed and a safe path from the bed to the bathroom. There is a need to provide a support/handhold for the patient when moving from sitting to standing from the bed. There is a need to provide rails and/or a walking frame for the patient who is moving unassisted to the bathroom. Such engineering/architectural developments would greatly decrease fall rates, providing support for the patient with poor balance and giving the nurse time to respond to the bed alarm.

20.7.3 Rails in Patients' Rooms

Hospitals provide miles of rails in corridors "to protect the walls." The rails are usually 10 in wide and flat, with a curved top that serves as a hand hold. Despite the extensive research of Maki and McIlroy (2006) on the dimensions and height of the rails, these commonly used rails do not meet their specifications and do not even have a place for a thumb grip to provide adequate support. In addition, often there are no rails in patients' rooms, forcing patients to grasp at other items on the walls for support—computer trays, thermostats, glove and mask boxes, and so forth. These items, acting as "substitute rails," have not been installed to bear the patient's falling weight, nor do they provide stable support.

20.8 Bathrooms

A large percentage of falls occur in the bathroom as a part of toileting or showering. In older hospitals in particular (those built before 1960), fixtures are installed for a person who is standing. Mirrors are too high for patients to use while sitting; rails are located in less than optimal positions to provide support when a patient moves around the room.

20.8.1 Floor/Standing Surfaces

The prevention of the initial foot slip is important in the reduction of falls in the bathroom. This can be accomplished through the use of floor materials that have a high coefficient of friction (CoF) (Rubenstein et al., 1996) and retain this high CoF when wet (Tideiksaar, 1989) and, if possible, even when soapy. Bowen (1993) found some floor materials that have a higher CoF with a bare foot when wet than when dry. Kim et al. (2009) found that slippery floors (OR = 12.130) and bathroom mats without rubber backing (OR = 3.564) were risk factors for slips for the elderly. The use of skid-resistant backing on bathroom rugs and skid-resistant adhesive appliqués can reduce slip potential (Rubenstein et al., 1996; Tideiksaar, 1989).

In an attempt to reduce injury in impact, Casalena et al. (1998) explored different floor surfaces, but surfaces that are both resilient enough to managed wheeled carts and beds and soft enough not to drag on patients' feet, and that can withstand daily wear while providing adequate absorption from fall impact, have yet to be developed.

20.8.2 Hand Rails

Because of the potential for slip and the presence of hard surfaces, hand rails or grab bars are particularly important in the bathroom. It has been found that when adequate hand rails are not available, people tend to use hazardous supports to facilitate bathing and toileting (Aminzadeh et al., 2000; Tideiksaar, 1989). Recommendations on the use of hand rails in the bathroom are ubiquitous and have existed for many years (Tideiksaar, 1989; Rubenstein et al., 1996; Tzeng and Yin, 2010; Woodson, 1981; Panero and Zelnik, 1979). When they are available, it is critical that bathroom handrails are secure. Loose or wobbly grab bars have been associated with a risk ratio of 7.83 for first falls in the elderly (Northridge et al., 1995).

20.9 Conclusions

Despite awareness of the human and economic cost of patient falls in institutions and administrators', caregivers', and researchers' efforts to reduce the risk of falling, we are still far from the goal of providing a safe yet therapeutic environment in hospitals. Research conducted for more than six decades has altered the pattern of patient falls but has not reduced the rate of falls and fall injuries. We can predict an anticipated physiological fall with some accuracy, but we still do not know how to prevent the fall from occurring. There is a need for large-scale research projects that develop a comprehensive and innovative approach to fall interventions.

We now recognize that hospitals should provide all patients with a safe route of egress that extends from the bed to the bathroom. Smart beds have been developed, with sensors to detect when occupied or unoccupied and automatically reset brakes. These features must be extended to automatically reset to the safest height for ingress and egress according to individual patient specifications. There is a need to develop an innovative room layout so that patients do not have to negotiate distances without handholds or other supports. Caregivers must be provided with sensors and alarms so they may monitor the location of patients, in particular those with unsteady or impaired gaits, hypovolemic incidences, or other physiological occurrences that may result in falling. These sensors should prompt caregivers to help with patient toileting and exercise needs and provide regular social contact. Caregivers must know where patients are, be alerted to their needs, and automatically record caregiver contacts.

In summary, most fall intervention research has been approached from the caregiver perspective: identifying the fall-prone patient, *preventing* the patient from falling, and *protecting* the patient from injury. Biomechanical and ergonomic researchers have explored lifts and mobility aids, gait, the mechanism of slips and falls, and fall injury causation. But these various branches of research have not been coordinated in a systematic review of all of the noted factors and implementation of research results into the design and use of patient care facilities.

Acknowledgments

This research was supported in part by AHRQ Grant: Linkages between the safety of the hospital bed, patient falls and immobility, AHRQ .1R01HS018953-01.

References

Aminzadeh, Faranak, Nancy Edwards, Donna Lockett, and Rama C. Nair. Utilization of bathroom safety devices, patterns of bathing and toileting, and bathroom falls in a sample of community living older adults. *Technology and Disability* 13 (2000): 95–103.

Barnett, Karen. Reducing patient falls in an acute general hospital. *The Foundations of Nursing Studies* 1, no. 1 (2002): 1–4.

Berry, Glenice, Rory H. Fisher, and Sandra Lang. Detrimental incidents, including falls, in an elderly institutionalized population. *Journal of the American Geriatrics Society* 29 (1981): 322–324.

Bourbonniere, Meg, Neville E. Strumpf, Lois K. Evans, and Greg Maislin. Organizational characteristics and restraint use for hospitalized nursing home residents. *Journal of the American Geriatrics Society* 51, no. 8 (2003): 1079–1084.

Bowen, Kyle M. Assessment of static coefficient of friction between barefeet and bathroom flooring surfaces under dry, wet, and soapy conditions. Unpublished M.S. Thesis, Salt Lake City, UT. 1993.

Bowers, Bonnie, John Lloyd, W. Lee, Gail Powell-Cope, and A. Baptiste. Biomechanical evaluation of injury severity associated with patient falls from bed. *Rehabilitation Nursing* 33, no. 6 (2008): 253–259.

Brush, Barbara L., and Elizabeth Capezuti. Historical analysis of siderail use in American hospitals. *Journal of Nursing Scholarship* 33, no. 4 (2001): 381–385.

Burlington, D. Bruce. FDA safety alert: Entrapment hazards with hospital bed side rails. 1995. http://www.fda.gov/MedicalDevices/Safety/AlertsandNotices/PublicHealthNotifications/ucm062884.htm (Downloaded 12 July 2014).

Butcher, Lola. The no-fall zone. *Hospitals and Health Networks/AHA* 87, no. 6 (2013): 26–30.

Cameron, Ian D., Geoff R. Murray, Lesley D. Gillespie, M. Clare Robertson, Keith D. Hill, Robert G. Cumming, and Ngaire Kerse. Interventions for preventing falls in older people in nursing care facilities and hospitals. *Cochrane Database of Systematic Reviews* 1, no. 1 (2010): CD005465.

Capezuti, Elizabeth, Barbara L. Brush, Stephen Lane, Hannah U. Rabinowitz, and Michelle Secic. Bed-exit alarm effectiveness. *Archives of Gerontology and Geriatrics* 49, no. 1 (2009): 27–31.

Capezuti, E., L. M. Wagner, B. L. Brush,, M. Boltz, S. Renz, and K. A. Talerico. Consequences of an intervention to reduce restrictive side rail use in nursing homes. *Journal of the American Geriatrics Society* 55, no. 3 (2007): 1334–41.

Casalena, J. A., A. Badre-Alam, T. C. Ovaert, P. R. Cavanagh, and D. A. Streit. The Penn State safety floor: Part II—Reduction of fall-related peak impact forces on the femur. *Journal of Biomechanical Engineering* 120, no. 4 (1998): 527–532.

Cho, Sung-Hyun, Shaké Ketefian, Violet H. Barkauskas, and Dean G. Smith. The effects of nurse staffing on adverse events, morbidity, mortality, and medical costs. *Nursing Research* 52, no. 2 (2003): 71–79.

Chrisman, M., J. Morse, C. Wilson, N. Godfrey, A. Doig, D. Bloswick, and A. Merryweather. Analysis of the influence of hospital bed height on kinetic parameters associated with patient falls during egress. *Science Direct*, (6th International conference on applied Human Factors and Ergonomics), (2015) 1–8.

Cohen, Linda, and Peggy Guin. Implementation of a patient fall prevention program. *Journal of Neuroscience Nursing* 23, no. 5 (1991): 315–319.

Cucchiara, Rita, Andrea Prati, and Roberto Vezzani. A multi-camera vision system for fall detection and alarm generation. *Expert Systems* 24, no. 5 (2007): 334–345.

DeGoede, Kurt M., and James A. Ashton-Miller. Biomechanical simulations of forward fall arrests: Effects of upper extremity arrest strategy, gender and aging-related declines in muscle strength. *Journal of Biomechanics* 36, no. 3 (2003): 413–420.

DeGoede, Kurt M., James A. Ashton-Miller, and A. B. Schultz. Fall-related upper body injuries in the older adult: A review of the biomechanical issues. *Journal of Biomechanics* 36, no. 7 (2003): 1043–1053.

Dekker, Dries, Sonja N. Buzink, Johan F.M. Molenbroek, and Renete de Bruin. Hand supports to assist toilet use among the elderly. *Applied Ergonomics* 38 (2007): 109–118.

Doig, Alexa K., and Janice M. Morse. The hazards of using floor mats as a fall protection device at the bedside. *Journal of Patient Safety* 6, no. 2 (2010): 68–75.

Donaldson, Nancy, Diane Brown, Carolyn E. Aydin, Linda Bolton, and Dana Rutledge. Leveraging nurse-related dashboard benchmarks to expedite performance improvement and document excellence. *Journal of Nursing Administration* 35, no. 4 (2005): 163–172.

Dykes, Patricia C., Diane L. Carroll, Ann Hurley, Stuart Lipsitz, Angela Benoit, Frank Chang, Seth Meltzer, Ruslana Tsurikova, Lyubov Zuyov, and Blackford Middleton. Fall prevention in acute care hospitals: A randomized trial. *JAMA* 304, no. 17 (2010): 1912–1918.

Forrest, George P., Eric Chen, Sara Huss, and Andrew Giesler. A comparison of the functional independence measure and Morse Fall Scale as tools to assess risk of fall on an inpatient rehabilitation. *Rehabilitation Nursing* 38, no. 4 (2013): 186–192.

Gajewski, Byron, Matthew Hall, and Nancy Dunton. Summarizing benchmarks in the National Database of Nursing Quality Indicators using bootstrap confidence intervals. *Research in Nursing and Health* 30, no. 1 (2007): 112–119.

Ganz, David A., Christina Huang, Debra Saliba, et al. Preventing falls in hospitals: A toolkit for improving quality of care. (Prepared by RAND Corporation, Boston University School of Public Health, and ECRI Institute under Contract No. HHSA290201000017I TO #1.) Rockville, MD: Agency for Healthcare Research and Quality, 2013. AHRQ Publication No. 13-0015-EF.

Garg, Arun, Suzanna Milholland, Gwen Deckow-Schaefer, and Jay Kapellusch. Justification for a minimal lift program in critical care. *Critical Care Nursing Clinics of North America* 19, no. 2 (2007): 187–196.

Garg, A., B. Owen, D. Beller, and J. Banaag. A biomechanical and ergonomic evaluation of patient transferring tasks: Bed to wheelchair and wheelchair to bed. *Ergonomics* 34, no. 3 (1991): 289–312.

Gatts, Strawberry K., and Marjorie Hines Woollacott. How Tai Chi improves balance: Biomechanics of recovery to a walking slip in impaired seniors. *Gait and Posture* 25, no. 2 (2007): 205–214.

Gillespie, Lesley D., M. Clare Robertson, William J. Gillespie, Sarah E. Lamb, Simon Gates, Robert G. Cumming, and Brian H. Rowe. Interventions for preventing falls in older people living in the community. *Cochrane Database of Systematic Reviews* 2, no. (2009): CD007146.

Grabiner, Mark D., Stephanie Donovan, Mary Lou Bareither, Jane R. Marone, Karrie Hamstra-Wright, Strawberry Gatts, and Karen L. Troy. Trunk kinematics and fall risk of older adults: Translating biomechanical results to the clinic. *Journal of Electromyography and Kinesiology* 18, no. 2 (2008): 197–204.

Healey, F., A. Monro, A. Cockram, V. Adams, and D. Heseltin. Using targeted risk factor reduction to prevent falls in older in-patients: A randomised controlled trial. *Age and Ageing*. 2004 Jul 1;33(4):390–5.

Healey, Frances, David Oliver, Alisoun Milne, and James B. Connelly. The effect of bedrails on falls and injury: A systematic review of clinical studies. *Age and Ageing* 37, no. 4 (2008): 368–378.

Hendrich, Ann L., Patricia S. Bender, and Allen Nyhuis. Validation of the Hendrich II Fall Risk Model: A large concurrent case/control study of hospitalized patients. *Applied Nursing Research* 16, no. 1 (2003): 9–21.

Hitcho, Eileen B., Melissa J. Krauss, Stanley Birge, William Claiborne Dunagan, Irene Fischer, Shirley Johnson, Patricia A. Nast, Eileen Costantinou, and Victoria J. Fraser. Characteristics and circumstances of falls in a hospital setting. *Journal of General Internal Medicine* 19, no. 7 (2004): 732–739.

Hubbartt, Beth, Sarah G. Davis, and Donald D. Kautz. Nurses' experiences with bed exit alarms may lead to ambivalence about their effectiveness (CE). *Rehabilitation Nursing* 36, no. 5 (2011): 196–199.

Inouye, Sharon K., Cynthia J. Brown, and Mary E. Tinetti. Medicare nonpayment, hospital falls, and unintended consequences. *New England Journal of Medicine* 360, no. 23 (2009): 2390–2393.

Joint Commission. National patient safety goals, 2009, Accreditation program: Hospital, 2009. Retrieved 28 April 2009 from http://www.jointcommission.org/GeneralPublic/NPSG/09_npsgs.htm

Kalyani, Rita Rastogi, Brady Stein, Ritu Valiyil, Rebecca Manno, Janet W. Maynard, and Deidra C. Crews. Vitamin D treatment for the prevention of falls in older adults: Systematic review and meta-analysis. *Journal of the American Geriatrics Society* 58, no. 7 (2010): 1299–1310.

Kayser-Jones, Jeanie Schmit. *Old, alone, and neglected: Care of the aged in the United States and Scotland*. Vol. 4. Berkeley, CA: University of California Press, 1990.

Keir, Peter J., and Christopher W. MacDonell. Muscle activity during patient transfers: A preliminary study on the influence of lift assists and experience. *Ergonomics* 47, no. 3 (2007): 296–306.

Kelly, Angela, and Maura Dowling. Reducing the likelihood of falls in older people. *Nursing Standard* 18, no. 49 (2004): 33–40.

Kilpack, Virginia, Judy Boehm, Nancy Smith, and Bridget Mudge. Using research-based interventions to decrease patient falls. *Applied Nursing Research* 4, no. 2 (1991): 50–56.

Kim, Kyu-Jung, and James A. Ashton-Miller. Biomechanics of fall arrest using the upper extremity: Age differences. *Clinical Biomechanics* 18, no. 4 (2003): 311–318.

Kim, J.Y., Y.W. Lee, and O.K. Ham. Factors related to falls in elderly patients with osteoporosis. *Korean Journal of Adult Nursing* 21, no. 2 (2009): 257–267.

Lake, Eileen T., and Robyn B. Cheung. Are patient falls and pressure ulcers sensitive to nurse staffing? *Western Journal of Nursing Research* 28, no. 6 (2006): 654–677.

Liu, Jian, and Thurmon E. Lockhart. Age-related joint moment characteristics during normal gait and successful reactive-recovery from unexpected slip perturbations. *Gait and Posture* 30, no. 3 (2009): 276–281.

Llewellyn, Jane, Barbara Martin, Maureen Shekleton, and Sharon Firlit. Analysis of falls in the acute surgical and cardiovascular surgical patient. *Applied Nursing Research* 1, no. 3 (1988): 116–121.

Lockhart, Thurmon E., James L. Smith, and Jeffrey C. Woldstad. Effects of aging on the biomechanics of slips and falls. *Human Factors: The Journal of the Human Factors and Ergonomics Society* 47, no. 4 (2005): 708–729.

Lockhart, Thurmon E., Jeffrey C. Woldstad, and James L. Smith. Effects of age-related gait changes on the biomechanics of slips and falls. *Ergonomics* 46, no. 12 (2003): 1136–1160.

Lui-Ambrose, Teresa, Meghan G. Donaldson, Yasmin Ahamed, Peter Graf, Wendy Cook, J. Close, Stephen Lord, and Karin Khan. Otago home-based strength and balance retraining improves executive functioning in older fallers: A randomized control trial. *JAGS* 56 (2008): 1821–1830.

Macintosh, S., K. Hill, K.J. Dodd, P. Goldie, and E. Culhan. Falls and injury prevention should be a part of every stroke rehabilitation plan. *Clinical Rehabilitation* 19 (2005): 441–451.

Maki, Brian E., and William E. McIlroy. Control of rapid limb movements for balance recovery: Age-related changes and implications for fall prevention. *Age and Ageing* 35, no. suppl 2 (2006): ii12–ii18.

Marras, William S., Kermit G. Davis, Bryan C. Kirking, and Patricia K. Bertsche. A comprehensive analysis of low-back disorder risk and spinal loading during the transferring and repositioning of patients using different techniques. *Ergonomics* 42, no. 7 (1999): 904–926.

Menéndez, M. D., J. Alonso, J. C. Miñana, J. M. Arche, J. M. Díaz, and F. Vazquez. Characteristics and associated factors in patient falls, and effectiveness of the lower height of beds for the prevention of bed falls in an acute geriatric hospital. *Revista de Calidad Asistencial* 28, no. 5 (2013): 277–284.

Merryweather, Andrew S., Janice M. Morse, Alexa K. Doig, Nathan W. Godfrey, Pierre Gervais, and Donald S. Bloswick. Effects of bed height on the biomechanics of hospital bed entry and egress. *WORK: A Journal of Prevention, Assessment and Rehabilitation* 52 (2015): 707–713.

Mion, Lorraine C., Sara Gregor, Margaret Buettner, Diane Chwirchak, Olga Lee, and Wilfredo Paras. Falls in the rehabilitation setting: Incidence and characteristics. *Rehabilitation Nursing* 14, no. 1 (1989): 17–22.

Morgan, Veronica R., Jerrell H. Mathison, Janet C. Rice, and Dorothy Iker Clemmer. Hospital falls: A persistent problem. *American Journal of Public Health* 75, no. 7 (1985): 775–777.

Morris, E.V., and Bernard Isaacs. The prevention of falls in a geriatric hospital. *Age and Ageing* 9 (1980): 1981–1985.

Morse, Janice M. *Preventing Patient Falls: Establishing a Fall Intervention Program.* (2nd ed.). New York: Springer, 2007.

Morse, Janice M. *Preventing Patient Falls: Establishing a Fall Prevention Program.* (2nd ed.). New York: Springer, 2009.

Morse, Janice M. The safety of safety research: The case of patient falls. *Canadian Journal of Nursing Research* 38, no. 2 (2006): 72–86.

Morse, Janice M., Colleen Black, Kathleen Oberle, and Patricia Donahue. A prospective study to identify the fall-prone patient. *Social Science and Medicine* 28, no. 1 (1989a): 81–86.

Morse, Janice M., Pierre Gervais, Charlotte Pooler, Andrew S. Merryweather, Alexa K. Doig, and Don Bloswick, (2015). The safety of hospital beds: Ingress, egress and in-bed mobility. *Global Qualitative Nursing Research*, 2, doi:10.1177/2333393615575321

Morse, Janice M., and Edna McHutchion. Releasing restraints: Providing safe care for the elderly. *Research in Nursing and Health* 14, no. 3 (1991): 187–196.

Morse, Janice M., Andrew S. Merryweather, Don S. Bloswick, Alexa K. Doig, Gary W. Donaldson, and Bob Wong. Linkages between the safety of the hospital bed, patient falls and immobility. Final report, Salt Lake City, UT: AHRQ, 2015.

Morse, Janice M., and Robert M. Morse. Calculating fall rates: Methodological concerns. *QRB: Quality Review Bulletin* 14, no. 12 (1988): 369–371.

Morse, Janice M., Robert M. Morse, and Suzanne J. Tylko. Development of a scale to identify the fallprone patient. *Canadian Journal on Aging/La Revue canadienne du vieillissement* 8, no. 4 (1989b): 366–377.

Morse, Janice M., Suzanne J. Tylko, and Herbert A. Dixon. Characteristics of the fall-prone patient. *The Gerontologist* 27, no. 4 (1987): 516–522.

Morse, Janice M., Suzanne J. Tylko, and Herbert A. Dixon. The patient who falls—and falls again: Defining the aged at risk. *Journal of Gerontological Nursing* 11, no. 11 (1985): 15–18.

Mott, Sarah, Julia Poole, and Marita Kenrick. Physical and chemical restraints in acute care: Their potential impact on the rehabilitation of older people. *International Journal of Nursing Practice* 11, no. 3 (2005): 95–101.

Myers, A.H., S.P. Baker, E.G. Robinson, H. Abbey, E.T. Doll, and S. Levenson. Falls in the institutionalized elderly. *Journal of Long-Term Care Administration* 17, no. 4 (1989): 12–16.

No Author. *The Hill Rom Difference.* Batesville, IN: Hill Rom Industries, (No date).

Northridge, Mary E., Michael C. Nevitt, Jennifer Kelsey, and Bruce Link. Home hazards and falls in the elderly: The role of health and functional status. *American Journal of Public Health* 85, no. 4 (1995): 509–515.

Nyberg, L., and Y. Gustafson. Fall prediction index for patients in stroke rehabilitation. *American Stroke Association* 28, no. 7 (1997): 716–721.

Oliver, David. Assessing the risk of falls in hospitals: Time for a rethink? *Canadian Journal for Nursing Research* 38, no. 2 (2006): 89–94.

Oliver, David, James B. Connelly, Christina R. Victor, Fiona E. Shaw, Anne Whitehead, Yasemin Genc, Alessandra Vanoli, Finbarr C. Martin, and Margot A. Gosney. Strategies to prevent falls and fractures in hospitals and care homes and effect of cognitive impairment: Systematic review and meta-analyses. *BMJ* 334, no. 7584 (2007): 82.

Oliver, David. Falls risk-prediction for hospital inpatients: Time to put them to bed? *Age and Ageing* 37I, no. 3 (2008): 248–250.

Oliver, David, M. Britton, P. Seed, F.C. Martin, and A.H. Hopper. Development and evaluation of evidence based risk assessment tool (STRATIFY) to predict which elderly inpatients will fall: Case-control and cohort studies. *BMJ* 315, no. 7115 (1997): 1049–1053.

Panero, Julius and Martin Zelnik. *Human dimension and interior space: A source book of design reference standards.* New York: Whitney Library of Design, 1979.

Papaioannou, Alexandra, William Parkinson, Richard Cook, Nicole Ferko, Esther Coker, and Jonathan D. Adachi. Prediction of falls using a risk assessment tool in the acute care setting. *BMC Medicine* 2, no. 1 (2004): 1.

Parker, Martyn J., William J. Gillespie, and Lesley D. Gillespie. Hip protectors for preventing hip fractures in older people. *Cochrane Database of Systematic Reviews* 3 (2005).

Raz, Tzvi, and Matthew F. Baretich. Factors affecting the incidence of patient falls in hospitals. *Medical Care* 25, no. 3 (1987): 185–195.

Reason, James. Human error: Models and management. *BMJ* 320, no. 7237 (2000): 768–770.

Robinovitch, Stephen N., Elizabeth T. Hsiao, Reuben Sandler, Jeff Cortez, Qi Liu, and Guy D. Paiement. Prevention of falls and fall-related fractures through biomechanics. *Exercise and Sport Sciences Reviews* 28, no. 2 (2000): 74–79.

Rubemstein, Laurence Z., Karen R. Josephson, and Dan Osterweil. Falls and fall prevention in the nursing home. *Clinics in Geriatric Medicine* 12, no. 4 (1996): 881–902.

Schultz, Albert B. Mobility impairment in the elderly: Challenges for biomechanics research. *Journal of Biomechanics* 25, no. 5 (1992): 519–528.

Schwendimann, René, Hugo Bühler, Sabina De Geest, and Koen Milisen. Characteristics of hospital inpatient falls across clinical departments. *Gerontology* 54, no. 6 (2008): 342–348.

Schwendimann, René, Hugo Bühler, Sabina De Geest, and Koen Milisen. Falls and consequent injuries in hospitalized patients: Effects of an interdisciplinary falls prevention program. *BMC Health Services Research* 6, no. 1 (2006): 69–76.

Silvia, Chris E., Donald S. Bloswick, Dean Lillquist, David Wallace, and Michael S. Perkins. An ergonomic comparison between mechanical and manual patient transfer techniques. *Work: A Journal of Prevention, Assessment and Rehabilitation* 19, no. 1 (2002): 19–34.

Sixsmith, Andrew, and Neil Johnson. A smart sensor to detect the falls of the elderly. *Pervasive Computing, IEEE* 3, no. 2 (2004): 42–47.

Tideiksaar, Rein. *Falling in Old Age: Its Prevention and Treatment.* New York: Springer, 1989.

Tinetti, Mary E., T. Franklin Williams, and Raymond Mayewski. Fall risk index for elderly patients based on number of chronic disabilities. *The American Journal of Medicine* 80, no. 3 (1986): 429–434.

Todd, J. Ferlo, Constance E. Ruhl, and Thomas P. Gross. Injury and death associated with hospital bed side-rails: Reports to the US Food and Drug Administration from 1985 to 1995. *American Journal of Public Health* 87, no. 10 (1997): 1675–1677.

Tzeng, Huey-Ming, and Chang-Yi Yin. Adding additional grab bars as a possible strategy for safer hospital stays. *Applied Nursing Research* 23, (2010): 45–51.

Tzeng, Huey-Ming, Chang-Yi Yin, and J. Grunawalt. Effective assessment of use of sitters by nurses in inpatient care settings. *Journal of Advanced Nursing* 64, no. 2 (2008): 176–183.

Udén, Giggi, Margareta Ehnfors, and Kerstin Sjöström. Use of initial risk assessment and recording as the main nursing intervention in identifying risk of falls. *Journal of Advanced Nursing* 29, no. 1 (1999): 145–152.

Vassallo, Michael, Raj Vignaraja, Jagdish C. Sharma, Roger Briggs, and Stephen C. Allen. Predictors for falls among hospital inpatients with impaired mobility. *Journal of the Royal Society of Medicine* 97, no. 6 (2004): 266–269.

Verhagen, Arianne P., Monique Immink, Annemieke van der Meulen, and Sita M.A. Bierma-Zeinstra. The efficacy of Tai Chi Chuan in older adults: A systematic review. *Family Practice* 21, no. 1 (2004): 107–113.

Vlahov, David, A. H. Myers, and M. S. Al-Ibrahim. Epidemiology of falls among patients in a rehabilitation hospital. *Archives of Physical Medicine and Rehabilitation* 71, no. 1 (1990): 8–12.

Von Rentein-Kruse, Von, and Tom Krause. Incidence of in-hospital falls in geriatric patients before and after the introduction of an interdisciplinary team–based fall-prevention intervention. *Journal of the American Geriatrics Society* 55, no. 12 (2007): 2068–2074.

Winter, David A., Aftab E. Patla, James S. Frank, and Sharon E. Walt. Biomechanical walking pattern changes in the fit and healthy elderly. *Physical Therapy* 70, no. 6 (1990): 340–347.

Wojcik, Laura A., Darryl G. Thelen, Albert B. Schultz, James A. Ashton-Miller, and Neil B. Alexander. Age and gender differences in peak lower extremity joint torques and ranges of motion used during single-step balance recovery from a forward fall. *Journal of Biomechanics* 34, no. 1 (2001): 67–73.

Woodson, Wesley E. *Human Factors Design Handbook*. New York: McGraw-Hill, 1981.

Yauk, S., A. Hopkins, C.D. Phillips, S. Terrell, J. Bennon, and M. Riggs. Predicting in-hospital falls: Development of the Scott and While Falls Risk screener. *Journal of Nursing Care Quality* 20, no. 2, (2005): 128–133.

Zijlstra, G. A., Jolanda Van Haastregt, Erik Van Rossum, Jacques Th M. Van Eijk, Lucy Yardley, and Gertrudis IJM Kempen. Interventions to reduce fear of falling in community-living older people: A systematic review. *Journal of the American Geriatrics Society* 55, no. 4 (2007): 603–615.

21

Slips, Trips, and Falls in the Firefighting Community

David Hostler and Gavin Horn

CONTENTS

ABSTRACT This chapter reviews the incidence, costs, and factors associated with slips, trips, and falls among firefighters. There are known extrinsic factors associated with firefighter injuries that result from slips, trips, and falls, including issues with the protective ensemble and the firefighting environment. Individual characteristics such as firefighter age, fitness, and body habitus may influence the risk of suffering a slip, trip, or fall and are primary areas for future investigation.

KEY WORDS: *firefighter, rescue, personal protective clothing, self-contained breathing apparatus, bunker gear, turnout gear.*

21.1 Introduction

Firefighting is an inherently dangerous occupation that inflicts physical and mental strain on the individual worker. Slips, trips, and falls are a common cause of injury among firefighters. While there have been studies examining the potential causes of slips, trips, and falls and their relationship with firefighting equipment, there has been little progress in reducing the incidence of slips, trips, and falls among firefighters. In this chapter, we provide the background on slips, trips, and falls in the fire service, and an overview of firefighters, their tools, and the fire environment (Section 21.1), what is known about the relationship between heat stress/fatigue, protective equipment, and the risk of slips, trips, and falls (Section 21.2), future areas of investigation still needed to reduce the incidence of slip, trip, and fall injuries in the fire service (Section 21.3), and a theoretical model of these injuries among firefighters (Section 21.4).

21.1.1 Slips, Trips, and Falls among Firefighters

Injuries suffered by a firefighter while wearing protective garments and breathing apparatus can be devastating and costly. Falls, jumps, and slips are typically the first or second largest category of firefighter injuries in the United States (Karter and Molis, 2013). For moderate and severe fireground injuries, this category accounts for the largest number, typically one out of every three injuries (Karter, 2013).

21.1.1.1 Incidence

The most recent reports from the National Fire Protection Association (NFPA) identified two fall-related fatalities (Fahy et al., 2013) and that falls, jumps, and slips comprised 23.2% of all firefighter injuries in 2012 (Karter and Molis, 2013). Fall-related fatalities are typically due to falling from a ladder or the sudden collapse of a structure with the firefighter working on the roof or on a disintegrating floor within (Hodous et al., 2004). Studies reporting injuries and fatalities typically use federal databases such as the National Fire Incident Reporting System (NFIRS) or local Workman's Compensation databases. It is likely that these, and similar databases, underestimate the true number of slips, trips, and falls among firefighters, since they do not include incidents that were not reported.

A survey of slip and fall experience among firefighters was conducted through the Illinois Fire Service Institute (IFSI) (Petrucci et al., 2012). For these respondents, approximately 75% of the sample had experienced a slip or fall, and 80% indicated that they had witnessed a fellow firefighter experience a slip or fall at some point in their career. Respondents were asked to provide examples of slips or falls that they had experienced or witnessed from fellow firefighters, and these responses were grouped and categorized. The most common cause was slips on ice and wet surfaces, followed by tripping over obstacles such as hose lines and objects on the ground. The third most common source was falling from apparatus or stairs.

21.1.1.2 Cost

The costs associated with an on-duty injury affect the firefighter and their family, the employer, and the insurer. As many as 20% of fall-related injuries result in missed work. One study examined an 8 year cohort of workman's compensation claims from a single insurer covering 77 municipalities (Walton et al., 2003). In a cohort of 13,680, 9.8% of the firefighters filed claims in the reporting period. While slips, trips, and falls only accounted for 13% of the total claims, the mean cost per claim was $8662, and the maximum claim was $174,394. Using these figures, eliminating this category of claim would save approximately $110 per covered firefighter each year.

21.1.2 Firefighting Environment

The firefighting environment provides ample opportunities for slips, trips, and falls among firefighters. While fire suppression is the activity most often perceived by the public when considering firefighters, the modern fire service includes caring for injured and ill patients, calls for public assistance (to check alarms, lift fallen citizens, etc.), hazardous materials mitigation, and technical and heavy rescue. In certain areas, firefighters may also be tasked with maritime fire suppression and rescue, and wildfire containment. While the total number of fires in the United States has declined significantly over the past 30 years, the injury rate has remained fairly constant at approximately 23 injuries per 1,000 fires. By comparison, the injury rate for non-fire emergencies is several orders of magnitude lower, approximately 0.42 per 1,000 incidents in 2012 (Karter and Molis, 2013).

In addition to emergency operations, firefighters must train for each of these activities using the same equipment and protective garments. While training activities are more controlled than emergency operations, injuries still occur (Thiel et al., 2003). Lastly, firefighters perform nonemergent duties such as building inspection, fire hydrant inspection, and equipment maintenance. Each of these activities requires the firefighter to be physically active and mobile, providing additional opportunities for slips, trips, and falls.

While injury rates have been reported to be similar among firefighters, law enforcement officers, and paramedics, the distribution of injury types differs among the agencies (Suyama et al., 2009). Incident-level risk factors associated with fireground injuries have also been reported (Fabio et al., 2002). Large fires (five or more alarms) (odds ratio [OR 3.85]; 95% confidence interval [CI], 3.32–4.48), structures higher than three stories (OR 2.49; 95% CI, 2.43–2.55), and the presence of at least one civilian injury (OR 3.69; 95% CI, 3.55–3.84) have each been associated with firefighter injury. Each of these risk factors is a relatively rare event for the individual firefighter, and may represent higher physical or emotional stress, which may predispose the firefighter to injury through either physical fatigue or cognitive strain.

21.1.3 Firefighting Personal Protective Equipment (PPE) and Tools

Although the progenitor of the modern fire helmet dates back to at least 1836, protective garments for firefighters changed little till World War II, when the NFPA first published documents that would evolve into the Standard on Protective Ensembles for Structural Fire Fighting and Proximity Fire Fighting (NFPA, 1971) (Lamb, 2014). Although structural firefighting gear is continuously evolving, the modern ensemble consists of a heavy pants/coat combination comprised of a flame-resistant outer layer, a moisture barrier, and an insulating layer to protect the wearer from heat, smoke, flames, and water (Figure 21.1). A flame-resistant hood is worn under an impact-resistant helmet to encapsulate the head and neck. The protective ensemble is completed with heavy steel-toed boots and thick fire-resistant gloves. This PPE is worn over a base layer that might vary significantly based on environmental conditions and departmental policies but can significantly impact the fit of the PPE, the range of motion limitations, and the development of heat stress during work.

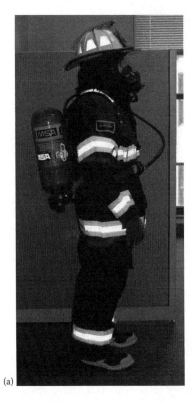
(a)

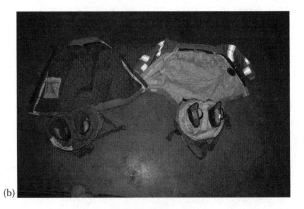
(b)

FIGURE 21.1
The firefighter protective ensemble: (a) breathing apparatus and (b) individual garments (coat, pants, boots).

Specifications for the firefighting PPE ensemble are completed following a complex risk–benefit analysis. Use of the PPE ensemble protects the firefighter from the environment but levies an important physiologic burden. While all PPE used by firefighters must comply with a standard set by the NFPA, some variation is allowed. Fire departments may specify an ensemble that emphasizes thermal protection. This gear will be thicker and bulkier, which inflicts additional metabolic strain while working and may reduce mobility. Reducing thermal protection to favor heat loss from within the ensemble may reduce bulk and metabolic load but exposes the wearer to higher ambient heat loads during fire suppression.

Multiple studies have reported adverse effects on mobility and performance when wearing the firefighting ensemble (Saul and Jaffe, 1955; Adams and Keyserling, 1993, 1995; Huck, 1988, 1991; Smith and Petruzzello, 1998; Coca et al., 2010). The full ensemble reduces exercise tolerance by as much as 56%, with the largest effect per kilogram of worn mass from the boots (Taylor et al., 2012). Use of firefighting PPE has been shown to alter gait and balance among firefighters (Turner et al., 2010; Park et al., 2011; Kong et al., 2012; Hur et al., 2013).

The most common form of respiratory protection worn with structural firefighting gear is the self-contained breathing apparatus (SCBA). The SCBA ensures a positive pressure air supply from a cylinder worn on a backpack-style frame to the firefighter's mask and is worn by the firefighter any time he or she is exposed to an immediately dangerous to life or health (IDLH) environment. Cylinder size varies, and work time typically ranges from

10 to 45 minutes on a single cylinder based on activity, cylinder size, and firefighter fitness. Commercially available systems are sold as "30 min," "45 min" and "60 min" cylinders (with a recent introduction of "75 min" cylinders) based on the assumed consumption rate of 42.5 L/min. Modern SCBA cylinders are constructed from carbon fiber wrapped around an aluminum core, but other material systems such as fiberglass, aluminum, and steel bottles are still in use. The air containment system is pressurized depending on the design of the SCBA system, with 4500 psi currently the most common.

Firefighters employ various tools during fire suppression and rescue, which may influence slips, trips, and falls (reviewed in Rosengren et al., 2014). Among the tools commonly used are striking tools (e.g., ax, maul) and prying tools (e.g., Halligan bar) to force entry into structures, cutting tools (e.g., power saw) to breach a roof and cut through structural members, long hooks to pull down ceiling and wall boards, and charged hose lines to extinguish fires. The typical mass of a tool varies from 3.5 to 11 kg. Common fire hose diameters used for extinguishment range from 2.5 to 6.4 cm. When pressurized, the hose lines are difficult to maneuver, often requiring—two or three firefighters to advance into a structure. Tools may have to be carried over long distances, up and down flights of stairs, and over and around many obstacles and slippery surfaces on the fireground. When carried, these items asymmetrically load the firefighter (both anterior–posterior and medial–lateral asymmetry) during deployment and potentially contribute to slips, trips, and falls.

21.1.4 Individual Firefighter Characteristics Related to Slips, Trips, and Falls

Among the individual characteristics typically studied in relation to risk of slips, trips, and falls among firefighters are age, experience, fitness, and body mass (reviewed in Kong et al., 2013). For each of these factors, there are relatively few studies among firefighters and little agreement between those experiments.

21.1.4.1 Age and Experience

Although this is not universal, age and experience tend to co-vary within the fire service. Experience per se has rarely been reported to be a factor associated with falls. One study of Polish firefighters reported that less than 1 year of fire service experience was associated with an increased risk of injury (Szubert and Sobala, 2002). It is not clear what proportion of those injuries were fall related, but we would hypothesize that less experience with heavy and bulky firefighting garments and tools could increase the risk of slips, trips, and falls among inexperienced firefighters. This is supported by a study demonstrating that firefighters are more reliable than non-firefighters in testing PPE with current test methods (Son et al., 2014).

Although there are more reports in the literature, the association between age and risk of falls among firefighters is equally unclear. One study that examined 1041 accident reports from a Canadian firefighter cohort reported that falls were most common among firefighters aged 40–44 years (Cloutier and Champoux, 2000). Liao et al. (2001) found that older firefighters suffered longer injury duration but were less likely to suffer a severe injury. On the other hand, a case–control study of 1200 firefighters failed to find any association between age and risk of falls when controlling for factors such as SCBA use, role on the fireground, and incident type (Heineman et al., 1989). Given the evolution of SCBA building materials, however, those findings may be less relevant 25 years later.

A study of Finnish firefighters reported that age was associated with postural sway but not functional balance (Punakallio et al., 2003). In a subsequent study by the same group, older firefighters experienced as many slips as their younger counterparts when walking on a contaminated surface, but their slips tended to be longer and more serious (Punakallio et al., 2005). The inconsistent findings among different tests and the lack of association between age and the risk of falls in the two studies by Punakallio et al. (2003, 2005) may be due, in part, to insufficient age differentiation between the younger (33–38 year) and older (43–56 year) groups.

21.1.4.2 Fitness

It has been reported that there are age-related changes in cardiovascular fitness, strength, and power among firefighters that are independent of body mass (Walker et al., 2014). The connection between fitness and risk of slips, trips, and falls is not clear. One study of functional balance among 23 male firefighters reported that subjects performing regular physical fitness training committed fewer errors on a test of functional balance and completed the task more quickly than sedentary firefighters (Kong et al., 2013). In contrast, another study using the same functional balance test failed to identify better performance among firefighters with greater muscular strength or muscular endurance (Punakallio et al., 2005).

21.2 What Is Known about Gait and Balance among Firefighters

Reports examining the causes of slips, trips, and falls in the fire service are sparse. It is generally accepted that slips, trips, and falls among firefighters are caused by perturbations of gait or balance and that alterations of gait and balance are the product of fatigue, heat stress, PPE, and the environment (Kong et al., 2013; Rosengren et al., 2014). While the fireground environment can be a significant contributor to slips, trips, and falls, it is the one component of the injury calculus that is difficult to control for on any given response. Therefore, studies examining gait and balance among firefighters have concentrated on physiology and PPE. The prospective studies in this area tend to be small or narrowly focused on a particular element of the ensemble. This section reviews those studies examining the role of heat stress and fatigue on gait and balance and the studies examining the protective ensemble.

21.2.1 Studies Directly Examining the Role of Heat Stress/ Fatigue in Firefighter Gait and Balance

Fire suppression results in cardiovascular strain and fatigue (Von Heimburg et al., 2006; Colburn et al., 2011; Fahs et al., 2011; Horn et al., 2011; Fernhall et al., 2012). Physical fatigue impairs balance control in healthy adults, as demonstrated by greater postural sway and measured by center of pressure (COP) displacements (Seliga et al., 1991; Pendergrass et al., 2003). Three studies have investigated various aspects of gait and balance following heat stress in the firefighting ensemble. Kong et al. (2010) investigated the effect of fatigue and hypohydration on gait characteristics during walking in the heat while wearing firefighter thermal protective clothing. In this study, the spatiotemporal variables, variability, and left–right symmetry of 19 subjects were compared at the beginning and end of a 50 min treadmill exercise in a heated room. Gait variability of the double-support time increased at the end of exercise, but no change was observed for other variables. It is possible that spatiotemporal gait characteristics and symmetry while wearing firefighting equipment are insensitive to physiological fatigue but prolonged walking in heat while wearing firefighting equipment increases gait variability and therefore the likelihood of a fall. Park et al. (2011) used an 8 m instrumented gait mat with a 30 cm obstacle in the path to measure gait parameters and obstacle-crossing safety before and after an 18 min bout of firefighting activities in a live-fire training structure. A significant reduction in obstacle clearance and an increase in obstacle-crossing errors were measured after completing the simulated firefighting activities, suggesting an increase in risk for trips after typical physiological fatigue that might be experienced on the fireground. Hur et al. (2013) employed a functional balance test based on that proposed by Punakallio (2004) and found that following this same simulated firefighting activity, the time to complete the task increased but the number of errors decreased, intimating that firefighters may trade off speed and accuracy depending on perceived threat to balance safety.

The effect of heat stress on balance and risk of falls among firefighters has only been sparsely addressed in the literature (Kong et al., 2010). Exercising in hot environments while wearing PPE leads to compromised physiological performance in a subsequent bout of work (Hostler et al., 2010a, 2010b; Selkirk and McLellan, 2004; Selkirk et al., 2004). Dehydration of approximately 1 kg has also been shown to occur after a relatively short period of exercise in PPE (Hostler et al., 2010b; Colburn et al., 2011; Horn et al., 2011). Exertional heat stress magnifies cardiovascular strain and worsens dehydration, but it is not known whether high body temperatures per se alter gait and balance. In aggregate, these data suggest that the risk of slips, trips, and falls among firefighters increases with the duration of the incident, as both fatigue and the magnitude of dehydration increase.

21.2.2 Studies Examining the Effect of the Protective Ensemble on Gait and Balance

There is a perception among firefighters that the protective clothing ensemble worn during fire suppression increases the risk of a slip, trip, or fall. In Petrucci et al. (2012), only 6% of surveyed firefighters indicated that they did not feel the gear had any effect, while 32% felt that firefighting PPE "severely affected" their balance. The respondents felt that the SCBA most severely hindered their ability to recover balance, but the protective clothing ensemble was rated as providing a slight hindrance. Responses to the effect of footwear had the largest variance, with more than 80% of the respondents indicating that their footwear had some effect (almost equally positive or negative) on their ability to regain balance.

21.2.2.1 Effect of Firefighting PPE on Biomechanics

Firefighting PPE also adds to the metabolic work that must be performed to complete a task, and interferes with heat dissipation because of encapsulation. Thus, wearing PPE compounds issues related to heat stress and fatigue when working in a hot environment. The specific design of firefighting PPE (bunker gear versus traditional long coat–style PPE) can influence thermal and cardiovascular strain in a laboratory setting and time to complete a firefighting task during a live-fire training evolution (Smith et al., 1995; Smith and Petruzzello, 1998). Other studies have investigated the effects of specific design elements of modern firefighting PPE, including the effect of conventional versus chem/bio prototype PPE (Coca et al., 2008; Williams et al., 2011).

Changes in balance due to wearing various types of PPE have been studied by quantifying postural sway during standing balance tests (Punakallio et al.,2003; Kincl et al., 2002; Sobeih et al., 2006; Hur et al., 2008); these studies have found mixed results when applied to firefighting PPE, as two studies reported an increase in postural sway on donning heavier firefighting PPE (Punakallio et al.,2003; Hur et al., 2008), while another study suggested a reduction in sway after donning PPE (Sobeih et al., 2006). Postural sway measurements may be less valuable than other tests when examining the effect of PPE on balance. One potential response to static balance in PPE would be to activate the lower limb and core muscles to compensate for the additional load, which could reduce postural sway in firefighters, especially if measured without SCBA. A functional balance test developed for firefighters (Punakallio, 2004) has also provided mixed results in the literature, but studies generally agree that adding SCBA to the PPE ensemble impairs functional balance (Punakallio et al., 2003; Kong et al., 2012). A similar functional balance test was employed to show a significant increase in the number of errors and time to complete the task after donning firefighting PPE when compared with completing the task wearing just base-layer clothing (Hur et al., 2013).

Data on the effects of wearing PPE on gait and mobility are clearer. Wearing PPE decreases both uphill walking speed and endurance (Louhevaara et al., 1995). Additionally, wearing PPE while walking on a slippery laboratory surface significantly increases fall risk (Punakallio et al., 2005) Park et al. (2011) reported an increased risk of tripping during obstacle crossing with firefighting PPE when compared with wearing just base-layer clothing. The increased risk for slips, trips, and falls may be attributed to a reduction in mobility caused by wearing PPE (Huck, 1991; Coca et al., 2010) and changes in firefighter center of mass caused by the additional weight and its distribution on the body (Hur et al., 2008).

21.2.2.2 Effect of Firefighting SCBA on Biomechanics

Wearing SCBA has been found to negatively impact physical performance (Louhevaara et al., 1984, 1985, 1995; Heineman et al., 1989; Huck, 1991; Hooper et al., 2001; Punakallio et al., 2003; Park et al., 2010; Kong et al., 2012). The addition of SCBA to the protective ensemble increases fatigue (Louhevaara et al., 1985), reduces maximal exercising time and maximal inclined walking speed (Louhevaara et al., 1995), and decreases postural and functional balance (Punakallio et al., 2003; Kong et al., 2012). Heineman et al. (1989) found that continual use of SCBA was significantly associated with fall occurrences among firefighters. The SCBA commonly used during that study period was considerably heavier than modern designs and this finding has not been reported again in the literature.

Louhevaara and coauthors suggest that it is most important to decrease the mass of SCBA to improve a firefighter's ability to safely conduct firefighting tasks (Louhevaara et al., 1995). To this end, several groups have studied the physiological effects of SCBA weight, showing that lightweight SCBA and novel harness designs result in lower energy expenditure during submaximal exercise (Hooper et al., 2001; Bakri et al., 2012). Results during live firefighting exercises, however, have been mixed. In one study, there was no difference in heart rates attained with lighter SCBA (Manning and Griggs, 1983). This may be due to the elevated heart rates commonly encountered during firefighting activity, or because energy expenditure during live firefighting activities is not reflected by the heart rate achieved. However, Manning and Griggs pointed out that the benefit of lighter SCBA is most likely to be seen as a reduced time to complete a given task as opposed to a reduced physiological load (Manning and Griggs, 1983). A more recent study examining a lighter SCBA paired with a novel rucksack design reported that simulated firefighting skills were performed more quickly with lower heart rates when wearing the new design (Griefahn et al., 2003).

Park et al. (2010) studied the effect of SCBA design in the context of carbon fiber versus aluminum cylinders and found that lighter designs result in lower anterior–posterior and vertical ground reaction forces and fewer obstacle contacts during obstacle-crossing trials, suggesting significantly reduced risk for slips and trips in lighter-weight SCBA (Park et al., 2010). Increased postural sway has also been reported with heavier SCBA cylinders when compared with lighter SCBA (Hur et al., 2008). Love et al. (1994) found that SCBA with a lower moment of inertia was rated as more comfortable based on questionnaire data. On the other hand, no difference was measured in any gait parameter (Park et al., 2010) or postural sway measure (Hur et al., 2008) between two different bottles of the same weight, yet different shapes that would significantly affect the center of mass.

21.2.2.3 The Effects of Firefighting Boot Design on Gait and Balance

It has been reported that under steady-state conditions, firefighting boots exert the greatest relative metabolic impact during walking and bench stepping when compared with the remainder of the PPE ensemble (Taylor et al., 2012). The magnitude of the effect was so large that the investigators reported that removing 100 g of mass from each boot would be metabolically equivalent to reducing the SCBA mass by 1.74 kg.

Fire boots approved for use in the United States tend to be 20–40 cm high, contain a steel toe, and are made of leather, rubber, aramid fibers such as Kevlar, or a hybrid combination of these materials (Figure 21.2). Leather/Kevlar boots are more expensive and more difficult to decontaminate/clean, but are lighter and believed to provide better support. A study of 25 men and 25 women comparing leather and rubber boots while exercising in PPE reported that increasing boot weight tended to increase minute ventilation, heart rate, oxygen consumption, and carbon dioxide production (Turner et al., 2010). The results were not entirely consistent across exercise conditions (treadmill walking vs. step climber) but overall indicated that heavier boots imparted higher metabolic costs that would decrease the allowable work interval due to increased SCBA air consumption. The magnitude of this effect was lower among female subjects. The investigators hypothesized that the larger burden of the entire ensemble (42% of the women's body mass versus 33% of the men's body mass) may have masked the effect of the boots among the female subjects. Another study comparing leather and rubber boots among 12 career firefighters performing a step mill test did not identify differences in heart rate or oxygen consumption responses

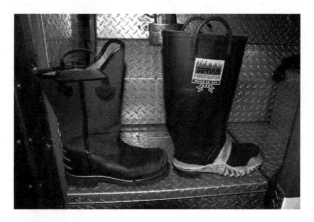

FIGURE 21.2
Hybrid leather/synthetic fire boot (left) compared with rubber fire boot (right).

between the two conditions (Huang et al., 2009). However, the subjects in that study wore a weight vest to simulate a load but did not wear any other portion of the PPE ensemble.

Heavier boots require greater muscular strength when stepping over obstacles. One study examined 13 female and 14 male firefighters who walked for 5 min, stepping over low and high obstacles while wearing a full firefighting PPE ensemble. Subjects wore leather, rubber, and hybrid (leather upper with rubber lower) boots with soles classified as more or less flexible (Chiou et al., 2012). Increased boot weight reduced trailing toe clearance when crossing the high (30 cm) obstacle and increased oxygen consumption. Lateral displacement of the foot increased near the end of the 5 min walk when compared with the beginning of the task. Lastly, more flexible soles decreased oxygen consumption.

21.3 Future Research Needs

The literature related to slip, trip, and fall risk and intervention studies in the fire service is relatively sparse. While data and information have been adopted from other occupational groups and the military and applied to the fire service, fire suppression is a unique scenario of aerobic and anaerobic physical exertion accompanied by heat stress, dehydration, and activation of the sympathetic nervous system. Most studies of gait and balance among firefighters have either manipulated the PPE ensemble or fatigued subjects wearing a standardized ensemble. Future studies should examine the interaction of heat stress and fatigue with PPE interventions such as modified SCBA or boot designs. The unique nature of firefighting activities also provides a set of challenges that must be studied in settings that replicate the fireground conditions using real firefighting equipment and tools.

21.3.1 Role of Physical Fitness and Training in Prevention

Despite the strenuous nature of firefighting operations, the average fitness level of a typical firefighter is not necessarily different from that of the general public who make up the fire service. The need to improve firefighter fitness has been identified as a necessity to reduce firefighter injuries (Storer et al., 2014). While the role of fitness in slip and fall risk has not been studied directly, it is promising that firefighters who report regular fitness training committed fewer errors on a functional balance task (Kong et al., 2012).

While many firefighters have suggested that training would improve their balance, only 16% of firefighter respondents of the Petrucci et al. (2012) survey indicated that they had received specific training to minimize slips and falls while wearing their PPE. Awareness-level training regarding the risks of slips and falls can be easily incorporated into recruit training to raise the level of understanding of the magnitude of this issue among firefighters. Other targeted interventions such as Tai Chi or strengthening specific muscle groups may provide useful in the context of injury prevention in the fire service (Ramachandran et al., 2007; Yang et al., 2007).

21.3.2 Ergonomics of SCBA and PPE

Changes to firefighting PPE technology and standards are often driven by the need for improved protection as well as the identified demand for reduction in heat stress.

Oftentimes, these improvements are considered individually and focusing on a specific concern without a holistic view of additional impacts. For example, there has recently been a significant increase in the purchase and use of larger SCBA air cylinders that hold more air. Anecdotally, this is attributed to concerns about running out of air, which may result in risk of asphyxiation. However, each year, more than an order of magnitude more firefighters are injured by slips, trips, and falls than by exposure to fumes, gases, or smoke (Karter, 2013). Louhevaara (1984) found that nearly all of the physiological strain caused by firefighting SCBA can be attributed to weight, which increases with the use of longer-duration SCBA cylinders, potentially increasing the risk for the former category of injuries.

There have been very few scientific studies on the interaction between firefighting activity and PPE or SCBA design on firefighter balance and gait. Thus, it is imperative to advance our understanding of the effect of PPE and SCBA design on slip, trip, and fall risk and safety of movement on the fireground.

21.3.3 Role of Situational Awareness in Slips, Trips, and Falls

Situational awareness can be defined as being aware of what is happening in the current scenario and understanding how one's actions may impact achieving a particular goal. Poor or inadequate situational awareness is thought to be a major factor in accidents attributed to human error (Hartel et al., 1991; Nullmeyer et al., 2005). It is important to understand how wearing PPE may influence decision-making as a firefighter operates on the fireground. Wearing PPE with different profiles will influence how effectively a firefighter moves about a cluttered and visually challenging environment. For example, it has been shown that individuals wearing SCBA often make contact with an overhead obstacle when they would not have done so without PPE, suggesting that they misjudged the size of the opening that they would be able to pass through (Hur et al., 2013) (Figure 21.3).Thus, safety on the fireground is significantly impacted by situational awareness. However, no research exists on the effect of metabolic stress and fatigue from firefighting activity on situational awareness and subsequent risks for slips, trips, and falls.

21.3.3.1 Role of Personality/Individual Traits in Slips, Trips, and Falls

The relationship between injury risk and personality traits may provide a fruitful area for future research. Firefighters must have a personality that is willing to accept a certain level of risk in their work environment due to the inherent nature of the job. That level of risk may change based on the situation (e.g., accepting greater risk to rescue a life vs. saving property). It is possible, however, that specific personality traits may predispose certain firefighters to experience more slips, trips, and falls. Liao et al. (2001) found that the psychopathic deviancy scores of the Minnesota Multiphasic Personality prospectively predicted higher rates of worker compensation claims over a 10 year period.

Understanding the role of personality traits in experiencing slips, trips, and falls in the fire service has several practical applications. Information about personality can be used to target training by focusing on those individuals who are more likely to experience slips, trips, and falls. Knowledge of the mediators of the relations between personality and work injury may also provide opportunities for targeted interventions that will decrease the likelihood of injury. Presumably, interventions targeted at these factors may help to inoculate certain individuals from experiencing slips, trips, and falls and therefore lead to a reduction in injuries.

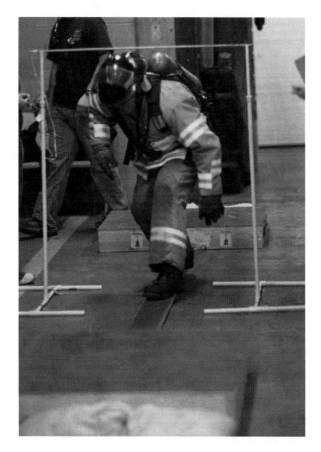

FIGURE 21.3
Test of overhead obstacle clearance while wearing protective clothing and breathing apparatus.

21.3.4 Role of Different "Firefighter" Tasks in Falls (Suppression and Non-Fire Activities)

While much can be learned from studying the effects of firefighting PPE on balance and gait in controlled laboratory conditions using functional balance tests, slip length measurements, and obstacle-crossing abilities, it is equally valuable to study the combined effects of firefighting PPE and firefighting activities on risk for slips, trips, and falls. The design of PPE and SCBA can significantly affect full body biomechanics and must be studied in a holistic manner. Furthermore, activities outside traditional firefighting must be considered, as more than half of firefighter injuries occur at locations other than the fireground.

21.4 Theoretical Model for Slips, Trips, and Falls among Firefighters

The current body of knowledge leads us to propose a model for the interaction of fatigue, equipment, and incident duration. It also allows investigators to thoughtfully design studies based on where in the model they are trying to affect.

We propose that there is a baseline risk for slips, trips, and falls. The connection between gear/boot design/SCBA configuration and slip, trip, and fall risk is clear even among rested individuals. The largest single contributor to baseline risk, in terms of gear, may be the SCBA and its effect on the center of gravity. Although lighter materials are being used to construct the SCBA cylinders, the basic design of modern SCBA is largely unchanged since its inception, and there is a secular trend for fire departments to purchase larger cylinders, negating the benefit of lighter materials. Future studies of SCBA design (e.g., worn weight distribution) and fitness to use breathing apparatus are needed. For example, studies have shown improved running endurance among athletes and improved performance among divers when using the related self-contained underwater breathing apparatus (SCUBA) after respiratory muscle training (Pendergast et al., 2006; Uemura et al., 2012; Held and Pendergast, 2014). Design of fire boots should be reconsidered with an emphasis on reducing boot mass, enhancing protection of the foot and ankle mortise, and increasing comfort.

The contributions of age, fitness, and experience to the baseline risk of slips, trips, and falls are less clear but theoretically should modify risk, based on work in other areas. Overweight and obese construction workers (body mass index [BMI] ≥ 26 kg m^{-2}) experience more frequent falls than their normal-weight counterparts (Chau et al., 2004). Obesity is also associated with reduced back and core muscular endurance in firefighters, which may increase the risk of musculoskeletal injuries, with a higher risk of job disability in firefighters (Soteriades et al., 2008; Poston et al., 2011; Mayer et al., 2012; Jahnke et al., 2013). Lastly, there is an association between obesity and ankle sprain severity, which is particularly concerning given the risk of slips, trips, and falls among firefighters (King et al., 2012).

Increasing age is associated with reduced performance and increased fall risk in age brackets well beyond the career of most firefighters (Maki et al., 1994; Vellas et al., 1997; Pajala et al., 2008). It is not known whether firefighters in their fourth and fifth decades suffer declines in balance when wearing protective garments. If decrements do occur in middle age, it is possible that physical fitness or balance training may compensate. Additional investigations in these areas are needed to determine their effect on slip, trip, and fall risk among firefighters and to identify appropriate interventions.

Risks for slips, trips, and falls on the fireground increase with the duration of the incident and are likely related to physical and cognitive fatigue. The baseline impediments created by boot mass, protective garments, SCBA, and asymmetric tool carriage may become more pronounced later in the incident as the firefighter continues to fatigue. The individual contributions of dehydration and hyperthermia are not well understood. Hydration status and core temperature can be partially corrected on the fireground, but physical and cognitive recovery may be delayed for hours (Hostler et al., 2010b; Horn et al., 2011; Morley et al., 2012; Greenlee et al., 2014). Physical fatigue may distract the firefighter, and cognitive fatigue may decrease situational awareness. If fatigue is a significant driver of slip, trip, and fall risk, it will be important to optimize recovery strategies or consider rotating crews more frequently during peak service times.

In conclusion, slips, trips, and falls remain a significant cause of injury and disability in the fire service. Few studies are available to advance our understanding of the cause for many slips, trips, and falls, making it difficult to formulate policies or drive changes in equipment design.

References

Adams PS, Keyserling WM. (1993) Three methods for measuring range of motion while wearing protective clothing: A comparative study. *Int J Ind Ergon* 12:177–91.

Adams PS, Keyserling WM. (1995) The effect of size and fabric weight of protective coveralls on range of gross body motions. *Am Ind Hyg Assoc J* 56(4):333–40.

Bakri I, Lee JY, Nakao K, Wakabayashi H, Tochihara Y. (2012) Effects of firefighters' self-contained breathing apparatus' weight and its harness design on the physiological and subjective responses. *Ergonomics* 55:782–91.

Chau N, Gauchard GC, Siegfried C, Benamghar L, Dangelzer JL, Français M, Jacquin R, Sourdot A, Perrin PP, Mur JM. (2004) Relationships of job, age, and life conditions with the causes and severity of occupational injuries in construction workers. *Int Arch Occup Environ Health* 77:60–6.

Chiou SS, Turner N, Zwiener J, Weaver DL, Haskell WE. (2012) Effect of boot weight and sole flexibility on gait and physiological responses of firefighters in stepping over obstacles. *Hum Factors* 54:373–86.

Cloutier E, Champoux D. (2000) Injury risk profile and aging among Québec firefighters. *Int J Ind Ergon* 25:513–23.

Coca A, Roberge R, Shepherd A, Powell JB, Stull JO, Williams WJ. (2008) Ergonomic comparison of a chem/bio prototype firefighter ensemble and a standard ensemble. *Eur J Appl Physiol* 104:351–9.

Coca A, Williams WJ, Roberge RJ, Powell JB. (2010) Effects of fire fighter protective ensembles on mobility and performance. *Appl Ergon* 41:636–41.

Colburn D, Suyama J, Reis SE, Morley JL, Goss FL, Chen YF, Moore CG, Hostler D. (2011) A comparison of cooling techniques in firefighters after a live burn evolution. *Prehosp Emerg Care* 15:226–32.

Fabio A, Ta M, Strotmeyer S, Li W, Schmidt E. (2002) Incident-level risk factors for firefighter injuries at structural fires. *J Occup Environ Med* 44:1059–63.

Fahs CA, Yan H, Ranadive S, Rossow LM, Agiovlasitis S, Echols G, Smith D, et al. (2011) Acute effects of firefighting on arterial stiffness and blood flow. *Vasc Med* 16:113–18.

Fahy RF, LeBlanc PR, Molis JL. (2013) Firefighter fatalities in the United States, 2012. *NFPA J* 107:65–73.

Fernhall B, Fahs CA, Horn GP, Rowland T, Smith D. (2012) Acute effects of firefighting on cardiac performance. *Eur J Appl Physiol* 112:735–41.

Greenlee TA, Horn G, Smith DL, Fahey G, Goldstein E, Petruzzello SJ. (2014) The influence of short-term firefighting activity on information processing performance. *Ergonomics* 57:764–73.

Griefahn B, Künemund C, Bröde P. (2003) Evaluation of performance and load in simulated rescue tasks for a novel design SCBA: Effect of weight, volume and weight distribution. *Appl Ergon* 34:157–65.

Hartel CEJ, Smith K, Prince C. (1991) Defining aircrew coordination: Searching mishaps for meaning. Paper presented at the 6th International Symposium on Aviation Psychology, Columbus, OH.

Heineman EF, Shy CM, Checkoway H. (1989) Injuries on the fireground: Risk factors for traumatic injuries among professional fire fighters. *Am J Ind Med* 15:267–82.

Held HE, Pendergast DR. (2014) The effects of respiratory muscle training on respiratory mechanics and energy cost. *Respir Physiol Neurobiol* 9;200C:7–17.

Hodous TK, Pizatella TJ, Braddee R, Castillo DN. (2004) Fire fighter fatalities 1998–2001: Overview with an emphasis on structure related traumatic fatalities. *Inj Prev* 10:222–6.

Hooper AJ, Crawford JO, Thomas D. (2001) An evaluation of physiological demands and comfort between the use of conventional and lightweight self-contained breathing apparatus. *Appl Ergon* 32:399–406.

Horn GP, Gutzmer S, Fahs CA, Petruzzello SJ, Goldstein E, Fahey GC, Fernhall B, Smith DL. (2011) Physiological recovery from firefighting activities in rehabilitation and beyond. *Prehosp Emerg Care* 15:214–25.

Hostler D, Bednez JC, Kerin S, Reis SE, Kong PW, Morley J, Gallagher M, Suyama J. (2010a) Comparison of rehydration regimens for rehabilitation of firefighters performing heavy exercise in thermal protective clothing: A report from the fireground rehab evaluation (FIRE) trial. *Prehosp Emerg Care* 14:194–201.

Hostler D, Reis SE, Bednez JC, Kerin S, Suyama J. (2010b) Comparison of active cooling devices with passive cooling for rehabilitation of firefighters performing exercise in thermal protective clothing: A report from the Fireground Rehab Evaluation (FIRE) trial. *Prehosp Emerg Care* 14:300–9.

Huang CJ, Garten RS, Wade C, Webb HE, Acevedo EO. (2009) Physiological responses to simulated stair climbing in professional firefighters wearing rubber and leather boots. *Eur J Appl Physiol* 107:163–8.

Huck J. (1988) Protective clothing systems: A technique for evaluating restriction of wearer mobility. *Appl Ergon* 19:185–95.

Huck J. (1991) Restriction to movement in fire-fighter protective clothing: Evaluation of alternative sleeves and liners. *Appl Ergon* 22:91–100.

Hur P, Rosengren KS, Horn GP, Schroeder T, Ashton-Szabo SE, Hsiao-Wecksler ET. (2008) Assessment of postural sway during multiple load and visual conditions. 17th Congress of the International Society of Electromyography and Kinesiology, Niagara Falls, Ontario, Canada.

Hur P, Rosengren KS, Horn GP, Smith DL, Hsiao-Wecksler ET. (2013) Effect of protective clothing and fatigue on functional balance of firefighters. *J Ergon* S2: 004.

Jahnke SA, Poston WS, Haddock CK, Jitnarin N. (2013) Obesity and incident injury among career firefighters in the central United States. *Obesity (Silver Spring)* 21:1505–8.

Karter Jr. MJ. (2013) Patterns of Firefighter Fireground Injuries. http://www.nfpa.org/~/media/files/research/nfpa%20reports/fire%20service%20statistics/ospatterns.pdf. Accessed 7 July 2014.

Karter Jr. MJ, Molis JL. (2013) U.S. Firefighter injuries in 2012. *NFPA J.* 107:60–7.

Kincl LD, Bhattacharya A, Succop PA, Clark CS. (2002) Postural sway measurements: A potential safety monitoring technique for workers wearing personal protective equipment. *Appl Occup Environ Hyg* 17:256–66.

King CM, Hamilton GA, Cobb M, Carpenter D, Ford LA. (2012) Association between ankle fractures and obesity. *J Foot Ankle Surg* 51:543–7.

Kong PW, Beauchamp G, Suyama J, Hostler D. (2010) Effect of fatigue and hypohydration on gait characteristics during treadmill exercise in the heat while wearing firefighter thermal protective clothing. *Gait Posture* 31:284–8.

Kong PW, Suyama J, Cham R, Hostler D. (2012) The relationship between physical activity and thermal protective clothing on functional balance in firefighters. *Res Q Exerc Sport* 83:546–52.

Kong PW, Suyama J, Hostler D. (2013) A review of risk factors of accidental slips, trips, and falls among firefighters. *Safety Sci* 60:203–9.

Lamb P. (2014) *The Fire Helmet.* www.petelamb.com/helmet/htm. Accessed 7 July 2014.

Liao H, Arvey RD, Butler RJ, Nutting SM. (2001) Correlates of work injury frequency and duration among firefighters. *J Occup Health Psychol* 6:229–42.

Louhevaara VA. (1984) Physiological effects associated with the use of respiratory protective devices. A review. *Scand J Work Environ Health* 10:275–81.

Louhevaara V, Ilmarinen R, Griefahn B, Künemund C, Mäkinen H. (1995) Maximal physical work performance with European standard based fire-protective clothing system and equipment in relation to individual characteristics. *Eur J Appl Physiol Occup Physiol* 71:223–9.

Louhevaara V, Smolander J, Tuomi T, Korhonen O, Jaakkola J. (1985) Effects of an SCBA on breathing pattern, gas exchange, and heart rate during exercise. *J Occup Med* 27:213–16.

Louhevaara V, Tuomi T, Korhonen O, Jaakkola J. (1984) Cardiorespiratory effects of respiratory protective devices during exercise in well-trained men. *Eur J Appl Physiol Occup Physiol* 52:340–5.

Love RG, Johnstone JBG, Crawford J, Tesh KM, Graveling RA, Ritchie PJ, Hutchison PA, Wetherill GZ. (1994) Study of the Physiological Effects of Wearing Breathing Apparatus, *Institute of Occupational Medicine Technical Memorandum* TM/94/05.

Maki BE, Holliday PJ, Topper AK. (1994) A prospective study of postural balance and risk of falling in an ambulatory and independent elderly population. *J Gerontol* 49:M72–84.

Manning JE, Griggs TR. (1983) Heart rates in fire fighters using light and heavy breathing equipment: Similar near-maximal exertion in response to multiple work load conditions. *J Occup Med* 25:215–18.

Mayer JM, Nuzzo JL, Chen R, Quillen WS, Verna JL, Miro R, Dagenais S. (2012) The impact of obesity on back and core muscular endurance in firefighters. *J Obes* 2012:729283.

Morley J, Beauchamp G, Suyama J, Guyette FX, Reis SE, Callaway CW, Hostler D. (2012) Cognitive function following treadmill exercise in thermal protective clothing. *Eur J Appl Physiol* 112:1733–40.

National Fire Protection Association (NFPA). (1971). *Standard on Protective Ensembles for Structural Fire Fighting and Proximity Fire Fighting.* 2013 Edition National Fire Protection Association: Quincy, MA 2013

Nullmeyer RT, Stella D, Montijo GA, Harden SW. (2005) Human factors in air force flight mishaps: Implications for change. Proceedings of the 27th Annual Interservice/Industry Training, Simulation, and Education Conference (paper no. 2260). Arlington, VA: National Training Systems Association.

Pajala S, Era P, Koskenvuo M, Kaprio J, Törmäkangas T, Rantanen T. (2008) Force platform balance measures as predictors of indoor and outdoor falls in community-dwelling women aged 63–76 years. *J Gerontol A Biol Sci Med Sci* 63:171–8.

Park K, Hur P, Rosengren KS, Horn GP, Hsiao-Wecksler ET. (2010) Effect of load carriage on gait due to firefighting air bottle configuration. *Ergonomics* 53:882–91.

Park K, Rosengren KS, Horn GP, Smith DL, Hsiao-Wecksler ET. (2011) Assessing gait changes in firefighters due to fatigue and protective clothing. *Safety Sci* 49, 719–26.

Pendergast DR, Lindholm P, Wylegala J, Warkander D, Lundgren CE. (2006) Effects of respiratory muscle training on respiratory CO_2 sensitivity in SCUBA divers. *Undersea Hyperb Med* 33:447–53.

Pendergrass TL, Moore JH, Gerber JP. (2003) Postural control after a 2-mile run. *Mil Med* 168:896–903.

Petrucci MN, Harton B, Rosengren K, Horn G, Hsiao-Wecksler E. (2012) What causes slips, trips, and falls on the fireground? A survey. In *36th Annual Meeting of the American Society of Biomechanics.* Gainesville, FL.

Poston WS, Jitnarin N, Haddock CK, Jahnke SA, Tuley BC. (2011) Obesity and injury-related absenteeism in a population-based firefighter cohort. *Obesity (Silver Spring)* 19:2076–81.

Punakallio A. (2004) Trial-to-trial reproducibility and test-retest stability of two dynamic balance tests among male firefighters. *Int J Sports Med* 25:163–9.

Punakallio A, Hirvonen M, Grönqvist R. (2005) Slip and fall risk among firefighters in relation to balance, muscular capacities and age. *Safety Sci* 43:455–68.

Punakallio A, Lusa S, Luukkonen R. (2003) Protective equipment affects balance abilities differently in younger and older firefighters. *Aviat Space Environ Med* 74:1151–6.

Ramachandran AK, Yang Y, Rosengren KS, Hsiao-Wecksler ET. (2007) Effect of Tai Chi on gait and obstacle crossing behaviors in middle-aged adults. *Gait Posture* 26:248–55.

Rosengren KS, Hsiao-Wecksler ET, Horn G. (2014) Fighting fires without falling: Effects of equipment design and fatigue on firefighters' balance and gait. *Ecol Psych* 26:167–75.

Saul EV, Jaffe J. (1955) The effects of clothing on gross motor performance. EP-12 US Army Quartermaster Research and Development Command (NTIS: AD-066 180).

Seliga R, Bhattacharya A, Succop P, Wickstrom R, Smith D, Willeke K. (1991) Effect of work load and respirator wear on postural stability, heart rate, and perceived exertion. *Am Ind Hyg Assoc J* 52:417–22.

Selkirk GA, McLellan TM. (2004) Physical work limits for Toronto firefighters in warm environments. *J Occup Environ Hyg* 1:199–212.

Selkirk GA, McLellan TM, Wong J. (2004) Active versus passive cooling during work in warm environments while wearing firefighting protective clothing. *J Occup Environ Hyg* 1:521–31.

Smith DL, Petruzzello SJ. (1998) Selected physiological and psychological responses to live-fire drills in different configurations of firefighting gear. *Ergonomics* 41:1141–54.

Smith DL, Petruzzello SJ, Kramer JM, Warner SE, Bone BG, Misner JE. (1995) Selected physiological and psycho-biological responses to physical activity different configurations of firefighting gear. *Ergonomics* 38:2065–77.

Sobeih TM, Davis KG, Succop PA, Jetter WA, Bhattacharya A. (2006) Postural balance changes in on-duty firefighters: Effect of gear and long work shifts. *J Occup Environ Med* 48:68–75.

Son SY, Bakri I, Muraki S, Tochihara Y. (2014) Comparison of firefighters and non-firefighters and the test methods used regarding the effects of personal protective equipment on individual mobility. *Appl Ergon* 45:1019–27.

Soteriades ES, Hauser R, Kawachi I, Christiani DC, Kales SN. (2008) Obesity and risk of job disability in male firefighters. *Occup Med (Lond)* 58:245–50.

Storer TW, Dolezal BA, Abrazado ML, Smith DL, Batalin MA, Tseng C-H, Cooper CB, the PHASER Study Group. (2014) Firefighter health and fitness assessment: A call to action. *J Strength Cond Res* 28: 661–71.

Suyama J, Rittenberger JC, Patterson PD, Hostler D. (2009) Comparison of public safety provider injury rates. *Prehosp Emerg Care* 13:451–5.

Szubert Z, Sobala W. (2002) Work-related injuries among firefighters: Sites and circumstances of their occurrence. *Int J Occup Med Environ Health* 15:49–55.

Taylor NA, Lewis MC, Notley SR, Peoples GE. (2012) A fractionation of the physiological burden of the personal protective equipment worn by firefighters. *Eur J Appl Physiol* 112:2913–21.

Thiel A, Stern J, Kimball J, Hankin N. (2003) U.S. Fire Administration/Technical Report Series Special Report: Trends and Hazards in Firefighter Training USFA-TR-100. http://www.usfa.fema.gov/downloads/pdf/publications/tr-100.pdf. Accessed 7 July 2014.

Turner NL, Chiou S, Zwiener J, Weaver D, Spahr J. (2010) Physiological effects of boot weight and design on men and women firefighters. *J Occup Environ Hyg* 7:477–82.

Uemura H, Lundgren CE, Ray AD, Pendergast DR. (2012) Effects of different types of respiratory muscle training on exercise performance in runners. *Mil Med* 177:559–66.

Vellas BJ, Wayne SJ, Romero L, Baumgartner RN, Rubenstein LZ, Garry PJ. (1997) One-leg balance is an important predictor of injurious falls in older persons. *J Am Geriatr Soc* 45:735–8.

von Heimburg ED, Rasmussen AK, Medbø JI. (2006) Physiological responses of firefighters and performance predictors during a simulated rescue of hospital patients. *Ergonomics* 49:111–26.

Walker A, Driller M, Argus C, Cooke J, Rattray B. (2014) The ageing Australian firefighter: An argument for age-based recruitment and fitness standards for urban fire services. *Ergonomics* 57:612–21.

Walton SM, Conrad KM, Furner SE, Samo DG (2003) Cause, type, and workers' compensation costs of injury to fire fighters. *Am J Ind Med* 43:454–8.

Williams WJ, Coca A, Roberge R, Shepherd A, Powell J, Shaffer RE. (2011) Physiological responses to wearing a prototype firefighter ensemble compared with a standard ensemble. *J Occup Environ Hyg* 8:49–57.

Yang Y, Verkuilen JV, Rosengren KS, Grubisich SA, Reed MR, Hsiao-Wecksler ET. (2007) Effect of combined Taiji and Qigong training on balance mechanisms: A randomized controlled trial of older adults. *Med Sci Monitor* 13: 339–48.

Section V

Fall Incident Investigation and Reconstruction

22

Fall Forensics: Principles and Applications

H. Harvey Cohen and Joseph Cohen

CONTENTS

ABSTRACT This chapter summarizes the rapidly emerging field of fall forensics. This field of consulting is really no different in its scientific and engineering methodologies from other applications, including perceptual-cognitive and biomechanical elements, with the sole exception being its application to the legal process, typically premises liability civil litigation. Some important terminology unique to forensics is covered, followed by a discussion of the process by which the forensic consultant is engaged to perform their work and the various generic tasks comprising that work. The chapter concludes with four actual case examples demonstrating such analyses as applied to the four most important types of falls in need of prevention.

22.1 Introduction

What is a forensic practice? The ancient Romans used the words *foris* or *foras* to refer to out of doors or outside. They built their communities around an open area in the center of their towns and villages. Much like the way they gathered in the atria of their homes, they gathered in and around their *fora* or town squares for the public aspect of their community life.

Since the town square was outside, they referred to that area as the *forum*. The forum was the center of commercial life, containing the community's markets as well as elements of their government, including tribunals. *Forensics* means *pertaining to the forum* and has come to have the specialized meaning of the art of argument, especially in legal proceedings. For the fall practitioner, forensics implies the application of both scientific and engineering principles to analyzing matters involved in legal proceedings.

22.2 The Nature of Forensic Practice

There have been disputes as to whether or not people who have been trained in an objective science should engage in the practice of forensics. The truth of the matter is that members of the scientific and engineering communities are engaging in forensics, and in ever-increasing numbers. When giving testimony, forensic consultants are giving reasoned presentations of their analyses and opinions, thus presenting arguments for their opinions and conclusions. They are not *advocating* the position of one side or the other. Rather, that is the job of the trial attorneys. They are there to present opinions within their areas of expertise, as well as the scientific/engineering bases or foundation for those opinions.

Is this a reasonable way for someone trained in the application of a scientific or engineering discipline to make a living? The courts prefer to think that when they use experts, they are not tapping people who make a living primarily as forensic practitioners. What they prefer to think they are doing is getting someone practicing in a field of endeavor and who is expert in that field to interrupt that practice to assist them in trying a matter of law.

We prefer to think of applied research and forensic consulting as being synergistic; that is, better applied research makes for better forensic consulting, and vice versa. We do not consider ourselves to be professional expert witnesses; rather, we consider ourselves to be both applied research scientists and practicing forensic consultants. The only thought the jury should have is that the forensic consultant is knowledgeable in their field (i.e., competent), and that their testimony would be the same no matter which side had retained their expertise (i.e., credible). Practicing as a forensic consultant should not be any different from any other type of consulting. In the case of our field, human factors–ergonomics (HFE), someone has a problem that involves a human engaged in some technological setting or built environment where something has gone wrong. We apply the same knowledge and tools as other practitioners in our discipline, namely, principles of analysis, design, and test and evaluation, to determine why and how a human error in a system occurred, as well as means for prevention of reoccurrence in the future.

For further information on forensic practice, the reader is referred to Rudov and Cohen (2009), for forensic principles related to HFE, to Cohen and Woodson (2005) and for the science-based forensic issues specifically related to the prevention and consequences of slips, trips, missteps, and falls, to Bakken et al. (2007) (3rd edition in press).

22.3 Some Basic Legal Concepts in Forensic Fall Practice

While from time to time forensic consultants involved in fall cases may get involved in other types of legal matters, such as criminal cases, the vast majority will likely involve a *tort*. A tort is a civil wrong resulting in damages, exclusive of contract. A wrong has allegedly been committed. This means that someone acted improperly (but not feloniously), either by doing something they should not have done (i.e., acts of commission) or by failing to do something they should have done (i.e., acts of omission). Such actions/inactions imply a relationship between that someone and the party or parties that was wronged. That relationship is called a *duty*. Typically, the legal *damages* are some form of bodily injury, monetary loss, and/or property damage. Finally, *exclusive of contract* means that there was neither a written nor an oral agreement that controlled the relationship between the two parties. In a court proceeding, the party (or parties) that claims damages is called the *plaintiff(s)*, and the party (or parties) that allegedly caused the damages is referred to as the *defendant(s)*.

A plaintiff's attorney, who bears the burden of proof of a tort, must establish four things to a court to prove that a tort was committed. The first point of proof is that a *duty* existed. If one party did not owe a duty to another party, a tort was not committed. Once the plaintiff's attorney has established that a duty was present, they next have to establish that the duty was breached. That is, they must prove that the defendant did something wrong by doing or not doing something required under the duty, for example, not providing a reasonably safe environment for patrons. This second point of proof is called *negligence*.

The third point of proof is *proximate cause*. For a tort to have been committed, there must be a causal relationship between the negligent act and the injury or other damages. A common example in fall cases is whether an alleged building code noncompliance had anything to do with the actual loss of balance and subsequent fall. The fourth point of proof is *damages*. In addition to personal injury, damages in matters related to falls may include a variety of economic losses, including, but not limited to, related medical costs, lost income, and in some cases, future earnings.

Finally, a court may find *contributory* and *comparative negligence*. That is, an award to a plaintiff may be diminished by a determination of apportioned or percentage of *fault*. For example, an award of $100,000 may result in only $70,000 to an injured party if the *trier of fact*, typically a jury (in the United States), determines that the plaintiff was 30% responsible for their injuries, for example, by not exercising reasonable care. Note that apportioning fault is the province of the jury, not the objective liability expert.

One further point is that the forensic fall expert will most likely be testifying in either a state (in the United States) or sometimes under the rules of a federal court. Even though somewhat similar, each jurisdiction has its own "rules of civil procedure" in discovery and "rules of evidence" during trial that a judge will ensure are followed. This may require, through what is called a *motion inlimine*, that the expert cannot testify about certain facts or evidence, most commonly that insurance coverage is involved, as that might bias the jury in their deliberations. Also, each jurisdiction has its own, often similar, generic jury instructions that the attorneys trying a particular case must tailor to address the specific facts they are attempting to prove.

22.4 The Forensic Process in Fall Incident Litigation

The forensic fall consultant analyzes situations involved in litigation and offers opinions that may support or refute the legal theories being pursued. Legal proceedings are an adversarial process in which lawyers represent opposing parties; in civil cases, as previously mentioned, they typically represent the plaintiff (injured party) or the defendant (the alleged injuring party). The role of the forensic fall consultant is to offer opinions in their field beyond the knowledge of the ordinary people comprising a jury. The process typically follows that outlined in Figure 22.1: consultation with client, review of information, inspection of premises, research, formulation of opinion(s), and expression of opinion(s) (Cohen and LaRue 2004).

22.4.1 Consultation with Client

The initial step in the forensic consulting process is discussion with the potential client, who usually is an attorney or insurance company representative but not the litigants. In this conversation, the client provides an initial description of the case and the issues involved. The forensic fall consultant can confirm that the issues in the case are ones that

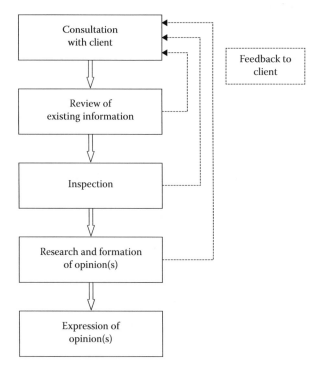

FIGURE 22.1
The forensic process in fall incident litigation.

fall within their area of expertise. The client will want to confirm that the consultant has appropriate experience and is qualified to be named to the court as an expert and offer opinions with respect to the issues in the case. An agreement on fees is generally tendered and signed at this stage (retention).

22.4.2 Review of Information

Similarly to any other scientific endeavor, the first true step is to review the existing information, which in the legal community is referred to as *discovery*. It is important for the forensic fall consultant to review all pertinent discovery to understand the relevant background facts of the case. In a typical lawsuit, a variety of information is available in the form of incident reports, statements, and medical records, as well as the complaint and other pleadings, and written and oral answers to legal questions in the form of interrogatories and depositions, respectively. Other important sources of information are witnesses to the incident, if any, and documents requested of and produced by defendants, such as related to prior similar incidents.

22.4.3 Inspection of Site

After reviewing the facts of the case, the forensic fall consultant will conduct an inspection of the location where the incident occurred. Unless the site has been dramatically altered or destroyed, an inspection is necessary to gather as much first-hand data as possible. At the inspection, photographs and/or video documenting the scene should be undertaken. It is also important to measure dimensions and conduct testing appropriate to the type of incident. If the fall incident involves a stairway, then measurements regarding the width, stair geometry (tread depths, riser heights, step nosings), and handrails must be gathered. Slip resistance tests are used to measure the traction of a surface for slip-and-fall cases. Other tests at the site can include illumination testing and walkway slope measurements.

22.4.4 Research and Formulation of Opinions

It is generally necessary to conduct research prior to developing a forensic opinion on a case. Research for falls can include scientific literature, building codes, industry standards, professional design guidelines, or even comparing how similar facilities through custom and practice have handled the design, construction, or maintenance issues in question.

The forensic fall consultant integrates all the information gathered from the legal discovery, inspection, and research with their knowledge and experience to form an opinion. The expert's opinions are strengthened when they can provide a sound authority as the basis for the opinion. The types of bases generally used and the strength of each are discussed in Section 22.5.

22.4.5 Expression of Opinions

After the forensic fall consultant, now the named expert, has formulated their opinions based on relevant case information, inspections, and research, an opinion may be rendered by several methods: reports, deposition, and testimony. An oral and/or written report is generally prepared for the client. The initial verbal report to the client should outline both strengths and weaknesses of the case. It is important that both sides of the case are presented, so that the client is aware of weaknesses in their possible arguments.

At this point, the client can decide whether they are interested in pursuing the case further, and the forensic fall consultant can determine whether they will agree to be named as an expert in the case. Increasingly, although this is not always required, a written report contains the results of the consultant's investigation along with their opinions and bases for the opinions.

A *deposition* is a formal question-and-answer session, with the same weight as courtroom testimony, in which the opposing attorney(s) have the opportunity to question the designated expert witness under oath. The topics covered at the deposition usually focus on the expert's qualifications (education and experience), their opinions regarding the case, and the bases for their opinions. The entire proceedings are typed by a court reporter and put into booklet form, where they become part of the case discovery.

If the case does not settle earlier in the legal process, it culminates with a trial before a judge and usually a jury (in the United States). At the trial, the expert witness will be sworn in and questioned by the retaining attorney (*direct examination*) and the attorney for the opposing side (*cross-examination*). The cross-examination is usually an attempt by the opposing attorney to impeach unfavorable testimony. Such questioning may be followed by *redirect* and *recross*, during which the attorneys are permitted only to ask desired clarifications to prior questions.

22.5 Basis for Forensic Fall Opinions

The forensic fall expert integrates the information gathered from the case discovery material, inspection of the incident site, and applicable research with their knowledge and experience to formulate opinions regarding the causation of the fall and subsequent injuries. The expert's opinions are strengthened when they can provide a sound authority as the basis of the opinion. These opinions may be supported by both facts (i.e., so-called factual bases) as well as based on a variety of authorities, some providing stronger support then others. These latter bases are illustrated in a hierarchical manner in Figure 22.2 according to their strength and the relative ease with which they can be supported (Cohen and LaRue 2006), as discussed in Sections 22.5.1 through 22.5.7.

22.5.1 Codes and Law

Codes and laws are legal requirements governing a particular jurisdiction. This basis is used when the expert opines that the situation does not meet the provisions of applicable codes or law. When a clear violation exists, an expert may also need to provide an opinion that the noncompliance has (or does not have) causal bearing on the incident. Examples of relevant codes and laws are the International Building Code (IBC) and the federal Americans with Disabilities Act (ADA), as well as many state-specific equivalents.

22.5.2 Voluntary Consensus Standards

Voluntary consensus standards are a group of requirements that have been developed by committees associated with standards-setting bodies through an industry consensus process. These standards are not legally binding, unless specifically cited within the codes,

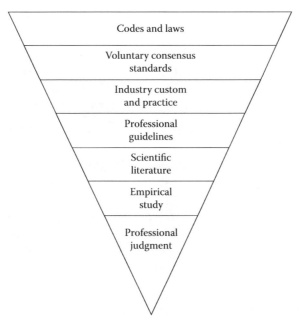

FIGURE 22.2
Basis for forensic fall opinions.

but are usually well known throughout the industry, as they describe design and safety features for the respective industry. Examples of these organizations are the American National Standards Institute (ANSI), American Society for Testing and Materials (ASTM) International, and the International Standards Organization (ISO).

22.5.3 Industry Custom and Practice

The way of doing business over the years within a particular industry is considered the industry custom and practice. The custom and practice is typically based on experience and is generally informal; it may not even be documented. In some cases, however, the practices may be formalized as written company policies and procedures. Often, such practices may have evolved from some type of rudimentary job analysis. These practices can be useful in forming an opinion, especially when evidence and/or research are available to support the practice.

22.5.4 Professional Guidelines

Most design-related professions have handbooks that offer criteria regarding proper and safe design. A citation from such an authoritative handbook may be appropriate. Examples commonly used by forensic fall experts include the Illuminating Engineering Society of North America's *Lighting Handbook* (IESNA 2000), *Human Factors Design Handbook* (Woodson et al. 1992), and *The Measure of Man and Woman* (Henry Dreyfuss Associates 1993). The major disadvantage of citing such an authority as the only opinion basis is that the source may not be widely known, especially by the party deemed responsible, such as the building manager or owner.

22.5.5 Scientific Literature

Due to their backgrounds as research scientists, many forensic fall experts feel most comfortable when citing scientific literature as the basis of their opinions. The primary drawback with using this type of literature as the sole basis of an opinion is that it is typically of very limited circulation. Consequently, citing scientific literature as the only opinion basis may represent information readily available only to other forensic fall experts.

22.5.6 Empirical Study

Sometimes, the specific issue is not significantly addressed by any documented authority and can only be addressed through original empirical research. In addition to the usual areas of possible impeachment of research studies (issues dealing with the appropriateness of experimental design, sample size, bias, confounding, and statistical power), this approach may not always be practical due to time and budget constraints. When feasible, however, research performed to answer specific issues not elsewhere addressed can be helpful in establishing a firm basis for expert opinions.

22.5.7 Professional Judgment

Sometimes, when no other foundational source is available, it becomes necessary for a forensic professional to base an opinion solely on their professional judgment. This opinion is more powerful when it is based on information extrapolated from previously encountered situations. Generally, the more similar the situations are to the current case, the more credible is the expert's opinion. An expert's opinion based solely on their judgment is only as powerful as their experience, credibility, and credentials. Such professional opinion alone is subject to attack, which may include impeachment of the expert's credentials, experience, and testimony in past similar cases. Consequently, though a legitimate and sometimes necessary basis for expert opinion, professional judgment alone is the most difficult to support.

22.6 Applications

This chapter closes with four case examples in fall forensics. These applications are based on actual tort litigation in the United States in which a plaintiff sought to recover monetary compensation for economic damages, such as lost wages, medical expenses, and pain and suffering caused by a fall. All four causes of actions were for general negligence and premises liability.

22.6.1 Trip-and-Fall

Lawyers representing a 44-year-old male plaintiff filed a complaint in a state court regarding a trip-and-fall incident he had had as a guest visiting a downtown building in a major metropolitan area. Plaintiff alleged that the property manager defendants, by and through duly authorized agents and/or employees, were negligent for (1) failing to maintain the entry to a men's restroom in a safe condition; (2) failing to warn the plaintiff of the dangerous condition; and/or (3) carelessly and negligently remodeling the restroom in such a way as to create a dangerous condition to anyone entering the restroom.

Plaintiff had sought to use the men's restroom in a common area of the 11th floor at the time of the incident. Entering the restroom required plaintiff to enter a numerical code on a keypad located next to the door handle. After entering the code, he turned the handle, pushed the door, and walked forward over the threshold. Plaintiff did not see a sign posted on the wall to his right that read "CAUTION: Step up." Moreover, he did not see the single step situated just beyond the inward swing of the door. Stumbling and falling forward, plaintiff's injuries occurred as he struck his right knee, shoulder, and side of his face on the tile floor.

An inspection of the area commissioned by plaintiff determined several significant observations by the retained expert. First, there was no visual contrast that would indicate the presence of the 15.24 cm elevation change posed by the step. Both the horizontal and vertical surfaces of the floor, including the step nosing, were the same tan color. Second, the sign posted on the wall inside the door warning plaintiff of the step was displayed perpendicularly to plaintiff's path of travel. Further, the colors of the letters and background of the sign matched that of the décor of the restroom, causing it to blend in with its surroundings, and lending it to being missed by restroom users.

In rebuttal, the property management defendants presented evidence that the step inside the restroom door was a necessary architectural feature to accommodate old plumbing lines in the building. There were several examples of single steps like it in restrooms on other floors of the building. Construction work to reroute the pipes and make the restroom floors flat was estimated to cost more than $2 million. Defendants also admitted that there had been more than a dozen fall incidents reported on the restroom steps in the building in the past 10 years, albeit only having occurred when guests were exiting the restrooms, not entering as in the present case. Nevertheless, defendants countered with a legal defense that plaintiff was negligent and his recovery of damages should be reduced accordingly.

The evidence according to the plaintiff's expert was consistent with the purported trip-and-fall incident. The same expert expressed an opinion that the step posed an unreasonable risk of harm because guests using the restroom would encounter it within a stride of clearing the door threshold. Plaintiff had to turn his head to his right to see the warning sign and back down to the step. But instead, plaintiff's relaxed line of sight was approximately 5.95 m ahead into the restroom. The unmarked step, meanwhile, was 82.55 cm in front of him, effectively outside his lower peripheral visual field, where acuity and sensitivity to contrast is diminished. Consequently, plaintiff had little time to perceive and react to the unexpected presence of the single step before tripping.

Prior to reaching a trial, all parties in this case entered into an agreement by which defendants paid financial compensation to the plaintiff for his injuries as well as pain and suffering.

22.6.2 Slip-and-Fall

Attorneys representing a defendant answered a complaint filed in state court by a plaintiff who allegedly sustained injuries from a fall on the ground floor of their medical plaza building. Plaintiff alleged that a wet concrete walkway was dangerously slippery due to rainwater runoff and was the proximate cause of her injuries. Also alleged was the defendant's failure to warn plaintiff, an invited guest, of the dangerously slippery condition.

Through discovery, it was revealed that the alleged fall occurred shortly before noon in February. There had been light rain in the area earlier that morning. Plaintiff was wearing rubber-soled shoes that were in nearly new condition at the time of the alleged slip-and-fall. The walkway was "flush, planar, and even" in accordance with the specifications of ASTM International's F1637-13 standard, *Standard Practice for Safe Walking Surfaces*. Defendants further understood that the plaintiff was walking straight ahead and not distracted in any way. There was no visible debris on the walkway.

An investigation by a defendant's expert determined that the walkway was constructed of Portland cement. It had a light "broom" finish and was located in an area of the property that received sunlight much of the day. On rainy days, a downspout attached to a roofline gutter shed water across the walkway in the area of plaintiff's fall. However, there was no visible evidence of any algae or other contaminant on the walkway in the area.

A subsequent inspection by defendant's expert included use of a tribometer to measure the slip resistance between a representative Neolite© test foot and the actual walkway, both dry and wet. The results indicated a "slip resistant" condition, with all tests exceeding the generally accepted .50 standard of care (ANSI/ASSE Technical Report TRA1264.3-07). Plaintiff's expert, based on a comprehensive analysis of the perceptual-cognitive and biomechanical aspects of the incident, concluded to a reasonable degree of scientific certainty that it was highly unlikely that plaintiff had slipped and fallen as she testified. There was little difference in both testing conditions, indicating that there was no need to warn of a sudden loss of traction.

This case was ultimately dismissed by a judge's order at a pretrial hearing. Plaintiff did not recover any monetary compensation for her purported damages.

22.6.3 Misstep-and-Fall

Attorneys filed a complaint in state court on behalf of a 60-year-old woman who fell inside a single-family residence. Plaintiff claimed that a dangerously designed, constructed, and maintained stairway on the premises caused her fall and resultant injuries. She demanded monetary compensation for her damages according to proof by trial in civil court. A defendant answered by claiming that the incident was caused by the plaintiff's own negligence and failure to exercise reasonable care in descending the stairway.

On a summer Friday evening, plaintiff went to the residence for a weekend stay with her extended family, as she had done previously on approximately 20 occasions. After entering the front door, with her suitcase, she ascended the only stairs in the house to the second-floor bedroom. Her sworn statements and deposition testimony follow that she then set down her suitcase in the bedroom and exited. As she descended the stairs back to the first floor, near the end of the flight, she "went to go to the next step, and there was nothing there." While testifying, she described a sensation of "flying in the air" before her knee and elbow struck the tile floor below.

An investigation by plaintiff's architect expert determined that the stairs were covered by pad and carpet. It was a so-called "8–9" stairway, meaning that the rise and run of the individual steps approximated 20.32 and 22.86 cm, respectively. The overall slope of the flight was 41.6°. Plaintiff's architect expert identified dimensional irregularities throughout the flight in violation of the International Building Code (IBC), with the riser heights varying up to 1.27 cm, and the tread lengths varying up to 1.11 cm. The handrail was likewise problematic from the perspective of both building code compliance and usability, as it was too low (74.93 cm above the tread nosing) and terminated before the bottom of the flight. It was further discovered that a 5.72 × 10.16 cm wood handrail had been placed over the existing metal rail from the original construction.

An expert who specializes in stairway use analyzed the circumstances of the fall. He reported that the irregularity in the step geometry was the primary cause. It was, further, his opinion that the plaintiff did not fall due to a loss of traction. Instead, the irregularity of the steps disrupted the rhythm of plaintiff's gait, causing her to misstep or overstep the third step from the bottom of the flight. The secondary causal factor of plaintiff's misstep was the retrofit wood handrail. He concluded that the handrail was 1) a misleading visual cue of the end of the flight; 2) a poor fit in hand (i.e., not "graspable" according to the building code) because it was too low and excessively wide; and 3) ineffective at providing a last clear chance for recovery after plaintiff misstepped.

After exchanging expert reports in this litigation, plaintiff reached a settlement with the homeowner defendant. The terms of the settlement remain confidential.

22.6.4 Fall From Elevation

This final case arises out of an 18-month-old child falling from a fire escape serving an apartment building in a metropolitan area. Through his father, the boy plaintiff brought suit against the property owner defendants. Plaintiff alleged that defendant failed to maintain a fire escape located on the front of the building because there was an unguarded opening and unsecured French doors. Defendant contended that responsibility for the incident was with the child's parents for their failure to properly supervise the child.

In discovery, a central factual dispute arose. Plaintiff's father testified that his son fell from a fire escape on the third floor of the building. The boy was under his supervision at the time. However, a handyman witness in the case, also working at the property at the time of the incident believed that the boy fell from the fire escape on the second floor while in the care of his mother in their second-floor apartment. He testified that he saw the boy's father cleaning outside in the back of the building while he was on his way back from the basement. Approximately 3–4 min later, he heard a noise that caught his attention, and he exited the front of the building. There, he found the boy on the ground under an opening in the second-floor fire escape, approximately .75 m from the building. However, the boy's father testified that he found the boy 2.5 m away from the building, and had moved him closer to the building prior to the handy man's arrival. In any event, the boy subsequently spent 3 days in a local hospital. He sustained a fractured femur and a chest contusion. There was no head injury.

To test the plausibility of the various accounts from witnesses, in separate analyses, the defendant's expert used mathematical expressions and basic assumptions about the boy's center of gravity and walking speed to model the boy's most probable path of travel had he fallen from the third or the second story. The second- and third-floor fire escapes are shown in Figure 22.3.

The third-floor fall scenario started at a height of nearly 7.6 m before passing through the opening in the third-floor fire escape. According to the model, less than a second later, the boy would have come into full contact with the ladder between the second and third floors. It was most probable that the ladder rail and its slope would have caused the boy to come to rest on the second-floor fire escape, not the ground floor near the street, as the boy's father had testified.

The second-floor fall scenario started at a height of nearly 2.5 m before passing through the opening in the second-floor fire escape. According to the model, the boy's feet would have hit the ground first before his upper body came crashing forward. Both the height of the fall from the second floor and the second impact of going forward onto to a nearby curb seemed to explain plaintiff's injuries. More importantly to defendant's case, the analysis

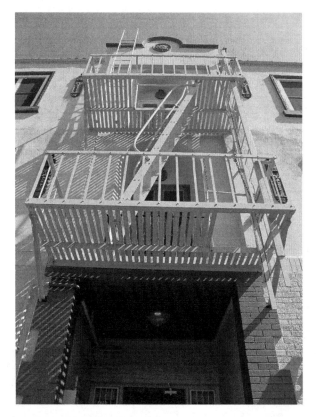

FIGURE 22.3
Photograph of the second- and third-floor fire escapes on the front of the building.

proved that the plaintiff's father's story was untrue, and that the parents had failed to supervise the boy at the time of his fall incident. It is unknown whether or not criminal charges were ever filed against the parents following the resolution of the case.

22.7 Conclusion

This chapter summarizes the rapidly emerging field of fall forensics. It starts by noting that this field of consulting is really no different in its scientific and engineering methodologies from other applications, including perceptual-cognitive and biomechanical elements, with the sole exception being its application to the legal process, typically premises liability civil litigation. Consequently, some important terminology unique to forensics is covered, followed by a discussion of the process by which the forensic consultant is engaged to perform their work and the various generic tasks comprising that work. The chapter concludes with four actual case examples demonstrating such analyses as applied to the four most important types of falls in need of prevention: slips, trips, missteps, and falls from elevation. The chapter shows that fall forensics, although relatively new, is an exciting and worthwhile field of endeavor for a variety of scientific and engineering disciplines, including that of the authors (HFE), interested in making immediate contributions to an important area of public health injury prevention.

References

American National Standards Institute/American Society of Safety Engineers. Technical Report TRA1264.3-07, Using variable angle tribometers (VAT) for measurement of the slip resistance of walkway surfaces, p. 12, New York, Des Plaines, IL.

ASTM International. F1637-13: Standard Practice for Safe Walking Surfaces. West Conshohocken, PA.

Bakken, Gary M., H. Harvey Cohen, Jon R. Abele, Alvin S. Hyde, and Cindy A. LaRue. *Slips, Trips, Missteps and Their Consequences.* 2nd Edition. Tucson, AZ: Lawyers & Publishing, 2007.

Cohen, H. Harvey, and Cindy A. LaRue. Forensic human factors/ergonomics. In *International Encyclopedia of Ergonomics and Human Factors*, Waldemar Karwowski (ed.). Boca Raton, FL: CRC Press, 2006.

Cohen, H. Harvey, and Cindy A. LaRue. Perceptual-cognitive and biomechanical factors in pedestrian falls. In *Handbook of Human Factors in Litigation*, Waldemar Karwowski and Y. Ian Noy (eds). Boca Raton, FL: CRC Press, 2004.

Cohen, H. Harvey, and Wesley E. Woodson. *Principles of Forensic Human Factors/Ergonomics.* Tucson, AZ: Lawyers & Judges Publishing, 2005.

Henry Dreyfuss Associates. *The Measure of Man and Woman: Human Factors in Design.* New York, NY: Whitney Library of Design, 1993.

Illuminating Engineering Society of North America. *The IESNA Lighting Handbook: Reference & Application.* 9th Edition. Edited by Mark Stanley Rea. New York, NY: Illuminating Engineering Society of North America, 2000.

Rudov, Melvin H., and H. Harvey Cohen. *Practice of Forensic Human Factors/Ergonomics and Related Safety Professions.* Tucson, AZ: Lawyers & Judges Publishing, 2009.

Woodson, Wesley E., Barry Tillman, and Peggy Tillman. *Human Factors Design Handbook.* 2nd Edition. New York, NY: McGraw-Hill, 1992.

23

Case Studies of Falls on Stairs

Daniel Johnson

CONTENTS

ABSTRACT   Many serious and fatal injuries occur as a result of falls on stairs. Falls associated with defects in the design, construction, and maintenance of the stairway, rather than the behavior of the user (which is difficult to control), are discussed. Some guiding human factors principles concerning adequate visual information, consistent step geometry, and adequacy of handrails are addressed.

KEY WORDS: *stairs, safety, top of flight flaw, bottom of flight illusion.*

23.1 Stairway Falls due to Defects in Construction and Maintenance

There are many reasons why a person may fall while walking up or down a stairway. But here we examine only those factors that stairway and handrail manufacturers, builders, inspectors, and owners would reasonably have control over.

John Archea et al. (1979) reported that in the United States in 1976, some 540,345 stair falls resulted in injuries serious enough to require emergency hospital treatment; about 4000 of those people died from their injuries. Pauls (2011) reports that in the United States and in many other countries, falling during stair use is the leading cause of injuries. In the United States, stair-related injuries led to about 1,300,000 hospital emergency room (ER) visits, with the great majority (85%–90%) occurring in homes. If the death:injury ratio that Archea et al. reported (4000:540,345) holds, then the number of current annual deaths among the 1,300,000 injuries in the United States would be about 9600.

Falls in public facilities have been drastically reduced compared with falls in homes, most likely because fear of litigation has resulted in building codes requiring safer stairs in public facilities than in homes, where lawsuits are less likely (e.g., Johnson and Pauls, 2012).

We realize that the person's own behavior may have been a prime cause of such a fall. A person may experience a misstep due to medications or imbibing too much alcohol, being distracted, or carrying too much in their hands. Even a small object, such as a set of keys, could interfere with the person's ability to use a handrail to prevent a fall. A person could also experience a misstep due to natural variability in foot placement or could be physically unable to arrest the fall after a misstep. But these causes could be considered to be due to idiopathic conditions that may not be readily remedied through improved design.

When a person falls on a stairway, one or more human factors design principles needed for successful stairway use may have been neglected:

- *Inadequate visual information*: Visual information must be adequate for the person to see the nosings (the foremost edge of each tread) for the foot to be accurately placed.
- *Inconsistent step geometry*: Step geometry must be consistent so as to conform to the person's expectations.
- *Inadequate handrails*: Handrails must be within reach and graspable so that the stair user can avert a fall following a misstep.

The following case studies demonstrate that when at least some of these design or maintenance principles are violated, serious injuries can result.

23.2 First Case: Top of Flight Flaw Causes Fall Down Stairs

A 62-year-old man was starting down a stairway for the first time at an apartment complex when he experienced a misstep. He fell to his left, hitting the handrail with the left side of his body. He slid on his buttocks nearly to the bottom of the nine-riser flight, incurring severe injuries.

23.2.1 Inadequate Visual Information

While the nosing of the top landing had a metal strip that was readily visible, the remaining nosings were not highlighted. Zietz et al. (2011) report that visually emphasized nosings have a beneficial effect on balance control in older adults, and when the nosings are not highlighted, the danger is increased. Further, Foster et al. (2014) experimented with placement of a high-contrast edge highlighter in the vicinity of the nosing. There could be no contrast highlighter, one that was flush with the nosing, or one that was either 10 mm (0.4 in.) or 30 mm (1.2 in.) back from the nosing. Subjects were either older adults or younger adults who were wearing lenses that simulated age-related cataracts. Measurements were taken of foot clearance during descent. The researchers concluded that high-contrast edge highlighters placed flush with the tread nosing resulted in greater foot clearance (i.e., less chance of a misstep) than when they were placed further from the nosing or when there was no high-contrast edge highlighter.

23.2.2 Inconsistent Step Geometry

A construction flaw at the top of the stairway results in what Pauls (2001) has called the top of flight flaw (TOFF), a dangerous condition, since it can cause a person to fall the full length of the stairs. Commonly, TOFF occurs where the first run (the dimension of a tread in the direction of travel) below a landing is larger than the remaining runs (Archea et al., 1979; Johnson and Pauls, 2010; Pauls and Harbuck, 2008). Typically, this is caused by non-uniform nosing projections for the top steps of a flight that induce a user to place a foot too far forward on the second or third tread down, thereby increasing the chance of a fall down the stairway. TOFF can also occur when the top riser is shorter than subsequent risers.

TOFF existed on this stairway. Investigation revealed that the first tread had a run of 302 mm (11.9 in.), whereas the second tread down had a run of only 201.2 mm (9.8 in.) (see Figure 23.1).

This 53 mm (2.1 in.) variation is disallowed by the local (state) building code, which allows only 9.6 mm (0.38 in.) of variation between runs or between risers in a flight. The first riser down was 198 mm (7.8 in.), while the second riser was only 175 mm (6.9 in.). This 20.6 mm (0.9 in.) variation is also disallowed by the code. Research has shown that excessive variations between risers or between runs are associated with falls on stairs (Cohen et al., 2009; Jones, 1963; Templer, 1992).

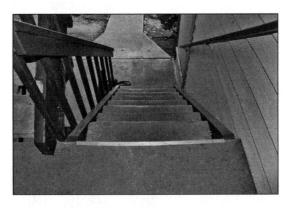

FIGURE 23.1
The top of flight flaw (TOFF) contributed to a fall on this stairway. The first run down was 53 mm (2.1 in.) larger than the next tread; there was also excess variation in risers, and the handrails were too low and too close to the supporting structures to grab.

23.2.3 Inadequate Handrails

Once the misstep occurred, the man's only chance of preventing a fall was to use a hand-rail. But the height of handrails above the treads on both sides of this stairway was, at 813 mm (32 in.), too short. According to Maki et al. (1984, 1985), the handrails should have extended 864–965 mm (34–38 in.) above the treads, a height that, they report, allowed users to exert greater force with which they could stabilize themselves in case of a misstep.

Further, the rails themselves were inadequate. The one to his right was as close as 19 mm (0.75 in.) to the supporting wall. The code requires at least twice that clearance, a minimum of 38 mm (1.5 in.). There is justification for this requirement: Openshaw and Taylor (2006) report that the 95th percentile male hand has a metacarpal thickness of 33 mm (1.3 in.). Even the 5th percentile female hand needs 20 mm (0.8 in.). Most adults would not have been able to grasp the right handrail with the power grip needed to stop a forward fall down the stairs.

The handrail to his left was even worse. There was zero clearance between it and the supporting structure. Further, it had a horizontal width of 89 mm (3.5 in.) and a vertical dimension of 127 mm (5 in.), a size that Maki (1985) found was not readily graspable. Even if he had been able to reach the rail, it is unlikely that he could have exerted adequate force to arrest his fall. The man suffered severe injuries to the left side of his body and his neck.

23.3 Second Case: Bottom of Flight Illusion Causes Fall Off Stairway

A 78-year-old lady was touring a model home and was descending the stairs when she fell near the bottom landing. Her fall was caused by what Johnson (2012) has referred to as the *bottom of flight illusion*, a situation that convinces the stair user she is stepping onto the bottom landing when, in reality, she is one or two treads above the landing.

23.3.1 Inadequate Visual Information

The view she had as she descended is approximated in Figure 23.2. Near the bottom, she turned to her right, stepped off onto what she thought was the bottom landing, and fell to the floor, fracturing her left proximal femur in the process. What she did not realize was that the bottom tread visually blended into the bottom landing.

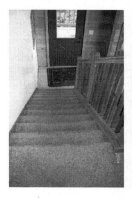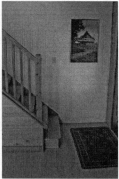

FIGURE 23.2
The bottom of flight Illusion was created by having the bottom tread of the same material and color as the bottom landing. Further, the handrail was too wide and did not extend to the bottom of the stairway as required.

23.3.2 Inadequate Handrails

Contributing to this bottom of flight illusion was a handrail that stopped 356 mm (14 in.) short of the bottom nosing, even though the building code (IRC, 2012) requires rails in private residences, as in this case, to extend to a point above the top and bottom nosings. This provision was not complied with. Further, the horizontal dimensions of the rail were, at 76 × 76 mm (3 × 3 in.), too large to be easily grasped. The code (IRC, 2012) called for the dimension to be no greater than 32 × 51 mm (1.25 × 2 in.).

23.4 Third Case: Variable Step Geometry Causes Misstep and Fall

A 48-year-old woman fell as she was descending the stairs from the apartment she had lived in for several years.

She had had no previous problems using the stairway. As she approached the intermediate landing, she experienced a misstep, fell forward, and impacted that landing. Her right foot ended up behind her, caught in the open riser between the second and third treads up from the landing. She fractured her right distal tibia and fibula.

23.4.1 Inadequate Visual Information

The nosings, as seen in Figure 23.3, were not highlighted, as required by the code, which had adopted ICC/ANSI A117.1. If the leading two nosings had been of high contrast, then, as Foster et al. (2014) found, she would have been more likely to place her feet accurately on the treads.

23.4.2 Inconsistent Step Geometry

In the section of the stairs where she started to fall, investigation revealed excessive variations of 43 mm (1.7 in.) between adjacent risers and 25.4 mm (1.0 in.) between adjacent runs. These variations most likely contributed to her misstep.

23.4.3 Inadequate Handrails

Although the code calls for handrails to be on both sides of the stairs, there was a handrail on one side only, and it was inadequate. It was only 787 mm (31 in.) above the treads, too

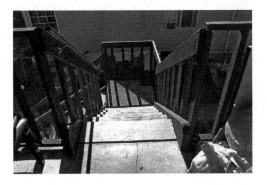

FIGURE 23.3
The woman was descending this flight when she experienced a misstep before reaching the intermediate landing. Irregular step geometry, lack of highlighting on the tread nosings, and inadequate handrails contributed to her fall.

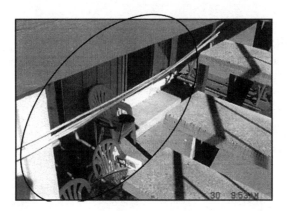

FIGURE 23.4
The opening through which the boy fell is circled. The loose electrical wires seen here were reportedly there on the day of the fall. The opening was such that a sphere 406 mm (16 in.) in diameter could have passed through it. The code calls for the opening to disallow a sphere 152 mm (6 in.) or larger to pass.

low to conform to the 864–965 mm (34–38 in.) height required by the code (IRC, 2012) and as recommended by research (e.g., Maki et al., 1984, 1985).

23.5 Fourth Case: Inadequate Guardrail Protection Allows Fall Off Stairway

On a mid-July day in 2002, a three-year-old boy, >1041 mm (41 in.) in height and weighing >17 kg (37 lb,) was sitting on a stairway of the apartment building where he lived when he fell through the open side of the stairway (see Figure 23.4). No one saw or heard him fall.

His 14-year-old aunt/guardian had briefly left him sitting on the 13th tread up from the concrete surface, a height of about 1956 mm (77 in.). She found him lying on the concrete off to the side of the stairway. He suffered a skull fracture with an epidural hematoma in the left occipital area. The fall reportedly caused a lasting brain injury with cognitive implications.

If a child's head can get through an opening, the child's body can also fit through that opening. The opening through which he fell would have allowed a sphere 406 mm (16 in.) in diameter to pass, more than enough to allow his body to fall through. But the code in existence at the time of the fall (1997 Uniform Building Code, Sec. 509.3) disallowed any side openings on stairs that would allow a sphere 152 mm (6 in.) or larger to pass. If the guardrail had met this specification, he would most likely not have fallen.

23.6 Fifth Case: Short Flight Causes Fall

Changes in level of only one to three risers can be hazardous unless they are in an expected location (e.g., curb–street transition). When approached from the lower level, such a change in level can cause a trip and fall forward. When approached from the upper level, a person can experience what has been called an *air step*, which occurs when a person who is on the upper level of a walking surface is unaware of a step down or depression in the walkway ahead and steps out into air (Thompson et al., 2005). While the foot that is in swing phase fails to land on the expected solid surface, the forward momentum of the upper torso continues to carry the person forward. But the forward foot lands later than expected and on a surface that is below what is expected.

When the forward foot lands on the lower level, the person's center of gravity may be too far forward to be supported by the forward foot. This can cause the person to continue moving forward and downward. A younger person may keep from falling to the ground by quickly moving the rearward foot forward for support. Older people, however, may be less likely to perform this feat.

23.6.1 Inadequate Visual Information

Just after dawn on a cloudy wet day in December, a 50-year-old bus driver was walking from a restroom toward external stairs leading down to the bus she was to operate as part of her employment. She had never walked this route before. As she approached the stairs, she encountered an unexpected and difficult-to-see single-riser step down that was not visually demarcated. She was focused on the handrail associated with the stairway beyond; there was no handrail for users of the single-riser step.

A national standard (ASTM F1637-95) had warned of the danger associated with flights of three or fewer risers and how the danger could be ameliorated. It was recommended that such short flights be avoided where possible and, if not possible, that

> obvious visual cues shall be provided to facilitate improved step identification. Handrails, delineated nosing edges, tactile cues, warning signs, contrast in surface colors, and accent lighting are examples of some appropriate warning cues. (ASTM F1637-95, Sec. 6.2)

Two years before her fall, the danger had been recognized by the county metro district that was in charge of the facility. A simple method for alleviating the danger (highlighting the step) was prescribed. Yet, no action was taken. On encountering this hazard, she fell forward, fracturing her right femur, right patella, and left thumb. She also sprained her left ankle and left knee, broke several teeth, and sustained a bloody forehead. If the top surface of the step had been highlighted, or if some other recommended action had been taken, then, more probably than not, this fall would have been prevented (Figure 23.5).

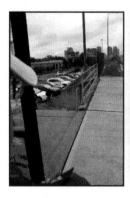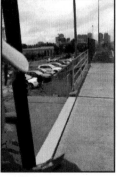

FIGURE 23.5
The left photograph, taken over the woman's right shoulder, shows the single riser tread and the lower level as it may have appeared to her before she fell. The right photograph shows the surface of the upper level after it was digitally "painted."

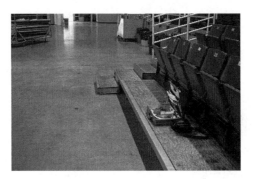

FIGURE 23.6
A woman was walking in front of the seated attendees when her view of the encroaching bottom tread of a stairway was blocked by her adult daughter. She tripped and fell over the tread. If the handrail had extended to the bottom of the stairs, as required, the chance of this fall occurring would have been greatly reduced.

23.7 Sixth Case: Encroaching Tread Causes a Trip and Fall

A 48-year-old woman was walking with her adult daughter toward the exit of an auditorium, while others, who were entering the auditorium, were coming from the opposite direction. This caused the two women to walk in single file next to the bleachers. The daughter then moved in front of her mother and walked around the encroaching tread in their path (see Figure 23.6).

There was adequate illumination inside the auditorium to see the encroaching tread, but her view of the tread was obscured by her daughter, who was only about 610–914 mm (24–36 in.) in front of her. The tread extended 41 mm (16 in.) into their path and protruded vertically 140 mm (5.5 in.), high enough to produce a significant trip hazard.

23.7.1 Inadequate Handrail

No handrail extended to the bottom of the stairway, although the code (1988 UBC Chapter 33, Sec. 3306) required at least one handrail to extend the full length of the stairs plus an additional 152 mm (6 in.). Even though the daughter saw and avoided the encroaching tread, her mother, without adequate preview time, did not see the tread before tripping over it. She incurred lacerations on her chin and right forearm and a hematoma on the right tibia area and fractured the head of her left tibia. If the handrail had extended to the bottom tread and beyond, as required by the code, she would more likely than not have seen it in time to avert tripping and falling.

23.8 Seventh Case: Broken Nosing

A large 45-year-old logger fell as he started to descend the external stairs outside an office when his right shoe was placed on the first tread down from the upper landing. His 338 mm (13.3 in.)-long shoe was placed on a step that had a run of 234 mm (9.2 in.) generally, but because of a defect, only 208 mm (8.2 in.) in the area where his foot landed in a 2.54 mm (1 in.) deep divot. The defect did not appear to be recent, indicating a lack of adequate maintenance.

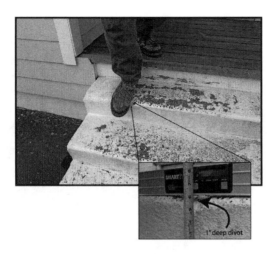

FIGURE 23.7
As the man stepped down, the sole of his right foot landed in a 1 in. deep divot in the nosing, which caused his shoe to twist unexpectedly, resulting in his fall. The fall could have been prevented if adequate maintenance had been performed on the steps and if a handrail had been placed within his reach.

23.8.1 Inconsistent Step Geometry

The small run of 208 mm (8.2 in.) violated building codes as far back as 1940. As he applied weight to his right foot, it pivoted over and then slipped off the nosing of the tread, and he fell backward, injuring his right shoulder and elbow as well as his back.

23.8.2 Inadequate Handrails

He might have been able to reduce the severity of injury had a handrail been on both sides of the stairway as required by the code. There was only one handrail, and it was out of his reach.

If the broken nosing had been repaired, and if there had been handrails within reach as required by the code, the probability of this fall occurring would have been greatly reduced (Figure 23.7).

23.9 Eighth Case: Slippery Nosing

A 42-year-old construction worker was descending a temporary stairway at a high-rise construction site when one of his feet slipped off the nosing of a tread near the top landing. He landed on his buttocks and, with both feet in front of him, bounced down several steps, causing injury to his back. Even though other workers had slipped on the wet metal stairs, and had notified management of the hazard, no actions had been taken to alleviate the danger.

Examination revealed extrusions in the metal surface. These extrusions were, when new, raised with sharp edges at the top. Such extrusions can increase the slip resistance of the surface unless they are worn smooth, as was the case in this incident (see Figure 23.8).

Further, the extrusions were placed over >2.54 mm (1 in.) back from the nosing. But to prevent the foot from pivoting over and slipping off a tread, slip-resistant surfaces must be closer to the nosing. The wet metal stairway where the man fell produced a slippery condition that is not allowed by code >(iBC 2012).

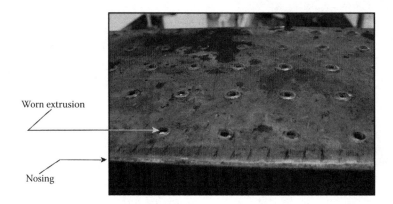

FIGURE 23.8
The nosing at the front of the tread is smooth. The extrusions nearest the nosing were worn smooth, so they no longer reduced slipperiness, thus contributing to the man's fall. If the step geometry had been consistent, and if the slip resistance of the stairs had been maintained, this fall most likely would have been averted.

23.9.1 Inconsistent Step Geometry

There was a variation of nearly 13 mm (0.5 in.) between runs at this location. If the step geometry had been consistent, and if the nosing had been slip resistant, this fall would have been averted.

23.10 Ninth Case: Unlit and Camouflaged Nosings

In the middle of a sunny afternoon, a man and his 52-year-old wife entered a theater to view a dance recital. It was their first time visiting this theater. They immediately climbed a well-lit stairway, which had handrails on both sides to an upper landing, and started down a darkened stairway toward their seating location. Only the stage lighting was up.

23.10.1 Inadequate Visual Information

The elapsed time from when they entered the theater until they were on the stairs where the fall occurred was 2 min or less. According to Lamb and Pugh (2006), the time it takes to recover dark adaptation for the rods and cones varies from 5 to 30 min. The woman would not have adapted to the dark by the time she started to descend the stairs toward their seats.

Further, as seen in Figure 23.9, the carpet pattern made it difficult to determine the locations of the nosings, a safety problem Templer (1992, p. 141) discusses. ASTM F1637 states that "Step nosings shall be readily discernable, slip resistant and adequately demarcated. Random, pictorial, floral geometric designs are examples of design elements that can camouflage a step nosing."

23.10.2 Inconsistent Step Geometry

The variation between the risers she encountered was a code-violating 20 mm (0.8 in.), and the runs in the vicinity of her fall *doubled* from an average of 267 mm (10.5 in.) to over 533 mm (21 in.).

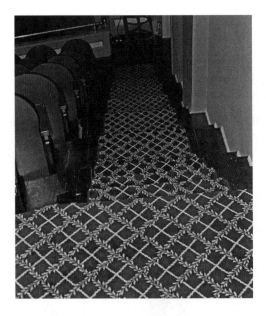

FIGURE 23.9
A woman was descending these stairs under low illumination and fell when she was about halfway down. The nosings were camouflaged, the step geometry was inconsistent, and there was no handrail she could use to stop herself falling after her design-induced misstep.

23.10.3 Inadequate Handrails

She had her right hand on the wall searching for a handrail (there was none) and was feeling with her feet for the front edges of the treads when she fell, fracturing her coccyx.

This fall would have been prevented if this stairway had been adequately illuminated, the treads had not been visually camouflaged but, instead, the nosings had been demarcated, the variation between the risers and between the runs had not been excessive, and a handrail had been in place.

23.11 Summary

These cases demonstrate that if building codes and safety standards were complied with, there would be fewer falls on stairs. Inadequate visual information was judged to have been a contributing factor in five cases (1, 2, 3, 5, and 9). Inadequate step geometry was a contributing factor also in five cases (1, 3, 7, 8, and 9). Inadequate handrails were a contributing factor in seven cases (1, 2, 3, 4 [guardrail], 6, 7, and 9). Lack of maintenance was a factor in two cases (7 and 8).

References

ASTM F 1637 - 95 (1995). Standard practice for safe walking surfaces. West Conshohocken, PA: ASTM International.

Archea, J., Collins, B. and Stahl, F. (1979). *Guidelines for Stair Safety. NBS Building Science Series 120.* Washington, DC: National Bureau of Standards. http://fire.nist.gov/bfrlpubs/build79/art002.html.

Cohen, J., LaRue, C. A., and Cohen, H. H. (2009). An ergonomics analysis of 80 cases. *Professional Safety,* 54, 27–41.

Foster, R.J., Hotchkiss, J., Buckley, J.G., and Elliott, D.B. (2014). Safety on stairs: Influence of a tread edge highlighter and its position. *Experimental Gerontology* 55(July), 152–158.

IBC, *International Building Code* (2012). Falls Church, VA: International Code Council.

ICC/ANSI A117.1-2003. (2004). Accessible and usable buildings and facilities. *International Code Council.* Falls Church, VA: International Code Council.

IRC, *International Residential Code for One- and Two-Family Dwellings* (2012). Falls Church, VA: International Code Council.

Johnson, D.A. (2012). Stair safety: Bottom of flight illusion. *Work: A Journal of Prevention, Assessment and Rehabilitation,* (41) Supplement 1/2012, 3358–3362. Presentation: The 18th World Congress on Ergonomics, Recife, Brazil. International Ergonomics Association.

Johnson, D.A. and Pauls, J. (2010). Systemic stair step geometry defects, increased injuries, and public health plus regulatory responses. In Anderson, M. (Ed.) *Contemporary Ergonomics and Human Factors.* Boca Raton, FL: CRC Press.

Johnson, D.A. and Pauls, J. (2012). Why should home stairs be less safe? *Trial News,* 47(8), 11–15. Seattle: Washington State Association for Justice.

Jones, R.A. (1963). New safety developments in home construction and equipment. *National Safety Council Transactions 6.* Itasca, IL: National Safety Council.

Lamb, T.D. and Pugh, E.N. (2006). Phototransduction, dark adaptation, and rhodopsin regeneration: The Proctor Lecture. *Investigative Ophthalmology and Visual Science,* 47(12), 5138–5152.

Maki, B.E. (1985). *Influence of Handrail Shape, Size and Surface Texture on the Ability of Young and Elderly Users to Generate Stabilizing Forces and Moments* (Contract No. 0SR84-00197). Ontario, Canada: National Research Council.

Maki, B.E., Bartlett, S.A., and Fernie, G. R. (1984). Influence of stairway handrail height on the ability to generate stabilizing forces and moments. *Human Factors,* 26(6), 705–714.

Maki, B.E., Bartlett, S.A., and Fernie, G.R. (1985). Effect of stairway pitch on optimal handrail height. *Human Factors,* 27(3), 355–359.

Openshaw, S. and Taylor, G. (2006). *Ergonomics and Design: A Reference Guide.* Downloaded April 1, 2014 from http://www.allsteeloffice.com/synergydocuments/ ergonomicsanddesignreferenceguidewhitepaper.pdf.

Pauls, J. (2001). Life safety standards and guidelines focused on stairways. In Preiser, W.F.E. and Ostroff, E. (Eds.) *Universal Design Handbook,* 23.1–23.20. New York: McGraw-Hill.

Pauls, J. (2011). *Injury Epidemiology.* Downloaded from http://stairusabilityandsafety.com/down-loads/ICSUS_Panel_Presentations/1%20ICSUS%20Summaries-REV.pdf.

Pauls, J.L. and Harbuck, S.C. (2008). *Ergonomics-Based Methods of Inspecting, Assessing and Documenting Environmental Sites of Injurious Falls.* Presented at American Society of Safety Engineers. Downloaded October 24, 2008 from www.asse.org/education/pdc08/show-session.php?id=704.

Templer, J. (1992). *The Staircase: Studies of Hazards, Falls and Safer Design. Vol. 2.* Cambridge, MA: MIT Press, 151–152.

Thompson, D. A. Cohen, H. H., Horst, D. P., Johnson, D.A., and Olsen, R.A. (2005). A guide to forensic human factors terminology. In W. Karwowski and I. Noy (Eds.) *Handbook of Human Factors in Litigation.* New York: Taylor & Francis Group.

Uniform Building Code. (1985). *UBC.* Whittier, CA: International Conference of Building Officials.

Zietz, D., Johannsen, L., and Hollands, M. (2011). Stepping characteristics and centre of mass control during stair descent: Effects of age, fall risk and visual factors. *Gait and Posture,* 34, 279–284.

24

Enhancing Safety Awareness among Roofing Workers

Yu-Hsiu Hung

CONTENTS

ABSTRACT One of the most hazardous sectors within the construction industry is the roofing industry. In this industry, falls from roof are the primary event source leading to fatal/nonfatal injuries. Research has shown that fall-prevention training is an effective measure to ensure that standard prevention practices are followed. However, standard prevention practices are poor among roofing subcontractors. To prevent falls through effective fall-protection training, in this chapter, we introduce two case studies that attempted to understand the deficiencies of the fall-prevention methods in the field and the field training needs among residential roofing subcontractors. The results of the two studies provide insight into the design of safety training interventions.

KEY WORDS: *fall, roof, safety training, fall protection.*

24.1 Introduction

The construction industry is a hazardous business. It leads all other private industries in the number of fatal injuries and represents about 21% of all work-related fatalities (US Bureau of Labor Statistics, 2009a). In residential construction, falls remain the leading cause of injuries and fatalities; the likelihood of roofing workers getting injured is higher than for workers in other trades. Although the Occupational Safety and Health Administration (OSHA) requires roofing employers to be responsible for providing workers with a place of employment that is free from hazards (US Bureau of Labor Statistics, 1999), such a general mandate becomes somewhat murky in the construction environment. The accident rate of roofing workers continues to be higher than for the average construction trades worker (US Bureau of Labor Statistics, 2009a). Developing safety measures to reduce fall injuries and accidents is becoming imperative.

Most fall accidents occur in situations where standard prevention practices and use of personal protective equipment are not in place (Lipscomb et al., 2004). Huang and Hinze (2003) concluded from their analysis of 10 years of construction accidents that the severity of fall hazards tends to be misjudged by workers—nor do workers' direct experiences with fall hazards seem to diminish accident occurrence. Huang and Hinze (2003) suggested that more training is needed to prevent falls, especially with respect to increased safety awareness. Similarly, research has confirmed that fall-prevention training is an effective measure to ensure that prevention practices are followed and to reduce falls.

Understanding roofing workers' training needs is an important step in the design of fall-protection training. However, knowing needs is inadequate to guarantee successful implementation of safety training. For safety training to be effective among roofing contractors, it is necessary to understand the methods that roofers typically use to prevent falls and how the deficiencies of the methods could be addressed by training courses and/or OSHA's safety training requirements. In fact, fall protection is the most frequently cited OSHA standard in construction (US Bureau of Labor Statistics, 2014), and fall-protection training has to be delivered in the languages roofing workers use (Hung et al., 2013). Only by reflecting the deficiencies of the fall-prevention methods in the field through training design can OSHA's safety training requirements be followed, and thus, falls be prevented. The goal of this chapter is to identify these deficiencies through Case Study 1. This chapter also includes Case Study 2 to understand roofers' field training needs (especially from the perspective of OSHA fall-protection training requirements). The two case studies were based on the notion that *understanding* roofing workers' fall-prevention methods and training needs for developing an "effective" training intervention was more important than simply having safety training programs in place.

24.2 Case Study 1: Understanding Current Fall-Prevention Methods among Residential Roofing Subcontractors

The construction industry consists primarily of small contractors (Hester et al., 2003), which represent 91% of the total number of construction establishments (US Census Bureau, 2008). The majority of these companies are associated with residential work—in fact, about five times more than those who work in the commercial sector (US Census Bureau, 2008). The aim of this case study was to identify (1) the deficiencies of the methods that roofers typically use to prevent injuries and falls and (2) the problems of current safety training (i.e., how safety training is wrongly practiced among residential roofing subcontractors). The results of this study would provide insight into the design of fall-protection training interventions.

24.2.1 Method: Semi-Structured Interview

24.2.1.1 Participants

Purposeful sampling (Patton, 1990) was employed to recruit participants. A total of 29 participants were recruited to participate in the semi-structured interview. The participants were from 29 small roofing companies in the rural and urban geographic regions in Virginia and North Carolina. Participants were required to be roofers working in a construction firm, because small construction firms represent most of the establishments (about 91% in 2008) in the roofing industry (US Census Bureau, 2008), and the accident rate among smaller firms is disproportionately higher than in larger firms (Holmes et al., 1999; Kines, 2003). In addition, one half of the participants were managerial personnel (including owners, supervisors, and foremen); the other half of the participants were employees. All participants had to be 18 years or older and to have had at least 1 year's work experience in the residential roofing industry. It should be noted that a research facilitator whose first language is Spanish was recruited and trained in advance to administer the questionnaire to Hispanic workers.

The sample demographics are shown in Table 24.1. Forty-five percent of the participants (13) were European–American workers, while 55% were Hispanic workers (16). The sampling structure (consisting of mainly European–American and Hispanic workers) reflected the ethnic distribution of the employed roofers (US Bureau of Labor Statistics, 2011b) and the fact that construction workers have differing "cultural" mindsets toward the perceptions of hazards (Brunette, 2004; Roelofs et al., 2011). Most of the participants had more than 10 years of work experience. In general, the managerial personnel tended to have more years of work experience.

24.2.1.2 Interview Questions and Procedure

The questions in the semi-structured interview were developed to identify methods roofers used to prevent falls and specific programmatic aspects that could potentially influence workers' willingness to use/implement OHSA's fall-protection training. Two main open-ended questions were used in this study:

1. Can you talk about your practices of fall prevention? In other words, what methods do you use to prevent falling off roof during work?
2. Can you talk about your needs for fall-protection training?

TABLE 24.1

Sample Demographics of the Semi-Structured Interview

Job	No.	Ethnicity		Work Experience (years)	
		European–American	Hispanic	1–10	>10
Managerial personnel	13	6	7	3	10
Worker	16	7	9	7	9
Total	29	13	16	10	19

The interview was conducted primarily during participants' lunch break. Before receiving the interview, participants signed an informed consent form, which included an assurance of confidentiality and anonymity. To prevent response bias, prior to the interview, the interviewer talked with the participants to put them at ease. The interviewer also ensured that participants understood the goals of the study and were comfortable with the process. This protocol helped the interviewer attain a certain level of trust and openness so that he could be accepted as nonjudgmental and nonthreatening. In addition to asking the participants the prepared questions, the interviewer also asked supplementary questions for clarification and to provide greater detail where necessary. All interviews with Hispanic workers were conducted in Spanish by the research facilitator recruited. Participants' responses were audio-recorded to support data analysis processes.

24.2.1.3 Content Analysis

The audio files of the interview (English and Spanish) were transcribed and translated into English by a professional transcription service company. Content analysis (Downe-Wamboldt, 1992) was carried out on the transcripts of the interview. Each piece of information (including participants' phrases, sentences, and paragraphs) related to the research questions was coded by two independent coders separately and without consultation. The independent coders had expertise in construction health and safety and human factors research. They created codes based on a Grounded Theory approach (Charmaz, 1995; Glaser and Strauss, 1977), whereby no presumptions were made on the participants' responses. Atlas.ti (ATLAS.ti Scientific Software Development GmbH, 2008), a qualitative data analysis software, was used to store text documents and support information coding.

24.2.2 Results and Discussion

Two major themes were generated from the content analysis in addressing the goals of this study: (1) current methods to prevent falls and injuries; and (2) problems of current safety training.

With respect to *Current methods to prevent falls and injuries*, participants highlighted differing methods/approaches they thought useful. These methods were coded and grouped into three areas in Table 24.2.

The first category was *Selfcare/Rely on coworker*, containing 11 codes related to self-control of risks and negative mentality toward injuries and accidents. Table 24.2 shows a high frequency of "rely on luck," "look out for each other," "self safety responsibility," "constant safety reminder," "pay attention," "complete trust in coworkers," "experienced workers give advice," and "experienced workers oversee the site." These codes show that in the participants' minds, paying attention will mean that they do not put themselves in danger. As indicated by a European–American worker, "If you get up there acting stupid, then you're going to fall, but if you get up there paying attention to what you're doing, those boards, then you ain't going to fall."

In addition, participants believed that coworkers or experienced workers would keep an eye on risks and hazards. Some participants thought that their health and safety would not be threatened by bad luck. For example, a Hispanic female worker commented: "They don't think that if they don't tie up themselves they are going to fall and they could die or they could get hurt in a way that they are going to be unable to work anymore." A similar comment was made by a European–American supervisor: "A lot of people think that they're—I guess they feel invincible, you know, that it's not going to happen to them."

TABLE 24.2

Current Methods to Prevent Injuries: Codes and Frequencies

Code	Frequency	%
Selfcare/Rely on Coworker	127	68.28
• Rely on luck	25	—
• Look out for each other	23	—
• Self safety responsibility	20	—
• Constant safety reminders	16	—
• Pay attention	16	—
• Complete trust in coworkers	11	—
• Experienced workers give advice	9	—
• Experienced workers oversee the site	4	—
• Follow standard work procedure	2	—
• Working in proper weather conditions to prevent problems	1	—
Personal Protective Equipment (PPE) Related	50	26.89
• Often check security of PPE on jobsite	28	—
• Employers provide PPE	8	—
• Always secures ladder	6	—
• Workers assimilate to uncomfortable PPE because it is important	5	—
• Daily equipment check	3	—
Worksite Safety Rules and Company Policy	9	4.84
• Drug and alcohol tests	3	—
• Assign new employees with less dangerous job	3	—
• Hires based on experience	2	—
• Safety sheet before work	1	—
Total	**186**	**100**

The second category was *personal protective equipment (PPE) related*, which encompassed the following five codes: "often check security of PPE on jobsite," "employers provide PPE," "always secures ladder," "workers assimilate to uncomfortable PPE because it is important," "daily equipment check." The frequency in this category was about one-half of that in the first category. It may mean that in the interview, proper use of PPE was the second thing that came into participants' minds to prevent falls. However, wearing/checking PPE (e.g., ladders and ropes) was important to prevent falls. As a European–American supervisor commented, "It's easy for a ladder to move, you know, if it's not set properly. And even if it is set properly, it can still move. So, umm, you know that's something, I think, most people should focus on a little bit more." A Hispanic supervisor echoed: "Yeah, yeah, that's the most important, have a rope, and never loose rope, which is tied to the trough. That's the one, you know, that's the main thing."

The third category was *worksite safety rules and company policy*, which contained four codes related to safety management and company policy to prevent falls: "drug and alcohol tests," "assign new employees with less dangerous job," "hires based on experience," "safety sheet before work." In fact, across all categories, this category was the least mentioned in the interview. The frequency of nine (4.84% of the total utterances) may mean that, for most participants (most with over 10 years of roofing experience), safety sheets/drug and alcohol tests, or even assigning less dangerous jobs to new workers and hiring

TABLE 24.3

Problems of Current Safety Training: Codes and Frequencies (Number of Utterances)

Code	Frequency	%
Poor Safety Training Climate	**65**	**67**
• No safety training at all	19	—
• Lack of formal training	18	—
• Safety meetings/training only for new information	11	—
• Low frequency of company safety meeting	9	—
• Vague training	8	—
Insufficient Safety Training at Work	**32**	**33**
• No training for experienced workers	12	—
• One-time safety training for new employees	6	—
• One-time training on safety equipment use	6	—
• Follow-up training if necessary	3	—
• Inappropriate safety training to senior workers	2	—
• Training depending on onsite work behavior	1	—
• No safety training for beginners	1	—
• Focus training on senior worker	1	—
Total	**97**	**100**

experienced workers, might not be the methods they commonly used to prevent injuries and falls.

With respect to *problems of current safety training*, participants targeted several areas. These were coded and grouped into two categories, shown in Table 24.3.

The first category was *poor safety training climate*, which included five codes indicating participants' shared perceptions on safety training practices – two of which received the highest frequencies: "no safety training at all" and "lack of formal professional training." According to participants, the problem was that safety training has been a missing piece on the construction site. As indicated by a European–American worker, "I don't think—we never really had no—this, other than they tell us where the harnesses are, and this stuff I get and that's it." A European–American supervisor also noted: "We don't have classes or groups or anything that…we don't do, you know, something every month or every week or what not, the safety meetings." Regarding the frequency of receiving formal safety training, a European–American supervisor responded: "I think that was three years ago… to get some uh—when you get that periodic stuff, and sit in health safety kinds of seminars that our whole company goes to, for example, for CPR and first aid."

In general, safety training was not perceived as a "must" by most participants. There might be safety training courses or seminars sporadically conducted by OSHA or insurance companies if rules or regulations changed. However, most participants felt vague about the new rules and course materials, as they might not necessarily reflect what they did or needed on the job.

The second category was *insufficient safety training at work*, which contained eight problems (codes) specifically about safety training practices on the site. The most frequently mentioned problem was that safety training was not provided to experienced workers. Sometimes, it was only provided once to new (i.e., inexperienced) workers and/or when new equipment arrived. Some companies preferred to provide safety training thoroughly at the beginning, but with no follow-ups unless necessary. In addition, safety training was sometimes not provided to beginners or even tailored to fit senior workers' needs. As a Hispanic supervisor commented, "I'm doing this for 12 years, for 15 years. And you're going to give me equipment on how to do this, you know, I will not be happy, because I know exactly what to do, and uh yeah, so, that's the main thing, really ... some companies will give you like a lot of stuff that you don't need." Additionally, safety training might only be held if the work crew demonstrated unsafe work practices. To make sure that most workers follow safety rules, it was also suggested that safety training should be delivered to senior workers. As indicated by a Hispanic supervisor, "They're going to be all day on the roof, and then they're going to stay all the time on the roof, and then all the employees. If you tell one, rest will follow, you know."

24.2.3 Conclusions: Deficiencies of the Field Fall-Prevention Methods

The results of the content analysis identified five primary methods that roofers used to prevent falls:

1. Count on coworkers or experienced workers to avoid risks and hazards
2. Push luck (health and safety would not be threatened by bad luck)
3. Pay attention to avoid danger
4. Wear/check PPE (e.g., ladder and rope setup)
5. Follow worksite safety rules and company policy (e.g., sign on safety sheets, receive drug and alcohol tests, assign less dangerous jobs to beginners, and hire experienced workers)

Among these five methods, the first two methods were actually the most frequently mentioned methods in the interview. However, they are the least reliable of the five identified methods and are not either encouraged or regulated by OSHA to prevent injuries and falls. Such deficiencies need to be addressed massively in fall-protection training.

In addition, the results of the content analysis also identified six major problems of current safety training:

1. Safety training was not perceived as a "must" at the jobsite.
2. Safety training was not provided to experienced workers.
3. Safety training was provided to senior workers because other workers would follow safety rules accordingly.
4. Formal safety training was typically vague.
5. Safety training might only be held if the work crew demonstrated unsafe work practices.
6. Safety training was conducted once at the beginning and only for beginners and/ or when new equipment arrived.

From the findings, safety training has been a work element generally ignored on the construction site. Roofing workers tended to accept the fact that safety training was not adequately conducted to benefit all workers. Thus, it is imperative to enhance safety awareness among roofing subcontractors through either formal or informal fall-protection training. Making workers perceive worksite safety as a top priority will be necessary to effectively prevent falls from roof.

24.3 Case Study 2: Understanding Fall-Protection Training Needs from the Perspective of OSHA's Safety Training Requirements

According to OSHA, of the top 10 most frequently cited workplace safety violations for fiscal year 2014, number one is fall protection (US Bureau of Labor Statistics, 2014). As fall-protection training may play a big role in decreasing the number of safety violations, this case study aimed to understand roofers' perceived fall-protection training needs, especially from the perspective of OSHA's safety training requirements. The results of this study would provide insight into the design of fall-protection training interventions.

24.3.1 Method: Questionnaire

24.3.1.1 Instrument Development Process

The questionnaire contained 10 close-ended items to understand workers' perceived fall-protection training needs, which were derived from OSHA's six fall-protection training requirements (US Bureau of Labor Statistics, 1999a). The response categories for the questionnaire items used a Likert scale format with anchors from 1 (strongly disagree) to 5 (strongly agree). The questionnaire items were:

Which piece of information should be added to your company's training program to avoid falls?

1. Identification of possible onsite fall hazards
2. Ways to minimize fall hazards for OSHA compliance
3. What to do when a safety monitoring system is in place
4. What to do in my company's alternative fall-protection plan when the use of traditional fall-protection systems is not feasible
5. Limitations of mechanical fall-protection systems used for roof work
6. Standard procedures for
   a. Maintaining, disassembling, and inspecting fall-protection systems
   b. Using fall-protection systems
   c. Handling and storing mechanical equipment used for work on low-sloped roofs
   d. Handling and storing roofing materials
   f. Putting up overhead protection systems

The development of the questionnaire was carried out through pre- (i.e., content validity) and post-data-collection assessment of reliability and construct validity, which were noted as requirements for creating a reliable instrument (Straub et al., 2004). To address the likelihood of non-English-speaking participants, a Spanish-language version of the questionnaire was created by an undergraduate student with research experience in construction safety and Spanish fluency. Both the English- and Spanish-language versions were then given to a professional Spanish translator for proofreading. The original English questionnaire and the Spanish questionnaire were then sent to two subject matter experts (SMEs) separately for proofreading. One SME had the same background as the developer of the Spanish questionnaire. Another SME was a specialist in construction health and safety and human factors theory. After reviewing the questionnaire, the two SMEs met with the principal investigator to finalize the Spanish-version questionnaire. Item finalization was based on group consensus.

24.3.1.2 Face and Content Validity

Face validity of the questionnaire was performed at the beginning by four SMEs with expertise in industrial and systems engineering, education, construction health and safety, and psychology, each of whom reviewed and commented on the wording of the questionnaire items. Content validity was performed using a quantitative approach to understand the extent to which a questionnaire item measures its given construct (Lawshe, 1975). First, a content validity questionnaire was generated, which included questionnaire items on a three-point scale: 1 = not necessary; 2 = useful but not essential; 3 = essential. Second, 11 SMEs were identified on the basis of their broad involvement with the research subject area, including experts in the fields of industrial and systems engineering, psychology, industrial management, education, design, construction health and safety, and computer science. After agreeing to participate in the study, the SMEs were given the instructions, a reference document explaining the constructs, and the content validity questionnaire. For each questionnaire item, the SMEs' responses indicating "Essential" were calculated.

The content validity ratio (CVR) for each item was estimated and evaluated with a significance level of 0.05. Items that were not significant were either removed or modified for reevaluation based on the SMEs' comments. Items that were not removed or reworded were considered to be effective in measuring their given constructs. All question items were reevaluated and modified till their CVR value was significant, which meant that its value was greater than 0.818—that is, a questionnaire item was rated "Essential" by at least 10 SMEs. The results of the content validity assessment showed that the CVR value was 0.96 (SD = 0.08), which suggested good content validity of the questionnaire. In addition, the Flesch–Kincaid readability test of the questionnaire was performed in Microsoft Word. The results showed that the reading level of the questionnaire was 7, meaning that the questionnaire could be easily understood by a seventh grader. To ensure that the questionnaire was understood by every roofing worker, this study also featured an informal pilot test, whereby a roofing manager checked the wording of the questionnaire items.

24.3.1.3 Participants

Purposeful sampling (Patton, 1990), a nonprobability sampling method used to select information-rich cases for in-depth studies, was employed to recruit participants. The sampling criteria and the time the questionnaire was administered were the same as those used in Study 1. The contact information of small roofing contractors was obtained through local business yellow pages and the phone book directory, from the Center for Innovation in Construction Safety and Health (CICSH) at Virginia Tech, and via information on local building permits. Roofing contractors were contacted and screened regarding their qualifications for this research. Appointments were made once roofing contractors agreed to participate in the study. A total of 128 participants from 29 small roofing companies in the rural and urban geographic regions in Virginia and North Carolina participated in the study. Of the 128 completed questionnaires (English or Spanish version), 24 were not used due to incomplete responses. Thus, 104 questionnaires were considered to be valid for data analysis.

24.3.2 Results and Discussion

Table 24.4 provides a demographic overview of the participants in the study. The majority of the participants were European–American workers (76%). Twenty-three percent were Hispanic workers, and 1% were Asian workers. Thirty-seven percent of the participants were managerial personnel; 63% were employees. The managerial personnel were more experienced and better educated than the employees.

A correlation analysis was performed to assess the reliability of the questionnaire items. The Cronbach coefficient alpha of *perceived fall-protection training needs* was $r_{alpha} = 0.96$, with an inter-item correlation r ranging from 0.54 to 0.88, $p < .05$. In addition, frequency analysis was performed on important demographic questions. The results showed that (1) about one tenth (12%) of the participants did not know whether their companies provided safety training; (2) 60% of the participants preferred informal training, whereas about 50% of the participants preferred training materials to be delivered as hard copies, such as documents created by lecturers, material safety data sheets (MSDSs) (e.g., adding information to the sheets for debris removal, single-ply roof system adhesives, and elastomeric coating materials), and notecards; (3) only a small portion (20%) of the participants preferred the materials to be delivered through technologies (e.g., computers and mobile devices). These results suggest that safety training is variable among roofing contractors. It may not have become an essential part of the organizational culture of most roofing companies. In addition, although participants preferred informal safety training on the site, they desired to be trained using formal portable training materials. In addition, although technological training materials may have been developed and/or proposed by scholars or safety services companies for some time, they did not get much attention from the participants when it came to safety training.

Figure 24.1 illustrates the descriptive statistics with respect to which piece of information should be added to a company's training program to avoid falls. The results showed that the average ratings for the 10 training need items were all above Neutral (3) and close to Agree (4). This suggests that participants wanted to receive more fall-protection training in every aspect required by OSHA, such as knowledge of minimizing and identifying fall hazards, limitations of mechanical fall-protection systems, and standard procedures for using, maintaining, and handling fall-protection systems.

24.3.3 Conclusions

The results of the study showed that, with respect to the fall-protection training areas, surprisingly, most participants thought that materials related to every aspect of OSHA training requirements should be covered (including fall hazard identification and

TABLE 24.4

Sample Demographics of the Questionnaire

Job	No.	Ethnicity			Work Experience (years)	
		European–American	Hispanic	Asian	1–5	>5
Managerial personnel	39	32	7	0	3	36
Worker	65	47	17	1	32	33
Total	104	79	24	1	35	69

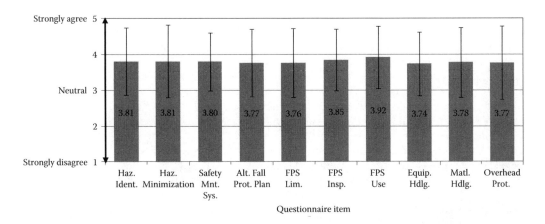

FIGURE 24.1
Participants' perceived fall-protection training needs. FPS denotes fall protection system.

minimization; safety management; limitations and inspection and use of fall-protection systems; handling of roofing materials and equipment; and overhead protection). The findings suggest that (1) there is a lack of fall-protection training among most roofing subcontractors; (2) most roofing workers desire to be trained well, and to be safe. In addition, regarding how fall-protection training should be delivered, workers would prefer it to be held in an informal setting (i.e., on the site) using formal and portable documentation covering hands-on and useful knowledge. Therefore, if fall-protection training is to be effective at reducing falls off roof in the residential sector, OSHA requirements and regulations should be modified to reflect the training needs of roofing workers.

References

ATLAS.ti Scientific Software Development GmbH. (2008). Atlas. Ti: Qualitative data analysis software. Retrieved March, 25, 2008, from http://www.atlasti.com/

Brunette, M. J. (2004). Construction safety research in the United States: Targeting the Hispanic workforce. *Injury Prevention* 10 (4), 244–248.

Charmaz, K. (1995). Grounded theory. In J. Smith, R. Harre, and L. V. Langenhove (Eds.), *Rethinking Methods in Psychology* (pp. 27–49). London: Sage.

Downe-Wamboldt, B. (1992). Content analysis: Method, applications, and issues. *Health Care for Women International*, 13 (3), 313–321.

Glaser, B., and Strauss, A. (1977). *The Discovery of Grounded Theory: Strategies for Qualitative Research.* Texas: Aldine.

Hester, J. L., John, M. D., Leiming, L., James, N., and Dennis, P. (2003). Work-related injuries in residential and drywall carpentry. *Applied Occupational and Environmental Hygiene*, 18 (6), 479–488.

Holmes, N., Lingard, H., Yesilyurt, Z., and Munk, F. D. (1999). An exploratory study of meanings of risks control for long term and acute effect occupational health and safety risks in small business construction firms. *Journal of Safety Research*, 30 (4), 251–261.

Huang, X., and Hinze, J. (2003). Analysis of construction worker fall accidents. *Journal of Construction Engineering and Management*, 129 (3), 262–271.

Hung, Y. H., Winchester, W., Smith-Jackson, T., Mills, T., Kleiner, B., and Babski-Reeves, K. (2013). Identifying fall-protection training needs for residential roofing subcontractors. *Applied Ergonomics*, 44 (3), 372–380.

Kines, P. (2003). Effects of firm size on risks and reporting of elevation fall injury in construction trades. *Journal of Occupational and Environmental Medicine*, 45 (10), 1074–1078.

Lawshe, C. H. (1975). A quantitative approach to content validity. *Personnel Psychology*, 28, 563–575.

Lipscomb, H. J., Glazner, J., Bondy, J., Lezotte, D., and Guarini, K. (2004). Analysis of text from injury reports improves understanding of construction falls. *Journal of Occupational and Environmental Medicine*, 46 (11), 1166–1173.

Patton, M. Q. (1990). *Qualitative Evaluation and Research Methods*. Newbury Park, CA: Sage.

Roelofs, C., Sprague-Martinez, L., Brunette, M., and Azaroff, L. (2011). A qualitative investigation of Hispanic construction worker perspectives on factors impacting worksite safety and risk. *Environmental Health* 10, 1–9.

Straub, D., Boudreau, M.-C., and Gefen, D. (2004). Validation guidelines for IS positivist research. *Communications of the Association for Information Systems*, 13, 380–427.

US Bureau of Labor Statistics (1999a). Plain Language Revision of OSHA Instruction STD 3.1, Interim Fall Protection Compliance Guidelines for Residential Construction. Retrieved April 5, 2008, from http://www.osha.gov/pls/oshaweb/owadisp.show_document?p_table=DIRECTIVES&p_id=2288

US Bureau of Labor Statistics (1999b). Safety and Health Regulations for Construction: 29 CFR 1926. Retrieved October 8, 2010, from http://www.osha.gov/pls/oshaweb/owastand.display_standard_group?p_toc_level=1&p_part_number=1926

US Bureau of Labor Statistics (2009a). 2009 Census of Fatal Occupational Injuries (preliminary data) – Industry by event or exposure. Retrieved November 8, 2010, from http://stats.bls.gov/iif/oshcfoi1.htm

US Bureau of Labor Statistics (2009b). Industry Injury and Illness Data: 2009 (Incidence rates – detailed industry level). Retrieved November, 8, 2010, from http://stats.bls.gov/iif/oshsum.htm#09Summary%20Tables

US Bureau of Labor Statistics (2011). Labor Force Characteristics by Race and Ethnicity, 2010. Retrieved July 26, 2012, from http://www.bls.gov/cps/demographics.htm

US Bureau of Labor Statistics (2014). Top 10 Most Frequently Cited Standards, 2014. Retrieved February 1, 2014, from https://www.osha.gov/Top_Ten_Standards.html

US Census Bureau (2008). Country Business Patterns (CBP). Retrieved November 8, 2010, from http://www.census.gov/econ/cbp/index.html

25

Case Studies on Fall from Elevated Devices among Fire Fighters

Timothy Merinar

CONTENTS

ABSTRACT   This chapter summarizes a number of incidents involving fire fighters falling from elevated devices such as aerial ladders and aerial platforms, from fire escapes, and from the top of fire apparatus. These incidents were investigated by the National Institute for Occupational Safety and Health (NIOSH) Fire Fighter Fatality Investigation and Prevention Program, Division of Safety Research, located in Morgantown, West Virginia.

KEY WORDS: *fire fighters, fire apparatus, aerial ladder, aerial platform, fall restraint, ladder belts, training.*

25.1 Fire Fighter Fatality Investigation and Prevention

The United States currently depends on approximately 1.1 million fire fighters to protect its citizens and property from losses caused by fire. Of these fire fighters, approximately 336,000 are career and 812,000 are volunteers. The National Fire Protection Association (NFPA) and the US Fire Administration (USFA) estimate that on average, 80–100 fire fighters die in the line of duty each year.

The NIOSH Fire Fighter Fatality Investigation and Prevention Program (FFFIPP) conducts independent investigations of selected fire fighter line-of-duty deaths. Investigations are conducted to provide recommendations to prevent future deaths and injuries. The FFFIPP is a public health practice investigation program. NIOSH investigations are not conducted to enforce compliance with state or federal job safety and health standards. NIOSH does not attempt to determine fault or place blame on fire departments or individual fire fighters.

The goal of FFFIPP is to learn from these tragic events and prevent future similar events. NIOSH has investigated approximately 40% of fire fighter deaths since the program began in 1998.

Fire fighters are exposed to the risks of falling from heights and from elevated firefighting equipment, ladders, and fire apparatus. This chapter presents nine case reports that describe firefighter falls from height with recommended control measures to reduce the likelihood of reoccurrence.

25.2 Career Fire Fighter Dies after Falling from Aerial Ladder during Training: Florida

On January 6, 2012, a 49-year-old male career fire fighter (the victim) died from injuries sustained after falling from the tip of a 105 ft aerial ladder during training. The aerial ladder was set up behind the victim's fire station so that personnel could climb the ladder for training purposes. Fire fighters were dressed in station or exercise attire. All fire fighters, including the victim, were wearing ladder safety belts as they ascended and descended the ladder. Some personnel included the ladder climb into a physical fitness exercise routine. Prior to the victim's second climb, he complained of his legs being wobbly and feeling out of shape. After reaching the tip of the ladder on his second climb, the victim failed to come back down immediately. The fire fighters on the ground did not think anything of it till they heard a noise and looked up to see the victim tumbling down the rungs of the ladder. The victim tumbled out of the protection of the ladder rails and struck the passenger-side rear outrigger. Lifesaving measures were taken by fire fighters on scene, but the victim succumbed to his injuries at the hospital. The victim was wearing a ladder belt, and the belt appeared to be intact at the time of the fall.

Key contributing factors identified in this investigation include aerial apparatus standard operating procedures (SOPs) not being fully developed and implemented to include measures to protect training participants from inadvertent falls and the safe and proper use of aerial apparatus; fire apparatus used as part of an unstructured training evolution and circuit training exercise; and a possible unknown medical problem experienced by the victim (NIOSH, 2012).

NIOSH investigators concluded that to minimize the risk of similar occurrences, fire departments should

- Ensure that SOPs regarding proper use and operation of aerial apparatus are developed, implemented, and enforced
- Ensure that a "safe discipline" is maintained at all times, including training
- Consider adopting a comprehensive wellness and fitness program, including annual medical evaluations consistent with NFPA standards and performing annual physical performance (physical ability) evaluations for all fire fighters

25.3 Volunteer Fire Fighter Dies after Falling From a Rope: Minnesota

On May 23, 2011, a 35-year-old male volunteer fire fighter (victim) died after falling from a rope he was climbing after the conclusion of a rope skills class. The department was conducting a ropes and mechanical advantage haul systems training session that consisted of classroom and practical skills training intended to provide the fire fighters with rope skills (Figure 25.1). The drill had concluded, and the students were in the process of breaking down the drill site and putting the equipment away. The victim and two fire fighters were standing in front of the tower ladder when the victim decided to climb one of two ropes suspended from the bottom of the tower ladder platform in an attempt to access the other suspended rope.

The victim was climbing up a rope, using a hand-over-hand technique that had been used to demonstrate rope haul systems, and attempted to grab another rope out of his reach. The victim likely lost his grip on the rope and fell to the asphalt pavement, striking his head. Emergency medical aid was administered by fellow fire fighters, and he was transported to a local hospital, where he died from his injuries. The medical examiner reported the cause of death as blunt force head trauma.

Key contributing factors identified in this investigation include lack of a safety officer, lack of proper personal protective equipment, and student to instructor ratio (NIOSH, 2011).

NIOSH investigators concluded that to minimize the risk of similar occurrences, fire departments should

- Ensure that a qualified safety officer (meeting the qualifications defined in NFPA 1521) is appointed in practical skills training environments
- Ensure that minimum levels of personal protective equipment are established for practical skills training environments (as defined in NFPA 1500)
- Ensure that sufficient instructors or assistant instructors are available for the number of students expected to participate in practical skills training evolutions

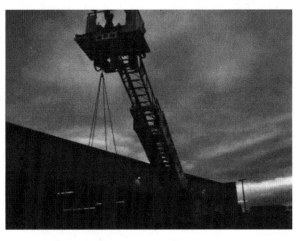

FIGURE 25.1
Training site. (Photo courtesy of Fire Department.)

Additionally, states, municipalities, and authorities having jurisdiction should

- Take steps to ensure that ropes and equipment used in emergency services practical skills training are inspected and records are kept on the purchase, use, and inspection of the ropes and equipment (as defined in NFPA 1500 4.6.5)

25.4 Two Career Fire Fighters Die after Falling from Elevated Aerial Platform: Texas

On January 25, 2009, two male career fire fighters, age 28 (Victim #1) and age 45 (Victim #2), died after falling from an elevated aerial platform during a training exercise in Texas. The fire fighters were participating in the exercise to familiarize fire department personnel with a newly purchased 95 ft mid-mount aerial platform truck. A group of four fire fighters were standing in the aerial platform, which was raised to the roof of an eight-story dormitory building at a local college (Figure 25.2). The platform became stuck on the concrete parapet wall at the top of the building. During attempts to free the platform, the top edge of the parapet wall gave way, and the aerial ladder sprang back from the top of the

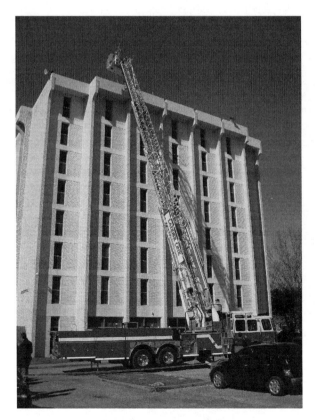

FIGURE 25.2
Aerial platform positioned at dormitory building to recreate incident scene. (Photo from NIOSH.)

building, then began to whip violently back and forth. Two of the four fire fighters standing in the platform were ejected from the platform by the motion. They fell approximately 83 ft to the ground and died from their injuries. None of the fire fighters in the elevated platform were wearing any type of fall restraint.

Key contributing factors identified in this investigation include the fire fighters being unfamiliar with the controls on the newly purchased aerial platform truck, training in a "high-risk" scenario before becoming familiar with new equipment, failure to use fall restraints, the design of the platform railing and integrated doors, and the location of the lifting eyes underneath the platform, which contributed to the platform snagging on the building's parapet wall (NIOSH, 2009).

NIOSH investigators concluded that to minimize the risk of similar occurrences, fire departments should

- Ensure that fire fighters are fully familiar with new equipment before training under "high-risk scenarios"
- Ensure that fall protection is used whenever fire fighters and other personnel are working in elevated aerial platforms
- Follow SOPs for training, including the designation of a safety officer
- Ensure that SOPs covering the operation and use of fire apparatus (including aerial platform apparatus) are developed and followed during training exercises as well as in fire suppression activities
- Provide fall protection belts with all aerial ladder and platform apparatus and ensure that fall protection is used in both training exercises and emergency response events

Fire apparatus manufacturers should

- Include the use of fall protection in both demonstration and training programs
- Ensure that aerial platforms and other aerial devices are designed to reduce or eliminate the potential for snagging on buildings or other elevated surfaces
- Ensure that aerial platform doors or gates are designed to prevent opening in the outward direction

25.5 Fire Fighter (Captain) Dies after Fall from Ladder during a Training Exercise: California

On June 16, 1999, a 38-year-old male fire fighter/captain (the victim) died after falling approximately 20 ft from the top of a ladder that had been previously raised to the second-story window of a fire building at a fire training center. On the morning of the incident, several fire departments were involved in a multijurisdictional, multicompany training exercise. The exercise was conducted by three divisions performing separate evolutions simultaneously. Division A demonstrated proper tactics and procedures during live fire-attack operations and proper search-and-rescue techniques within a simulated single-family residential occupancy. Division B demonstrated proper search-and-rescue techniques

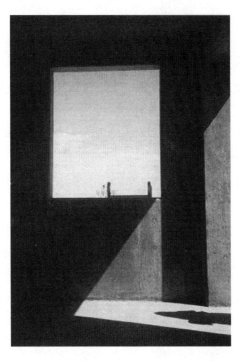

FIGURE 25.3
Forty-two inch window sill and ladder tip. (Photo from NIOSH.)

and ladder-rescue operations from a second-story elevated platform and/or window, and Division C demonstrated proper tactics and procedures for advancing a fire-attack hose-line to gain access to a third-floor fire by entering a second-floor window via a ladder and extending the hoseline up a stairwell to the fire (Figure 25.3). The evolutions were to be performed twice a day over a 3 day period (Session #1 in the morning and Session #2 in the afternoon). The incident occurred near the end of Session #1 on the first day of training. The victim, who was acting as a proctor for the training exercise and monitoring Division C, was positioned on the second floor of the training facility with Division C, who had just completed their evolution when the incident occurred. The victim and fire fighters from Division C were assembled on the second story when the air horn sounded to evacuate the building, as previously planned. At that time, and for unknown reasons, the victim announced that he was going to attempt a new procedure he had learned previously at a rescue intervention training course, which was referred to as the *bail out*. The new procedure involved a headfirst advance over the top of the ladder, hooking an arm through a ladder rung, and grasping a side rail, swinging the legs around to the side of the ladder and sliding down the ladder to the ground. Without hesitation or comment, the victim, who was about 3 ft away from the top of the ladder, took one step and leaped over the top of the ladder. The victim was unable to adequately hook the ladder rungs or grasp a ladder side rail and fell about 20 ft headfirst to the concrete landing. The victim received immediate attention from fire fighters and medics in the area and was transported to the local hospital, where he was pronounced dead about 40 min after the incident.

Key contributing factors identified in this investigation include the lack of an incident safety officer and an unpracticed emergency bailout procedure (NIOSH, 1999).

NIOSH investigators concluded that to minimize the risk of similar occurrences, fire departments should

- Ensure that all new training programs undergo a comprehensive review prior to the implementation of the program
- Collaborate with other fire-related organizations regarding the feasibility of all new training procedures before the programs are implemented
- Ensure that all aspects of safety are adhered to per established standards and recommendations while training is being conducted
- Designate individual safety officers at all significant training exercises to observe operations and ensure that safety rules and regulations are followed

25.6 Volunteer Fire Fighter Dies after Ten-Foot Fall from Engine: Ohio

On July 24, 2007, a 38-year-old male volunteer fire fighter (victim) died after falling from the top of an engine. The victim had returned to the fire station after working a structure fire and was preparing the engine for future fire calls. Following the reloading of hose on the engine, the victim climbed on the driver's side of the engine to adjust and secure a vinyl hose bed cover (Figure 25.4). While attempting to adjust the cover, the victim slipped and fell onto the station's concrete apron. The victim landed on his head and lay supine

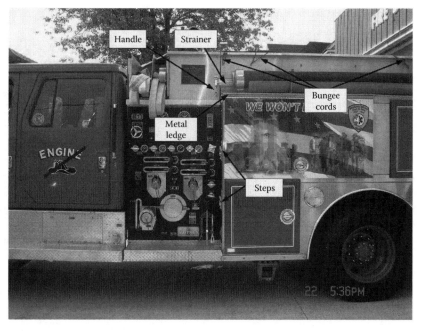

FIGURE 25.4
Side of the engine where the victim ascended and the incident occurred. (Photo from NIOSH.)

on the ground. The victim was transported to an area hospital, where he received medical care and was pronounced dead.

Key contributing factors identified in this investigation include the design of the engine, which introduced numerous potential fall risks when loading the hose bed and securing the vinyl protective cover; fire department practices in loading the hose bed and securing the vinyl hose bed cover, which were unwritten and inadequately addressed fall hazards; and damage to the mounting system of snaps, which made securing the vinyl hose bed cover more cumbersome (NIOSH, 2007a).

NIOSH investigators concluded that to minimize the risk of similar occurrences, fire departments should

- Develop and implement SOPs on the correct procedures/safe methods for reloading hose and securing hose bed covers
- Consider requiring the use of a ladder when servicing items that are out of reach from ground level on the fire apparatus
- Ensure that hose bed covers on fire apparatus are maintained in good physical condition or are replaced when needed
- Consider, when purchasing a new fire apparatus, that it be equipped with available safety features to assist with hose loading and covering the hose bed (e.g., a hose bed that hydraulically lowers, or hose bed covers that are hydraulic, roll-up, or hinged metal)

Although it was difficult to substantiate the actual level of lighting when the incident occurred, NIOSH concluded that as a matter of prudent safe operations, fire departments should

- Ensure adequate exterior lighting for activities outside the fire station

---

25.7 Career Fire Fighter Dies from Fall off Fire Escape Ladder: Illinois

On August 9, 2010, a 31-year-old male career fire fighter (the victim) died from a fall while climbing a fire escape ladder. Crews were responding to an alarm at a four-story mixed occupancy structure. When crews arrived at 00:31, they noticed sparks being emitted from the top of the roof near an external exhaust duct that originated in a street-level restaurant. The victim and three other fire fighters were using an exterior fire escape to access the roof (Figure 25.5). At the fourth-floor landing, the victim started to ascend the vertical ladder to the roof carrying a 63 lb hand pump in his right hand while being supported by a fire fighter on the landing. When out of reach of the supporting fire fighter, the victim lost his grip on the ladder, falling 53 ft to the pavement. The victim was transported to the local medical center, where he was pronounced dead.

Key contributing factors identified in this investigation include using a fire escape to access the roof, rather than a safer means such as an aerial ladder or interior stairway, and the victim being unable to maintain a three-point contact with the vertical portion of the fire escape due to carrying the hand pump (NIOSH, 2010).

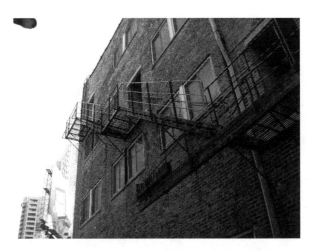

FIGURE 25.5
Fire escape post incident. The access ladder from which the victim fell can be seen at the upper left corner.
(Photo from NIOSH.)

NIOSH investigators concluded that to minimize the risk of similar occurrences, fire departments should

- Ensure that standard operating guidelines (SOGs) on the use of fire escapes are developed, implemented, and enforced
- Ensure that tactical-level accountability is implemented and enforced
- Ensure that companies are rigorously trained in safe procedures for roof operations and climbing ladders of any type
- Ensure that fire fighters are rigorously trained in safe procedures for carrying and/or hoisting equipment when ascending or descending elevations
- Evaluate the fire prevention inspection guidelines and process to ensure that they address high-hazard occupancies, such as restaurants, and incorporate operational crew participation

25.8 Career Fire Fighter Dies in Fall from Roof at Apartment Building Fire: New York

On June 21, 2007, a 23-year-old male career fire fighter (the victim) died after falling from the roof at a four-story apartment building fire. When fire fighters arrived on scene, light smoke and fire were showing from a fourth-floor window. The victim had just climbed the truck ladder to the roof bulkhead and was attempting to lower himself to the main roof when he fell (Figure 25.6). The roof saw (slung on the victim's back) shifted, causing the victim to lose his balance and fall to the ground. Fire fighters had been on scene less than 3 min when the victim fell. The victim was transported to a metropolitan hospital, where he succumbed to his injuries.

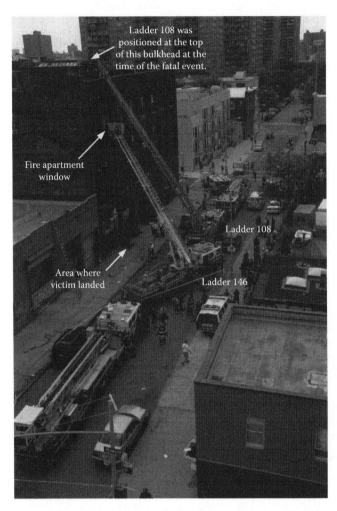

FIGURE 25.6
Aerial view of incident scene. (Photo courtesy of Fire Department.)

Key contributing factors identified in this investigation include the judgment of the fire fighter in deciding on a riskier means of moving from the roof bulkhead to the main roof; the placement of the ladder against the roof bulkhead rather than the main roof, which introduced additional fall risks for fire fighters; the hazardous task of climbing a ladder while laden with tools and equipment; and the method by which the saw was carried, which allowed the shifting saw to put the fire fighter off balance (NIOSH, 2007b).

NIOSH investigators concluded that to minimize the risk of similar occurrences, fire departments should

- Stress to fire fighters the importance of exercising caution when working at elevation
- Consider the location and placement of aerial ladders to prevent fire fighters from climbing from different elevations during fireground operations

- Consider the use of portable scissor ladders to facilitate access from an aerial ladder to the roof
- Ensure that fire fighters communicate any potential hazards to one another and ensure that team continuity is maintained during roof operations
- Evaluate the manner in which equipment is harnessed or carried by fire fighters to prevent loss of balance
- Consider reducing the amount of equipment that fire fighters must carry while climbing ladders

Manufacturers of fire service saws should

- Consider ergonomic design principles to reduce the weight of ventilation saws
- Consider developing improved carrying slings

25.9 Volunteer Training/Safety Officer Dies from Injuries Received in Fall from Pick-Up Truck Following Training Exercise: Tennessee

On May 18, 2003, a 28-year-old male volunteer training/safety officer (the victim) was seriously injured when he fell from a moving pick-up truck. He had completed a 3 day training course and at the time of the incident was being transported within the training grounds. The victim was riding on the lowered tailgate of a moving pick-up truck when he fell onto the road. He suffered severe head trauma and was treated at the scene by fellow fire fighters/emergency medical technicians (EMTs) and on-site emergency medical services. The victim was transported by medical helicopter to a local trauma center, where he died from his injuries on May 24, 2003.

Key contributing factors identified in this investigation include sitting on the open tailgate of a moving pickup truck and possible underlying medical conditions (NIOSH, 2003).

NIOSH investigators concluded that to minimize the risk of similar occurrences, fire departments should

- Ensure that all personnel being transported when on duty be securely seated and restrained in approved vehicle passenger compartments

Although it is unclear whether a medical or physical condition contributed to this fatal incident, fire departments should consider implementing these safety and health recommendations based on the physical demands and medical requirements of fire fighting:

- Provide mandatory preplacement and annual medical evaluations, consistent with NFPA 1582, for all fire fighters to determine medical fitness for duty and training exercises
- Conduct periodic physical capabilities testing to ensure that fire department personnel meet the physical requirements for duty and training exercises

25.10 Volunteer Fire Fighter Dies after 9 ft Fall
      from Ladder: Pennsylvania

On January 17, 2000, a 53-year-old male volunteer fire fighter (the victim) died from injuries received the previous day after the extension ladder he was descending slipped out from under him while he was performing maintenance work (Figure 25.7). On the previous day (January 16, 2000), the victim had been working on replacing a garage door opener in the middle bay of the fire station. Access to the door opener was gained by placing a 14 ft fireground aluminum extension ladder against the side of a fire rescue truck (see Figure 25.7), climbing the ladder to the roof of the fire rescue truck, and then accessing the garage door opener. The victim had removed the existing door opener and was in the process of going to assist in getting the new door opener ready for installation. While he was descending the extension ladder, the ladder slipped out from under him, and the victim fell headfirst to the concrete floor. Another fire fighter, who was assisting the victim in the replacement of the door opener, saw the victim fall and immediately jumped down to the ground from the roof of the rescue truck to assist the victim. He summoned a civilian, who was on the ground putting the new opener together, to help. The fire fighter who had jumped from the roof of the rescue truck ran to a nearby house to inform the victim's wife, while the civilian called 911. Within a few minutes, paramedics and a police officer arrived on the scene. The victim was intubated

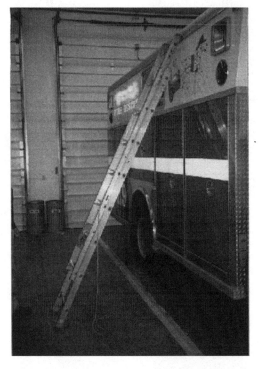

FIGURE 25.7
Fire rescue truck with ladder. (Photo from NIOSH.)

and transported via a helicopter to the local hospital, where he died the next day from his injuries.

Key contributing factors identified in this investigation include failure to properly position the ground ladder in a safe manner, use of the incorrect type of ladder, and failure to size up the work area to consider potential safety issues (NIOSH, 2000).

NIOSH investigators concluded that to minimize the risk of similar occurrences, fire departments should

- Ensure that ladders are used in accordance with existing safety standards
- Designate an individual as the fire station safety officer for all in-house maintenance to identify potential hazards and ensure that those hazards are eliminated
- Consider the use of mobile scaffolding, personnel lifts, scissor lifts, or boom lifts, instead of the top surface of a fire truck

25.11 Summary

Fire fighters are at risk of falling from elevated devices such as aerial ladders and aerial platforms, ladders, and fire escapes and from the top of fire apparatus when performing their normal job duties. Fire fighters often have to carry hand tools such as axes, halogen tools, fire extinguishers, ventilation saws, and other heavy objects while climbing. Fire fighters cannot wear body harnesses or fall restraint systems as construction workers, roofers, and other workers do, because fire fighters must wear heavy turnout clothing and self-contained breathing apparatus. Fire fighters are required to wear ladder belts that are secured to attachment points while working in elevated aerial platforms, but it is not practical for fire fighters to tie off to an attachment point while climbing ladders.

To reduce the possibility of injury and death, fire departments and fighters should take the following actions:

- Develop, implement, and enforce SOPs regarding the proper use of safety equipment and procedures when climbing ladders and working at elevated heights
- Ensure that fall protection is used whenever fire fighters and other personnel are working in elevated aerial platforms
- Ensure that fire fighters are fully familiar with new equipment before training in high-risk scenarios
- Ensure that qualified incident safety officers are designated and in place at all practical skills training environments and at all incidents where fire fighters are working at height
- Ensure that fire fighters are trained and exercise caution when working at height

Fire departments, authorities having jurisdiction, equipment manufacturers, and researchers should consider ways to reduce the amount of equipment that fire fighters must carry while climbing ladders and working at height, where they are at risk of falling.

References

NIOSH (1999). Fire fighter (captain) dies after fall from ladder during a training exercise—California. Morgantown, WV: US Department of Health and Human Services, Centers for Disease Control and Prevention, National Institute for Occupational Safety and Health, Fatality Assessment and Control Evaluation (FACE) Report 99-25. http://www.cdc.gov/niosh/fire/pdfs/face9925.pdf

NIOSH (2000). Volunteer fire fighter dies after nine-foot fall from ladder—Pennsylvania. Morgantown, WV: US Department of Health and Human Services, Centers for Disease Control and Prevention, National Institute for Occupational Safety and Health, Fatality Assessment and Control Evaluation (FACE) Report F2000-07. http://www.cdc.gov/niosh/fire/pdfs/face200007.pdf

NIOSH (2003). Volunteer training/safety officer dies from injuries received in fall from pick-up truck following training exercise—Tennessee. Morgantown, WV: US Department of Health and Human Services, Centers for Disease Control and Prevention, National Institute for Occupational Safety and Health, Fatality Assessment and Control Evaluation (FACE) Report F2003-17. http://www.cdc.gov/niosh/fire/pdfs/face200317.pdf

NIOSH (2007a). Volunteer fire fighter dies after ten-foot fall from engine—Ohio. Morgantown, WV: US Department of Health and Human Services, Centers for Disease Control and Prevention, National Institute for Occupational Safety and Health, Fatality Assessment and Control Evaluation (FACE) Report F2007-27. http://www.cdc.gov/niosh/fire/pdfs/face200727.pdf

NIOSH (2007b). Career fire fighter dies in fall from roof at apartment building fire—New York. Morgantown, WV: US Department of Health and Human Services, Centers for Disease Control and Prevention, National Institute for Occupational Safety and Health, Fatality Assessment and Control Evaluation (FACE) Report F2007-19. http://www.cdc.gov/niosh/fire/pdfs/face200719.pdf

NIOSH (2009). Two career fire fighters die after falling from elevated aerial platform—Texas. Morgantown, WV: US Department of Health and Human Services, Centers for Disease Control and Prevention, National Institute for Occupational Safety and Health, Fatality Assessment and Control Evaluation (FACE) Report F2009-06. http://www.cdc.gov/niosh/fire/pdfs/face200906.pdf

NIOSH (2010). Career fire fighter dies from fall off fire escape ladder—Illinois. Morgantown, WV: US Department of Health and Human Services, Centers for Disease Control and Prevention, National Institute for Occupational Safety and Health, Fatality Assessment and Control Evaluation (FACE) Report F2010-25. http://www.cdc.gov/niosh/fire/pdfs/face201025.pdf

NIOSH (2011). Volunteer fire fighter dies after falling from a rope—Minnesota. Morgantown, WV: US Department of Health and Human Services, Centers for Disease Control and Prevention, National Institute for Occupational Safety and Health, Fatality Assessment and Control Evaluation (FACE) Report F2011-12. http://www.cdc.gov/niosh/fire/pdfs/face201112.pdf

NIOSH (2012). Career fire fighter dies after falling from aerial ladder during training—Florida. Morgantown, WV: US Department of Health and Human Services, Centers for Disease Control and Prevention, National Institute for Occupational Safety and Health, Fatality Assessment and Control Evaluation (FACE) Report F2012-01. http://www.cdc.gov/niosh/fire/pdfs/face201201.pdf

Section VI

Knowledge Gaps, Emerging Issues, and Recommendations for Fall Protection Research and Fall Mitigation

26

Accident Causes and Prevention Measures for Fatal Occupational Falls in the Construction Industry

Chia-Fen Chi

CONTENTS

ABSTRACT Accident analysis is an important source of information for developing prevention strategies and making decisions. This chapter is based on the author's previous work on the accident analysis of occupational fatal falls. In the most recent study (Chi et al. 2014), each fatality was analyzed based on individual factors (i.e., age, gender, and experience), falling site, falling height, company size, and the accident causes. Each of these contributing factors was derived from accident reports of 411 work-related fatal falls occurring during 2001–2005. Given that most fatal accidents involved multiple events, our previous study coded up to a maximum of three causes for each fall fatality and applied a fault tree analysis to represent the causal relationships among events and the causes. After the Boolean algebra and minimal cut set analyses, accident causes associated with each falling site can be presented as a fault tree to provide an overview of the basic causes that could trigger fall fatalities in the construction industry. Graphical icons were designed for each falling site along with the associated accident causes to illustrate the fault tree in a graphical manner. A graphical fault tree can improve interdisciplinary discussion of risk management and the communication of accident causation to first-line supervisors. Primary and secondary prevention measures can be used to prevent falls or to mitigate the consequences of falls and are suggested for each type of accident. Primary prevention measures would include fixed barriers, such as handrails, guardrails, surface opening protections (hole coverings), crawling boards/planks, and strong roofing materials. Secondary protection measures would include travel restraint systems (safety belts), fall arrest systems (safety harnesses), and fall containment systems (safety nets).

KEY WORDS: *graphical fault tree, Boolean algebra, minimal cut set, graphical icon.*

26.1 Introduction

The construction industry has been identified as one of the most hazardous industries in many parts of the world, and falls from height are a leading cause of fatalities in construction operations (Sorock et al. 1993). In the United States, construction had the highest count of fatal injuries in 2012, while agriculture, forestry, and the fishing and hunting sector had the highest fatal work injury rates (US Bureau of Labor Statistics 2014). In Taiwan, Chi and Wu (1997) showed that falls contributed to more than 30% (377) of 1230 work-related fatalities. Effective strategies for preventing fatal falls must be developed based on the in-depth analysis of accident scenarios associated with these fatal falls. One of our previous studies (Chi et al. 2005) developed a classification scheme and categorized 621 fatal falls during 1994–1997 in terms of the cause of the fall, the falling site, individual factors, and company size to derive effective prevention strategies. However, in that particular study, only one primary cause was identified for each fall fatality. Given that most fatal accidents involve multiple events, our subsequent study coded a maximum of three accident causes for each fall fatality (Chi et al. 2009) and applied fault tree analysis and Boolean algebra to reduce accident causes while presenting the results as a graphical fault tree (Chi et al. 2014b). This chapter is an extensive review of the author's previous studies and discusses all relevant issues on fatal occupational falls in the construction industry.

26.1.1 Classification Scheme

In seeking to understand the causes of fatal fall incidents, epidemiological analyses are of value in revealing the factors associated with fatal injuries. However, care is needed with the choice of classification scheme for the analysis, as this can materially affect the outcome (Chi and Wu 1997). Appropriately defined classification categories are also important in forming the basis for effective accident prevention programs (Hinze et al. 1998). Chi et al. (2014b) presented a coding system to facilitate the categorization of fatal falls in terms of the cause of the fall, the fall location, individual factors, and company size, to determine the importance of contributing factors and to derive effective protection strategies. A total of 411 fatal falls were coded based on the classification scheme in Chi et al. (2014b).

26.1.2 Cause of Fall

Causes of accidents are not easy to isolate, especially in fatal accidents (Cattledge et al. 1996). Drury and Brill (1983) derived hazard scenarios in terms of the actors (individuals), the prop (the tools, instruments, and equipment), the scene (environment), and the action (task) from incident reports. They emphasized that each scenario suggested at least one feasible and effective intervention, but such an intervention strategy was appropriate only to that scenario. Chi et al. (2014b) adopted Drury and Brill's (1983) scenario analysis to characterize the causes of work-related fatal falls in terms of (1) unsafe behavior, (2) unsafe machines and tools, and (3) unsafe environment, as in Chi et al. (2005, 2009). For unsafe behavior, these studies included bodily action, poor work practices, improper use of personal protective equipment (PPE), overexertion, insufficient capacities, unsafe climbing, being pulled down (pulled by a heavy object, pulled by a hoist, or pulled by a wheelbarrow), and improper use of PPE. Unsafe machines and tools were further divided into unsafe ladders or tools, and mechanical failure. Unsafe environment included lack of complying scaffold (improper scaffolds, improper platform, or improper guardrails), inappropriate protection (unfixed floor cover, insecure warning barrier, ineffective safety net, and lack of attachment point for safety harness), harmful environment (poor weather, bumpy and restricted walkway, and poor lighting), and other unsafe environments. These categories were chosen to link directly to obvious and useful prevention measures. Each accident report was reviewed several times to itemize the detailed causes of fall under each factor.

Similarly to our previous coding of electrocution fatalities (Chi et al. 2009), a parsimony of coding was taken into consideration to reduce the number of redundant fatal fall causes and minimize complexities in the statistical analysis. For workers who fall from a scaffold due to unsafe climbing of a scaffold, the root cause could be that employers failed to provide an access ladder or equivalent safe access. In such cases, we choose to code only the primary cause of unsafe climbing. Weak supporting structure was coded for the following two types of fatalities: for workers who fell from a scaffold due to the scaffold being unstable to support the worker and the intended load, and for workers who fell through a roof surface due to weak roofing material or a lack of secured platforms (Chi et al. 2014b).

Another concern is the difficulty in differentiating between the following three types of accident causes: bodily action, overexertion, and poor work practices. After combining the most similar cases, we came to the following suggestion. For bodily action, workers often took up an unsafe posture, such as standing with their back toward an unguarded opening, while overexertion emphasized that the material-handling activity (such as lifting, carrying, or disassembly) caused the worker's loss of balance. Lastly, for poor work practice, workers used an incorrect procedure (Chi et al. 2014b).

26.1.3 Falling Site

The US Department of Labor (2003) has 11 categories to classify the falling site for fatal falls. These include (1) falls from stairs or steps, (2) falls through existing floor openings, (3) falls from ladders, (4) falls through roof surfaces (including existing roof openings and skylights), (5) falls from roof edges, (6) falls from scaffolds or staging, (7) falls from building girders or other structural steel, (8) falls while jumping to a lower level, (9) falls through existing roof openings, (10) falls from floors, docks, or ground level, and (11) other nonclassified falls to lower levels. These categories were used directly in this study.

26.1.4 Individual Factors

Age was coded as in our previous study (Chi and Wu 1997). Worker's experience was classified after Butani (1988) into six different levels to compare the relative risk of injuries for different levels of experience. These levels were $0 < \text{to} \leq 1$, $1 < \text{to} \leq 5$, $5 < \text{to} \leq 10$, $10 < \text{to} \leq 15$,

15 < to ≤ 20, and >20 years. Company size was coded according to the categories used by the Directorate General of Budget, Accounting and Statistics (1997).

26.1.5 Fault Tree Analysis of a Database

As Ale et al. (2006) suggested, causal modeling is a powerful tool for gaining insight into the interdependencies between the constituent parts of a complex system. It enables policies and inspection regimes to be tailor made to the vulnerabilities in systems and to those activities that pose the most risk (Ale et al. 2006). Fault tree analysis has been applied to the analysis of catastrophic events, for example, the Schoharie Creek bridge collapse (LeBeau et al. 2007), and a complicated system, for example, a power system (Volkanovski et al. 2009). Construction of a fault tree normally begins with the top event and proceeds in a top-down manner (Harms-Ringdahl 2001). The AND- and OR- gates are used to provide logical connections between the basic events. The multiple events that cause a fatality can be described graphically using a fault tree diagram. The fault tree symbol OR-gate, which is equivalent to the Boolean symbol +, represents the union of the events attached to the gate. One or more of the input events must occur to cause the event above the OR-gate to occur. The fault tree symbol AND-gate, which is equivalent to the Boolean symbol •, represents the intersection of the events attached to the gate. All the input events attached to the AND-gate must exist for the event above the gate to occur (Vesely et al. 1981).

Given that fatal falls can be caused by more than one cause combination, the integration of all possible cause combinations can be regarded as the union of these cause combinations. Since these cause combinations have redundancies, when the same event appeared more than once, a minimal cut set (MCS) was applied to reduce the redundancy of basic events. By examining the MCS, the smallest combination of root causes, an analyst can prioritize prevention measures to prevent the top event from occurring (Doytchev and Szwillus 2009). Our previous study applied the fault tree analysis to present the causal relationships among events and causes that contributed to work-related fatal fall in terms of MCSs. These MCSs can be compared in terms of their relative frequencies to prioritize their importance for prevention measures (Chi et al. 2014b).

26.2 Materials and Methods

26.2.1 Accident Reports of Fatal Falls

In Taiwan, the Occupational Safety and Health Act requires that the employer report any occupational fatality to the appropriate inspection agency within 24 h. Trained inspectors must inspect the workplace and file a formal accident report soon after they are notified. Each formal accident report covers the type of industry; the age, gender, and experience level of the victim; the source of the injury; the company size, measured by the number of workers; the accident type; and any other factors that are judged to be relevant. The accident report can be used as legal evidence against the employer for any violation of the Occupational Safety and Health Act. Inspection agencies, all over Taiwan, must report all occupational fatalities to the Ministry of Labor on a monthly basis. The Ministry of Labor collects and publishes all occupational fatalities on a monthly and yearly basis to alert employers to pay special attention to similar accident scenarios and renew their inspection policy. Most of our previous studies extracted age, gender, experience, falling site, falling height, company size, and the causes from these accident reports for further analysis.

26.2.2 Standardized Mortality Ratios (SMRs)

An SMR for each stratified gender, age, and occupational group was calculated using the whole working population as the reference group (Fisher and Belle 1993; Chi and Chen 2003). The SMR for each stratified gender, age, and company size group was calculated, along with 95% confidence intervals (Kelsey et al. 1996), using the working population of the Taiwanese construction industry in 2001–2005 (Directorate General of Budget and Accounting Statistics 2001–2005) as the reference group for the calculations. Using the same reference population can aid in making a direct comparison of the SMRs among different demographic segments.

26.2.3 Fault Tree Analysis and Boolean Algebra Representation

A fault tree can always be translated into entirely equivalent MCSs, which can be considered as the root causes for these fall fatalities (Vesely et al. 1981). Our fault tree analysis begins by identifying multiple-cause combinations for each fatality. These multiple-cause combinations can be connected by an AND-gate (for two-cause and three-cause combinations), indicating that these two or three events contributed simultaneously to these fatal falls. The integration of all possible cause combinations for each falling site can be regarded as the union (connected with an OR-gate) of these cause combinations. Fundamental laws of Boolean algebra (Whitesitt 1995) (see Table 26.1) were applied to reduce all possible cause combinations to the "smallest" cut set (Vesely et al. 1981) that could cause the top event to occur. Eventually, all cause combinations associated with each falling site can be simplified and presented in a fault tree diagram.

26.3 Results

26.3.1 Frequency Analysis

A frequency analysis was performed on each coded variable. The analysis indicated that the majority of victims were male (387, 94.2%), were between 25 and 44 years old (220, 53.5%), worked for companies with fewer than 30 workers (367, 89.3%) (see Table 26.2), and had less than 1 year of working experience (308, 74.9%) (see Table 26.3). The SMR analysis of various population segments (gender, age, and company size) was taken to be significantly

TABLE 26.1

Boolean Algebra Fundamental Laws

Laws	Formula
Commutative laws	$X+Y=Y+X$
Associative laws	$X+(Y+Z)=(X+Y)+Z$
Distributive laws	$XY+XZ=X(Y+Z)$
Laws of absorption	$X+XY=X$

TABLE 26.2

Frequency Distribution and SMR for Stratified Gender, Age, and Company Size, together with SMR Groupings Derived from the Statistical Analysis

Factor	Frequency	%	SMR	95% CI	SMR Groupings
Gender					
Male	387	94.2	1.64	(1.29–2.04)	B
Female	18	4.4	0.11	(0.03–0.29)	A
Unknown	6	1.4	—	—	—
Age					
15–24	26	6.3	0.60	(0.20–1.39)	A
25–34	102	24.8	0.86	(0.53–1.33)	A
35–44	118	28.7	0.97	(0.62–1.46)	AB
45–54	101	24.6	1.16	(0.71–1.79)	AB
≥ 55	57	13.9	1.64	(0.83–2.91)	B
Unknown	7	1.7	—	—	—
Company size					
<5	153	37.2	1.87	(1.27–2.66)	E
5–9	117	28.5	1.01	(0.64–1.51)	D
10–29	97	23.6	1.48	(0.89–2.31)	C
30–49	11	2.7	0.44	(0.06–1.49)	BC
50–99	11	2.7	0.48	(0.06–1.66)	B
100–499	9	2.2	0.25	(0.02–0.97)	AB
≥ 500	4	0.9	0.24	(0.00–1.57)	A
Unknown	9	2.2	—	—	—

Source: Chi, C-F. et al., *Accident Anal. Prev.*, 72, 359–369, 2014.
CI, confidence interval.

different when the 95% confidence intervals of their SMRs did not overlap (Chi and Chen 2003). Significant differences in SMR are indicated by alphabetical letters (Table 26.2).

The SMR indicated that males are more likely to be victims of fatal falls in the construction industry. Our previous analysis, which was a national and cross-sectorial study of occupational fatalities, indicated that female workers in high-risk industries, such as construction, mining, and quarrying, have a lower fatality rate than their male counterparts (Chi and Chen 2003). Possible reasons for the difference may be that female workers work fewer hours (Messing et al. 1994) and that females are seldom employed in outdoor jobs or in jobs with extreme conditions (Lucas 1974).

A significant rising trend was found between age and SMR, indicating that age had an aggravating effect on accident risk, mainly caused by a functional decline with age (Laflamme and Menckel 1995; Chi and Wu 1997). Aging workers (aged 45 and above) had reduced visual and auditory capability, physical strength, and flexibility (Charness 1985). In the United States, fatal work injury rates, by age group, in 2012 indicated that fatal work injury rates for workers 45 years of age and older were higher than the overall US rate, and the rate for workers 65 years of age and older was around three times the rate for all workers (US Bureau of Labor Statistics 2014). Besides age, there was a significantly increasing SMR with decreasing company size ($p < 0.001$) (Buskin and Paulozzi 1987). Possible reasons for the greater risk with decreasing company size might be due to smaller companies' inability to afford safety programs and personnel, or because smaller companies are

TABLE 26.3

Frequency Distributions of Worker Experience, Falling Height, and Falling Sites

Factors	Frequency	%
Experience		
Under 1 year	308	74.9
1–15 years	79	19.2
Over 15 years	8	1.9
Unknown	16	4
Falling height		
0–2.0 m	24	5.8
2.1–3.0 m	24	5.8
3.1–10.0 m	200	48.7
10.1–30.0 m	119	29
>30 m	30	7.3
Unknown	14	3.4
Falling sites		
Falls from scaffolds	98	23.8
Falls from building girders or steel	78	19
Falls through existing floor opening	56	13.6
Stepping through roof surface	49	11.9
Falls from ladders	37	9
Falls from roof edge or opening	29	7.1
Falls from dock or floor edge	26	6.3
Falls from scaffolds with wheels	12	2.9
Falls from deck or balcony	9	2.2
Others (falls from construction vehicle, falls down stairs, collapsing material or structure)	17	4.1

Source: Chi, C-F. et al., *Accident Anal. Prev.*, 72, 359–369, 2014.

less likely to be inspected by relevant government agencies and often perform inherently riskier work (Buskin and Paulozzi 1987).

In terms of the falling site, out of the 411 cases analyzed, 23.8% (98 cases) of the fatalities were classified as falling from scaffolds or from a building girder or other steel structure (78 cases, 19.0%), falling through an existing floor opening (56 cases, 13.6%), stepping through a roof surface (49 cases, 11.9%), falling from a ladder (37 cases, 9.0%), falling from the roof edge or opening (29 cases, 7.1%), falling from the dock or floor edge (26 cases, 6,3%), falling from a scaffold with wheels (12 cases, 2.9%), falling from a deck or balcony (9 cases, 2.2%), and other falling sites (17 cases, 4.1%) (see Table 26.3).

Table 26.4 shows the frequency distribution of accident causes, given that multiple causes were identified for each fatality. Table 26.5 shows all cause combinations (single, two-cause, and three-cause) for the 411 cases in terms of unsafe behavior, unsafe machines and tools, and unsafe environment. There were 179 single-cause cases, 217 cases of two-cause combinations, and 15 cases of three-cause combinations. Overall, these 411 fatality cases can be described by 91 distinctive combinations of accident causes, and 90.8% of these fatalities were associated with unsafe behavior and unsafe environment. About 48% of fatalities were caused by unsafe behavior, of which improper use of PPE (28.9%), bodily action (5.8%), and unsafe climbing (4.3%) were the most common causes. An unguarded

TABLE 26.4

Frequency Distribution of Accident Causes

Accident Cause	Chi et al. (2014b)		Chi et al. (2005)	
	Frequency	%	Frequency	%
Unsafe behavior	**315**	**47.9**		
Bodily action	38	5.8	62	10.0
Poor work practices	26	4.0	44	7.1
Overexertion	11	1.7	16	2.6
Insufficient capacities	2	0.3	11	1.8
Unauthorized access	0	0	5	0.8
Unsafe climbing	28	4.3	—	—
Being pulled down	20	3.0	—	—
Pulled by heavy object	8	1.2	24	3.9
Pulled by hoist	7	1.1	9	1.4
Pulled by wheelbarrow	5	0.8	6	1.0
Improper use of PPE	190	28.9	35	5.7
Unsafe machines and tools	**36**	**5.5**		
Unsafe ladders or tools	26	4.0	7	1.1
Mechanical failure	10	1.5	3	0.5
Unsafe environment	**215**	**32.7**	—	—
Unguarded opening	60	9.1	104	16.7
Weak roofing material	59	9.0	—	—
Removal of protection measure	16	2.4	15	2.4
Unfixed floor cover	1	0.2	15	2.4
Improper platform	41	6.2	58	9.3
Improper guardrails	18	2.7	113	17.2
Improper scaffolds	20	3.0	—	—
Harmful environment	**92**	**14.0**		
Poor weather	8	1.2	13	2.1
Bumpy and restricted walkway	14	2.1	7	1.1
Poor lighting	4	0.6	3	0.5
Hit by falling objects	2	0.3	22	3.5
Other unsafe environments	0	0	6	1.0
Lack of attachment for safety harness	35	5.3	1	0.2
Ineffective safety net	29	4.4	2	0.3
Unknown	0	0	40	6.4

opening and weak roofing (supporting) structure were the most frequent unsafe environmental situations; each contributed to 9.1% and 9% of the falls, respectively. On the other hand, an unsafe ladder (4%) was the most common unsafe tool.

26.3.2 Falling Height and Posture

Working height is one of the most hazardous aspects in a construction site (Hu et al. 2011). As stated by Hammer (1989), falls do not have to be of a great height to be fatal. A head injury is the most serious and frequent trauma from a fall. However, most occupational

TABLE 26.5

Cause Combination of Falling Fatality

Accident Cause ($N=411$)	Frequency
Single cause	**179**
Unsafe environment	83
Unsafe behavior	73
Unsafe machines and tools	23
Two-cause	**217**
Unsafe behavior–Unsafe environment	120
Unsafe behavior–Unsafe behavior	51
Unsafe environment–Unsafe environment	32
Unsafe machines and tools–Unsafe environment	12
Unsafe behavior–Unsafe machines and tools	2
Three-cause	**15**
Unsafe behavior–Unsafe behavior–Unsafe environment	7
Unsafe behavior–Unsafe environment–Unsafe environment	4
Unsafe environment–Unsafe environment–Unsafe environment	2
Unsafe behavior–Unsafe behavior–Unsafe behavior	1
Unsafe behavior–Unsafe machines and tools–Unsafe environment	1

Source: Chi, C-F. et al., *Accident Anal. Prev.*, 72, 359–369, 2014.

safety and health regulations protect workers at heights greater than 2 m (in Taiwan and in Australia). The United States has similar Safety and Health Standards for the construction industry. The Occupational Safety and Health Administration (1996) stated that "each employee on a walking/working surface with an unprotected side or edge which is 6 ft (1.8 m) or more above a lower level shall be protected from falling by the use of guardrail systems, safety net systems, or personal fall arrest systems." According to the US Bureau of Labor Statistics (2014), falls to a lower level accounted for 570 fatal work injuries in 2012. Ten percent of falls to a lower level involved falls of 6 ft or less. Our statistics indicated that 24 victims (about 5.8% of all 411 fatalities) (see Table 26.3) fell from heights of less than 2 m, where workers may ignore the risk of falling. In these cases, most of these victims were not wearing a helmet and fell backward, hitting the back of their head. More than half (14 of 24 cases) of these cases were falls from ladders. The other falls from less than 2 m included falls from scaffolds (three cases), from a building girder or steel (two cases), through a floor opening (three cases), and from scaffolds with wheels (two cases).

26.3.3 Boolean Algebra Simplification

Taking as an example the 35 distinctive cause combinations associated with the 98 falls from scaffold cases (see Table 26.6), of these 98 cases, 24 cases were caused by eight single causes, with improper use of PPE (eight cases) as the most frequent single cause. Seventy cases were caused by 23 two-cause combinations, with improper scaffolds and improper use of PPE (16 cases) as the most frequent combination. Lastly, four cases of falling from scaffold were caused by a three-cause combination. According to the fault tree analysis, two-cause and three-cause combinations would be connected by the AND-gate, as shown at the bottom layer of Figure 26.1. The union of the 35 distinctive cause combinations can be connected with an OR-gate. In terms of Boolean algebra, accident causes associated

TABLE 26.6

Cause Combinations of Falling from Scaffold

Cause Combinations	Frequency	Subtotal
Improper use of PPE	8	**24**
Poor work practices	4	
Lack of attachment point for safety harness	3	
Unsafe climbing	3	
Improper scaffolds	2	
Unsafe tools	2	
Bodily action	1	
Removal of protection measure	1	
Improper use of PPE · improper scaffolds	16	**70**
Improper use of PPE · improper guardrails	11	
Improper use of PPE · improper platform	10	
Improper use of PPE · unsafe climbing	5	
Improper use of PPE · poor work practices	4	
Improper platform · ineffective safety net	4	
Improper scaffolds · ineffective safety net	2	
Improper use of PPE · weak supporting structure	2	
Lack of attachment point for safety harness · improper scaffolds	2	
Improper use of PPE · bodily action	1	
Improper use of PPE · hit by falling objects	1	
Improper use of PPE · mechanical failure	1	
Improper use of PPE · removal of protection measure	1	
Improper use of PPE · unsafe tools	1	
Improper platform · bumpy and restricted walkway	1	
Improper platform · unsafe climbing	1	
Improper scaffolds · bodily action	1	
Lack of attachment point for safety harness · ineffective safety net	1	
Improper guardrails · unsafe climbing	1	
Unsafe tools · being pulled down	1	
Unsafe tools · unsafe climbing	1	
Overexertion · improper guardrails	1	
Weak supporting structure · ineffective safety net	1	
Being pulled down · improper platform · improper use of PPE	1	**4**
Bodily action · improper scaffolds · improper use of PPE	1	
Improper guardrails · bumpy and restricted walkway · improper use of PPE	1	
Unsafe climbing · improper scaffolds · improper use of PPE	1	
Total	98	**98**

Source: Chi, C-F. et al., *Accident Anal. Prev.*, 72, 359–369, 2014.

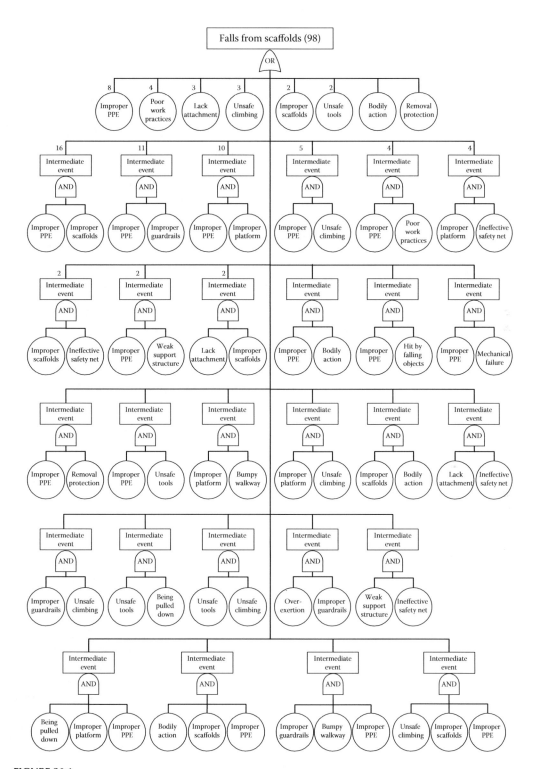

FIGURE 26.1
Fault tree illustration for falling from scaffold before the MCS analysis. (From Chi, C-F. et al., *Accident Anal. Prev.*, 72, 359–369, 2014.)

TABLE 26.7

Abbreviations of Boolean Representation for Accident Cause

Act: bodily action	Exert: overexertion
Attach: lack of attachment for safety harness	Platform: improper platform
Capacity: insufficient capacities	PPE: improper use of PPE
Climb: unsafe climbing	Remove: removal of protection measure
Cover: unfixed floor cover	Practice: poor work practices
Guard: improper guardrails	Pull: being pulled down
Light: poor lighting	Structure: weak roofing material or supporting structure
Mechanical: mechanical failure	Scaffold: improper scaffolds
Net: ineffective safety net	Tool or ladder: unsafe ladders or tools
Objects: hit by falling objects	Bumpy: bumpy and restricted walkway
Open: unguarded opening	Weather: poor weather

Source: Chi, C-F. et al., *Accident Anal. Prev.*, 72, 359–369, 2014.

with falling from scaffold can be presented as follows. (Abbreviations of these Boolean representations are summarized in Table 26.7.)

$$
\begin{aligned}
& 8\text{PPE} + 4\text{Practice} + 3\text{Attach} + 3\text{Climb} + 2\text{Scaffold} + 2\text{Tool} + \text{Act} + \text{Remove} \\
& + 16(\text{PPE} \cdot \text{Scaffold}) + 11(\text{PPE} \cdot \text{Guard}) + 10(\text{PPE} \cdot \text{Platform}) + 5(\text{PPE} \cdot \text{Climb}) \\
& + 4(\text{PPE} \cdot \text{Practice}) + 4(\text{Platform} \cdot \text{Net}) + 2(\text{Scaffold} \cdot \text{Net}) + 2(\text{PPE} \cdot \text{Structure}) \\
& + 2(\text{Attach} \cdot \text{Scaffold}) + \text{PPE} \cdot \text{Act} + \text{PPE} \cdot \text{Object} + \text{PPE} \cdot \text{Mechanical} \\
& + \text{PPE} \cdot \text{Remove} + \text{PPE} \cdot \text{Tool} + \text{Platform} \cdot \text{Bumpy} + \text{Platform} \cdot \text{Climb} \\
& + \text{Scaffold} \cdot \text{Act} + \text{Attach} \cdot \text{Net} + \text{Guard} \cdot \text{Climb} + \text{Tool} \cdot \text{Pull} + \text{Tool} \cdot \text{Climb} \\
& + \text{Exert} \cdot \text{Guard} + \text{Structure} \cdot \text{Net} + \text{Pull} \cdot \text{Platform} \cdot \text{PPE} + \text{Act} \cdot \text{Scaffold} \cdot \text{PPE} \\
& + \text{Guard} \cdot \text{Bumpy} \cdot \text{PPE} + \text{Climb} \cdot \text{Scaffold} \cdot \text{PPE}
\end{aligned}
\tag{26.1}
$$

Subsequently, the absorption law in the MCS analysis was applied to reduce the cause combinations by absorbing a secondary cause with a primary cause. For example, 11 falling from scaffold fatalities were caused by the combination of improper use of PPE and improper guardrails. Because improper use of PPE itself can cause falling from scaffold fatalities, while improper guardrails cannot, improper use of PPE and improper guardrails would be regarded as primary and secondary, respectively. Improper use of PPE would absorb improper guardrails and become the only accident cause presented in the fault tree after the MCS analysis. For other two-cause or three-cause combinations in which each accident cause alone can contribute to a fatality, such causes would be regarded as primary. Each such primary cause would absorb the total number of cases divided by the number of primary causes of the same combination. For example, five falling from scaffold fatalities were caused by the combination of improper use of PPE and unsafe climbing. Given that improper use of PPE and unsafe climbing each can cause falling from scaffold fatalities, we assumed that improper use of PPE and unsafe climbing each absorbed 2.5 cases out of these five two-cause fatalities. For cases in which none of the causes in a multiple-cause combination had caused the fatality by itself, the absorption law would not be applied, and the multiple-cause combination would remain in its original format. One last possibility for the three-cause combination is that two causes are primary and one is secondary. In this case, the number of cases associated with the secondary cause would be absorbed equally by the other two primary causes. For example, falling from a building girder was caused by the combination of bodily action (primary), mechanical failure (primary), and improper use of PPE (secondary); the improper use of PPE would be absorbed equally by the other two primary causes and give 0.5 bodily action + 0.5 mechanical failure. This consideration allows us to keep track of the fatality frequency after applying the MCS analysis.

Eventually, all cause combinations associated with fall from scaffold can be simplified as follows:

$$49.67 \text{ PPE} + 14.17 \text{ Scaffold} + 8.33 \text{ Climb} + 6 \text{ Practice} + 5 \text{ Attach} + 4 \text{ Tool} + 2.33 \text{ Act}$$
$$+ 1.5 \text{ Remove} + 4 \text{ Platform} \cdot \text{Net} + \text{Platform} \cdot \text{Bumpy} + \text{Exert} \cdot \text{Guard} + \text{Structure} \cdot \text{Net} \quad (26.2)$$

The original fault tree of 35 distinctive accident causes associated with falling from a scaffold (see Figure 26.1) can be reduced to a logically equivalent fault tree consisting of 12 MCSs connected by an OR-gate beneath the top event (see Figure 26.2). Each MCS can be a basic event (denoted by a circular shape) or an intermediate event (denoted by a rectangular shape) consisting of multiple basic events connected by an AND-gate that causes the top event to occur. Similarly, the same MCS analysis can be applied to other falling sites to derive logically equivalent fault trees for further development of prevention measures (see Table 26.8). All the MCSs are necessary and sufficient to cause the fall from a scaffold fatalities.

26.4 Discussion

26.4.1 Fall Protection Measures

Manitoba Labor and Immigration Division (MLID) (2003) suggested six categories of fall protection measures in their *Fall Protection Guidelines*: (1) surface protections (nonslip flooring), (2) fixed barriers (handrails and guardrails), (3) surface opening protections (removable covers and guardrails), (4) travel restraint systems (safety line and belt), (5) fall arrest systems (safety line and harness), and (6) fall containment systems (safety nets). Bobick et al. (1994) classified protective measures as either primary or secondary. The first three categories of protection measures were considered active or primary, because they physically prevent falls to a lower level from occurring. The last three categories were referred to as passive or secondary, since they inhibit or minimize injury after an already-initiated fall to a lower level. MLID (2003) stated that it is preferable to provide a fixed barrier to prevent a worker from falling than to provide PPE (such as a safety harness and lifeline), and the selection of the particular fall protection measure is dependent on the circumstances and the job task.

As shown in Table 26.8, the accident causes associated with each falling site can be reduced to the MCSs of accident causes; each accident cause corresponded to at least one feasible and effective intervention (Drury and Brill 1983). Instead of discussing each prevention measure by its cause or falling site, these prevention measures can be elaborated by the categories of unsafe behavior, unsafe environment, and unsafe machines and tools.

To improve the recognition of hazards and the enforcement of fall protection systems, unsafe behaviors (for example, insufficient capacities, improper use of PPE, unsafe climbing, poor work practice, overexertion, and being pulled down) can be eliminated or reduced by proper selection and safety training for the workers. For these accident causes and prevention measures, relevant research can be found to eliminate each accident cause

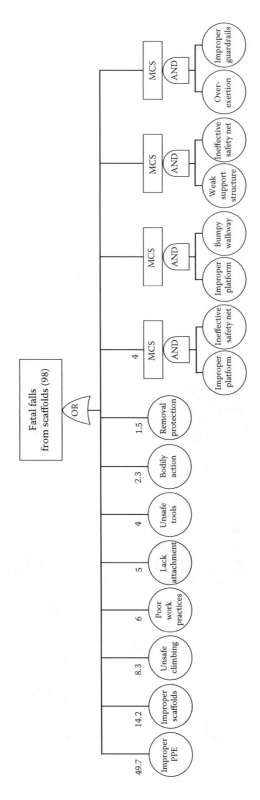

FIGURE 26.2
Fault tree illustration for falling from scaffold in terms of the MCSs. (From Chi, C-F. et al., *Accident Anal. Prev.,72*, 359–369, 2014.)

TABLE 26.8

Original Cause Combinations and Simplified Result by Applying Boolean Algebra

Falling Site (Frequency)	Accident Causes Combinations	MCS
Scaffolds (98)	8PPE + 4Practice + 3Attach + 3Climb + 2Scaffold + 2Tool + Act + Remove + 16(PPE · Scaffold) + 11(PPE · Guard) + 10((PPE · Platform) + 5(PPE · Climb) + 4(PPE · Practice) + 4(Platform · Net) + 2(Scaffold · Net) + 2(PPE · Structure) + 2(Attach · Scaffold) + PPE · Act + PPE · Object + PPE · Mechanical + PPE · Remove + PPE · Tool · Platform · Bumpy · Platform · Climb + Scaffold · Act + Attach · Net + Guard · Climb + Tool · Pull + Tool · Climb + Exert · Guard + Structure · Net + Pull · Platform · PPE + Act · Scaffold · PPE + Guard · Bumpy · PPE + Climb · Scaffold · PPE	49.67PPE + 14.17Scaffold + 8.33Climb + 6Practice + 5Attach + 4Tool + 2.33Act + 1.5 Remove + 4Platform · Net + Platform · Bumpy + Exert · Guard + Structure · Net
Building girders (78)	10PPE + 4Attach + 3Climb + 2Scaffold + Act + Open + Pull + Structure + 6(Climb · PPE) + 5(PPE · Net) + 4(Structure · PPE) + 4(Scaffold · PPE) + 3(Act · PPE) + 3(Open · PPE) + 2(Open · Attach) + 2(PPE · Weather) + 2(Remove · PPE) + 2(PPE · Scaffold) + Act · Bumpy + Act · Open + Attach · Net + Bumpy · PPE + Climb · Weather + Cover · PPE + Guardrail · PPE + Mechanical · PPE + Practice · PPE + Object · PPE + Practice · Attach + Pull · PPE + Pull · Attach + Pull · Net + Pull · Guard + Scaffold · Attach + Structure · Net + Act · Mechanical · PPE + Act · Platform · Weather + Climb · Attach · Net + Climb · PPE · Net + Structure · Attach · Net	37.5PPE + 9Attach + 8Climb + 5.5Act + 5.5Scaffold + 4.5Structure + 4Open + 4Pull
Floor opening (56)	11Open + 6Practice + 5Remove + 2Attach + PPE + Structure + Tool + 7(Open · PPE) + 4(Pull · PPE) + 3(Act · Open) + 2(Act · PPE) + 2(Mechanical · PPE) + Act · Guard + Exert · Attach + Exert · Guard + Open · Exert + Open · Light + PPE · Net + Remove · Exert + Remove · PPE + Structure · Attach + Exert · Pull · Attach + Pull · Open · Attach	20Open + 14PPE + 6.5Remove + 6Practice + 5Attach + 1.5Structure + Tool · Guard · Act + Guard · Exert
Roof surface (49)	40Structure + Open + 5 Structure · PPE + Act · Structure + Open · Net + Open · PPE	46 Structure + 3Open
Ladders (37)	16Ladder + 5PPE + 3Act + Bumpy + Capacity + Climb + Exert + Scaffold + 2(Act · PPE) + 2(Ladder · PPE) + Act · Ladder + Open · Attach + Open · PPE + Practice · Ladder	18.5Ladder + 8PPE + 4.5Act + Bumpy + Capacity + Climb + Exert + Scaffold + Open · Attach
Roof edge or opening (29)	5PPE + 3Attach + Open + Pull + 3(Open · PPE) + 2(Act · PPE) + Attach · Net + Bumpy · PPE + Exert · Open + Exert · PPE + Open · Attach + Open · Bumpy + Open · Net + Open · Weather + PPE · Net + Pull · PPE + Scaffold · PPE + Weather · Attach + Open · Bumpy · Attach + Practice · Pull · PPE	13.5PPE + 7.5Open + 6Attach + 2Pull
Floor edge (26)	4PPE + 2Open + Bumpy + Scaffold + 3(Open · PPE) + 2(Open · Net) + Act · PPE + Act · Pull + Exert · PPE + Open · Attach + Open · Weather + PPE · Net + Practice · PPE + Pull · PPE + Remove · PPE + Remove · Weather + Scaffold · PPE + Exert · Guard · PPE	13PPE + 8.5Open + 1.5Scaffold + Bumpy + Act · Pull + Remove · Weather
Scaffolds with wheels (12)	3Mechanical + 2Act + Act · Light + Act · PPE + Bumpy · Guard + Climb · Bumpy + Climb · Net + Practice · Pull + Act · Remove · Light	5Act + 3Mechanical + Bumpy · Guard + Practice · Pull + Climb · Bumpy + Climb · Net
Deck or balcony(9)	3Practice + Open + Act · PPE + Practice · Attach + Practice · PPE + Practice · Scaffold + Remove · PPE	6Practice + Open + PPE · Act + PPE · Remove
Others (17)	2Act + 2Bumpy + 2Open + Mechanical + PPE + 2Scaffold · PPE + Capacity · PPE + Climb · Structure + Mechanical · PPE + Open · Weather + PPE · Net + Pull · PPE + Remove · Bumpy	6.5PPE + 3Bumpy + 3Open + 2Act + 1.5Mechanical + Climb · Structure

and effectively implement prevention measures. MLID (2003) suggested that only workers wearing a whole-body safety harness with a lifeline secured to a proper anchorage should have access to unprotected openings more than 2.5 m above a lower floor. For proper use of PPE, to reduce the risk of worker injury resulting from poor fit, Hsiao et al. (2007) suggested an alternative system of two sizes for women and three sizes for men over the current four sizes for unisex. For the design of a more widely adopted training program, Hung et al. (2013) conducted semi-structured interviews with 29 residential roofing subcontractors to derive some effective delivery means and design features for the implementation of fall protection training. The training should focus on the proper use of fall prevention equipment, safety awareness, and the consequences of safety violations and should encourage engagement and participation by giving workers opportunities "to talk to learn, not to learn from talk." Prevention measures are useful only if they are implemented by the company and applied by the workers. Thus, safety performance measures of the company, for example, unsafe working behavior, as in Haslam et al. (2005), should be collected and monitored for motivation and feedback. Besides these measures, the inspection and testing of protection systems and tools, the inspection of the facility and the environment, and other administrative interventions should not be neglected (Janicak 1998).

For unsafe environment, including improper scaffolds, unguarded openings, weak roofing material or supporting structure, and others, the general suggestion is to protect workers from falling by the use of guardrail systems, safety net systems, or personal fall arrest systems (Occupational Safety and Health Administration 1996). Helander (1984) suggested that the number of fall accidents could be reduced dramatically by using guardrails. However, prior to the installation of guardrails, and even after their installation, safety harnesses and an independent lifeline should be properly secured to an adequate anchor and used by those who may be exposed to any open edge or risk of falling (MLID 2003). Safety nets should be used in places where it is difficult or impossible to install guardrails or to provide a proper anchoring and lifeline system for fall arrest. Also, visual markings such as warning signs or warning tape should be used to mark off the hazard area for places where a guardrail is temporarily removed (MLID 2003).

Regarding unsafe machines and tools, the majority of fatal falls were contributed to by unsafe ladders and construction vehicles. For accidents resulting in part from unsafe ladders, Cohen and Lin (1991) suggested three major approaches for prevention: (1) choosing the right equipment, (2) safe use of ladders, and (3) regular inspection and maintenance of the ladders. Regarding fatal falls contributed to by construction vehicles, either some part of the vehicle was broken or a risky driving maneuver was involved. The risky driving maneuvers included driving a mobile crane or forklift from a flat platform into a building, which resulted in a fall because of a missed link between the flatbed and the building floor; or the mobile crane tipped over when leaning forward or lifting a heavy load with an extended boom; or the material (H beams) picked up by a forklift rolled over and struck other workers. Other cases caused by unsafe construction vehicles involved some poor work practice on the part of the workers. For example, cases could happen because construction workers were standing on top of the lifting load or clump weight and fell with the load when a cable or boom broke. Only a very small number of accidents involving unsafe construction vehicles can be directly related to a broken machine (a broken operator cage). As suggested by Roberts (1989), good crane safety practice, such as operating the crane on a firm footing, in a slow, controlled, cautious manner, should be followed. The personnel platform may be designed by a qualified engineer or a non-engineer with a structural design experience and welded by a qualified welder who is familiar with weld grades, types, and materials specified (Roberts 1989). The platform must be capable of supporting its own weight and five times the intended load, while the load lines must be able to suspend seven times the maximum intended load (Roberts 1989). A plate or permanent marking must show the weight of the platform and its rated capacity or maximum intended load (Roberts 1989).

Other prevention measures regarding unsafe environment are related to a specific falling site. For preventing falls through existing floor openings and through existing roof openings, the openings must be protected with guardrails or adequate coverings: for example, secured wood or metal covers that are capable of supporting subjected loads, and warnings indicating that there is an opening below (MLID 2003). For preventing falls down stairs or steps, MLID (2003) suggested the use of proper handrails on open sides of stairs, ramps, and other similar means of access. These not only act to prevent falls from open sides, but also serve as a support to workers moving up and down the access way. To prevent falls through roof surfaces, various researchers have suggested a fundamental approach. This includes the suggestion that manufacturers should use roofing material that is strong enough not only to support workers and equipment (Helander 1981) but also the dynamic loading during walking, falling against, or sitting on the material (Bobick et al. 1994). Wide and properly secured support platforms (crawling boards and planks) should be provided for any roof under construction.

26.4.2 Proportion of Unsafe Behavior

One interesting observation is the proportion of the causes of falls in terms of unsafe acts and unsafe mechanical or physical conditions, as defined in Heinrich et al. (1980). In our previous study (Chi et al. 2005), by analyzing each fatal fall with a single cause, if unknown and other unclassified causes are excluded, unsafe acts including bodily action, poor work practices, improper use of safety equipment, overexertion, distraction, insufficient capacities, unauthorized access, being pulled down, and removal of protection measures accounted for only 35.6% of the total number of fatal falls. In a recent study (Chi et al. 2014b), by analyzing each fatal fall with multiple causes, the number of single and multiple-cause combinations with unsafe behaviors accounted for a significantly greater proportion (63%; 259 cases) of the total number of fatal falls. This 63% is much closer to the 88% suggested by Heinrich et al. (1980). The difference between our two studies (Chi et al. 2005, 2014b) and Heinrich et al. (1980) can be attributed to the focus on liability litigation from the insurance company in Heinrich et al. (1980) versus our focus on accident prevention.

26.4.3 Why a Graphical Fault Tree?

Based on focus group discussions to investigate why accidents still happen in the construction industry, Haslam et al. (2005) found that construction supervisors frequently have little safety awareness and a poor understanding of accident causation and prevention. Similarly, Hung et al. (2013) explored fall protection training needs through 29 semi-structured interviews among residential roofing subcontractors with respect to recommendations for the design of fall protection training. In general, it was found that pictures work better than words, especially in communicating with foreign (Hispanic) workers. Including as many pictures as possible on safety materials can increase their effectiveness and the workers' engagement (Hung et al. 2013). Fault trees can be very effective in creating an overview of a complex occurrence and in communicating our research findings of potential accident causes and scenarios to construction workers (Svedung and Rasmussen

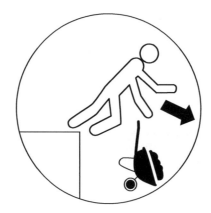

FIGURE 26.3
Graphical icon designed for the accident cause "being pulled down." (From Chi, C-F. et al., *Accident Anal. Prev.*, 72, 359–369, 2014.)

2002). To improve effectiveness in communication of accident causation, pictures depicting features of the real-world object or concept they represent (Dewar 2004) (graphical icons) were incorporated into our fault tree analysis. Graphical icons were designed for each falling site scenario and associated accident cause, to illustrate the fault tree in a graphical manner so that accident causation can be easily understood by construction workers who may not read English (or Chinese).

As an example, Figure 26.3 shows the icon designed for representing the accident cause "being pulled down." Based on the concept of image-related icons (Chi and Dewi 2014a), the icon was created based on the accident scenario found in the database that workers could be pulled down while dumping a wheelbarrow filled with heavy materials. Other considerations include that all graphical icons should have borders to make icons appear orderly, consistent, and uniform (Campbell et al. 2004). Also, icons should be legible and comprehensible by the viewers (meaningful) (Dewar 2004). Following the standard format of fault tree analysis, icons representing different falling site scenarios are designed to have rectangular borders, while icons indicating accident causes have circular borders. As examples, graphical fault trees, as shown in Figures 26.4 and 26.5, were developed for falling through roof surface and falling from a roof edge or opening, to support interdisciplinary discussion of risk management (Svedung and Rasmussen 2002) and facilitate the communication of accident causation to first-line supervisors (Hung et al. 2013).

Similar figures were found in Drury and Brill (1983) to describe commonly seen accident patterns related to consumer product usage or the 18 lifesaving rules developed by the International Association of Oil and Gas Producers (OGP) to mitigate risk and reduce fatalities (International Association of Oil and Gas Producers 2013) (see Figure 26.6). Each OGP lifesaving rule consists of a simple icon and descriptive text, with additional detailed guidance to explain why the rule is important and what aspects workers and supervisors should focus on (International Association of Oil and Gas Producers 2013).

26.4.4 Qualitative and Quantitative Application of Fault Tree Analysis

As described in Section 25.1.5, fault tree models can be analyzed qualitatively or quantitatively. Qualitative analysis leads to the determination of the MCSs contributing to a fatality. For quantitative analysis, Khakzad et al. (2011) suggested presenting

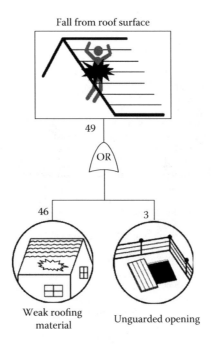

FIGURE 26.4
Graphical fault tree for fatal fall from roof surface. (From Chi, C-F. et al., *Accident Anal. Prev.*, 72, 359–369, 2014.)

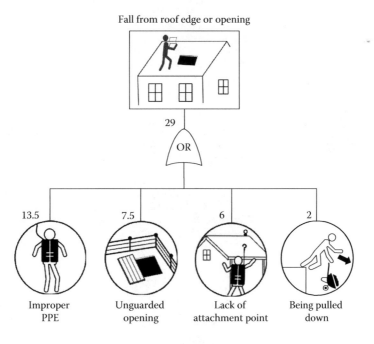

FIGURE 26.5
Graphical fault tree for fatal falls from roof edge or opening. (From Chi, C-F. et al., *Accident Anal. Prev.*, 72, 359–369, 2014.)

Icon and primary text	Additional guidance
Protect yourself against a fall when working at height.	**Use fall protection equipment when working outside a protective environment where you can fall over 1.8 m (6 ft) to keep you safe.** A protective environment includes approved scaffolds, stairs with handrails, and man lifts. You should: ➤ Have authorisation to work at height outside a protective environment. ➤ Be aware of what fall protection equipment to use and how to use it. ➤ Check equipment before using it. ➤ Always tie off when at height outside of a protective environment. If you are the supervisor or person in charge of the work, you should ➤ Confirm that it is safe to start work at height.
Do not walk under a suspended load	**Working or walking immediately under a suspended load is unsafe as the load can fall on you.** A suspended load is an object that is temporary lifted and hangs above the ground (rig floors are excluded from this rule). You should ➤ Never cross a barrier controlling an area with a suspended load without authorisation. ➤ Follow the instructions of the flagman or the person in charge of the lift. If you are the person in charge of the lift you should ➤ Mark the unsafe area and put barriers in place. Ensure that nobody walks under a suspended load.
  permit Work with a valid work permit when required	**A work permit describes what you must do to stay safe.** You should: ➤ Understand the work permit and follow it. ➤ Confirm that the work permit is valid. ➤ Confirm with the supervisor or the person in charge of the work that it is safe to start work. If you are the supervisor or person in charge of the work you should: ➤ Confirm if a work permit is required for this work. ➤ Confirm that the workplace has been inspected before work starts. ➤ Explain how the work permit keeps you safe. ➤ Confirm the work permit is signed. ➤ Confirm that it is safe to start work. ➤ Get a new work permit when the work or the situation changes. confirm that the work is completed.
 Prevent dropped objects	**There is a significant risk of dropped objects when using tools and portable equipment at height. Preventing objects from falling keeps you and people working below you safe.** You should: ➤ Secure all tools and equipment to prevent them from falling/being dropped. ➤ Put barriers around areas where there is a potential for dropped objects. ➤ Always wear head protection where required. If you are the supervisor or person in charge of the work you should ➤ Create awareness of the risk of dropped objects and understanding of what actions need to be taken (for example during team/toolbox meetings). ➤ Regularly inspect the site to ensure that precautions are taken to prevent objects from falling from height (e.g., Hand tools are tied off, no loose objects, no holes in grating, toe boards are in place, barriers are in place where necessary, head protection is worn where required, etc.).

FIGURE 26.6

Example of the OGP lifesaving rules. (From International Association of Oil & Gas Producers, *OGP Life-Saving Rules*, Report No. 459 version 2, 2013. www.iogp.org.)

the probability of the top event in terms of the occurrence probability of MCS events. However, one problem in this respect is the denominator: the population or exposure data, such as the total number of events in which a certain fraction led to a fault, are rarely available (Ale et al. 2006). For example, our previous study on occupational fatalities (Chi and Chen 2003) focused only on the controllable demographic factors (e.g., age, gender, and industry). Other factors, such as working experience, company size, and source of injury, could not be analyzed, because a working population with a similar background was not available.

Although the probability of a top event in terms of probability of MCS events cannot be derived without the exposure data as the denominator, the frequency of the MCSs can still be prioritized to indicate the importance of the cause(s) and can be used to customize the construction site inspection to improve the utility of human inspectors (Chi and Chen 2003). Through fault tree and MCS analyses on 411 fatal falls, MCSs associated with each falling site can be presented as a fault tree, as shown in Figure 26.7, to guide the inspection agency or the construction company to conduct safety audits focusing on these basic causes.

A limitation of the study is that the fatalities considered occurred several years ago, during the period 2001–2005. However, the reuse of the coding scheme proved that even though construction methods and practices may have developed during the intervening period, the essence of the accident causation remains the same. The results nevertheless give a useful cross-sectional indication of the patterns of fatal falls and their causation in construction operations. Fall incidents caused by unguarded openings, inappropriate usage of a safety harness, and poor communication with the work team were also reported in Haslam et al. (2005). Accident cases published by the Occupational Safety and Health Administration (OSHA) and the National Institute for Occupational Safety and Health (NIOSH) also indicated that the scenario for fatal falls associated with each falling site in the US construction industry during 2010–2013 has a similar nature (see Table 26.9). It is also argued that the classification scheme and analytical approach used by the study, mostly based on existing literature and an American National Standards Institute (ANSI) standard, has relevance for the analysis of fatal falls more widely.

26.5 Conclusion

Our study applied a fault tree analysis to represent the causal relationships among events and causes that contributed to fatal falls in the construction industry. The causes for the falls and the nature of the accident events were classified and coded with the same coding scheme as in Chi et al. (2005). Boolean algebra was applied for these 411 fall fatalities to derive MCSs associated with each falling site. Eventually, all 411 accident causes can be presented in a fault tree to provide an overview of all accident causes for fall fatalities included in this study. Also, the relative frequency of the MCSs can be prioritized to customize the construction site inspection to improve the utility of human inspectors. Furthermore, icons representing different falling site scenarios and accident causes were designed to illustrate the fault tree analysis to support an interdisciplinary discussion of risk management and improve effectiveness in communication of accident causation to first-line supervisors.

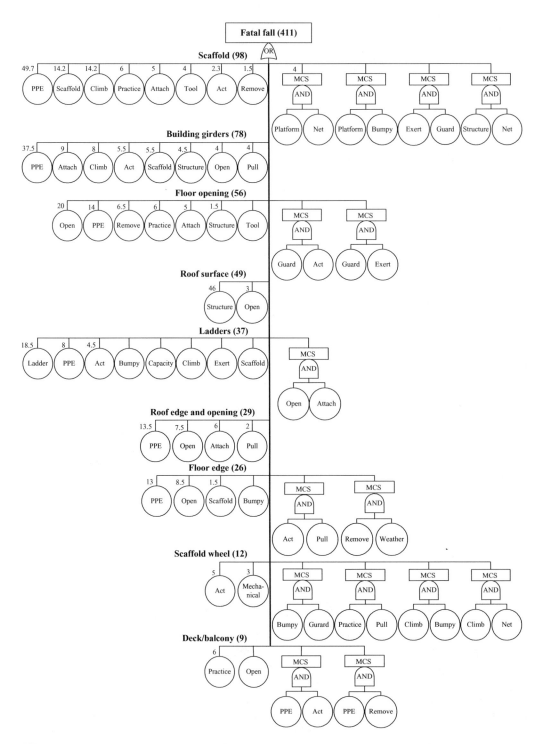

FIGURE 26.7
A complete fault tree of fatal falls for all falling sites. (From Chi, C-F. et al., *Accident Anal. Prev.*, 72, 359–369, 2014.)

TABLE 26.9

Examples of Similar Fatal Fall Scenarios in the United States during 2010–2013

Date and Falling Site	Event Description
Date: July 24, 2012 Falling site: scaffold Source: OSHA	The victim was working from a job-built wooden scaffold constructed on the fourth-floor exterior balcony walkway. A wooden guardrail system was in place along the length of the fourth-floor balcony and along the exterior side of the elevated scaffold platform. The victim unsecured the end of the top guardrail, nearest the work being performed, and let it drop down onto the scaffold while the opposite end of the guardrail was still attached. This created an unprotected open area along the exterior side of the scaffold. He was on one knee, along the unprotected edge of the scaffold, and proceeded to strike the block with his hammer. On the final strike, the block came free. The victim's momentum and force while swinging the hammer caused him to pitch forward through the open unprotected space. He fell about 36–40 ft to the asphalt below.
Date: March 27, 2011 Falling site: scaffold Source: NIOSH	A male municipal custodian was fatally injured while painting an interior section of a school lobby. Although the incident was unwitnessed, it appears that the victim was on mobile scaffolding when he fell from the scaffolding, landing on the lobby floor.
Date: January 4, 2013 Falling site: tower (building girders) Source: OSHA	A communications worker was on a cellular communications tower, at a position more than 25 m above the ground, when he fell. Although he was using a PPE, the anchorage he was using failed.
Date: May 21, 2012 Falling site: walk board (floor opening) Source: OSHA	An employee was engaged in residential framing work from a walk board 8 ft above the ground while relocating the end truss, which had been placed in the wrong location. The employee fell from the walk board to the concrete surface below, suffering a concussion.
Date: September 25, 2012 Falling site: roof Source: OSHA	The owner of a roofing and repair company was working on the roof of a three-story hotel. The owner, while installing a tarp, stepped close to the roof's eave. The eave collapsed, and he fell 26 ft to the parking lot.
Date: October 10, 2012 Falling site: ladder Source: NIOSH	The three-man crew of a construction business were removing shingles to reroof a private recreation facility. The victim carried a tarp up an extension ladder to the roof so that the owner could cover the roof in anticipation of impending rain. He fell an estimated 10–12 ft to the foundation retaining wall. A stabilizer bar attached to the ladder had come apart from the ladder, and a nylon tie-down strap used to secure the stabilizer bar to the roof had broken when the ladder slid sideways.
Date: October 11, 2012 Falling site: decking (roof edge and opening) Source: OSHA	The victim and a coworker were covering an open-air atrium with a 24 by 45 ft piece of rolled polyplastic sheeting. They were told to install the rolled polyplastic over the existing plastic from the second floor and roof deck. They were pulling the plastic over the open atrium when the victim fell. The victim was wearing a full body harness with a retractable lanyard device, but his fall was not arrested, due to the failure of the anchors, and he fell 20 ft from the roof atrium opening onto the floor.
Date: September, 2010 Falling site: highway bridge (floor edge) Source: NIOSH	A worker fell from a highway bridge in the process of levelling jacks for concrete forms. Wearing a fall protection harness with an attached lanyard, he stepped outside the lifeline onto a 10″ × 2″ wooden board to verify that the jacks were level. As he stepped over the lifeline, he did not attach the lanyard, and fell approximately 28 ft onto the railroad tracks below.
Date: September 22, 2012 Falling site: scissor lift (scaffold with wheels) Source: OSHA	The victim was using an upright scissor lift on the forks of a forklift to access light fixtures. The scissor lift was extended to a height of 22.33 ft. As he went to change a bulb, the scissor lift tilted and fell off the forks. The victim fell to the asphalt parking lot.
Date: October 18, 2012 Falling site: unguarded opening (deck/balcony) Source: OSHA	A male carpenter was working on the overhead archway on a balcony of a wood-framed residential house when he fell more than 14 ft to the ground from an unguarded second-story opening. The victim was not wearing or using any type of fall protection at the time of the fall.

Source: Chi, C-F. et al., *Accident Anal. Prev.*, 72, 359–369, 2014.

References

Ale, B. J. M., L. J. Bellamy, R. M. Cooke, L. H. J. Goossens, Andrew Richard Hale, A. L. C. Roelen, and Euan Smith. Towards a causal model for air transport safety: An ongoing research project. *Safety Science* 44, no. 8 (2006): 657–673.

Bobick, T. G., L. S. Ronald, T. J. Pizatella, P. R. Keane, and D. L. Smith. Preventing falls through skylights and roof openings. *Professional Safety* 39, no. 9 (1994): 33.

Buskin, S. E., and L. J. Paulozzi. Fatal injuries in the construction industry in Washington State. *American Journal of Industrial Medicine* 11, no. 4 (1987): 453–460.

Butani, S. J. Relative risk analysis of injuries in coal mining by age and experience at present company. *Journal of Occupational Accidents* 10, no. 3 (1988): 209–216.

Campbell, J. L., J. B. Richman, C. Carney, and J. D. Lee. *In-Vehicle Display Icons and Other Information Elements. Volume I: Guidelines.* No. FHWA-RD-03–065, 2004.

Cattledge, G. H., A. Schneiderman, R. Stanevich, S. Hendricks, and J. Greenwood. Nonfatal occupational fall injuries in the West Virginia construction industry. *Accident Analysis and Prevention* 28, no. 5 (1996): 655–663.

Charness, N. *Aging and Human Performance.* Vol. 5. Wiley, 1985.

Chi, C-F., T-C. Chang, and H-I. Ting. Accident patterns and prevention measures for fatal occupational falls in the construction industry. *Applied Ergonomics* 36, no. 4 (2005): 391–400.

Chi, C-F., and C-L. Chen. Reanalyzing occupational fatality injuries in Taiwan with a model free approach. *Safety Science* 41, no. 8 (2003): 681–700.

Chi, C-F., and R. S. Dewi. Matching performance of vehicle icons in graphical and textual formats. *Applied Ergonomics* 45, no. 4 (2014a): 904–916.

Chi, C-F., S-Z. Lin, and R. S. Dewi. Graphical fault tree analysis for fatal falls in the construction industry. *Accident Analysis and Prevention* 72 (2014b): 359–369.

Chi, C-F., and M-L. Wu. Fatal occupational injuries in Taiwan: Relationship between fatality rate and age. *Safety Science* 27, no. 1 (1997): 1–17.

Chi, C-F., C-C. Yang, and Z-L. Chen. In-depth accident analysis of electrical fatalities in the construction industry. *International Journal of Industrial Ergonomics* 39, no. 4 (2009): 635–644.

Cohen, H. H., and L-J. Lin. A scenario analysis of ladder fall accidents. *Journal of Safety Research* 22, no. 1 (1991): 31–39.

Dewar, R. E. Design and evaluation of public information symbols. In *Visual Information for Everyday Use: Design and Research Perspectives.* Zwaga, H., Boersema, T., and Hoonhout, H. (Eds.). Boca Raton, FL, CRC Press, 2004.

Directorate-General of Budget, Accounting and Statistics. *The Report on 1996 Industry, Commerce and Service Census Taiwan area.* Executive Yuan, 1997.

Directorate-General of Budget, Accounting and Statistics. *Annual Bulletin of Manpower Statistics Taiwan area.* Executive Yuan. 2001–2005.

Doytchev, D. E., and G. Szwillus. Combining task analysis and fault tree analysis for accident and incident analysis: A case study from Bulgaria. *Accident Analysis and Prevention* 41, no. 6 (2009): 1172–1179.

Drury, C. G., and M. Brill. Human factors in consumer product accident investigation. *Human Factors: The Journal of the Human Factors and Ergonomics Society* 25, no. 3 (1983): 329–342.

Fisher, L. D., and G. V. Belle. *Biostatistics: A Methodology for the Health Sciences.* Hoboken, NJ, Wiley, 1993.

Hammer, W. *Occupational Safety Management and Engineering.* 4th Edition. NJ: Prentice Hall, 1989.

Harms-Ringdahl, L. *Safety Analysis: Principles and Practice in Occupational Safety.* New York, Taylor & Francis, 2001.

Haslam, R. A., S. A. Hide, A. G. F. Gibb, et al. Contributing factors in construction accidents. *Applied Ergonomics* 36, no. 4 (2005): 401–415.

Heinrich, H. W., D. Petersen, and Nestor Roos. *Industrial Accident Prevention.* New York: McGraw-Hill, 1980.

Helander, M. (Ed.). Safety in construction. In *Human Factors/Ergonomics for Building and Construction.* New York: Wiley, 1981.

Helander, M. A review of research on human factors and safety in building/construction. In *Proceedings of the 1984 International Conference on Occupational Ergonomics*, pp. 95–104. 1984.

Hinze, J., C. Pedersen, and J. Fredley. Identifying root causes of construction injuries. *Journal of Construction Engineering and Management* 124, no. 1 (1998): 67–71.

Hsiao, H., J. Whitestone, and T-Y. Kau. Evaluation of fall arrest harness sizing schemes. *Human Factors: The Journal of the Human Factors and Ergonomics Society* 49, no. 3 (2007): 447–464.

Hu, K., H. Rahmandad, T. Smith-Jackson, and W. Winchester. Factors influencing the risk of falls in the construction industry: A review of the evidence. *Construction Management and Economics* 29, no. 4 (2011): 397–416.

Hung, Y-H., W. W. Winchester, T. L. Smith-Jackson, B. M. Kleiner, K. L. Babski-Reeves, and T. H. Mills. Identifying fall-protection training needs for residential roofing subcontractors. *Applied Ergonomics* 44, no. 3 (2013): 372–380.

International Association of Oil and Gas Producers. *OGP Life-Saving Rules.* Report No. 459 version 2, 2013. www.iogp.org.

Janicak, C. A. Fall-related deaths in the construction industry. *Journal of Safety Research* 29, no. 1 (1998): 35–42.

Kelsey, J. L., A. S. Whittemore, A. S. Evans, and W. D. Thompson. *Methods in Observational Epidemiology.* Vol. 26. New York: Oxford University Press, 1996.

Khakzad, N., F. Khan, and P. Amyotte. Safety analysis in process facilities: Comparison of fault tree and Bayesian network approaches. *Reliability Engineering and System Safety* 96, no. 8 (2011): 925–932.

Laflamme, L., and E. Menckel. Aging and occupational accidents: A review of the literature of the last three decades. *Safety Science* 21, no. 2 (1995): 145–161.

LeBeau, K. H., and S. J. Wadia-Fascetti. Fault tree analysis of Schoharie Creek Bridge collapse. *Journal of Performance of Constructed Facilities* 21, no. 4 (2007): 320–326.

Lucas, R. E. B. The distribution of job characteristics. *The Review of Economics and Statistics* (1974): 530–540.

Manitoba Labour and Immigration Division. *Fall Protection Guidelines*, 2003. (http://www.oshforeveryone.org/wsib/default.html).

Messing, K., J. Courville, M. Boucher, L. Dumais, and A. M. Seifert. Can safety risks of blue-collar jobs be compared by gender? *Safety Science* 18, no. 2 (1994): 95–112.

Occupational Safety and Health Administration. *Safety and Health Standards for the Construction Industry.* OHSA 3129, 1996.

Roberts, C. A. *OSHA's New Rules for Crane-Suspended Personnel Platforms.* Boston, MA, The Aberdeen Group, 1989.

Sorock, G. S., E. O'Hagen Smith, and M. Goldoft. Fatal occupational injuries in the New Jersey construction industry, 1983 to 1989. *Journal of Occupational and Environmental Medicine* 35, no. 9 (1993): 916–921.

Svedung, I., and J. Rasmussen. Graphic representation of accident scenarios: Mapping system structure and the causation of accidents. *Safety Science* 40, no. 5 (2002): 397–417.

US Bureau Labor Statistics. Census of Fatal Occupational Injuries Charts, 1992–2012 (revised data), 2014. Retrieved July 12, 2014 from http://www.bls.gov/iif/oshcfoi1.htm#charts.

US Department of Labor, Bureau of Labor Statistics. *Occupational Injury and Illness Classification Manual: Section 2*, 2003. http://www.bls.gov.

Vesely, W. E., F. F. Goldberg, N. H. Roberts, and D. F. Haasl. *Fault Tree Handbook.* Washington: US Government Printing Office, 1981.

Volkanovski, A., M. Čepin, and B. Mavko. Application of the fault tree analysis for assessment of power system reliability. *Reliability Engineering and System Safety* 94, no. 6 (2009): 1116–1127.

Whitesitt, J. E. *Boolean Algebra and Its Applications.* Mineola, NY, Courier Dover Corporation, 1995.

27

Knowledge Gaps and Emerging Issues for Fall Control in Construction

G. Scott Earnest and Christine M. Branche

CONTENTS

ABSTRACT This chapter reviews the history and ongoing multidisciplinary research to address the prevention of falls from elevation in the construction industry. It touches on both personal and environmental factors that affect construction falls, as well as their often devastating consequences, including the number of people affected and businesses impacted. It outlines issues, often difficult, related to falls from roofs, ladders, and scaffolds. Because falls involve a complex combination of safety controls, safety culture and management, and worker behavior, this chapter covers each. The chapter addresses efforts toward sustainable solutions, ranging from education, training, and behavior to engineering, controls, and prevention through design, in addition to administrative issues. Because it has brought a lot of attention to the issue of falls in construction and effective ways to prevent them, the chapter also covers the national falls prevention campaign. Finally, research needs and gaps are presented, with the goal of advancing the science of preventing construction falls.

KEY WORDS: *construction, safety, falls, ladders, roofing, scaffolds, towers, lifts, prevention, training, campaign.*

Disclaimer

Mention of any company or product does not constitute endorsement by the National Institute for Occupational Safety and Health (NIOSH). In addition, citations to Web sites external to NIOSH do not constitute NIOSH endorsement of the sponsoring organizations or their programs or products. Furthermore, NIOSH is not responsible for the content of these Web sites.

27.1 Introduction

Falls from elevation are the leading cause of construction industry injuries and deaths in the United States. According to 2010 data from the Bureau of Labor Statistics (BLS), falls to a lower level accounted for 251 of 751 deaths in construction, just under half (49%) of the total number of falls in all private industry that year (www.bls.gov/iif/oshwc/cfoi/cftb0258.pdf). Most construction fatalities occurred when workers fell from roofs, ladders, and scaffolds. According to a study by the Center for Construction Research and Training (CPWR), small construction companies (with 10 or fewer employees) had the highest percentage of fatal falls (64%). In addition, laborers, carpenters, and roofers were the construction workers with the largest number of fatal falls. Furthermore, workers with less than a year in the industry accounted for 56% of fatal falls (Dong, 2010).

Construction workers are more likely to die on the job than workers in any other industry, and falls from elevation (often one story or higher) take the heaviest toll (Dong et. al., 2014). Approximately 4400 occupational fatalities occurred in 2012 (BLS, 2013), and about 18% of these were in the construction industry. More than a third of the construction fatalities that year were caused by falls, of which 35% were from a roof. Half of the workers fell from the roof edge, and the others fell through an existing roof hole, skylight, or collapsing roof surface. Details on the causes of these falls are often unreported.

The costs of fatal falls and injuries in construction are high, including heavy burdens on workers, families, employers (often small businesses), and the broader society in general. Even when workers survive, many have significant nonfatal injuries, such as traumatic brain injuries for example, or other issues requiring lengthy rehabilitation. These place enormous emotional, medical, and financial burdens on their families. Falls also result in significant costs to employers, including lost productivity, loss of skilled workers, and increased workers' compensation costs.

Because of the tremendous toll of these injuries and deaths on the nation's workforce, their families, employers, and society, extensive research has been conducted and is continuing to address this problem, to better understand their causes, and to design technologies and methods for advancing their prevention, with the ultimate goal of eliminating falls in construction. Researchers are assessing gaps in knowledge and are encouraging the development and adoption of new technologies and procedures. Studies with a wide range of methods have examined many factors involved in falls, including the populations affected and the situations and tasks most commonly associated with them. Additional research has focused on different approaches to reducing the severity and likelihood of construction falls. Despite these substantial efforts, however, more studies are needed for progress to continue. The following pages describe recent work and emerging issues, as well as some ideas on where research is headed in this important area of construction safety and health.

27.2 Gaps and Emerging Issues

27.2.1 Risk Factors Influencing Falls

Many studies have focused on the factors associated with falls in construction. These factors can generally be placed into two categories: environmental factors (relating to the worker's surroundings) and personal factors (relating to the individual who suffered the fall). Much of the information available on both factors is based on surveillance and epidemiological studies of falls in construction.

27.2.1.1 Environmental Factors

Environmental risk factors associated with construction falls include surface properties (e.g., strength, stability, and slippage), incline and restrictions of the support surface, and visual elements. Surface properties involve issues such as the coefficient of friction between the worker's shoes and the walking surface (Hanson et al., 1999). In roofing, other surface factors that may be consequential are unstable elements such as roof shingles, as well as potential obstructions or uneven surfaces, which are all tripping hazards. Another surface property risk is posed by fragile materials that can cause falls through the surface. Shoe style also affects workers' walking stability at elevation (Simeonov et al., 2008). Challenging work environments, such as narrow walking surfaces, result in modified walking for balance control, which points to the potential role of footwear in loss of balance. Weather conditions (e.g., rain, wind, or even dew), furthermore, can affect the walking surface. A study in Hong Kong showed that the highest percentage of falls occurred in August, which is the hottest month and has the most rainfall (Wong et al., 2005). The fewest falls occurred during February, one of the driest months of the year in that city.

Although some roofs are flat, many have pitch for drainage. In general, low-sloped roofs have a pitch ratio of <4–12 (vertical to horizontal), and for steep-sloped roofs, the ratio is >4–12. As roof pitch increases, the likelihood of slipping rises, because higher coefficients of friction are needed between the roof and the worker's shoes. Finally, a considerable amount of research has been conducted on visual aspects that influence falls. Hsiao and Simeonov (2001) reported that worker balance, as well as depth perception and detection of obstacles or other potential hazards, is affected by elevation.

TABLE 27.1

Types of Falls and Related Activities

Fall Type	Associated Activity
Falls through floors	Unguarded openings or inadequate fall protection
Falls from girders or structural steel	Bodily action or improper use of PPE
Falls from roof edge	Bodily action or being pulled down by heavy objects
Falls through roofs	Noncompliance with scaffold standards
Falls from ladders	Overexertion or use of unsafe ladders and tools

Chi et al. (2005) studied over 600 fatal construction falls, using accident reports to determine each victim's age, gender, experience, and use of personal protective equipment (PPE); the fall site; and the company size. Approximately 92% of the fall victims were men. Also, for a variety of reasons, the risk of falling was higher for small businesses, and over 80% of the fatal falls were of workers with less than 1 year of experience. Falls from scaffolding (30% of falls) were associated with violating government standards and bodily action (i.e., climbing, walking, or leaning against something). The associations between types of falls and specific associated activities found by Chi and colleagues are provided in Table 27.1.

Primary fall prevention measures that were discussed in Chi et al. included handrails, guardrails, surface opening protections, crawling boards/planks, and stronger roofing material. Secondary prevention measures included travel restriction, fall arrest, and fall containment systems.

Fong et al. (2005) investigated lower-extremity kinematics of walking on slippery simulated construction surfaces. Variations in footwear, flooring, and contaminants were tested. The dynamic coefficient of friction was measured for each condition. Fifteen men wearing fall harnesses walked and avoided slips. Their movements were measured with a motion analysis system. Recommendations to prevent slips included increased stance and stride time, shortened strides, decreased speed, and gentle heel strike. Hanson et al. (1999) studied friction and gait biomechanics for actual slips and falls. The goal was to develop a method for estimating the probability of slips and falls. Subjects wearing safety harnesses walked down a ramp at various angles (0°, 10°, and 20°) on either a tile or carpeted surface under dry, wet, or soapy conditions. The dynamic coefficient of friction of shoe, floor surface, and contaminant interfaces was measured. Friction was assessed by examining the foot forces during walking when no slips occurred. Slips were recorded and categorized to develop a model of the probability of a slip or fall. Slips and falls increased as the difference between the required coefficient of friction and the measured dynamic coefficient of friction increased.

Finally, another environmental factor that impacts construction falls is the worksite safety culture and safety climate. Safety culture is associated with deeply held beliefs, attitudes, and values within an organization. Safety climate is closely related to safety policies and procedures within the organization. Some of the important elements that influence safety climate within an organization include worker participation, management commitment, leadership, training, communication, and trust. Each of these elements can play a significant role in reducing the likelihood of falls in construction (CPWR, 2013).

27.2.1.2 Personal Factors

Dong et al. (2009) studied trends in fatal falls from roofs in US construction from 1992 to 2009. Their analysis of data from the BLS Census of Fatal Occupational Injuries (CFOI) and the Current Population Survey showed that falls from roofs accounted for one third of fatal falls in construction during the period. Approximately 67% of deaths from roof falls occurred in small construction businesses (i.e., having 10 or fewer employees). Roofers, ironworkers, roofing contractors, and residential construction workers were most at risk for fatal roof falls. Elevated rates of roof fatalities were found also among workers aged under 20 years old or more than 44 years old, Hispanics, and immigrants (Dong et. al., 2013). Dong (2010) recommended that prevention strategies target these high-risk workers.

Hispanics represent over 25% of US construction workers and are more likely to experience fatal falls than non-Hispanics. Approximately 17% of the US population is Hispanic. The proportion of fatal falls among Hispanic construction workers increased from approximately 37% of all fatal falls annually during 1992–2002 to 40% of all fatal falls in 2006. The risk of fatal falls is higher for Hispanic workers who were not born in the United States. Nearly 80% of the Hispanic workers who died from falls in 2003–2006 were foreign born, and many were young and inexperienced. Nearly 65% of Hispanic workers who died—compared with about 53% of white, non-Hispanic workers who died—had been employed for less than a year (Dong et al., 2009). These differences in fall rates could be related to factors such as employers' failure to train these workers adequately in relation to their pre-employment education or attainment of job skills; difficulties in understanding or implementing training due to lower English language proficiency; and assignment of these workers to jobs with higher exposures to fall risks.

In another study, Chau et al. (2004) compared job, age, and life conditions with the causes and severity of occupational injuries among 880 male construction laborers. All had at least one occupational injury involving sick leave. For each injury, a questionnaire was completed by an occupational physician and the worker. The researchers found that worker risk was related to age, body mass index, hearing ability, and sporting activities (which could be a surrogate for physical fitness). Certain types of injuries were correlated with specific jobs. Data showed that the risk for falls and injuries from handling of objects or hand tools was similar for all construction workers, but the risk of injury from moving objects was highest for masons, plumbers, and electricians. Carpenters, roofers, and civil-engineering workers were most at risk for injury from construction machinery and devices. Being overweight was related to falls from the same or a lower level.

Other personal risk factors associated with construction falls and reported in the scientific literature include age, gender, strength, general health, fatigue, behaviors and attitudes, and (in many cases) training or job experience (Hsiao and Simeonov, 2001). Unfortunately, many of these factors can be directly related to each other (collinear) and may be sources of confounding, such as age, health, and experience. For example, as persons age, they are more likely to suffer from instability, which can lead to falls. Inherent in the aging process is a gradual decline in vision, physical strength, range of motion, and flexibility. Dong et al. (2012) found that older construction workers have a higher risk of fatal falls than younger workers, and that falls from roofs and ladders are a particular concern.

Visual performance is another personal factor that commonly decreases with age, which can increase the likelihood of a fall. For working at height, visual performance is related to elevation, changes in depth perception, and the ability to recognize potential hazards on the basis of training and experience (Hsiao and Simeonov, 2001). Simeonov et al. (2003) reported that standing postural instability is related to the effects of slope and elevation. Lastly, novice workers who lack training and experience may be more susceptible to falling because they are less familiar with the work environment and have less experience with maintaining balance in some conditions. Lack of worker training also may relate to environmental factors involving leadership, management commitment, and corporate culture.

27.2.2 Falls from or through Ladders

Falls from ladders are the second leading cause of fall fatalities in construction. Most of the ladder-related injuries and fatalities that occur in construction involve the use of extension ladders or stepladders. Extension ladders have several connected telescopic lengths, come in four duty ratings, and are often between 32 and 72 ft long. Stepladders are hinged in the middle, form an inverted V when locked in place, and are typically shorter, ranging from 3 to 20 ft long.

A Swedish study showed that of 114 ladder accidents in 1 year, 73% involved extension ladders, 20% involved stepladders, and 7% involved fixed or stationary ladders (Bjornstig and Johnnson, 1992). Falls from ladders in construction are often related to worker activities rather than ladder design; however, it is unclear how often best practices are used. Overreaching or slipping on the rungs is a common cause of ladder falls. Because of ladder safety concerns, some construction companies have implemented administrative controls through policies that discourage ladder use unless all other options have been exhausted.

Dennerlein et al. (2009) developed and tested an audit tool that assesses compliance with best practices for step- and extension ladder use in construction. The audit tool consists of checklists for ladder conditions (length, ratings, etc.), setup (proper angle, secure top, dry surface, etc.), and moving and working on a ladder (three points of contact, tied off, etc.). Individuals trained to use the tool scored a set of photographs and videos of ladder conditions, setups, and users working on them. The assessment tool has good agreement across users and provides a method to quantify ladder best practices and conduct safety evaluations.

Falls from extension ladders are caused by the ladder base slipping; the ladder tipping; the worker slipping while on the ladder or while transitioning from it to a surface at height; and failure of the ladder itself. Although engineering control measures are available, four actions are needed to advance ladder safety: research on visual indicators for setting up ladders at the proper angle; developing and evaluating methods to simplify moving from a ladder to a surface at height; integrating ladder safety accessories to ease carrying, assembly, and storage; and developing simple guidance for safe ladder use, maintenance, and inspection (Hsiao et al., 2008).

When setting up an extension ladder, the traditional approach involves grasping the rung in front with outstretched arms. NIOSH researchers have demonstrated a better method: grasping the side rails of the ladder instead of a step (Simeonov et al., 2012a; OSHA, 2013). This change provides a more natural placement of the outstretched hands and a safer ladder angle. NIOSH researchers (Simeonov et al., 2010) have also evaluated the use of electro-adhesion technology to help stabilize extension ladders at either end. Electro-adhesion technology uses electrostatic forces between surfaces, such as a wall and electro-adhesive pads on a ladder, to increase stability. A small battery pack provides power to each adhesive pad. A patent application has been submitted for using electro-adhesion technology with an extension ladder.

Simeonov developed a patented engineering solution to help extension ladder users position them at the proper angle. The indicator provides user feedback with visual, auditory, and vibration signals when the correct angle (75.5°) is reached (Simeonov et al., 2013). Without feedback, users tend to set up ladders at a shallower angle than needed. The NIOSH Ladder Safety Phone App has an angle-of-inclination indicator and is available free of charge through the NIOSH website (http://www.cdc.gov/niosh/topics/falls/), the Apple App Store, and Google Play.

27.2.3 Falls from or through Roofs

Working on roofs is a high-risk activity that has resulted in serious workplace injuries and deaths from falls. Roofers and their employers need help to better manage and prevent falls from heights. Roof work is laborintensive, and it requires climbing and walking at different inclinations (Fredericks et al., 2005). Roofers install roofing materials and siding and work with sheet metal; their jobs also can involve inspections, repairs, cleaning, and other maintenance activities. It is important that the fall hazards associated with roofing are recognized and understood by all stakeholders.

Critical considerations for working safely on roofs include planning the work; being aware of fall hazards at various stages of the work; and using fall control measures, administrative controls, and PPE. Employers and workers should be able to identify the risks involved with roofs; choose proper access equipment for the job; understand and determine appropriate measures for risk control; and develop a plan to prevent falls during roof work.

Commercial and residential roofing are the two major roofing sectors. Commercial roofing typically involves low-pitched roofs that rise 4 in. per horizontal foot or less, whereas most residential buildings have steep-slope roofs that rise more than 4 in. per horizontal foot (Choi, 2007). According to NIOSH (2004), the rate of nonfatal work-related injuries was 1.1–1.8 times greater among roofers than among construction workers overall from 1992 to 2001. In addition, the rate of fatal work-related injuries was 1.6–2.8 times higher for roofers than for construction workers overall (Sa et al., 2009).

Falls from roofs depend on many factors, including the roof type or profile; roof slope and height; and duration and frequency of work. The potential fall hazards of roofing include falling over an unprotected edge; falling through a fragile or unstable roof surface (e.g., a skylight or rotted board); falling through openings on the roof; and slipping on roof surfaces, especially on pitched roofs. Falls can occur while accessing the roof, working on the roof, and transferring materials onto the roof.

Openings on roofs can also lead to fatal falls. Sometimes, the openings are created during work on roofs. Secured and marked rigid objects may be used to cover roof openings or fragile walking and working surfaces. The covers should support at least twice the maximum load and have full edge bearing on all sides. Falls through fragile roofs are problematic in both roof and building maintenance work, and cause half of the fatal falls. Fragile roof surfaces are areas that are not designed to bear loads. Persons standing on fragile and brittle roof surfaces are at risk if the roof gives way. These roofs are often made from molded or fabricated synthetic materials. The following are likely to be fragile: skylights (Figure 27.1), glass, fiberglass, polycarbonate roofing, old ceramic tiles, corroded metal roof sheets, and rotting wood.

Current measures to reduce falls from roofs focus mainly on fall protection, such as covers, guardrails, safety nets, and personal fall arrest systems, or the application of warning-line systems, safety monitoring systems, and fall protection plans. In many instances, these procedures are not practical for the industry, and current regulations allow the use of alternative means of fall protection, such as slide guards (Hsiao and Simeonov, 2001).

NIOSH has studied guardrail systems used to prevent falls through roofs (Bobick et al., 2010). Commercial edge-protection products were evaluated when used as perimeter guarding around a hole. Installations of the commercial products were compared

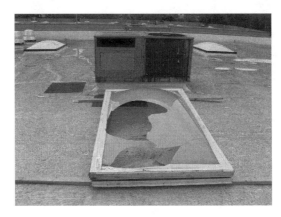

FIGURE 27.1
Skylight on a roof that had a fall through.

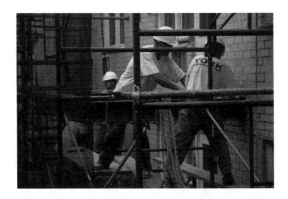

FIGURE 27.2
Construction workers using scaffolding on the side of a building.

with job-built guardrails made of 2×4 in lumber. The Occupational Safety and Health Administration (OSHA) requires that the top rail of a guardrail system be able to support 200 lb. Laboratory tests were developed using a 200 lb manikin, nine test subjects, and five guardrail configurations. All configurations met the 200 lb OSHA requirement. Bobick et al. found that the two edge-protection products can be used as perimeter guarding, and it highlights the importance of using proper materials and fasteners to construct guardrails. A follow-up laboratory study evaluated the strength of job-built guardrails made of lumber and nails (2×4 in and 16 penny nails). This work resulted in a patented guardrail system for use on roofs, stairs, and floors to prevent falls from holes or unguarded edges (Bobick and McKenzie, 2011).

27.2.4 Falls from and through Scaffolds

Scaffolds are temporary structures used to support workers and material during building repairs and construction (Figure 27.2). Scaffolds are typically built from metal pipes or tubes, horizontal boards, and couplers. Falls from scaffolds accounted for 21% of fatal construction falls reported from 1974 to 1978 (OSHA, 1979). Similarly, falls from scaffolds during 1980–1985 accounted for 17% of all fatal falls from elevations, second only to falls from buildings (Bobick et al., 1990; NIOSH, 1991). The high rate of scaffold-related injuries caused OSHA to revise their scaffold safety standards in the late 1980s.

Suspended scaffolds were involved in 30% of the falls from scaffolds. Of the 25 falls from suspended scaffolds, 17 (68%) involved equipment failure. Personal fall protection equipment was used in only three of these incidents, but in each case it was not properly used. In one incident, a worker fell out of his improperly fastened safety belt. In the other two incidents, excessively long lanyards broke or separated after victims fell.

Halperin and McCann (2004) studied safe scaffolding practices at over 100 construction sites in the eastern United States and recommended improvements. A checklist was used to evaluate scaffold safety practices. Approximately 32% of the evaluated scaffolds were near collapse or were missing planks, guardrails, or adequate access. There was a strong correlation between structural problems and fall protection hazards. A correlation was shown among safe scaffold practices and competent persons with scaffold safety training, use of scaffold erection contractors, and scaffolds that were not simple frames. The authors recommended that construction firm managers outsource scaffolding assembly to specialized companies (many have lower accident rates) and that all scaffolding be checked prior to the start of work.

Yassin and Martonik (2004) conducted a similar study by evaluating regulatory changes from 1996 related to the design and assembly of scaffolding in the United States. The study examined the impact of those changes on the accident rate and failure to comply with standards. The study compared records for 5 years prior to the regulatory changes and for 4 years after passage. Although no distinctions were made related to the kind of scaffolding (suspended, mast climbing, or based on the ground), the study showed that the regulations produced a significant decrease in accident rates and the associated costs.

Falls from scaffolds are associated with a lack of compliance in scaffold design and construction as well as bodily action (Chi et al., 2005). Accidents involving temporary scaffolds represent a large percentage of construction injuries (Whitaker et al., 2003). Overexertion and fall injuries represent the largest categories of injuries to scaffold workers (Cutlip et al., 2002). The presence of guardrails or safety handrails on scaffolds could prevent slipping or falling if balance is lost; however, special training in maintaining postural balance at elevation is needed for inexperienced workers.

27.2.5 Falls from and through Telecommunication Towers

The number of telecommunication towers (Figure 27.3) in the United States has increased dramatically over the past 30 years. This increase has closely followed the greater use of cell phones, especially smartphones, and other wireless devices, and the demand they make, subsequently, for faster speeds and more data capacity. Similarly, more workers are needed to upgrade existing towers, which presents unique risks.

In 2013, 13 workers died after falling from telecommunication towers, and a similar number of fatal falls has continued into 2014. Some of the fatalities involved structural collapses. According to OSHA, a telecommunication tower worker has a 25–30 times greater risk of becoming a workplace fatality than the average US worker (Bukowski, 2014). Several of the 2013 fatalities involved workers who were not tied off or who had little or no experience climbing up to 200 ft to perform maintenance.

NIOSH reviewed BLS CFOI data from 1992 to 1998 and found 118 deaths associated with work on telecommunication towers. The fatalities included 93 falls, 18 telecommunication tower collapses, and four electrocutions (NIOSH, 2001). These incidents suggest that employers, workers, tower owners, manufacturers, and wireless service carriers may not

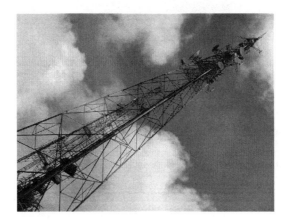

FIGURE 27.3
Construction worker using an aerial lifts near structural steel.

fully recognize the serious hazards associated with the construction and maintenance of telecommunication towers. Safe work practices should be followed, including the use of 100% fall protection (at all times).

Telecommunication towers are often manufactured in sections and constructed on-site by hoisting each section into place using cranes and bolting the sections together. Some smaller towers are self-erecting. Unfortunately, many of the older towers do not have embedded safety features such as permanent horizontal or vertical lifelines or anchor points to attach safety harnesses. NIOSH (2001) found the following factors in fatal falls from telecommunication towers: hoist failures, hoists not rated to hoist workers, truck-crane failures, inadequate fall protection, inadequate training, improper use of or incompatibility of lanyards, and worker fatigue. Although additional research is needed to fully understand how best to prevent these falls, some significant factors have been identified, including use of fall protection systems compatible with the tower being climbed, daily equipment inspections, and improved worker training on safe climbing and use of hoists.

27.3 Fall Solutions That Have Their Own Risks

27.3.1 Aerial Lifts

Ladder-related falls can be reduced through more frequent use of aerial lifts (Figure 27.4). Aerial lifts include vehicle-mounted "bucket trucks," boom lifts, and scissor lifts. Scissor lifts are well suited for smooth finished floors in manufacturing. Rugged-terrain boom lifts are used on construction projects. When aerial lifts are extended, they can present stability issues, and they are complex systems that can fail because of mechanical issues or operator error.

Fall hazards associated with aerial lifts are well recognized (Burkart et al., 2004). McCann (2003) studied construction fatalities related to aerial lifts from 1992 to 1999. Of the 339 deaths reported in the BLS CFOI data, 42% involved boom lifts, 19% involved scissor lifts, and 7% involved other types of unapproved lifts. The main causes of lift-related deaths

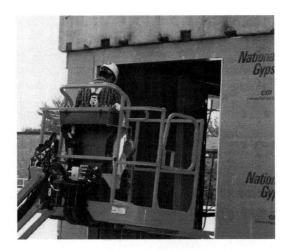

FIGURE 27.4
Construction workers using several aerial lifts near structural steel.

were falls (36%) and collapses or tip-overs (29%), followed by electrocutions (21%). Most of the deaths were among electrical workers.

In a similar study, Pan et al. (2007) analyzed 306 fatalities related to aerial lifts (228 boom lifts and 78 scissor lifts) that occurred between 1992 and 2003. The researchers found that lift height and the vertical position of the worker correlated with fatalities. Tip-overs accounted for 44%–46% of boom lift falls and 56%–59% of scissor lift falls. Height accounted for 72% of the scissor lift fatalities in the BLS CFOI data. Falls, collapses, and tip-overs were involved in 83% of cases investigated by OSHA and the NIOSH Fatality Assessment and Control Evaluation (FACE) Program in all industries between 1990 and 2003.

Approximately 72% of scissor lift fatalities occurred in construction, yet the use of fall protection equipment on scissor lifts is not universally accepted as effective by safety experts. Pan and his colleagues showed that for a significant percentage of falls (82% per OSHA and NIOSH investigation data), existing fall protection systems were not used. NIOSH (Pan et al., 2012) conducted a laboratory study using a commercially available 19 ft electric scissor lift. Manikin drop tests were used to study fall arrest systems from a fully extended scissor lift. A computer model simulated movements, falls, and biomechanical impact. The study showed that fall arrest systems can provide effective fall protection on scissor lifts. However operators could suffer significant force to the lower neck during impact. When a fall arrest system is used on a lift, it must be anchored to the floor of the lift rather than to a railing (Harris et al., 2010).

27.3.2 Mast Climbing Work Platforms

A mast climbing work platform (MCWP) is a power-driven work scaffolding surface that climbs a vertical tower mast, allowing both work at height and the carrying of larger loads to higher elevations compared with traditional scaffolds. MCWPs are often used by masonry workers because they increase efficiency, save time, and are considered safer than traditional scaffolding. They potentially reduce the risk of musculoskeletal injuries to workers, because the platforms can be adjusted to an optimal height. The 22,000 MCWPs functioning in the United States are used by nearly 50,000 workers. When installed and used correctly, mast climbers are considered to be as safe as other scaffolds.

When they fail, however, deaths and serious injuries may occur, but the actual rate is not well documented.

Up to 80% of the MCWPs are anchored or tied to an adjacent structure. Even though they are considered to be safer than conventional scaffolding, from 2005 to 2007, MCWPs were involved in an average of three serious incidents, and multiple fatalities occurred each year. OSHA has documented 18 deaths and numerous serious injuries on MCWPs from 1990 to 2010 (CPWR, 2012). In addition, incidents involving near-misses, nonfatal injuries, and multiple fatalities have been recorded and investigated over the past decade. The greater loads that are possible on MCWPs can expose masons to falls and trips and increase the potential for collapse and falls. This risk is related to moving and carrying loads on unstable, confined platforms and the need to work using unbalanced postures.

CPWR established a diverse work group to examine problems associated with MCWPs and to discuss solutions to improve safety. The work group developed recommendations that have been directed to regulators and to persons or entities responsible for specifying and contracting construction work for mast climbers. A CPWR "white paper" indicated concern over the risk of fatalities (CPWR, 2010).

27.4 Fall Solutions Aimed at Prevention

27.4.1 Hierarchy of Controls

The traditional hierarchy of controls is widely used to eliminate or minimize occupational health hazards. The hierarchy includes, in preferential order, the use of (1) substitution or elimination, (2) engineering controls (such as local exhaust ventilation and process enclosure), (3) administrative controls (such as exposure limitations, training, and work practices), and (4) personal protective equipment (PPE) (such as respiratory protection and gloves).

To prevent falls in construction, a similar hierarchy should be followed. This hierarchy involves five levels, beginning with eliminating the risk by avoiding work at height where possible (Weisgerber and Wright, 1999). The five levels of the hierarchy of fall protection are outlined in Table 27.2.

27.4.2 Fall Protection Measures

In general, three types of conventional fall protection equipment are widely used in construction: guardrails, safety nets, and personal fall arrest systems (typically used as part of a comprehensive fall protection plan).

TABLE 27.2

The Five Levels of Hierarchy for Fall Protection in Construction

Level	Measure
1	Work on the ground or on a solid construction
2	Use a passive fall protection device (such as guardrails)
3	Use a work positioning system (such as fall restraints)
4	Use a fall injury prevention system (such as safety nets)
5	Work from ladders or implement administrative controls

Source: Adapted from Weisgerber, F. and Wright, M., *Elements of a Fall Safety through Design Program: Implementation of Safety and Health on Construction Sites*, Balkema, Rotterdam, 1999.

27.4.2.1 Personal Fall Arrest and Restraint Systems

Personal fall arrest systems (PFAs) are designed to protect a worker in the event of a fall (Figure 27.5), and fall restraint systems are designed to prevent a fall (Figure 27.6). PFAs consist of an anchor, connectors, a deceleration device, and a body harness. These systems stop a fall (OSHA, 1998) by preventing the worker from contacting a surface below through deceleration. PFAs must be inspected for wear damage and deterioration before each use.

Fall protection harnesses (Figure 27.7) are an integral part of PFAs; however, for many years, little was known about how well they fit workers. Early harnesses were designed based on parachute harnesses for men in the military rather than the more diverse construction populations, including women. At times, suspension trauma injuries after a fall have been attributed to poor harness fit. Hsiao et al. (2003) evaluated the fit of body harnesses for approximately 100 male and female construction workers. Their body sizes and shapes were measured with a laser scanner while they were suspended (with a harness) and standing (with and without a harness). Analysis determined that the current sizing selection scheme by height and weight was acceptable. However, redesign of harness components was needed for approximately 40% of those evaluated while standing or suspended. Fifteen body models for standard harnesses were identified.

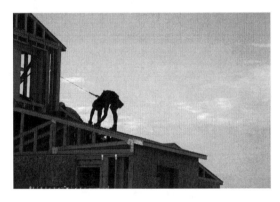

FIGURE 27.5
Roofer using a fall arrest system.

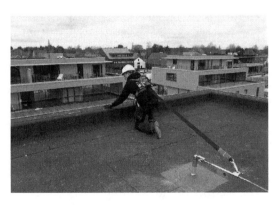

FIGURE 27.6
Worker using a fall restraint system.

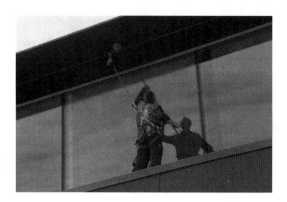

FIGURE 27.7
Worker wearing a body harness and fall arrest system.

Hsiao et al. (2007, 2009) evaluated harness sizing schemes and anthropometric data for workers. Three-dimensional torso scans and human–harness interfaces were evaluated for over 200 men and women. A model was developed and tested to classify over 96% of participants for best-fitting sizes. The authors recommended two sizes for women and three sizes for men over the current unisex system. The study suggested that thigh-strap angle and back D-ring locations could be used with static-fit testing to improve and reduce the risk of injury during a fall.

Fall protection for high steel and commercial construction is challenging, and workers are often forced to anchor at their feet. PFAs are designed to stop workers from free-fall. However, even after the PFA engages, the worker may continue to fall and could strike an object. The distance a worker falls includes the free-fall distance, the lifeline stretch from the force of the fall, and (if the worker uses a PFA or deceleration energy-absorbing device) the distance involved in absorbing shock. In its regulation (OSHA, 1998), OSHA limits free falls to 6 ft or less, and lifeline stretch and deceleration distance cannot exceed 3.5 ft. Therefore, a worker wearing a PFA system could fall up to 9.5 ft before stopping. Longer free-fall distances increase the chance of swing falls. Swing falls are especially hazardous, because the worker can hit an object or a lower level during the pendulum motion.

Fall restraint systems prevent workers from going over the unprotected edge of a walking or working surface by restricting movement (OSHA, 1998). They differ from PFA systems in that they consist of a body harness or belt attached to a tether, which is then attached to one or multiple anchor points (they do not include a deceleration device). Although these systems are not addressed by the OSHA Fall Protection Standards, some states require them. Guardrails are also a type of fall restraint system.

27.4.2.2 Guardrails and Slide Guards

Guardrails (Figure 27.8) are barriers to prevent employees from falling to lower levels (OSHA, 1998). They should be used when work is expected to take place at elevations of 6 ft (1.8 m) or higher. OSHA requires that guardrails be constructed from 2×4 in. lumber ranging from 39 to 45 in above the working surface. They are often mounted on the roof as joists or attached to the wall or roof of the building.

Slide guards consist of 2×6 in. or 2×8 in. pieces of lumber supported at the ends by metal brackets or lumber. They are intended to prevent workers from sliding down a roof

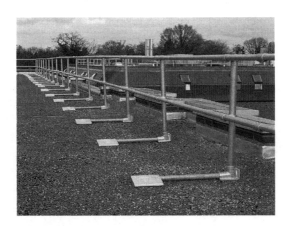

FIGURE 27.8
Guardrail system near the edge of a roof.

if they lose their balance. Slide guards were the primary means of fall protection in residential construction when the Interim Fall Protection Standards were in effect from 1996 to 2012. In 2012, OSHA rescinded the Interim Standards and required Subpart M, 29 CFR 1926 Section 500, which states that slide guards provide a minimum level of protection for certain roofing applications, but they primarily provide a means of precaution for specific limiting criteria. Therefore, slide guards may now be used with other fall protection techniques but cannot be used alone. More research is needed on their effectiveness.

27.4.2.3 Safety Nets

Safety net systems are placed under the work surface to prevent employees from contacting a lower level during a fall. OSHA regulates safety net systems to ensure safe and accurate performance of the net. When workers are at high elevations, the systems should be installed no more than 30 ft below the working surface and should have sufficient clearance to avoid contact with lower-level surfaces. Mesh sizes are limited to 6 by 6 in, and nets should be properly secured to prevent enlargement of mesh openings during a fall (OSHA, 1998).

27.5 Other Interventions

27.5.1 Training and Experience

In construction, falls from heights are more common among inexperienced workers. Studies have shown that well-developed safety training programs can be effective administrative controls to prevent falls (Kaskutas et al., 2009, 2010). In the US residential construction industry, employers often lack the specific safety knowledge to conduct adequate fall protection training. This problem can be more acute for small businesses, which often lack the significant resources and expertise of larger companies, and often results in higher injury rates (McVittie et al., 1997). Common sources for fall protection training include OSHA, insurers, unions, on-site mentors, and construction vendors.

Fall safety in the residential construction industry lags well behind that in the commercial and industrial sectors. Kaskutas et al. (2010) evaluated gaps in residential fall prevention training for apprentice carpenters. Trainers and researchers worked collaboratively to revise training and to fill the gaps. Evaluation and feedback from apprentices were used to improve the curriculum. Most apprentices worked at heights prior to training but did not commonly use fall protection. The revised training addressed safe ladder habits, truss setting, scaffold use, guarding floor openings, and using PFAs. New apprentices were targeted to ensure that training occurred before they began working. Hands-on experiences were emphasized in the training by using a fabricated residential construction site to practice fall protection. The revised curriculum was delivered consistently, and apprentice feedback was favorable. Needs assessment results were used to make further revisions, and researchers worked closely with the instructors to tailor the learning experiences. The researchers found that all these changes and adaptations made for positive results. Improving the quality of training and education in construction is important, and more work is needed to assess the impact of training efforts.

The analysis by Kaskutas et al. revealed two problems with formal safety training programs: (1) instructors are not always knowledgeable about application principles; and (2) safety training taught in class may be different from what is practiced on-site. According to study participants, these problems made them feel disengaged from safety training.

Fall prevention programs and equipment are necessary but are less effective without adequate training. Many Hispanic construction workers lack English proficiency (CPWR, 2008), which could impact their understanding of proper working procedures. Lipscomb et al. (2008) studied residential fall prevention through a series of focus groups with union apprentice carpenters at various levels of training. Their findings indicate that apprentices often do not apply safety principles they are taught to their work, a circumstance which illustrates how training alone can fall short. The findings also demonstrate the importance of measuring more than just knowledge when evaluating training effectiveness.

27.5.2 Prevention through Design

Prevention through design (PtD) is the concept of reducing occupational hazards by designing them out. PtD builds on the existing, traditional hierarchy of controls and moves it to a place earlier in the process. PtD is a viable intervention to improve worker safety that has gained momentum globally (Gambatese et al., 2005), but it has been slow to take root in the United States. In US construction, many barriers detract from its wider use, and design professionals have not embraced it as standard practice.

Many safety professionals feel that hazards are inadvertently "designed into" construction projects but could be eliminated with more focused PtD efforts. In fact, studies have shown a link between the PtD concept and a reduction in construction fatalities. Approximately 230 fatalities in NIOSH FACE reports were reviewed to determine whether they could be linked to the lack of PtD. The results showed that 42% of the fatalities could have been prevented if PtD had been used (Behm, 2005). For example, installing parapet walls or permanent guardrails on roofs can effectively prevent falls (NIOSH, 2014a).

The most important design issue identified was lack of embedded safety features. Behm, however, offered existing or new designs that could have prevented the fatalities. Embedded safety features on roof perimeters to aid in fall protection (NIOSH, 2014b) can include concrete straps, anchor points for use with appropriate PFA systems and lifelines, and guardrail supports. Another example is the use of prefabricated structures that are subsequently lifted into place rather than constructed at elevation. Design professionals (i.e., architects and design engineers) are in decision-making positions and influence construction safety. It is easier to reduce hazards when safety is considered earlier in the project life cycle. This concept is in contrast to the common methods of planning for construction site safety, which occurs shortly before construction begins, when the ability to positively influence safety is limited.

Unfortunately, in the United States, there are few motivating forces (legal, economic, or regulatory) to encourage designers to adopt PtD. In traditional construction procurement, legal precedent precludes a designer from considering construction safety during the design process. Many design decisions are driven by the client's needs alone and a desire to reduce costs. The latter is based on a fallacious notion that increasing the safety of the workers will drive up construction costs. Construction contracts and the regulatory requirements of OSHA place the responsibility of worker safety on the construction firm or employer. For this reason, architects and design engineers often do not consider hazards during the design phase. In addition, they may be concerned about being responsible for future safety incidents, although it is unlikely that considering safety would put them at increased risk of legal liability. The lack of consideration of hazard prevention in the design phase also could relate to the common lack of training in construction safety and health early in their design and engineering education and careers. More research is needed in this area, but it is fairly clear that broader adoption and implementation of PtD principles could significantly reduce the risk of falls in construction.

27.5.2.1 Building Information Modeling (BIM)

There is significant interest in improving worker safety through safer design and the use of building information modeling (BIM) (Chi et al., 2012). BIM allows constructors to visually assess jobsite conditions and recognize hazards by using a virtual three-dimensional computer model during the design and engineering phases of construction (Azhar et al., 2012). BIM can allow the user to link construction management to safety-related activities. The use of BIM technologies can improve occupational safety by linking the safety issues more closely to construction planning; providing better site layout and safety plans; providing methods for managing and visualizing up-to-date plans and site status; and supporting safety communication, such as informing site staff about safety arrangements in response to a particular risk or warning. The use of BIM also encourages partners to conduct risk assessment and planning (Sulankivi et al., 2012).

Rajendran and Clarke (2011) outlined areas in which safety and health professionals can use BIM technologies: (1) designing for safety; (2) safety planning (job hazard analysis and pre-task planning); (3) worker safety training; (4) accident investigation; and (5) facility and maintenance phase safety. For these tasks, safety and health professionals can use three-dimensional renderings generated from the BIM models and walk-through animations. In addition, four-dimensional phasing simulations focused on the safety procedures can be generated to show how temporary safety elements and areas of concern transition during a project. A by-product of integrating safety with BIM is safety-related training videos, which help workers understand project conditions in a format that crosses language barriers (Azhar et al., 2012).

27.5.3 National Fall Prevention Campaign

A national campaign to prevent falls in construction began in April 2012 (NIOSH, 2013a). The campaign focuses on reducing the number and severity of falls from ladders, scaffolds,

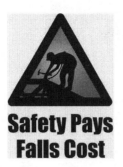

FIGURE 27.9
Image used for the National Falls Prevention Campaign.

and roofs. The motto of the campaign is "Safety Pays, Falls Cost" (Figure 27.9). The campaign is co-sponsored by OSHA, NIOSH, and CPWR. The idea for the campaign originated from discussions among multiple stakeholders through the National Occupational Research Agenda (NORA) Construction Sector program, which is managed by NIOSH. Those stakeholders included internal NIOSH researchers and external organizations, such as universities, large and small businesses, worker organizations, professional societies, and other government agencies. The campaign is using a variety of strategies to reach the construction industry through the three-part message *Plan, Provide, and Train*: plan ahead to get the job done safely; provide the right equipment for workers; and train everyone to use the equipment safely.

Materials and resources are available on the campaign websites www.stopconstructionfalls.com, hosted by CPWR; http://www.osha.gov/stopfalls/; and http://www.cdc.gov/niosh/construction/stopfalls.html.

The first few years of the national campaign have been a success. Over 1 million people have been touched by it, and the research supporting the campaign received the prestigious 2012 Thoth Award from the Public Relations Society of America. An evaluation of the early months of the campaign indicated that information was not reaching small construction contractors, the primary target audience. Since then, reaching them has been a key focus. In 2013, the target of the campaign was expanded to preventing falls in all types of construction. Over 7000 construction employers and over two million construction employees have participated in some form of the campaign. Dozens of participants remain committed to this endeavor, and continued success is expected in the future.

The broad array of almost 70 campaign partners reflects the firm commitment of government, industry, labor, trade groups, and professional stakeholder organizations to end falls from heights, and so far the results are promising. The campaign is based on solid research analysis, organized by NIOSH and conducted by the NORA Construction Sector Council.

27.6 Discussion and Conclusions

Unlike others, the construction industry is difficult to study because of its complexity and the diversity of job tasks and employers, the prevalence of small companies, and variations in workforce skills, weather conditions, and work environments. Many construction projects are characterized by temporary and transitory work. A typical construction workplace changes daily, and the type of work varies greatly, from new construction, repairs or renovations, and demolition to cleanup and reconstruction. One of the challenges inherent in construction is that the restructuring of work practices cannot be accomplished in individual workplaces or with individual workers. Turnover of workers is relatively high. Construction workers are employed by many contractors during their lifetimes, and industrywide changes are needed. Because the industry is so complex, this challenge will not be accomplished easily.

Why workers are injured and how physical hazards and behavior play a role are not well understood, partly because accident reporting details are not completely clear. Relatively simple hazard controls may prevent some injuries, however. Examples of such measures include perimeter protection for roofs and floor edges, correct ladder placement and anchorage, guarding of floor openings, housekeeping, inspection and maintenance of ladders, and proper scaffold erection.

Novice workers and those working for small companies are at greatest risk of fatal falls. Reasons for the greater risk in small companies may relate to a lack of resources for safety programs and personnel, owners' lack of knowledge of safety principles, the possibility that such companies are less likely to be inspected by government agencies, and their performance of inherently riskier work. As expected in a male-dominated industry, most victims are male. Older workers are represented disproportionately among fatalities, and declining physical and sensory capabilities likely play a role (Dong et al., 2012). Prevention measures are available to mitigate many of the falls. Although these are relatively simple, significant commercial and cultural barriers must be addressed to achieve broad acceptance and adoption of the measures.

The relationship of any particular variable with falls in many studies does not necessarily mean that its impact is great. However, it is helpful to summarize the major factors that minimize the risk of falls: dry, stable working surfaces; safety training with proper supervision and guidance; fall arrest systems and other PPE; a safety culture and climate; and worksite ergonomics. Other circumstances can have a negative effect on safety: poor weather, industry, and psychological issues; fatigue; and individual, organizational, and cultural factors.

Performing multidisciplinary research and addressing pertinent practices—involving engineering and design, education and training, behavioral and visual performance, and administrative issues—will offer the best chance of achieving meaningful, sustained results. Future fall prevention research should consider the main effects and interactions of the environmental, task-related, and personal factors that affect workers' balance. Improvements in the work environment, construction materials and methods, and work procedures and practices may improve safety and reduce falls (Hsiao and Simeonov, 2001; Hsiao et al., 2008).

Finally, the frequency of deaths and injuries related to roofs, scaffolds, and ladders should mandate dedicated efforts to develop intervention programs and evaluate their effectiveness. For example, incentive systems, work organization, and other managerial and organizational issues related to falls have not received significant attention and could be opportunities for study. Few studies have evaluated fall intervention programs in the real world. Although feasibility and study design require researchers to simplify this complex picture, the research should provide a holistic picture to evaluate interventions. A dynamic model for fall prevention is needed to provide feedback for construction stakeholders to aid in safety planning and fall prevention.

References

Azhar, S., Khalfan, N., Maqsood, T. (2012). Building information modeling: Now and beyond. *Australasian Journal of Construction Economics and Building, 12*(4), 15–28.

Behm, M. (2005). Linking construction fatalities to the design for construction safety concept. *Journal of Safety Research, 43*, 589–611.

Bjornstig, U., Johnnson, J. (1992). Ladder injuries: Mechanisms, injuries, and consequences. *Journal of Safety Research, 23*, 9–18.

BLS (2013). Bureau of Labor Statistics. 2003–2012 Census of Fatal Occupational Injuries. Retrieved from http://www.bls.gov/iif/.

Bobick, T.G., Bell, C.A., Stanevich, R.L., Smith, D.L., Stout, N.A. (1990). Analysis of selected scaffold-related fatal falls, in *Proceedings of the Human Factors Society 34th Annual Meeting.* Orlando, FL. October 8–12.

Bobick, T.G., McKenzie, E.A. (2011). Construction guardrails: Development of a multifunctional system. *Professional Safety, 56*(1), 48–54.

Bobick, T.G., McKenzie, E.A., Kau, T.-Y. (2010). Evaluation of guardrail systems for preventing falls through roof and floor holes. *Journal of Safety Research, 41*(3), 203–211.

Bukowski, T.J. (2014). Communication tower safety. *Safety and Health, 189*(6), 51–53.

Burkart, M.J., McCann, M., Paine, D.M. (2004). *Aerial Work Platforms: Elevated Work Platforms and Scaffolding.* New York: McGraw-Hill, 239.

Chau, N., Gauchard, G.C., Siegfried, C., Benamghar, L., Dangelzer, J.-L., Français, M., Jacquin, R., Sourdot, A., Perrin, P.P., Mur, J.-M. (2004). Relationships of job, age, and life conditions with the causes and severity of occupational injuries in construction workers. *International Archives of Occupational and Environmental Health, 77*(1), 60–66.

Chi, C.-F., Chang, T.-C., Ting, H.-I. (2005). Accident patterns and prevention measures for fatal occupational falls in the construction industry. *Applied Ergonomics, 36*(4), 391–400.

Chi, S., Hampson, K., Biggs, H. (2012). Using BIM for smarter and safer scaffolding and formwork construction: A preliminary methodology, in *Proceedings of 2012 CO CIB W099 International Conference on Modeling and Building Safety*, Singapore.

Choi, S. (2007). Opportunities for improving productivity in roofing construction. *International Journal of Construction Education and Research, 3*(1), 67–77.

CPWR (2008). *The Construction Chart Book* (4th ed.). CPWR—The Center for Construction Research and Training. Silver Spring, MD.

CPWR (2010). *Reaching higher: Recommendations for the safe use of mast climbing work platforms.* CPWR—The Center for Construction Research and Training.

CPWR (2012). *CPWR Impact: Reaching higher for the safe use of mast climbing work platforms.* CPWR—The Center for Construction Research and Training.

CPWR (2013). *Safety culture and climate in construction: Bridging the gap between research and practice.* CPWR—The Center for Construction Research and Training.

Cutlip, R., Hsiao, H., Garcia, R., Becker, E., Mayeux, B. (2002). Optimal hand locations for safe scaffold end-frame disassembly. *Applied Ergonomics, 33*(4), 349–355.

Dennerlein, J.T., Ronk, C.J., Perry, M.J. (2009). Portable ladder assessment tool development and validation: Quantifying best practices in the field. *Safety Science, 47*(5), 636–639.

Dong, X.S. (2010). Trends in fatal falls in construction, 1992–2008, in *The Construction Research Center (CPWR) Presentation*, Silver Spring, MD.

Dong, X.S., Choi, S.D., Borchardt, J.G., Wang, X., Largay, J.A. (2013). Fatal falls from roofs among U.S. construction workers. *Journal of Safety Research, 44*, 17–24.

Dong, X.S., Fujimoto, A., Ringen, K., Men, Y. (2009). Fatal falls among Hispanic construction workers. *Accident Analysis and Prevention, 41*(5), 1047–1052.

Dong, X.S., Largay, J.A., Wang, X. (2014). New trends in fatalities among construction workers. *CPWR Data Brief, 3*(2).

Dong, X.S., Wang, X., Daw, C. (2012). Fatal falls among older construction workers. *Human Factors: The Journal of the Human Factors and Ergonomics Society, 54*(3), 303–315.

Fong, D.T.-P., Hong, Y., Li, J.X. (2005). Lower-extremity gait kinematics on slippery surfaces in construction worksites. *Medicine and Science in Sports and Exercise, 37*(3), 447–454.

Fredericks, T.K., Abudayyeh, O., Choi, S.D., Wiersma, M., Charles, M. (2005). Occupational Injuries and fatalities in the roofing contracting industry. *Journal of Construction Engineering and Management, 131,* 1233–1240.

Gambatese, J., Behm, M., Hinze, J. (2005). Viability of designing for construction worker safety. *Journal of Construction Engineering and Management, ASCE 131*(9), 1029–1036.

Halperin, K.M., McCann, M. (2004). An evaluation of scaffold safety at construction sites. *Journal of Safety Research, 35*(2), 141–150.

Hanson, J.P., Redfern, M.S., Mazumdar, M. (1999). Predicting slips and falls considering required and available friction. *Ergonomics, 42*(12), 1619–1633.

Harris, J.R., Powers, J.R., Pan, C., Boehler, B. (2010). Fall arrest characteristics of a scissor lift. *Journal of Safety Research, 41,* 213–220.

Hsiao, H., Bradtmiller, B., Whitestone, J. (2003). Sizing and fit of fall-protection harnesses. *Ergonomics, 46*(12), 1233–1258.

Hsiao, H., Friess, M., Bradtmiller, B., Rohlf, F.J. (2009). Development of sizing structure for fall arrest harness design. *Ergonomics, 52*(9), 1128–1143.

Hsiao, H., Simeonov, P. (2001). Preventing falls from roofs: A critical review. *Ergonomics, 44*(5), 537–561.

Hsiao, H., Simeonov, P., Pizatella, T., Stout, N., McDougall, V., Weeks, J. (2008). Extension-ladder safety: Solutions and knowledge gaps. *International Journal of Industrial Ergonomics, 39*(11–12), 959–965.

Hsiao, H., Whitestone, J., Kau, T.-Y. (2007). Evaluation of fall arrest harness sizing schemes. *Human Factors, 49,* 447–464.

Kaskutas, V., Dale, A.M., Lipscomb, H., Gaal, J., Fuchs, M., Evanoff, B. (2010). Changes in fall prevention training for apprentice carpenters based on a comprehensive needs assessment. *Journal of Safety Research, 41*(3), 221–227.

Kaskutas, V., Dale, A.M., Nolan, J., Patterson, D., Lipscomb, H.J., Evanoff, B. (2009). Fall hazard control observed on residential construction sites. *American Journal of Industrial Medicine, 52*(6), 491–499.

Lipscomb, H.J., Dale, A.M., Kaskutas, V., Sherman-Voellinger, R., Evanoff, B. (2008). Challenges in residential fall prevention: Insight from apprentice carpenters. *American Journal of Industrial Medicine, 51*(1), 60–68.

McCann, M. (2003). Deaths in construction related to personnel lifts, 1992–1999. *Journal of Safety Research, 34,* 507–514.

McVittie, D., Banikin, H., Brocklebank, W. (1997). The effects of firm size on injury frequency in construction. *Safety Science, 27*(1), 19–23.

NIOSH (1991). *National Institute for Occupational Safety and Health (NIOSH) alert: Request for assistance in preventing electrocutions during work with scaffolds near overhead power lines.* Cincinnati, OH: US DHHS, (NIOSH) Publication no. 91-110. 1991.

NIOSH (2001). *National Institute for Occupational Safety and Health (NIOSH) alert: Preventing injuries and deaths from falls during construction and maintenance of telecommunication towers.* Cincinnati, OH: US DHHS, (NIOSH) Publication No. 2001-156.

NIOSH (2004). *National Institute for Occupational Safety and Health (NIOSH) alert: Preventing falls of workers through skylights and roof and floor openings.* Cincinnati, OH: US DHHS, (NIOSH) Publication No. 2004-156.

NIOSH (2013a). *National Institute for Occupational Safety and Health (NIOSH) Campaign to Prevent Falls in Construction* (http://www.cdc.gov/niosh/construction/stopfalls.html).

NIOSH (2013b). *National Institute for Occupational Safety and Health (NIOSH) Fatality Assessment and Control Evaluation Program* (http://www.cdc.gov/niosh/face/).

NIOSH (2014a). *National Institute for Occupational Safety and Health (NIOSH) Workplace Design Solutions: Preventing falls through the design of roof parapets.* Publication No. 2014-108.

NIOSH (2014b). *National Institute for Occupational Safety and Health (NIOSH) Workplace Design Solutions: Preventing falls from heights through the design of embedded safety features.* Publication No. 2014-124.

OSHA (1979). *Occupational fatalities related to scaffolds as found in reports of OSHA fatality/catastrophe investigations.* Washington, DC: US Department of Labor, Occupational Safety and Health Administration, Office of Statistical Studies and Analysis.

OSHA (1998). *Fall protection in construction.* (OSHA 3146.) Washington, DC: US Department of Labor, Occupational Safety and Health Administration.

OSHA (2012). *OSHA guidance document: Fall protection in residential construction.* Washington, DC: US Department of Labor, Occupational Safety and Health Administration. Retrieved from http://www.osha.gov/doc/guidance.pdf.

OSHA (2013). *OSHA Factsheet: Reducing falls in construction - safe use of extension ladders.* (OSHA 3146.) Washington, DC: US Department of Labor, Occupational Safety and Health Administration.

Pan, C.S., Hoskin, A., McCann, M., Lin, M.L., Fearn, K., Keane, P. (2007). Aerial lift fall injuries: A surveillance and evaluation approach for targeting prevention activities. *Journal of Safety Research, 38,* 617–625.

Pan, C.S., Powers, J.R., Hartsell, J.J., Harris, J.R., Wimer, B.M., Dong, R.G., Wu, J.Z. (2012). Assessment of fall-arrest systems for scissor lift operators: Computer modeling and manikin drop testing. *Human Factors, 54*(3), 358–372.

Rajendran, S., Clarke, B. (2011). Building Information Modeling: Safety benefits and opportunities. *Professional Safety, 2011,* 44–51.

Sa, J., Seo, D.-C., Choi, S.D. (2009). Comparison of risk factors for falls from height between commercial and residential roofers. *Journal of Safety Research, 40,* 1–6.

Simeonov, P., Hsiao, H., Dotson, B.W., Ammons, D.E. (2003). Control and perception of balance at elevated and sloped surfaces. *Human Factors, 45*(1), 136–147.

Simeonov, P., Hsiao, H., Kim, I., Powers, J.R., Kau, Y. (2012a). Factors affecting extension ladder angular positioning. *Human Factors, 54*(3), 334–345.

Simeonov, P., Hsiao, H., Powers, J., Ammons, D., Amendola, A., Kau, T.-Y., Cantis, D. (2008). Footwear effects on walking balance at elevation. *Ergonomics, 51*(12), 1885–1905.

Simeonov, P., Hsiao, H., Powers, J., Kim, I.J., Kau, T.Y., Weaver D. (2013). Research to improve extension ladder angular positioning. *Applied Ergonomics,* (44) 496–502.

Simeonov, P., Prahlad, H., Hsiao, H., Pelrine, R. (2010). Application of electro-adhesion technology for improving extension ladder stability. *International Conference on Fall Prevention and Protection.* Morgantown, WV.

Sokas, R.K., Jorgensen, E., Nickels, L., Gao, W., Gittleman, J.L. (2009). An intervention effectiveness study of hazard awareness training in the construction building trades. *Public Health Reports, 124*(Suppl. 1), 161–168.

Sulankivi, K., Teizer, J., Kiviniemi, M., Eastman, C.M., Zhang, S., Kim, K. (2012). Framework for integrating safety into Building Information Modelling. *Proceeding of the CIB W099 International Conference on "Modelling and Building Health and Safety,"* September 10–11, 2012. Singapore, 93–100.

Weisgerber, F., Wright, M. (1999). *Elements of a Fall Safety through Design Program: Implementation of Safety and Health on Construction Sites.* Rotterdam: Balkema, 867–874.

Whitaker, S.M., Graves, R.J., James, M., et al. (2003). Safety with access scaffolds: Development of a prototype decision aid based on accident analysis. *Journal of Safety Research, 34*(3), 249–261.

Wong, K.W.F., Chan, A.P.C, Yam, M.C.H., Wong, E.Y.S., Tse, K.T.C., Yip, K.K.C. (2005). *A Study of the Construction Safety in Hong Kong: Accidents Related to Fall of Person from Height.* Hong Kong: The Hong Kong Polytechnic University.

Yassin, A.S., Martonik, J.F. (2004). The effectiveness of the revised scaffold safety standard in the construction industry. *Safety Science, 42*(10), 921–931.

28

Taking a Human Factors Systems Approach to Slips, Trips, and Falls Risks in Care Environments

Sue Hignett, Laurie Wolf, and Ellen Taylor

CONTENTS

28.1 Introduction

As human factors/ergonomics (HFE) becomes more embedded in healthcare (National Quality Board, 2013), there is an opportunity to consider one of the more intransigent safety problems: slips, trips, and falls (STFs). This chapter will first, consider the risks for STF within (a) an HFE design model and (b) a new healthcare architecture risk assessment tool, and secondly, reflect on staff and patient engagement in quality improvement (Lean and Six Sigma) projects to reduce both the number of STFs and associated injuries.

We start by offering an inclusive definition for healthcare HFE by extending the International Ergonomics Association (IEA) definition (2000) to include concepts of clinical performance from Catchpole et al. (2010):

> Scientific discipline concerned with the understanding of interactions among humans [patients and staff] and other elements of a [healthcare] system [with the vision of enhancing human experience in a collaborative, inclusive partnership].
>
> HFE professionals apply theoretical principles, data and methods to design to optimize human well-being and overall system performance. [Approaches include the study of tasks, equipment, workspace, culture, teamwork and organization in clinical care and treatment settings].

This introduces theoretical models by describing the discipline of HFE in terms of systems and professional practice applications in terms of design.

28.2 Context

Donaldson et al. (2014) describe STFs in hospitals as "seemingly intractable" in a review of patient deaths due to unsafe care. STFs were the second most frequently occurring incident type (after failure to act on or recognize deterioration, and equal to healthcare-associated infection) but have not received the same national priority as infection, deep vein thrombosis, and pressure sore risks. The incident rate for STFs is approximately three times higher in hospitals and nursing homes than in community-dwelling older people (American Geriatrics Society, 2001). It has been suggested that this may be due to a combination of extrinsic risk factors (relating to the environment), for example, unfamiliar setting and wheeled furniture, combined with intrinsic risk factors (relating to the patient) such as confusion, acute illness, and balance-affecting medication (Tinetti, 2003; Salgado et al., 2004; Tinker, 1979; Kannus et al., 2006). These have been categorized in Figure 28.1 as assessment, communication, monitoring, modify patient, and modify environment (Hignett, 2010).

The main users of hospitals are older people, with people over 65 accounting for 62% of total bed days in hospitals in England and 68% of emergency bed days (Imison et al., 2012). In 2013, the National Institute for Clinical Excellence (NICE, 2013) summarized the research evidence on STFs in hospitals and recommended that all people admitted to hospital over the age of 65 years should automatically be considered to be at high risk of STF. This means that a detailed individual assessment is no longer required, and more time/resources can be focused on, for example, interventions with ward-specific STF run-charts, reducing environmental hazards, providing personal alarms, and communicating patient risk across multidisciplinary teams (Oliver et al., 2010; Donaldson et al., 2014).

In the United States, STFs with trauma in hospital are a "Never Event," with no reimbursement for associated costs (investigation, treatment, and additional duration of stay) so there is considerable motivation to reduce (eliminate) the total numbers of both STFs and injuries (National Quality Forum, 2007). This has resulted in STF interventions being prioritized and financially supported, with the outcome that STF rates are generally reported at lower rates in the United States (2.0–7.74 falls per 1000 patient bed days) and associated injuries at less than 0.5 per 1000 patient bed days (Wolf et al., 2013; Bouldin et al., 2013; Hempel et al., 2013) compared with the United Kingdom (2.1–9.0 per 1000 patient bed days; National Patient Safety Agency, 2010) with variations due to reporting mechanisms, clinical specialty, and acuity. However despite numerous best-practice interventions, STFs remain one of the major patient safety and preventable harm issues.

28.3 HFE Design Model for STF: DIAL-F

The Systems Engineering Initiative for Patient Safety (SEIPS) model has been widely used as an intervention framework in healthcare (Carayon et al., 2006, 2014). It describes the process of care and treatment as five components in an interdependent work system, in which the care provider (people factor) performs various tasks using tools and technology in a given environment within an established organization to achieve patient and hospital outcomes. We suggest that SEIPS 1.0 (Carayon et al., 2006) perpetuated the passive role of patients as care recipients in a minimum-risk environment, described by Miller and

Assessment

Communication

Staff education
Educate patient (and family) to ask for help
Educate patient (and family) on use of equipment e.g. nurse call, lighting, bed controls, bathroom facilities
Signs for staff, patients, families
Staff handover
Post fall huddles
Labels on patients (wristbands, socks)
Labels on patient notes

Monitoring

Move closer to nursing station/toilet
Assist patient with transfers at all times
Regular visits/rounding (hourly/2–4 hourly at night)
Shared accommodation (informal monitoring)
Patient sitters (family, volunteers)
CCTV cameras
Stay with patient during elimination (bathroom)
Alarms (bed, chair, sock)

Modify Patient

Medication (poly pharmacy)
Continence management (regular toileting, condom catheter)
Strength/balance (exercises, physical therapy)
Falls training (how to get up from the floor)
Walking aids
Impact protection (hip protectors, helmets)
Vision (review and treatment)
Podiatry/foot wear/anti-skid socks

Modify Environment

Bed height
Restraints (bed rails, enclosed bed, wrist/body)
Decrease impact (anti-slip mats, flooring, cushions)
Remove obstacles (de-clutter)
Clear (and marked) pathway between bed and toilet
Keep items (water, call bell, telephone) within reach
Commode next to bed
Grab rails in bedroom and bathroom
Toilet height
Maintain equipment/environment
Close doors to decrease noise
Lighting
Design of room/ward (inappropriate door openings, layout)

FIGURE 28.1
Interventions for inpatient falls. (From Hignett, S., *Healthcare Environments Research and Design Journal*, 3(4), 62–84, 2010.)

Gwynne (1972) as the "warehousing model of care" (passive), in contrast to a more stimulating, riskier (active) environment described as the "horticultural model of care." In 2013, Holden et al. introduced SEIPS 2.0 with modifications to more clearly articulate the role of the patient in the system as "patient work." This is very welcome but, we suggest, implies a compliant role whereby patients engage with the system and follow instructions to deliver their "work." For STF, where over 70% of incidents are unwitnessed (Healey et al., 2008), we suggest that a model relying on patient engagement in the system is less applicable. Many unwitnessed STFs will be associated with an independently initiated activity (e.g., feeding, grooming, bathing, dressing, bowel and bladder care, and toilet use) without calling or waiting for assistance (Hignett et al., 2014).

To address this theoretical gap, we have developed an HFE design model for STF to consider which interventions are likely to be the most sustainable and embedded within the care/treatment system. The DIAL-F model (Figure 28.2; Hignett et al., 2013; Hignett, 2013) describes system elements in terms of stability or transience (duration of action/involvement). The building design (layouts, decor, signage, lighting levels, etc.) is at the core as the least frequently changing element requiring a major project for either refurbishment or new build. Organizational policies and procedures (defining the organizational culture) of the hospital or care facility will probably be modified/updated on an annual basis. Technology is likely to change more frequently, either through the introduction of new equipment, furniture, and medical devices or by being moved between wards and departments.

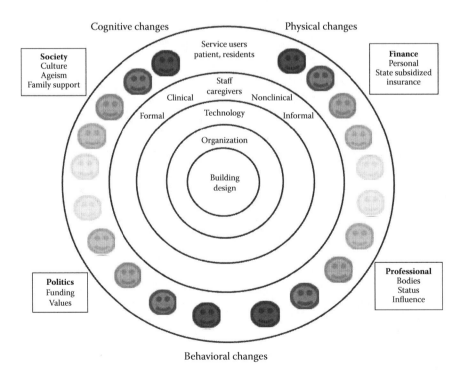

FIGURE 28.2
DIAL-F. (From Hignett, S., et al., *Proceedings of the International Symposium of Human Factors and Ergonomics in Healthcare*, 2(1), 99–104, 2013.)

The staff layer includes clinical, nonclinical (including contractors), formal, and informal (visitors, family) caregivers. Clinical staff may vary between shifts and areas in the organization in terms of their permanence, number on duty, knowledge, skills, and competencies. The patient is the most transient element of the system and is represented in the outer layer, in contrast to more usual person-centered HFE models (Bogner, 2005). The external factors (society, finance, politics, and professional bodies) impact throughout the system on patient expectations, staff terms and conditions, and organizational policies.

Patients are described as *personas*—fictitious representations used in design to describe groups of archetypal (rather than actual) people (Adlin and Pruitt, 2010). Personas have been used to describe patients with physical changes at five levels of functional mobility, ranging from "independent for activities of daily living with or without a mobility aid but susceptible to fatigue," through to "wheelchair users with some or no ability to stand and sit without support," and finally, to "fully dependent patients (bed bound) to describe terminal stages of care" (ArjoHuntleigh, 2012). However, these personas do not include cognitive or behavioral changes; a systematic review of risk factors for falls in dementia identified eight categories, including visual and functional impairments (Härlein et al., 2009), which could be used to develop a wider range of personas.

The DIAL-F model was used to discuss the results from an STF audit, which confirmed the role of the active patient, whereby significantly more patients needing mobility assistance than expected indicated that they would mobilize independently to the toilet. Building design and technology risks were identified, with only 24% of bedside areas having no obstacles/hazards (Hignett et al., 2014). The STF risks were found to vary with patient characteristics, with two distinct groups identified: patients needing mobility assistance (frail) and patients with cognitive changes (confused), with only a small overlapping population.

28.4 Safety Risk Assessment (SRA) Tool for Healthcare Architecture

The design process for healthcare architecture is notable for its ability to address complexity but traditionally follows a lengthy and complex process that balances scope, schedule, and budget, which often results in conflicting goals (silos) for service, care, and long-term efficiency. As the ramifications of healthcare facility design are felt for the next 30–50 years or more, the integration of research evidence is very important. Over the lifespan of the building (and sometimes the life cycle of a project), priorities will change, models of care will change, staff and patients will change, and technology will change. So, a building design requires systems thinking that addresses physical, cognitive, and organizational issues, and design teams must navigate from simple "functions" to a more complete understanding of the user actions that the building has to support (Attaianese and Duca, 2012). To promote a proactive process, there is a need to understand the integration of hazard and risk reduction; for example, many emergency events are not entirely unexpected and could be reasonably mitigated (Bosher et al., 2007). The built environment has the potential to be an enduring and viable approach to improving outcomes but requires new perspectives to encourage innovative design solutions (Steinke et al., 2010).

To address this gap, the Center for Health Design (CHD) is developing a proactive SRA tool based on the premise that the built environment is a critical component of the healthcare system (Taylor et al., 2014). The goal was to create safer healthcare environments by developing a toolkit to enable careful consideration of built environment factors that impact safety proactively, during the design and construction of healthcare facilities.

The first stage (the Delphi process; Gallagher et al., 1993) constructed evidence statements to link research evidence (Ulrich et al., 2008; Quan et al., 2011) with guidelines (Facility Guidelines Institute, 2014). These were developed, were tested, and achieved consensus for six safety issues: healthcare-associated infection, patient movement and handling, falls and immobility, medication safety, security, and behavioral health (Taylor et al., 2014; Figure 28.3).

Items were indexed and reviewed for setting (e.g., hospital, ambulatory care), hospital department (e.g., nursing unit, diagnostic and treatment), unit (e.g., emergency, medical/surgical, intensive care unit [ICU]), population (e.g., elderly, rehabilitation), built environment design category (e.g., building envelope, room layout) and a subset of conditions leading to the built environment hazard (e.g., acoustical environment, visibility). The consensus process used an online survey in which participants evaluated both inclusion and wording of a statement (Figure 28.4). Any unresolved statements (less than 70% agreement) were reviewed in a second consensus round, after which any residual unresolved statements were included in the nominal group technique (NGT; Gallagher et al., 1993) workshop.

For the falls and immobility group, 36 evidence statements were reviewed by 15 participants in the Delphi process (online) with 32 statements (as design questions) finally included at the NGT workshop by eight participants. The risks are mapped into six categories: environmental hazards (e.g., slippery floors), ergonomics (physical interactions, anthropometry), interior layout (family-friendly environment, proximity), light quality/levels and noise, and accessibility and visibility (Figure 28.5).

These design questions have been tested in three design projects and multiple hypothetical scenarios, and the final SRA toolkit is available from the Center for Health Design (http://www.healthdesign.org/). This provides an evidence-based resource in building design to both integrate and support the elements in the DIAL-F model.

28.5 Staff and Patient Engagement in STF Risk Management through Quality Improvement (QI) Projects

This section describes two projects on oncology wards using Lean and Six Sigma to introduce interventions by engaging patients and staff in the risk management process. The results will be discussed using the DIAL-F model to consider the sustainability of interventions using QI methods.

28.5.1 QI and HFE

Although Lean and Six Sigma methodologies began in other industrial sectors, they have been implemented in healthcare for over ten years. The most common uses of Lean and Six Sigma have involved throughput, length of stay, resource use, and patient safety (Graban and Prachand, 2010).

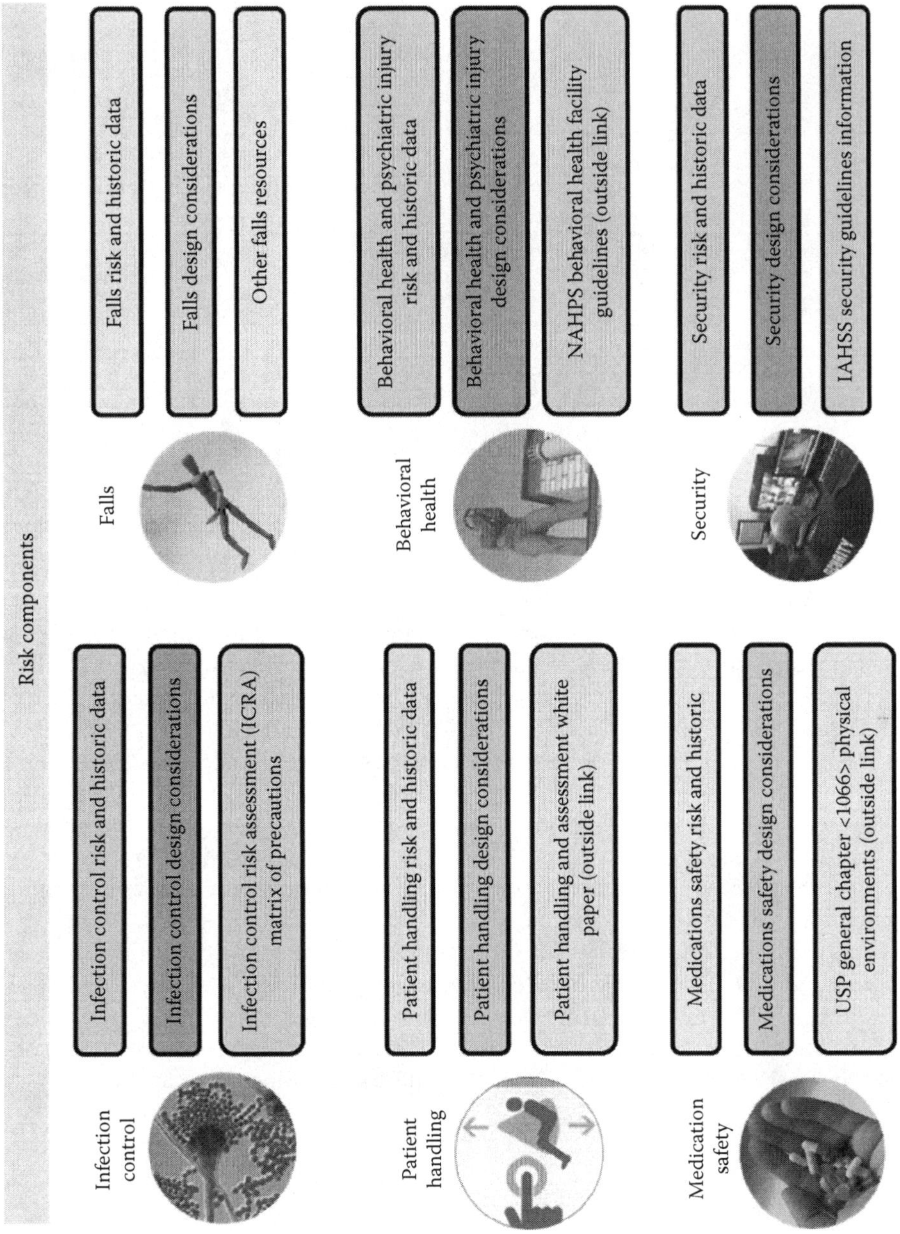

FIGURE 28.3
Safety risk assessment components. (Reproduced with permission of CHD.)

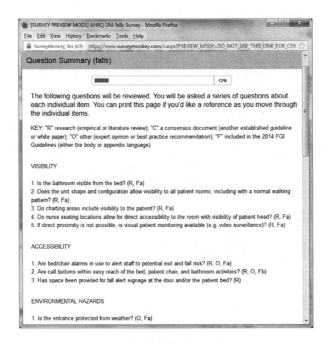

FIGURE 28.4
Delphi process.

Lean is a QI method that requires employee engagement to solve problems by eliminating waste. The fundamental concepts include focusing on the process, respecting every individual (employees, partners, suppliers), quality assurance at the source, continually seeking perfection, embracing scientific thinking (value stream analysis, problem-solving), transparency, standardizing tasks, and going to the source of work and observing all the tasks (Liker, 2004).

Six Sigma is a systematic, fact-based, data-driven, problem-solving QI process that aims to increase business performance by reducing defects (unexpected outcomes) and process variation (inconsistent methods and results) (Junewick, 2002). It is comprised of five phases (Define–Measure–Analyze–Improve–Control [DMAIC]) and focuses on strong leadership tools and an emphasis on bottom-line financial results (Benbow and Kubiak, 2005).

The definitions of HFE and QI overlap substantially with the design of work, workplace, and work environment leading to quality deficiencies, human error, and physical/cognitive harm (Eklund, 1997). Wolf (2013) compared Lean, Six Sigma, and HFE approaches using the dimensions of philosophy, focus, data-collection strategies, improvement tools, techniques for understanding tasks and workflow, data transparency, and analysis:

- Each approach has a unique philosophy (epistemology), but all share a common goal of improving the process for the user, with a safer, more efficient system.
- The focus for all three approaches is to develop a process that matches the needs of the human (supplier, customer, user/operator) who will use it or benefit from the output of the process.
- Six Sigma and HFE are more closely aligned than Lean to data-collection strategies. Lean projects typically collect data with a quick (hourly or daily) snapshot in time and may not include the impact of long-term issues.

1. Is the bathroom door clearly identifiable from the bed?
2. Does the unit layout allow staff to easily see the patient head in all rooms from work stations or a routine circulation pattern?
3. Does the design maximize the ability of staff to view patients?
4. If direct visibility is not possible, is additional patient monitoring available (e.g., video surveillance, alarms)?
5. Are all call button/systems accessible and usable?
6. Is there space for safety alert signage at the patient room entrance and/or the patient bed?
7. Is the entrance protected from weather?
8. Does the room layout provide clear and unobstructed paths of travel?
9. Is space provided on the opening side of the patient toilet room door to facilitate the use of equipment and/or assistive devices?
10. Are the use of unnecessary restraints minimized (including the use of bilateral full-length bed rails)?
11. Does furniture selection/specification support independent mobility?
12. Are there smooth transitions in walking surfaces or between flooring types to avoid surface irregularities leading to trips?
13. Does selection/specification of floor materials and pattering accurately convey the floor conditions (level floor vs. stair/threshold)?
14. Does the design (e.g., flooring, lighting, windows) minimize glare?
15. Is contrast designed to differentiate between the floors and walls and minimize transitions between colours and/or materials?
16. Are mats, rugs and carpeting secured to the floor?
17. Are floors slip-resistant in potential wet areas (e.g., bathrooms, entrances, kitchens) and on ramps and stairs?
18. Are grab bars and hand rails located to support patients while ambulating to the toilet?
19. Are grab bars located on either side of the toilet to support patients getting up and down toileting?
20. Are grab bars and hand rails in the bathroom mounted to support people of different heights?
21. Are lifts being used to assist staff in performing transfer of patients?
22. Have beds been selected to afford low height positions and brakes?
23. Has ergonomic design been considered in furniture selection?
24. Has toilet accessibility been considered (e.g., height)?
25. Are flooring and subflooring materials selected to mitigate injury in the event of a fall?
26. Is there space for families to be present in the patient room to encourage communication with caregivers about falls and increase the level of patient surveillance?
27. Has lighting been designed to eliminate abrupt changes in light levels?
28. Is low-level lighting available in night time/dark conditions?
29. In areas where lighting needs to be dimmed for treatment purposes, is there sufficient light to navigate safely?
30. Are call and communication systems designed to minimize public noise?
31. Is noise controlled through the design (e.g., material selection)?
32. Is the bathroom located in close proximity to the bed?

FIGURE 28.5
Preliminary included statements (design questions) for falls and immobility.

- There is evidence of transfer of improvement tools, with the greatest overlap between Lean and Six Sigma (value stream mapping, standard work, and voice of the customer).
- Techniques for understanding tasks and workflow are similar, but each has a different complexity level. For example, a Lean spaghetti diagram will simply illustrate where a worker travels along a floor plan by linking one location to the next, whereas in HFE, a task analysis can be very complex, with added meaning (weighting or importance) to each link.
- Lean typically uses very simple, visual process control charts which can easily be updated throughout the day to provide timely feedback. Six Sigma and HFE tend to use more complex quantitative and qualitative data analyses.

28.5.2 Lean

The first project used Lean techniques on three oncology wards (97 beds; 71 single rooms) with the aim of reducing patient STFs and associated injuries (Wolf et al., 2013). STFs in oncology wards were often found to involve patients who would not call for help (even when instructed to do so) and specific risk factors associated with medications (i.e., ben-zodiazepines, sedatives/hypnotics) and disease-associated pathologies that could cause altered elimination (frequent urination or diarrhea).

A systematic, data-driven process was used, starting with a 3 day Rapid Improvement Event (RIE). There was excellent leadership support from hospital and unit-level management, which allowed front-line nursing staff to attend the RIE as well as other members of the multidisciplinary team (physical and occupational therapy, pharmacy, physicians, information systems, low bed equipment vendor, and clinical operations). The hospital leadership performed a SIPOC (Supplier/Input/Process/Output/Customer) to select the roles to be represented in the RIE, and a key stakeholder assessment was conducted to identify potential areas of support and resistance.

The current state was documented in a process map with swim lanes for each ward using traditional Lean methods to resolve issues, such as fist-to-five, silent voting, affinity diagramming, and brainstorming round-robin techniques to ensure input from all participants, and was subsequently verified by direct observation. The initial gap analysis found that assessments for gait and mental status were not being carried out in a consistent manner, and that there were delays in implementing interventions (e.g., bed alarm or low bed). The future state map included

- STF risk assessment to be completed every shift (and when patient condition changed) including gait and mental status assessment using the Get-Up-and-Go test (GUG; Currie, 2008) and Short Portable Mental Status Questionnaire (SPMSQ; Pfeiffer, 1975)

- Implementation using an intervention algorithm (Figure 28.6) based on a linking evaluation and practice (LEAP) grid and the Johns Hopkins risk assessment methodology (Poe et al., 2007) to assist nursing staff in linking the risk assessment results to the selection of appropriate interventions

- Collection of incident data within 60 min following an STF (post-incident huddle) followed by a more detailed investigation by the advanced practice nurse (APN)

- Data transparency (post-incident) for all staff with a wall-mounted fall tracker board (FTB) to display data from the post-fall huddle and APN investigation

The algorithm was used, for example, with a patient having an "altered gait" (failed GUG test) with recommended interventions to use a low bed, floor mat, bedside commode, and gait belt and to request physical and occupational therapy. If the same patient also had altered elimination (frequent toileting), no additional interventions would be required. However, if this patient subsequently became confused (missed three or more questions on the SPMSQ), the algorithm would recommend bed and chair alarms as additional interventions.

The action lists (e.g., educational materials, standard work processes, training for approximately 150 nurses, and communication to the multidisciplinary team) from the RIE took approximately 4 weeks to prepare before "Go Live." Each action plan complied with the W-W-W methodology (WHAT action is needed—WHEN must it be completed—WHO is responsible).

Various problems and barriers were encountered during implementation, including training provision (resolved by using nurse champions), acceptance of SPMSQ (withdrawn and replaced with the existing mental status assessment questions), use of low beds and bed alarms (addressed by increasing availability and reducing delivery time), and documentation of gait and mental status data in the electronic medical record (EMR; added as free text).

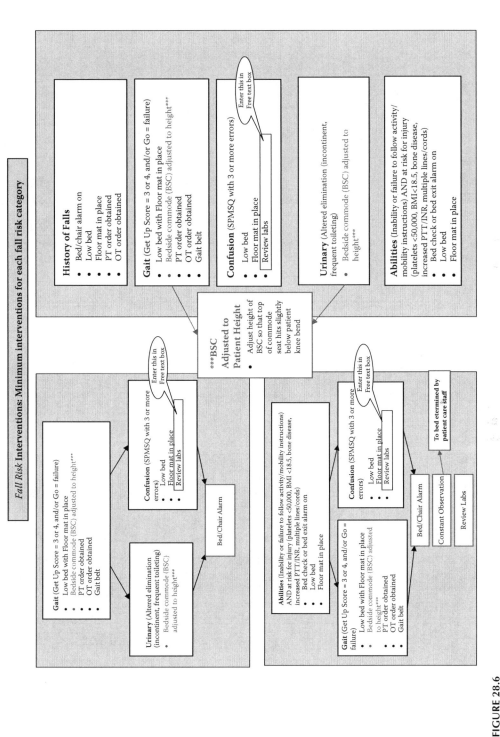

FIGURE 28.6
Algorithm for linking fall risk assessment to appropriate intervention.

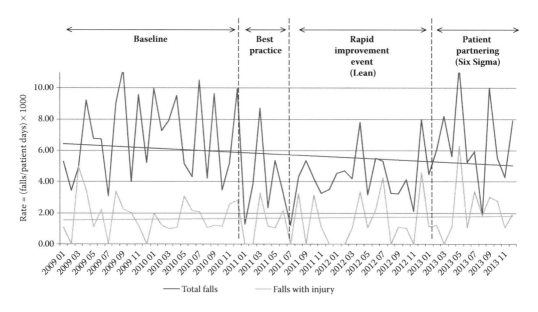

FIGURE 28.7
Rates of falls and falls with injury in oncology from 2009 to 2013. (Wolf, L., et al., *Proceedings of the HFES 2014 International Symposium on Human Factors and Ergonomics in Health Care*, Chicago, IL, 2014.)

Initially, the reported STFs decreased by 26%, and associated injuries decreased by 38%; however, the success was not sustained after 9 months (Figure 28.7). There were benefits through increased staff engagement with newsletters, practice updates, feedback to leadership, and improved data from the FTB and EMR, and based on this heightened engagement, one of the wards was selected to participate in a collaborative Six Sigma project with the Joint Commissions Center for Transforming Healthcare (DuPree et al., 2014).

28.5.3 Six Sigma

The second project used Six Sigma on one oncology ward over 12 months with a 1 year post-intervention period to investigate the root causes of enduring risk factors such as unassisted toileting and continuously changing patient conditions (Wolf et al., 2014). The intervention was conducted with 87 high–fall risk patients, of whom 6% ($n = 5$) experienced a fall.

The five phases in the DMAIC process were

1. *Define.* The issues were defined using the SIPOC and solution tree (affinity diagram) methods to collect the voice of the customer (equipment, environment, call lights, communication, staffing, staff education and awareness, patient assessment, patient education, and family education).
2. *Measure.* A cause–effect matrix was used to determine the most critical factors and represented on fishbone diagrams to determine root causes, which were then investigated in more detail.
3. *Analyze.* Additionally, five common issues were recorded and analyzed: call light response time; patient activity and behavior at the time of the STF; and medications given and changes in patient condition in the preceding 24 h. Failure mode effects analysis (FMEA; Ashley et al., 2010) was used to explore possible barriers

or failure routes using the impact matrix technique for likelihood and severity. These included no power to hold staff accountable; turnover (with 100% change in ward management during the project); lack of APN time (initially, the daily report preparation required 1 h, but this was reduced to 30 min with data from the EMR); and lack of nursing engagement.

4. *Improve.* The chosen intervention was "Patient Partnering," to encourage patients to call for help and participate in preventing their own STF risks. The APN reviewed all patients at risk and mentored nurses to partner with patients with the aim of empowering patients to seek assistance when moving about in the room, especially during toileting activities. This included a video and demonstrating and practicing the call bell with the patient (with follow-up review after 2 h).

5. *Control.* The intervention was disseminated through staff meetings and individual coaching. It was found that nurses would cooperate with the APN in patient partnering, but did not initiate the partnership themselves due to the perceived additional time requirement.

28.5.4 Did the QI Projects Sustain an Embedded Impact?

Although the 16 months after the RIE showed 33% improvement in total STF rate, 10 months after the completion of the Six Sigma project, the total STFs dropped to only 6% improvement over baseline (Figure 28.7); however, STFs with minor injuries increased after Project 2. The percentage of STFs with serious injury decreased from 10% in 2010 to 6% in 2011, and there were no STFs with serious injury in 2013.

It was concluded that a deeper understanding of patient and staff perceptions was needed to create more sustainable solutions.

28.6 Discussion

The use of QI approaches was very popular in the 2000s, with multimillion-dollar projects. In England, the Productive Ward initiative was based on Lean, with the aim of increasing "the proportion of time nurses spend on direct patient care, to improve experiences for staff and patients, and to make structural changes to the use of ward spaces to improve efficiency" (National Nursing Research Unit and NHS Institute for Innovation and Improvement, 2010, 2011). Pockets of success were reported, but despite positive bias in the evaluation, there were reports of difficulties in sustaining change (Wright and McSherry, 2013; National Nursing Research Unit and NHS Institute for Innovation and Improvement, 2011). This has also been identified as a problem for Six Sigma; for example, Christopher et al. (2014) highlighted the difficulty in maintaining "longevity of these strategies ... [and] a sustainable process to prevent falls" despite heightened staff awareness and engagement. For STF risk management, there is some evidence of short-term success with expensive (labor-intensive) solutions that increase staffing (Veluswamy and Price, 2010). However, as these QI programs matured, compliance waned, possibly due to a failure to achieve the culture shift required to achieve a sustained impact. So, a simultaneous drawback and benefit of using QI methods is that they require a culture change in every employee (Radnor et al., 2012), and healthcare workers, as an industrial sector, are susceptible to change fatigue (National

Nursing Research Unit and NHS Institute for Innovation and Improvement, 2010) due to the frequent shifts in initiatives (Ferlie and Shortnell, 2001).

These problems can be described in terms of the DIAL-F model, whereby initiatives focusing on the outer layers (patient partnering, staff training) have failed to impact on the more central organizational layer. Dy et al. (2011) compared STFs with other patient safety events using 11 dimensions (regulatory versus voluntary; setting; feasibility; individual activity versus organizational change; temporal (one-time vs. repeated/long-term); pervasive versus targeted; common versus rare events; maturity of patient safety practices; degree of controversy/conflicting evidence; degree of behavioral change required for implementation; and sensitivity to context). They describe STF initiatives as previously having been based on individual activity (patient assessment) rather than organizational change. However, the QI projects described in this chapter have attempted to impact on organizational (and safety) culture with limited success.

Dy et al. (2011) continue by describing the research for patient safety practices relating to STF risk management as conflicting and controversial, with a high need for behavioral change (described as *human factors*). We suggest that a more comprehensive interpretation and application of HFE is needed, based on the IEA (2000) definition to "apply theoretical principles, data and methods to design in order to optimise human well-being and overall system performance." The DIAL-F model seeks to achieve this by locating the more sustainable element (building) as the central component in the design of the system for STF risk management. We contend that if the design of the physical (micro) environment (core element) is intrinsically unsafe, then no amount of improvement interventions at staff (meso) or organizational (macro) levels will produce an embedded reduction in STF risks.

References

Adlin, T., Pruitt, J. (2010). *The Essential Persona Lifecycle*. San Francisco, CA: Morgan Kaufmann.

American Geriatrics Society (2001). Guideline for the prevention of falls in older persons. *Journal of the American Geriatrics Society*, 49(5), 664–672.

ArjoHuntleigh (2012). *Residents Mobility Gallery*. www.arjohuntleigh.com/Pageasp?PageNumber=2/ (Accessed April 9, 2013).

Ashley, L., Armitage, G., Neary, M., Hollingsworth, G. (2010). A practical guide to failure mode and effects analysis in health care: Making the most of the team and its meetings. *The Joint Commission Journal on Quality and Patient Safety*, 36(8), 351–358.

Attaianese, E., Duca, G. (2012). Human factors and ergonomic principles in building design for life and work activities: An applied methodology. *Theoretical Issues in Ergonomics Science*, 13(2), 187–202.

Benbow, D.W., Kubiak, T.M. (2005). *The Certified Six Sigma Black Belt Handbook*. Milwaukee, WI: ASQ Quality Press.

Bogner, M.S. (2005). There is more to error in healthcare than the care provider. *Proceedings of the Human Factors and Ergonomics Society Annual Meeting*, 49, 952–954.

Bosher, L., Carrillo, P., Dainty, A., Glass, J., Price, A. (2007). Realising a resilient and sustainable built environment: Towards a strategic agenda for the United Kingdom. *Disasters*, 31(3), 236–255.

Bouldin, E.L.D., Andresen, E.M., Dunton, N.E., Simon, M., Waters, T. M., Liu, M., Daniels, M.J., Mion, L., Shorr, R. (2013). Falls among adult patients hospitalized in the United States: Prevalence and trends. *Journal of Patient Safety*, 9(1), 13–17.

Carayon, P., Hundt, A.S., Karsh, B.T., Gurses, A. P., Alvarado, C.J., Smith, M., Flatley Brennan, P. (2006). Work system design for patient safety: The SEIPS model. *Quality and Safety in Health Care*, 15(Suppl. I), i50–i58.

Carayon, P., Wetterneck, T.B., Rivera-Rodriguez, A.J., Schoofs Hundt, A., Hoonakker, P., Holden, R., Gurses, A. (2014). Human factors systems approach to healthcare quality and patient safety. *Applied Ergonomics*, 45, 14–25.

Catchpole, K.R., Dale, T.J., Hirst, D.G., Smith, J.P., Giddings, T.A. (2010). A multi-center trial of aviation-style training for surgical teams. *Journal of Patient Safety*, 6(3), 180–186.

Christopher, D.A., Trotta, R.L., Strong, J., Dubendorf, P. (2014). Using process improvement methodology to address the complex issue of falls in the inpatient setting. *Journal of Nursing Care Quality*, 29(3), 204–214.

Currie, L. (2008). Fall and injury prevention. In R. Hughes (Ed.), *Patient Safety and Quality: An Evidence-Based Handbook for Nurses*. Rockville, MD: Agency for Healthcare Research and Quality, US Department of Health and Human Services.

Donaldson, L.J., Panesar, S.S., Darzi, A. (2014). Patient-safety-related hospital deaths in England: Thematic analysis of incidents reported to a national database, 2010–2012. *PLOS Medicine*, 11(6), e1001667.

DuPree, E., Fritz-Campiz, A., Musheno, D. (2014). A new approach to preventing falls with injuries. *Journal of Nursing Care Quality*, 29(2), 99–102.

Dy, S.M., Taylor, S.L., Carr, L.H., Foy, R., Pronovost, P.J., Øvretveit, J, Wachter, R.M., Rubenstein, L.V., Hempel, S., McDonald, K.M., Shekelle, P.G. (2011). A framework for classifying patient safety practices: Results from an expert consensus process. *BMJ Quality and Safety*, 20, 618–624.

Eklund, J. (1997). Ergonomics, quality and continuous improvement—conceptual and empirical relationships in an industrial context. *Ergonomics*, 40(10), 982–1001.

Facility Guidelines Institute (2014). *2014 FGI Guidelines for Design and Construction of Hospitals and Outpatient Facilities*. Dallas, TX: ASHE.

Ferlie, E.B., Shortell, S.M. (2001). Improving the quality of healthcare in the United Kingdom and the United States: A framework for change. *The Millbank Quarterly*, 29(2), 99–102.

Gallagher, M., Hares, T., Spencer, J., Bradshaw, C., Webb, I. (1993). The nominal group technique: A research tool for general practice? *Family Practice*, 10(1), 76–81.

Graban, M., Prachand, A. (2010). Hospitalists: Lean leaders for hospitals. *Journal of Hospital Medicine*, 5(6), 317–319.

Härlein, J., Dassen, T., Halfens, J.G., Heinze, C. (2009). Fall risk factors in older people with dementia or cognitive impairment: A systematic review. *Journal of Advanced Nursing*, 65(5), 922–933.

Healey, F., Scobie, S., Oliver, D., Pryce, A., Thomson, R., Glampson, B. (2008). Falls in English and Welsh hospitals: A national observational study based on retrospective analysis of 12 months of patient safety incident reports. *Quality and Safety in Health Care*, 17, 424–430.

Hempel, S., Newberry, S., Wang, Z., Booth, M., Shanman, R., Johnsen, B., Shier, V., Saliba, D., Spector, W.D., Ganz, D.A. (2013). Hospital fall prevention: A systematic review of implementation, components, adherence and effectiveness. *Journal of the American Geriatrics Society*, 61, 483–494.

Hignett, S. (2010). Technology and building design initiatives in interventions to reduce the incidence and injuries of elderly in-patient falls. *Healthcare Environments Research and Design Journal*, 3(4), 62–84.

Hignett, S. (2013). *Why Design Starts with People*. The Health Foundation: Patient Safety Resource Centre. http://patientsafety.health.org.uk/sites/default/files/resources/why_design_starts_with_people.pdf (Accessed June 10, 2013).

Hignett, S., Griffiths, P., Sands, G., Wolf, L., Costantinou, E. (2013). Patient falls: Focusing on human factors rather than clinical conditions. *Proceedings of the International Symposium of Human Factors and Ergonomics in Healthcare*, 2(1), 99–104.

Hignett, S., Youde, J., Reid, J. (2014). Using the DIAL-F systems model as the conceptual framework for an audit of in-patient falls risk management. *Proceedings of the HFES 2014 International Symposium on Human Factors and Ergonomics in Health Care*, 3(1), 112–116. Chicago.

Holden, R.J., Carayon, P., Gurses, A.P., Hoonakker, P., Schoofs Hundt, A., Ant Ozok, A., Joy Rivera-Rodriguez, A. (2013). SEIPS 2.0: A human factors framework for studying and improving the work of healthcare professionals and patients. *Ergonomics*, 56(11), 1669–1686.

IEA (2000). *International Ergonomics Association, Triennial Report*. Santa Monica, CA: IEA, 5.

Imison, C., Thompson, J., Poteliakhoff, E. (2012). *Older People and Emergency Bed Use: Exploring Variation*. London: The King's Fund. Available at www.kingsfund.org.uk/publications/older-people-and-emergency-bed-use (Accessed May 20, 2013).

Junewick, M.A. (2002). *LeanSpeak: The Productivity Business Improvement Dictionary*. Portland, OR: Productivity.

Kannus, P., Khan, K.M., Lord, S.R. (2006). Preventing falls among elderly people in the hospital environment. *Medical Journal of Australia*, 184(8), 372–373.

Liker, J.K. (2004). *The Toyota Way: 14 Management Principles from the World's Greatest Manufacturer*. New York: McGraw-Hill.

Miller, E.J., Gwynne, G.V. (1972). *A Life Apart: A Pilot Study of Residential Institutions of Physically Handicapped and the Young Chronic Sick*. London: Tavistock.

National Nursing Research Unit and NHS Institute for Innovation and Improvement (2010). *The Productive Ward: Releasing Time to Care. Learning & Impact Review*. Warwick: NHS Institute for Innovation and Improvement.

National Nursing Research Unit and NHS Institute for Innovation and Improvement (2011). *Improving Healthcare Quality at Scale and Pace Lessons from the Productive Ward: Releasing Time to Care Programme*. Warwick: NHS Institute for Innovation and Improvement.

National Patient Safety Agency (2010). *Slips Trips and Falls Data Update*. London: NPSA. www.nrls.npsa.nhs.uk (Accessed January 27, 2014).

National Quality Board (2013). *Human Factors in Healthcare*. http://www.england.nhs.uk/wp-content/uploads/2013/11/nqb-hum-fact-concord.pdf (Accessed April 9, 2014).

National Quality Forum (2007). *Serious Reportable Events in Healthcare 2006 Update. A Consensus Report*. Washington, DC: National Quality Forum.

NICE (2013). *Falls: Assessment and Prevention of Falls in Older People. Clinical Guidance 161*. National Institute for Health and Care Excellence. http://guidance.nice.org.uk/CG161 (Accessed October 25, 2013).

Oliver, D., Healey, F., Haines, T. (2010). Preventing falls and fall-related injuries in hospitals. *Clinics in Geriatric Medicine*, 26, 645–692.

Pfeiffer, E. (1975). A short portable mental status questionnaire for the assessment of organic brain deficit in elderly patients. *Journal of the American Geriatrics Society*, 23, 433–441.

Poe, S.S., Cvach, M., Dawson, P.B., Straus, H., Hill, E.E. (2007). The Johns Hopkins Fall Risk Assessment Tool: Post-implementation evaluation. *Journal of Nursing Care Quality*, 22(4), 293–298.

Quan, X., Jospeh, A., Malone, E., Pati, D. (2011). *Healthcare Environmental Terms and Outcome Measures: An Evidence-Based Design Glossary*. Concord, CA: Center for Health Design.

Radnor, Z., Holweg, M., Waring, J. (2012). Lean in healthcare: The unfilled promise? *Social Science and Medicine*, 74, 364–371.

Salgado, R.I., Lord, S.R., Ehrlich, F., Janji, N., Rahman, A. (2004). Predictors of falling in elderly hospital patients. *Archives of Gerontology and Geriatrics*, 38, 213–219.

Steinke, C., Webster, L., Fontaine, M. (2010). Evaluating building performance in healthcare facilities: An organizational perspective. *Healthcare Environments Research and Design Journal*, 3(2), 63–83.

Taylor, E., Joseph, A., Quan, X., Nanda, U. (2014). Designing a tool to support patient safety: Using research to inform a proactive approach to healthcare facility design. *Proceedings of the 3rd International Conference on Human Factors and Ergonomics in Healthcare/5th International Conference on Applied Human Factors and Ergonomics*. Krakow, Poland. July 21–25.

Tinetti, M. (2003). Clinical practice: Preventing falls in elderly persons. *New England Journal of Medicine*, 348(1), 42–49.

Tinker, G.M. (1979). Accidents in a geriatric department. *Age Ageing*, 8(3), 196–198.

Ulrich, R.S., Zimring, C., Zhu, X., DuBose, J., Seo, H.B., Choi, Y.S., Joseph, A. (2008). A review of the research literature on evidence-based healthcare design. *Healthcare Environments Research and Design Journal*, 1(3), 61–125.

Veluswamy, R., Price, R. (2010). I've fallen and I can't get up: Reducing the risk of patient falls. *Physician Executive*, 36(3), 50–53.

Wolf, L. (2013). *Implementing Quality Improvement and Human Factors Engineering Strategies in Healthcare: Risk Management of In-Patient Falls.* Unpublished internal report. Loughborough Design School, Loughborough University.

Wolf, L., Costantinou, E., Limbaugh, C., Rensing, K., Gabbart, P., Matt, P. (2013). Fall prevention for inpatient oncology using lean and rapid improvement event techniques. *Healthcare Environments Research and Design Journal*, 7(1), 85–101.

Wolf, L., Hignett, S., Costantinou, E. (2014). Ending the vicious cycle of patient falls. *Proceedings of the HFES 2014 International Symposium on Human Factors and Ergonomics in Health Care.* Chicago. March 9–11, 2014.

Wright, S., McSherry, W. (2013). A systematic literature review of Releasing Time to Care: The Productive Ward. *Journal of Clinical Nursing*, 22, 1361–1371.

29

Prevention of Slips, Trips, and Falls among Hospital Workers

James W. Collins, Jennifer L. Bell, and Christina Socias

CONTENTS

29.1 Fall Injuries in the Health Care and Social Assistance Industry Sector

Health Care and Social Assistance (HCSA), with over 18 million workers, is one of the largest industry sectors in the United States and is rapidly growing (Bureau of Labor Statistics, 2015). In 2013, HCSA workers, who include workers in hospitals and other patient care settings, incurred more nonfatal work-related injuries than workers in the construction and mining industries combined (Bureau of Labor Statistics, 2013a). Private employers in the HCSA industry reported that slips, trips, and falls (STFs) accounted for 24% ($n = 39,630$) of the total work-related injuries requiring at least 1 day away from work (Bureau of Labor

Statistics, 2013b). The incidence of STFs in hospitals was considerably higher than the STF incidence for the overall HCSA industry sector (Bureau of Labor Statistics, 2013c). The Bureau of Labor Statistics (2013c) also reported that the incidence of lost-workday injuries from same-level STFs in hospitals was 32.9 per 10,000 full-time equivalent (FTE) workers, nearly 32% greater than the STF incidence for all other private industries combined (25 per 10,000 FTE). STF injuries resulted in nine HCSA industry worker deaths in 2013 (Bureau of Labor Statistics, 2013d).

Ensuring safe, effective, and quality healthcare is a nationwide public health priority (Institute of Medicine, 1999). Extensive research, resources, and prevention efforts have been directed at preventing patient falls in healthcare settings (Wolf et al., 2013; Hignett et al., 2015). However, a key factor contributing to the delivery of quality healthcare to patients is maintaining the health and safety of healthcare workers. Although the rate of injurious STF events is excessively high among healthcare workers (Drebit et al., 2010; Bell et al., 2013; Gomaa et al., 2015), there have been relatively few research projects or systematic efforts to develop evidence-based guidance for preventing STFs for workers in healthcare settings. Historically, STF incidents have been considered largely nonpreventable and attributed to the carelessness of the fall victim (Lacroix and Dejoy, 1989; Sotter, 2000; Lehane and Stubbs, 2001).

The focus of this chapter is on understanding how to reduce STF hazards and subsequently reduce injuries. Research conducted by the Centers for Disease Control and Prevention (CDC) and the National Institute for Occupational Safety and Health (NIOSH) demonstrated that a comprehensive STF prevention program can significantly reduce same-level fall injuries among hospital staff (Bell et al., 2008). From this research, prevention strategies were evaluated empirically and implemented in the workplace.

29.2 Principal Research into Work-Related STF Injury in Hospitals

A multidisciplinary research team comprised of government, private, and university researchers collaborated to conduct laboratory and field research to identify risk factors for STF injuries among healthcare workers and evaluate the impact of that STF prevention program in three hospitals (Lombardi et al., 2007; Bell et al., 2008; Collins et al., 2008, 2010). Researchers worked with hospital staff to identify risk factors and design, implement, and evaluate a comprehensive STF prevention program over a 10 year period from 1996 through 2005. This comprehensive study included the following multiple concurrent components: (1) a descriptive analysis of 6 years of historical worker's compensation STF incident data; (2) an epidemiologic risk factor study; (3) laboratory evaluations of flooring and footwear; (4) on-site hazard assessments; and (5) a field study of prevention strategies to evaluate an STF prevention program.

29.2.1 Descriptive Analysis

During the ten year study period, a dynamic cohort of 16,900 individual employees worked 80,506,017 h, representing 40,253 worker-years across three acute-care hospitals representing approximately 6700 hospital workers. A total of 2263 workers' compensation claims were filed, and 21% ($n = 472$) involved STFs, resulting in 1.2 workers' compensation injury claims attributed to STF incidents per 100 FTEs.

The three hospitals' total STF workers' compensation claims incidence declined by 58% from a pre-intervention incidence of 1.66 claims per 100 FTEs to a post-intervention STF injury incidence of 0.76 claims per 100 FTEs (Bell et al., 2008). Worker's compensation record analysis may be limited to reported injuries and may not capture some injuries that were treated outside the worker's compensation system; however, it provides a basis for understanding which injuries and risk factors are most important to target in an STF prevention program.

29.2.1.1 Occupations

The comprehensive prevention program included an analysis of injury records to identify common causes of STFs, including changes to housekeeping procedures and products, changes to ice- and snow-removal procedures, and campaigns to highlight the importance of STF prevention among hospital workers. Most hospitals have a food service department on the premises that provides meals around the clock for patients, visitors, and staff, and high rates of workers' compensation claims overall have been found for food service workers in the healthcare sector (Alamgir et al., 2007). According to Bell et al. (2008), food-service workers in the hospital suffered the highest rate of STF workers' compensation claims, with 4.0 claims per 100 FTEs (Table 29.1). Nursing staff incurred most STF claims ($n = 141$), but because they comprised the largest proportion of the total work hours (33.6%), they had a much lower claim rate (1.0 STF workers' compensation claim per 100 FTEs). In the Lombardi et al. (2007) study, 50% of the participants worked in an occupation that provided direct care to hospital patients, with a distribution similar to those in the Bell et al.

TABLE 29.1

Pre- and Post-Intervention Slip, Trip and Fall (STF) Workers' Compensation Claims Rates and Rate Ratios by Select Job Groups

	Person-Time (Hours)	STF Claims (*n*)	Unadjusted Rate per 100 FTEs[a]	Adjusted Rate Ratio (95% CI)	*p*-Value
Food Services, Kitchen					
Pre-intervention	1,035,298	30	5.8	0.33 (0.14, 0.75)	<0.01
Post-intervention	933,035	10	2.1		
Custodial, Housekeeping					
Pre-intervention	1,406,566	19	2.7	0.39 (0.15, 0.95)	0.04
Post-intervention	1,304,651	7	1.0		
Nursing and Nursing-Related					
Pre-intervention	9,283,525	72	1.5	0.34 (0.21, 0.55)	<0.01
Post-intervention	8,443,803	26	0.5		
Medical, Laboratory and Other Technologists/Technicians					
Pre-intervention	3,074,882	23	1.5	0.27 (0.10, 0.70)	<0.01
Post-intervention	2,935,526	7	0.4		
Office/Administrative					
Pre-intervention	6,560,805	47	1.4	0.42 (0.25, 0.70)	<0.01
Post-intervention	7,223,896	23	0.6		

Source: Bell et al., *Ergonomics*, 51(12), 1906–1925, 2008.

[a] FTE = full-time equivalent worker, 2000 h worked per year.

(2008) study. Table 29.1 lists pre- and post-intervention STF workers' compensation claims and rate ratios for occupations with the highest frequencies and rates of STF incidents.

29.2.1.2 Body Part and Nature of Injury

According to an analysis of worker's compensation claims for the whole time period of the study, the most commonly injured body part from STF events was a lower extremity (44.9%), followed by an upper extremity (17.7%), multiple body parts (16.7%), back/trunk (16.2%), and head/neck (4.5%) (Bell et al., 2008). The nature of the injury was most often sprains, strains, dislocations, and tears (48.1%). STF injuries were significantly more likely to result in fractures, multiple injuries, and bruises, contusions, and concussions than non-STF injuries, and were less likely to result in cuts, lacerations, punctures, and abrasions than non-STF injuries ($\chi^2 = 213.1$, $p < 0.0001$). Lower extremities were much more likely to be injured by an STF incident than by a non-STF incident, and upper extremities were less likely to be injured after an STF injury than after a non-STF injury ($\chi^2 = 404.0$, $p < 0.0001$).

29.2.1.3 Age Group, Length of Employment, and Gender

STF injury rates were nearly twice as high for females, older workers, and those employed for less than 6 months. Bell et al. (2008) showed that 88% of the total STF claims ($n = 412$) occurred to females, and the STF claims rate for females (1.27 per 100 workers, unadjusted) was significantly higher than for males (0.77 per 100 workers, unadjusted). Workers employed for <6 months experienced the highest claims rate (2.0 STFs per 100 workers), followed by workers employed ≥6 months and <1 year (1.7 STFs per 100 workers); both of these groups had significantly greater STF claim rates than workers employed ≥1 year (1.1 STFs per 100 workers). STF claim rates were significantly greater for employees >45 years of age (1.6 STFs per 100 workers) than for employees ≤45 years (1.0 STFs per 100 workers). Older employees of both genders had higher STF claims rates compared with younger employees (Figure 29.1), and no interaction between age and length of employment was found (Bell et al., 2008).

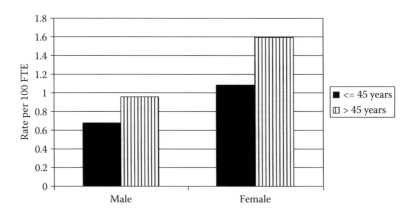

FIGURE 29.1
STF claim rates by age group and gender. (Adapted from Bell et al., *Ergonomics*, 51(12), 1906–1925, 2008.)

29.2.1.4 Circumstances of STFs

Of the 472 STF incidents, 85% ($n = 405$) were same-level STFs, and 15% ($n = 70$) were falls from elevation, which primarily occurred on stairs or from stepstools, ladders, or hospital shuttle buses (Bell et al., 2008). STFs due to liquid contamination (water, grease, ice, soapy detergent, floor stripper, or wax) were the most common cause of STF incidents. In the food services department, the most common slippery conditions consisted of food and grease on the floor in food preparation and cooking areas, spilled drinks and ice in food-serving areas, and soapy detergent on the floor in dishwashing areas.

Courtney et al. (2001) reported that slipperiness or slipping was found to contribute to between 40% and 50% of fall-related injuries across a variety of industries, and similar numbers were found specific to the hospital industry, where workers reported slipping (55%) more frequently than tripping (33%) (Lombardi et al., 2007). The direction of the fall was reported, and 41% of workers indicated that they fell forward, 23% fell to the side, and 21% fell backward. Workers who fell most often cited the hands, knees, or buttocks as the primary points of impact with the floor or ground, and the back, knees, and ankles/feet were the most frequently injured body parts. Forty-four percent of workers described the walking surface where they experienced their STF as clean and dry, while 53% reported the presence of some type of contaminant, including water, ice, or body fluids. Sixty-four percent of STFs occurred at a transitional area—wet to dry or dry to wet (32%), from one floor type to another (20%), or involving uneven surfaces (15%). Overall, 114 workers reported 228 injuries as a result of their STF event, an average of two injuries per event. Only 7% ($n = 8$) of study participants were not injured in the fall incidents. The results highlight the importance of managing surface contamination and surface transitions in hospitals (Lombardi et al., 2007).

29.2.2 Risk Factor Study

Collaborators from the Liberty Mutual Research Institute for Safety also conducted a case-crossover study of employees in seven hospitals to identify risk factors for STFs. This study is a type of epidemiology study in which the cases become their own control due to changes in exposures over time. In this case, hospital workers with injuries became their own control because they were not always exposed to STF hazards. The researchers interviewed a total of 153 hospital employees who had been injured by a work-related STF (both indoors and outdoors) to describe STF circumstances and risk factors. The respondents had a mean age of 46 (range = 19–67) years, the majority were women (86%), and they had worked for the hospital for an average of 9.3 years (Lombardi et al., 2007). The findings from this study indicate that transient, modifiable risk factors, specifically contaminated flooring, were most frequently associated with STF injuries.

29.2.3 Friction Characteristics of Footwear and Flooring

The coefficient of friction between the footwear and the floor is affected by the footwear material, the floor, and contamination conditions (Chang and Matz, 2001; Li and Chen, 2004; Li et al., 2004; Verma et al., 2011). While the slip-resistance characteristics of safety shoes and general footwear have been studied (Leclercq et al., 1995; Grönqvist, 1995), footwear commonly worn in hospital settings has not been systematically evaluated. The slip-resistance characteristics of footwear and flooring are one of the significant considerations regarding fall prevention (Collins et al., 2008, 2010; Thorpe et al., 2007).

The CDC/NIOSH study to prevent falls among hospital workers included laboratory analysis of the friction characteristics of footwear and flooring to evaluate the slipperiness of shoes commonly worn by hospital workers, slip-resistant shoes, and hospital flooring. Simulations were conducted to test footwear and floor surfaces under normal, "soapy," and "oily" conditions, as commonly encountered in food service areas of hospitals (Collins et al., 2008). The laboratory testing used a slipmeter apparatus that closely simulated the movements of a human foot and the forces applied between the shoe sole and the floor during heel strike in normal gait (Grönqvist et al., 1989). The dynamic coefficient of friction (DCOF) was computed during the time interval 100–150 ms from heel strike, which represents a critical moment for a slip and fall under conditions of level walking (Grönqvist et al., 1989). A DCOF >0.30 indicates slip resistance; ≥0.20–0.30 indicates moderate slip resistance; and <0.20 indicates slippery.

Seven shoe types were first pretested on a stainless steel surface (roughness Rz 1.6 µm) under test conditions "new" (intact heel and sole) and "abraded" (after abrasion, as stipulated in the standard [European Standard EN 13287: 2004] Section 9 [preparation of the sole]). Ten different flooring surfaces were also tested using two shoe types that were determined to have significantly different slip-resistance characteristics, including separate trials for "new" and "abraded" shoe conditions.

The laboratory study identified the combination of slip-resistant shoes and flooring that performed optimally under soapy and oily conditions. Slip-resistant shoes with laces performed better than athletic shoes, nursing clogs, or other types of commonly worn shoes. This study confirmed previous results (Grönqvist, 1995) showing that heel and sole abrasion significantly improved slip resistance. Quarry tile was the only flooring tested that was slip resistant with both test shoes under all contaminant conditions.

29.2.4 Identifying STF Hazards

A review of historical injury records, on-site hazard assessments, and investigations of fall incidents can identify conditions, circumstances, locations, occupations, and patterns of work-related STF incidents. Incident investigations should interview workers who have fallen to identify potential "hot spots," or locations where multiple STF incidents have occurred. Details of STF incidents among hospital employees often reveal risk factors that can be targeted to prevent STF injuries (Collins et al., 2008).

A comprehensive hazard assessment can identify conditions that might increase the risk of STFs and includes multiple components. The hazard assessment should evaluate specific conditions such as walkway surfaces, walkway levelness, objects and contaminants on the floor, projecting objects, cords, lighting, handrails, and drains (watch for standing water where drainage is not functioning properly) both inside and outside the hospital. Areas inside the hospital that should be inspected include the hospital's entrances, stairs, ramps, operating rooms (ORs), the emergency room, scrub sink areas, nursing stations, the pharmacy, the histology laboratory, hallways, the kitchen (including dishwashing areas and the cafeteria), patient rooms (including bathrooms), surgical instrument decontamination areas, laundry rooms, engineering and carpenter shops, and the morgue. Areas outside the hospital should also be examined, including parking areas, streets, handicap ramps, and sidewalks. A comprehensive hazard assessment in combination with interviews and historical records can help target areas with the highest STF risk.

29.2.5 Prevention Strategies

The descriptive analysis, combined with the information from the risk factor study, the friction testing of the footwear and flooring, and the hazard assessment, provided the foundation to implement a comprehensive STF prevention program. The three hospital's total STF workers' compensation claims incidence declined by 58% from a pre-intervention incidence of 1.66 claims per 100 FTEs to a post-intervention STF injury incidence of 0.76 claims per 100 FTEs (Bell et al., 2008).

The following prevention strategies developed during this comprehensive study may help reduce STF incidents in other hospitals. Hospital safety and health staff, housekeepers, and all hospital staff can use this information to take preventive action to mitigate hazardous environmental conditions in and around their hospitals and to minimize STF hazards to their coworkers. Additionally, visitors and patients can benefit from many of the elements of a comprehensive STF prevention program (Department of Health and Human Services, Centers for Disease Control and Prevention, National Institute for Occupational Safety and Health, 2010). This section presents a variety of strategies to reduce the risk of STF injuries in hospital settings.

29.2.5.1 Create a Written Housekeeping Program

A written housekeeping program should be provided to all employees to help ensure the quality and consistency of housekeeping procedures. The program should describe

- Procedures for routine floor care
- Procedure to contact the housekeeping department so that spills or other contaminants on floor surfaces can be cleaned up promptly
- Storage of cleaning materials and housekeeping products
- Use and storage of "wet floor" signs and barriers
- Cleaning schedules
- Appropriate cleaning methods and procedures

29.2.5.2 Maintain Floors Clean and Dry

Contaminants such as water, body fluids, spilled drinks, and grease are the most common hazards that make walking surfaces slippery and lead to STF incidents for hospital employees. These hazards primarily occur at building entrances, where rain and snow are tracked in; in food service areas, such as the kitchen, cafeteria, serving line, freezers, and dishwashing areas; and near sinks, ice machines, soap dispensers, and water fountains. Floors can also be wet in areas where surgical instruments are decontaminated. Most walking surfaces are slip resistant when they are clean and dry. The following prevention strategies can help keep floors clean and dry.

- Encourage workers to cover, clean, or report spills promptly.
- Advertise telephone/pager numbers for housekeeping through e-mails, posters, and general awareness campaigns, so that all hospital staff know the number to call to have spills cleaned up quickly.
- Conveniently locate wall-mounted paper towels or other cleanup materials throughout the hospital (near elevators, in nursing stations, outside the cafeteria, by water fountains) so that all employees have easy access to cleanup materials.

- Conveniently locate pop-up warning signs so that staff can quickly place them over a spill while waiting for housekeeping to clean up the spill. For large spills, it is important to block off the area rather than just place unconnected cones that may be ignored by pedestrians.

- Optimal floor-cleaning procedures can prevent slips and falls. Research by Quirion et al. (2008) found that damp mopping alone is not the best floor-cleaning method. A two-step immersion mopping process was found to be superior to damp mopping. In the two-step process, (1) cleaning solution is applied to a section of the floor with a dripping mop and (2) after a few minutes, the cleaning solution is removed with a wrung mop, before the solution has had a chance to dry.

- Not all floor-cleaning products are equally effective. Make sure the product used is suited to the environmental contamination conditions.

- Make sure cleaning products are mixed according to the manufacturer's recommendations, including water and product temperature.

- Effective procedures to degrease floors should be implemented in areas where food is prepared, cooked, and served. The appropriate degreaser/cleaner should be used, and the manufacturer's instructions should be carefully followed. Common mistakes include not letting the cleaner stay on the floor for the proper length of time, not using a stiff deck brush to loosen contaminants, and not providing a thorough clean rinse (for cleaning products that require it).

- Place umbrella bags by building entrances to prevent water from dripping on the hospital floor.

- Provide a sufficient number of water-absorbent walk-off mats with beveled edges at hospital entrances. The mats should be large enough for multiple steps to fall on the mat and wide enough to cover the entire doorway. As a general rule, when a person steps off the last mat, the soles of their shoes should not leave tracks on the floor. During inclement weather, it may be necessary to add additional mats or replace mats that have become saturated.

29.2.5.3 Prevent Pedestrian Access to Wet Floors

Mopping, disinfecting, stripping, and waxing floor surfaces in hallways, patient rooms, med rooms, bathrooms, kitchens, and cafeterias create slipping hazards for hospital staff. Simple steps to reduce this risk include

- Barrier signs (tension rod across bathroom doorways, cones with chains, hallway barriers) can be effective for blocking access to public bathrooms in the hospital during cleaning.

- Use high-visibility, taller "wet floor" caution signs/cones that can be joined by plastic chains or warning ribbons/tape to warn pedestrians of slippery conditions. Cordon off slippery areas, and direct pedestrian traffic to a clear dry lane. Cones alone are not effective for keeping pedestrians off wet floors.

- "Wet floor" signs should be promptly removed after the floor is clean and dry to prevent staff from becoming complacent about the sign's intended warning.

- Completely block off pedestrian access when stripping or applying wax.

29.2.5.4 Use Slip-Resistant Shoes

Slip-resistant shoes are an important component of a comprehensive STF prevention program, and staff who work on walking surfaces that are continually wet, greasy, or slippery may benefit from slip-resistant shoes. Job classifications at highest risk of an STF injury that may benefit from slip-resistant shoes are food service workers, housekeepers, custodians, maintenance workers, dishwashers, and instrument-decontamination workers. Because nursing personnel suffer the highest total number of STF claims in hospital settings (Bell et al., 2008), they should also be included in a slip-resistant footwear program. Specialized shoes, designed to reduce the risk of slipping while stripping or applying wax, should be provided to housekeeping staff.

Anecdotal evidence suggests that use of slip-resistant shoes by employees is enhanced when the employer provides either the shoes or a payroll deduction for approved shoe purchases. Shoe fit, comfort, and style are important factors that determine whether employees will wear slip-resistant shoes. It may be useful for employees to have the opportunity to try on shoes to obtain the proper fit before purchasing. Some shoe vendors will make periodic site visits so that employees may try on shoes at their workplace to ensure a proper fit. Slip-resistant shoes are a low-cost way to provide slip resistance to staff.

29.2.5.5 Minimize Tripping Hazards

Exposed cords stretched across walkways and under workstations can catch an employee's foot and lead to a trip and fall incident. Clutter in walkways, storage areas, and hallways can potentially lead to a trip and fall incident. The following should be considered to minimize tripping hazards inside the hospital:

- Keep hallways, work areas, and walkways clear of objects and clutter.
- Use cord organizers to bundle and secure loose cords and wires under nursing stations, computer workstations, and patient rooms.
- Reroute cords so that they do not cross walking paths.
- Organize ORs to minimize equipment cords across walkways.
- Consider retractable cord holders on phones in patient rooms and nursing stations.
- Replace or restretch loose or buckled carpet.
- Replace mats with curled or ripped edges; secure edges with carpet tape.
- Remove, patch underneath, and replace indented or blistered floor tiles.
- Patch or fill cracks in walkways greater than a quarter inch in width (¼").
- Create visual cues for pedestrians by highlighting changes in walkway elevation with yellow warning paint or tape.
- Consider replacing smooth flooring materials with rougher-surfaced flooring with a higher coefficient of friction when renovating or replacing hospital flooring.

To minimize tripping hazards outside hospitals, the following strategies should be considered:

- Patch and repair holes, deep grooves, and cracks greater than ½" in cement, asphalt, or other surfaces in parking areas and sidewalks.

- For adjoining walkway surfaces with changes in walkway level greater than ¼", bevel the surface by providing a ramp, or provide a visual cue by painting uneven floor surfaces a bright contrasting color (i.e., yellow).

29.2.5.6 Safer Operating Rooms

Although STFs occur throughout a hospital, the OR is of special interest, because a fall in the OR can cause direct patient injury, disrupt the surgical procedure, contribute to surgical errors, or delay future surgeries (Brogmus et al., 2007). The following features of a well-designed OR may reduce the risk of STFs:

- Slip-resistant flooring
- Procedures to control contaminants
- Proper floor-cleaning methods
- Minimized tripping hazards through securing and routing walking paths with cords
- Preplanned placement of low-profile equipment and supplies so that equipment and supplies remain off the floor and are accessible from mobile utility booms
- Use of slip-resistant absorptive mats to control contaminants, and removal of mats when they become saturated
- An unobstructed view of the walking pathways in the OR
- Use of enhanced OR lights so that general lighting corresponds to the lighting level needed at the surgical site
- Efficient placement of equipment and supplies to minimize the walking distance to obtain instruments and supplies and to access waste containers
- Ample waste receptacle systems and contaminant cleanup materials placed in strategic locations
- Mandated planning briefings to discuss cleanup duty assignments and equipment and tube arrangement and routing to ensure OR team efficiency
- Minimized fatigue by ensuring all OR personnel are well rested for each procedure and receive scheduled time off and breaks during the work shift
- Participative architectural design; have architects, engineers, builders, and hospital administrators collaborate on OR-design decisions with end users such as surgeons, circulating nurses, and scrub technicians
- Policies and procedures to investigate fall incidents

29.2.5.7 Facilitate Ice and Snow Removal

The most important aspect of controlling risks during winter weather is to remove snow and ice as soon as possible after they have accumulated. According to Drebit and colleagues (2010), in their study of falls among workers in the HCSA sector, weather was a consistent contributor to employee falls across all healthcare subsectors, with the greatest number of weather-related falls in the community health subsector. Hospital administrators should work with their snow removal staff or vendors to ensure frequent removal when needed. In addition:

- Encourage employees to report icy conditions; prominently display phone or pager numbers for staff to report icy conditions.
- Provide ice cleats or slip-resistant shoe covers for home health workers, maintenance workers, and other workers who work outdoors.
- Distribute winter weather warnings by e-mail when ice and snow storms are predicted.
- Conveniently place bins containing ice-melting chemicals near the top and bottom of outdoor stairways, parking garage exits, and heavily traveled walkways that are prone to refreezing, so that any employee can apply ice-melting chemicals when they notice icy patches.
- Provide a sufficient number of water-absorbent walk-off mats with beveled edges at hospital entrances. The mats should be large enough for multiple steps to fall on the mat and wide enough to cover the entire doorway. As a general rule, when a person steps off the last mat, the soles of their shoes should not leave tracks on the floor. During inclement weather, it may be necessary to add additional mats or replace mats that have become saturated.
- When renovating exterior entrances, build well-lit, well-draining, covered walkways leading to entrances to provide walk-off areas that allow water, snow, and other contaminants to be removed from footwear before entering the building.

29.2.5.8 Ensure Adequate Lighting

Inadequate lighting impairs vision and ability to see hazards. The hazard can occur anywhere, but particular attention should be paid to lighting levels in parking structures, storage rooms, hallways, and stairwells. Adequate lighting helps to illuminate areas, which makes walking safer and easier and allows employees to see their surroundings. Prevention strategies include

- Installing more light fixtures in poorly lit areas
- Verifying that light bulbs have an appropriate brightness
- Installing light fixtures that emit light from all sides

29.2.5.9 Increase Safety of Stairs and Handrails

Uneven and poorly marked stairs can lead to missteps and can cause employees to trip and fall. Handrails that are not of the appropriate height or poorly maintained can also lead to a fall. Prevention strategies should

- Confirm that all handrails are up to code (34″–38″ from flooring)
- Ensure that discontinuous handrails are of a consistent height
- Paint the edge (nosing) of each step, including the top and bottom, to provide a visual cue of a change in elevation
- Ensure that stairwells and steps have adequate lighting

29.3 Conclusion

STF events can cause serious injuries to hospital staff and are one of the leading causes of workers' compensation claims in hospital settings. Little emphasis has been placed on fall prevention among hospital staff because of the widespread perception that these incidents are not preventable. However, examination of the details surrounding STF incidents among hospital staff indicates that many of these incidents are preventable. Research provides evidence that implementation of a comprehensive STF prevention program can significantly reduce STF injury claims involving diverse hospital staff. Because STFs result from a wide variety of circumstances, a coordinated effort is required by the safety department, the housekeeping staff, and essentially every hospital staff member to prevent STF incidents.

In addition to all the products and procedures that can be implemented to reduce known hazards, one of the key components of a successful STF prevention program is to raise awareness regarding the importance of STF prevention among hospital staff and to empower every employee to share in the responsibility of eliminating STF hazards. Whether this involves cleaning spills, applying ice-melting chemicals to icy patches in parking areas or sidewalks, or cordoning off an area to alert fellow employees while waiting for housekeeping staff to arrive, a successful STF program requires that all hospital staff share the responsibility for prevention. Implementing a comprehensive STF prevention program in combination with other safety programs can lead to a significant reduction in workers' compensation costs and improve the well-being of our healthcare workforce.

29.4 Disclaimer

The findings and conclusions in this chapter are those of the author and do not necessarily represent the views of the National Institute for Occupational Safety and Health (NIOSH). Mention of company names or products does not constitute endorsement by NIOSH.

References

Alamgir H, Swink H, Yu S, Yassi A. 2007. Occupational injury among cooks and food service workers in the healthcare sector. *American Journal of Industrial Medicine* 50:528–535.

Bell JL, Collins JW, Tiesman HM, et al. 2013. Slip, trip, and fall injuries among nursing care facility workers. *Workplace Health & Safety* 61:147–152.

Bell JL, Collins JW, Wolf L, et al. 2008. Evaluation of a comprehensive slip, trip and fall prevention programme for hospital employees. *Ergonomics* 51(12):1906–1925.

Brogmus G, Leone W, Butler L, Hernandez E. 2007. Best practices in OR suite layout and equipment choices to reduce slips, trips, and falls. *AORN Journal* 86(3):384–398.

Bureau of Labor Statistics. 2013a. Incidence rate and number of nonfatal occupational injuries by industry and ownership. Accessed February 4, 2015, http://www.bls.gov/iif/oshwc/osh/os/ostb3966.pdf.

Bureau of Labor Statistics. 2013b. Occupational injuries and illnesses and fatal injuries profiles. Case and demographic numbers for health care and social assistance industry. Accessed February 4, 2015, http://data.bls.gov/gqt/InitialPage.

Bureau of Labor Statistics. 2013c. Occupational injuries and illnesses and fatal injuries profiles. Case and demographic incidence for health care and social assistance industry. Accessed February 4, 2015, http://data.bls.gov/gqt/InitialPage.

Bureau of Labor Statistics. 2013d. Occupational injuries and illnesses and fatal injuries profiles. Fatal injuries numbers for health care and social assistance industry. Accessed February 4, 2015, http://data.bls.gov/gqt/.

Bureau of Labor Statistics. 2015. Health care and social assistance: NAICS 62. Accessed October 15, 2015, http://www.bls.gov/iag/tgs/iag62.htm.

Chang WR, Matz S. 2001. The slip resistance of common footwear materials measured with two slipmeters. *Applied Ergonomics* 32:540–558.

Collins JW, Bell JL, Grönqvist R. 2010. Developing evidence-based interventions to address the leading causes of workers' compensation among healthcare workers. *Rehabilitation Nursing* 35(6):225–235, 261.

Collins JW, Bell JL, Grönqvist R, et al. 2008. Multi-disciplinary research to prevent slip, trip, and fall (STF) incidents among hospital workers. *Contemporary Ergonomics* 2008:693–698.

Courtney TK, Sorock GS, Manning DP, et al. 2001. Occupational slip, trip, and fall-related injuries: Can the contribution of slipperiness be isolated? *Ergonomics* 44:1118–1137.

Department of Health and Human Services, Centers for Disease Control and Prevention, National Institute for Occupational Safety and Health. 2010. Bell JL, Collins JW, Dalsey E, Sublet V. Slip, trip, and fall prevention for healthcare workers. DHHS (NIOSH) Publication Number 2011–123.

Drebit S, Sharjari S, Alamgir H, Yu S, Keen D. 2010. Occupational and environmental risk factors for falls among workers in the healthcare sector. *Ergonomics* 53:525–536.

European Standard EN 13287. 2004. Personal protective equipment: Footwear—Test method for slip resistance.

Gomaa AE, Tapp LC, Luckhaupt SE, et al. 2015. Occupational traumatic injuries among workers in health care facilities—United States, 2012–2014. *Morbidity and Mortality Weekly Report* 64(15):405–410.

Grönqvist R. 1995. Mechanisms of friction and assessment of slip resistance of new and used footwear soles on contaminated floors. *Ergonomics* 38(2):224–241.

Grönqvist R, Roine J, Järvinen E, Korhonen E. 1989. An apparatus and method for determining the slip resistance of shoes and floors by simulation of human foot motions. *Ergonomics* 32:979–995.

Hignett S, Wolf L, Taylor E, Griffiths P. 2015. Firefighting to innovation: Using human factors and ergonomics to tackle slip, trip, and fall risks in hospitals. *Human Factors: The Journal of the Human Factors and Ergonomics Society* 57:1195–1207.

Institute of Medicine. 1999. *To Err Is Human: Building a Safer Health System*. Washington, DC: Institute of Medicine of the National Academies, http://www.iom.edu/Reports/1999/To-Err-is-Human-Building-A-Safer-Health-System.aspx.

Lacroix D, Dejoy D. 1989. Causal attribution to effort and supervisory response to workplace accidents. *Journal of Occupational Accidents* 11:97–109.

Leclercq S, Tisserand M, Saulinier H. 1995. Assessment of slipping resistance of footwear and floor surface. Influence of manufacture and utilization of the products. *Ergonomics* 38:209–219.

Lehane P, Stubbs D. 2001. The perceptions of managers and accident subjects in the service industries towards slip and trip accidents. *Applied Ergonomics* 32:119–126.

Li KW, Chang WR, Leamon TB, Chen CJ. 2004. Floor slipperiness measurement friction coefficient, roughness of floors, and subjective perception under spillage conditions. *Safety Science* 42(6):547–565.

Li KW, Chen CJ. 2004. The effect of shoe soling tread groove width on the coefficient of friction with different sole materials, floors, and contaminants. *Applied Ergonomics* 35(6):499–507.

Lombardi DA, Courtney TK, Verma SK, et al. 2007. Risk factors for slips, trips, and falls: A case-crossover study of U.S. health care workers. *Oral Presentation at the Annual Meeting of the American Public Health Association*, Washington, DC, November 3–7, 2007.

Quirion F, Poirier P, Lehane P. 2008. Improving the cleaning procedure to make kitchen floors less slippery. *Ergonomics* 51(12):2013–2029.

Sotter G. 2000. *Stop Slip and Fall Accidents*. Mission Viejo, CA: Sotter Engineering Corporation.

Thorpe S, Loo-Morrey M, Houlihan R, Lemon P. 2007. Slip and fall accidents in workplace environments – the role of footwear. *Presented at the International Conference on Slips, Trips, and Falls Research to Practice*, Hopkinton, MA, August 23–24, 2007.

Verma SK, Chang WR, Courtney TK, et al. 2011. A prospective study of floor surface, shoes, floor cleaning and slipping in US limited-service restaurant workers. *Occupational and Environmental Medicine* 68:279–285.

Wolf L, Costantinou E, Limbaugh C, Rensing K, Gabbart P, Matt P. 2013. Fall prevention for inpatient oncology using lean and rapid improvement event techniques. *Health Environment Research & Design Journal* 7:85–101.

Author Index

A

Abeysekera, J., 298
Adams, P. S., 372
Adisesh, A., 115
Adkin, A. L., 133
Adlin, T., 495
Agashivala, N., 32
Alamgir, H., 511
Alexander, B. H., 19
Allcott, G. A., 201
Anderson, J. T., 46
Archea, J. C., 198, 404, 405
Aschan, C., 184
Ashley, L., 502
Aven, T., 160
Azhar, S., 485

B

Bakri, I., 376
Bariod, J., 110, 114
Barquins, M., 177
Bauby, C. E., 123
Bauer, J. M., 33
Becker, C., 30
Begg, R., 149
Behm, M., 484
Bell, J. L., 511, 512, 513, 515, 517
Benbow, D. W., 498
Benolken, M. S., 11, 123
Bentley, T. A., 170, 458, 459
Berry, S. D., 32, 347
Berthoz, A., 66, 123
Beschorner, K. E., 192
Bidanda, B., 180, 182
Bjornstig, U., 474
Black, A. A., 7, 51, 65, 66, 68, 69
Bles, W., 7, 122, 124
Bobick, T. G., 455, 459, 475, 476
Bogner, M. S., 495
Bosher, L., 495
Bouldin, E. L. D., 492
Braithwaite, R. S., 22
Brandt, T., 7, 122
Brinkley, J. W., 110

Brocklehurst, J. C., 67
Brogmus, G., 332, 518
Brown, L. A., 122, 133
Bukowski, T. J., 476

C

Caetano, M. J. D., 133
Calvert, G. M., 161
Cameron, I. D., 34, 35, 354
Campbell, A. J., 67, 70, 460
Capezuti, E., 349, 352
Carayon, P., 492
Carpenter, M. G., 133
Carson, D. H., 198, 201, 209, 404, 405
Casalena, J. A., 361
Catchpole, K. R., 491
Chaffin, D. B., 258
Cham, R., 177
Chambers, A. J., 299
Chang, W.-R., 143, 148
Chateauroux, E., 296
Chau, N. A., 381, 473
Chiou, S. S., 378
Choi, M., 34, 51, 475
Chrisman, M., 358
Christopher, D. A., 503
Clark, M., 11
Clarke, J. C., 122, 485
Clift, L., 247, 248, 251, 257, 261
Close, J., 71
Cloutier, E., 373
Cohen, H. H., 201, 203, 252, 292, 347, 390, 392, 394, 405, 458
Coleman, A. L., 67, 68, 69, 178, 183
Coleman, V., 67, 68, 69, 178, 183
Collins, J. W., 510, 514
Commissaris, D. A., 11
Corlett, E. N., 161, 215, 251
Cotnam, J. P., 293, 295
Crocker, T., 35
Cruz-Jentoft, A. J., 32, 33
Cumming, R. G., 71
Cummings, S. R., 67
Currie, L., 500
Cutlip, R., 477

Subject Index